Cholera

ALSO BY S.L. KOTAR AND J.E. GESSLER
AND FROM MCFARLAND

Smallpox: A History (2013)

Ballooning: A History, 1782–1900 (2011)

The Rise of the American Circus, 1716–1899 (2011)

*The Steamboat Era: A History of Fulton's Folly on
American Rivers, 1807–1860* (2009)

Cholera

A Worldwide History

S.L. KOTAR *and*
J.E. GESSLER

McFarland & Company, Inc., Publishers
Jefferson, North Carolina

Library of Congress Cataloguing-in-Publication Data

Kotar, S. L., author.
Cholera : a worldwide history / S.L. Kotar and J.E. Gessler.
        p.   cm.
Includes bibliographical references and index.

ISBN 978-0-7864-7242-0 (softcover : acid free paper) ∞
ISBN 978-1-4766-1364-2 (ebook)

1. Cholera—History.   I. Gessler, J. E., author.   II. Title.
RA644.C3K68 2014   614.5'14—dc23   2014000864

British Library cataloguing data are available

On the cover: (*front*) 19th century line drawing, "Protections Against
Cholera"; (*left*) advertisement for the Chamberland-Pasteur water filter
(*The Colonies & India*, London, June 18, 1886); (*right*) advertisement
for Bromo-Chloralum (*Defiance Democrat*, Ohio, July 26, 1873)

Manufactured in the United States of America

*McFarland & Company, Inc., Publishers
Box 611, Jefferson, North Carolina 28640
www.mcfarlandpub.com*

This work is lovingly dedicated to Josephine Campbell,
known as "Aunt Jo" to her nieces and nephews,
who have always looked to her for guidance, inspiration
and as a second mother.

Table of Contents

Preface

To the philanthropist, the statesman, and the philosopher—to the sagacious enquirer into abstruse and distant causes, and the acute observer of present and practical effects—the new and fatal disease by which this country is now afflicted, is a subject for careful observation and deep and serious reflection. The origin, the former course, and the probable future progress of the malady—the means of prevention, and the mode of cure—the effect that has been, and will hereafter be, produced upon commercial intercourse and political combinations—these are objects which demand the profound consideration of the most powerful intellects. They afford abundant matter for the searching eye of speculative inquiry in the present day, and will in future times be the subjects of the curious and minute investigation of the historian who shall record the occurrences of this eventful period.[1]

In 2007, we had the honor to attend the 25th anniversary of the Jimmy and Rosalynn Carter Center in Atlanta. Among the seminars given during this four-day celebration was an update on the center's work in eliminating river blindness caused by the Guinea worm. The presentation was so stimulating and the accomplishments so inspiring that we left Atlanta filled with pride and awe that so much had been achieved by the application of scientific methods and plain hard work.

For the past 36 years our professional work has been in cardiology—more specifically, the monitoring, interpretation and study of arrhythmia. We have participated in several national and international research studies, published papers, written a book on the subject and finally contributed, in a small way, to Dr. Preben Bjerregaard's investigations into Short QT Syndrome. Coupled with a lifelong fascination with the 19th century, we decided to turn our attention to those diseases that most plagued the people of the 1800s.

Cholera was a natural choice. Although cholera has its roots in antiquity, the first recognized global epidemic occurred in 1817. Until the turn of the next century, five major pandemics were recorded, decimating hundreds of thousands of individuals. Statistics alone were dire enough to fill a book, but what we wanted to achieve was a view of the disease through the eyes of those who lived during the speculations, missteps, sidetracks, impending doom and ultimately the advancements of the 1800s and then carry this through the 20th and into the 21st centuries. Relying as little as possible on hindsight, this work presents the slow (at times excruciatingly laborious) march through the unknown toward the discovery of causation and ultimately the successful treatment of symptoms.

How did cholera originate? No one knows for certain. But tracing the deadly path of this acute diarrheal disease from the Ganges Basin of the Indian subcontinent throughout Europe, the Americas and around the globe, the science of epidemiology was born. In the beginning, cholera had many names, but perhaps the "King of Terrors" serves better than any to describe its consequences. In 1847, during the Second Pandemic, a writer for the Pennsylvania newspaper *Tioga Eagle* (November 10, 1847) put in words what the world was experiencing:

1

The Cholera.—The great Scourge of humanity, a scourge more awful than ATILA and his Huns— more terrible than the eruptions of a volcano—more devastating than the throes of an earthquake— the Great Scourge of the Cholera is at this moment advancing towards us with silent but indomitable rapidity if we may believe the intelligence received almost daily from the frontiers of the Russian empire. Its course is described as being northwesterly, and is said to have penetrated into the interior of Europe. GOD defend us from the agonies which desolated the world in 1832!

By the time this was penned, physicians had experimented with intravenous saline injections to restore life. Within the next ten years, Dr. John Snow would demonstrate how cholera was spread through water dispensed by the Broad Street pump in Golden Square, London. But people were slow to abandon old ideas. Miasma, temperature, ozone and elevation remained higher on the list of causes. Cathartics and myriad bowel treatments, mercurial medicines and alcohol-laced nostrums prevailed in the treatment. Politicians quarreled over responsibilities, businessmen fought contagionists over the effectiveness of quarantines and mobs caused havoc in the belief they were being poisoned by authorities. The belief in visitations from an avenging God went hand in hand with superstition. Governments were overburdened with costs, orphans crowded charity houses and immigrants were always the first target of established communities. African slaves and Native Americans suffered in horrific numbers, staggering casualties in India were reported alongside the price of tea and every household had its own "cure" that did not cure anything at all.

Cholera was a disease of filth and it represented the wide spectrum of human disgust and loathing of its own waste products while accentuating the fear of death, burial and the putrid disintegration of the body. But investigation into its root causes by determined individuals led to the international sanitary movements of the 19th century and was pivotal in the establishment of Boards of Health. In the process of eradicating cholera, water supplies of established and emerging nations were vastly improved, down to the introduction of chlorine in public drinking water.

It is tempting to say that cholera is a disease of the past but this is not so. The natural disasters of our present age have rekindled its fires, triggering the 7th pandemic between the years 1961 and 2008. Sporadic outbreaks occur after tsunamis and earthquakes in the present day, forcing a reevaluation of established thought. Although there are no definitive answers yet, modern researchers have made the case that this complex disease does not originate from within Homo sapiens, but from warm seas harboring genetically unstable organisms.[2]

Seeking answers for the betterment of the human condition is a complex process that involves human hearts as well as brains. Into the mix is woven creativity, daring, surrender to accepted principles, personal and worldwide pathos and the occasional spice of humor. By projecting the story prospectively, we have followed the chronology of cholera as it happened, interjecting as little hindsight as possible so the reader can experience events as they happened in the words of those who lived through those harrowing times. At times we have emphasized the trivial over the traumatic as a means of putting everyday life into context. Disease, after all, is not a series of numbers, but one of heartbeats and heartbreaks that ultimately create the human whole. One particular story, insignificant in history, perhaps best summarizes the whole.

In the middle of the 19th century the city of Sandusky, Ohio, comprised immigrants who had come by water and rail to enjoy personal freedom and industrial independence. In 1849, a young man traveling from New Orleans to Cincinnati arrived in Sandusky. He was suffering from cholera, and the disease quickly spread to the community. In two short days, July 28 and 29, sixty persons were buried in one grave; ultimately, 357 persons perished. Over the years, the cemetery fell into disrepair; many bodies were removed to Oakland Cemetery and the markers lost or recycled for other purposes. In 1920, a rather lilting article appeared in the *Sandusky Star-Journal* (September 21, 1920) advising citizens that the city commissioners were considering a grant to the Kiwanis club to use the abandoned cholera cemetery on Harrison Street for a high school football field. The legislation was expected to pass on the first reading.

On November 17, 1924, the same newspaper printed a very different article, somber and respectful in tone. In it, the reporter described the dedication of a new monument erected at the Harrison Street cemetery. Former mayor John Molter's remarks included these:

> We have gathered here to pay an all too long delayed tribute to the memory of the victims of that terrible scourge, cholera, who are filling the unmarked graves of this much neglected cemetery, all the victims of this dreadful epidemic; and also to pay homage to those men and women who through all that dreadful period, stood bravely and heroically by, with helping hands, willing to work for humanity's sake.

To remember and to seek. To pay homage to those who lived and those who died; to honor the individuals who questioned and the men and women who enlightened the world. That is the story of cholera we hope to have captured in this book.

SLK   JEG
St. Louis, Missouri

1

"Water, water, every where,
Nor any drop to drink"

Day after day, day after day,
We stuck, nor breath nor motion;
As idle as a painted ship
Upon a painted ocean.

Water, water, every where,
And all the boards did shrink;
Water, water, every where,
Nor any drop to drink ...

About, about, in reel and rout
The death-fires danced at night;
The water, like a witch's oils,
Burnt green, and blue, and white....

Ah! well-a-day! what evil looks
Had I from old and young!
Instead of the cross, the Albatross
About my neck was hung.[1]

The *Rime of the Ancient Mariner*, Samuel Taylor Coleridge's brilliant poem, vividly described images of desiccation and death at the hands of a terrifying and all-encompassing sea. In the year it was published (1798), people across the globe might have linked his two evils—water and the symbol of impending doom—to a far more tangible and terrifying killer that was known as the "King of Terrors," with its life-threatening symptoms of diarrhea and shock.

The Centers for Disease Control and Prevention describe cholera (also known as "Asiatic cholera," or "epidemic cholera") as "an acute intestinal infection causing profuse watery diarrhea, vomiting, circulatory collapse and shock." The disease is caused by toxigenic *Vibrio cholerae* O-group 1 or O-group 139. These strains, reported to the World Health Organization (WHO) as "cholera," are responsible for widespread epidemics. Two biotypes of *Vibrio cholerae*, Classical and El Tor, have two distinct serotypes, Inaba and Ogawa. Symptoms of infection between the two are indistinguishable, although those with the El Tor biotype are asymptomatic or suffer only mild illness. The classical biotype *Vibrio cholerae* O1 is now rare, limited to areas in Bangladesh and India.[2]

Vibrio cholerae

Kingdom:	Bacteria
Phylum:	Proteobacteria
Class:	Gamma Proteobacteria
Order:	Vibrionales
Family:	Vibrionaceae
Genus:	Vibrio
Species:	Vibrio cholerae

The genus Vibrio consists of gram-negative straight or curved rods, capable of spontaneous movement by means of a single flagellum, as well as respiratory and fermentative metabolism. Vibrios are related to enteric bacteria (found in the small intestines) but share some properties with pseudomonads, as well. Of all the vibrios that are clinically significant to humans, Vibrios cholerae, the agent of cholera, is the most important. It acts noninvasively in the small intestines through secretion of an enterotoxin; a second bacteria, Vibrio parahaemolyticus, is an invasive organism affecting the colon. A third, Vibrio vulnificus, is an emerging pathogen (a microorganism capable of producing a disease[3]) of humans, causing wound infections, gastroenteritis, or "primary septicemia." Vibrios are typically marine organisms and are one of the most common found in surface waters around the globe. They thrive in both salt- and freshwater, and in association with fish and other marine life.[4]

The most common cause of *Vibrio cholerae* is ingestion of water or food contaminated by fecal matter. It is not contagious, per se, but may be transmitted, for instance, if a person touches contaminated material or waste products, getting *V. cholerae* on their hands. If the hands are left unwashed and the fingers touch food or are brought to the mouth, the disease may take hold. The natural reservoir of the organism is unknown. Researchers have assumed it to be human, but some current evidence indicates an aquatic environment.[5] There are no known animal hosts, but the bacteria easily attach to the chitin-containing shells of crabs, shrimps and other shellfish, spreading to humans when eaten raw or undercooked. As proof of its continuing devastation to human populations, in 2009, 45 countries reported 221,226 cases and 4,946 cholera-related deaths to WHO, of which 99 percent originated from Africa.

Other serogroups of *Vibrio cholerae*, with or without the cholera toxin gene, cause cholera-like symptoms, as does the O1 and O139 serogroups. Unlike smallpox (variola major and minor), where recovery from the disease offers lifetime protection from recurrence and vaccination prevents the disease, currently available vaccines for cholera offer only incomplete protection. No multivalent vaccines are available for O139 infections.[6] As an example of how little cholera was understood, one American physician in 1855 maintained that sores of any kind acted as a preventative, and he accordingly believed that inoculation by caustic issue would prevent the disease.[7]

There is no explanation why certain persons suffer fatal attacks of cholera while others are only mildly affected. According to bacteriologist Kenneth Todar, PhD, one hypothesis is that individuals differ in the availability of intestinal receptors for cholera vibrios or their toxin. Some immunity by persons having once experienced cholera is suggested by the fact that in heavily endemic regions such as Bangladesh, the preponderance of cases are seen in children. In nursing children, the incidence of cholera is lower, presumably due to antibodies in the mother's milk.

Recurrent infections among adults are rare, probably due to the immune system's secreting antibodies onto the surface of the intestinal mucosa. After natural infection by Vibrio cholerae, these circulating antibodies can be detected working against cholera antigens, including the toxin. Those directed against Vibrio O antigens are called "vibriocidal" antibodies. They reach a peak 8–10 days after the onset of cholera and then decrease, returning to baseline in 2–7 months. Additionally, victims develop toxin-neutralizing antibodies. But Todar relates there is no positive correlation between antitoxic antibody levels and the incidence of disease in cholera zones.[8]

Differing from smallpox, that great disease killer of the 19th century, cholera is not typically spread through contact with an infected person. Those suffering from the "Speckled Disease" quickly passed it to others, while those inoculated (as opposed to those undergoing vaccination) became carriers, an equally dangerous threat. During the 19th century, the most significant argument over cholera centered on whether the disease was contagious or noncontagious. The answer hinged on how it was spread and, since the cause was not definitively proven until Robert Koch identified the comma-shaped bacillus in 1883, linking it to the germ theory and contaminated water, speculations varied widely. Because the answer held serious medical, financial and political connotations, supporters of both theories drafted literally hundreds of thousands of studies, pamphlets and letters. Dr. Edward Jenner proved smallpox was contagious: but if cholera was caused by miasma or impurities in the soil, temperature or "local conditions," the answer was less clear. German physician Jeremias Lichtenstaedt gravely noted, "the non-infectivity of cholera ... belongs in the category of the most dangerous errors of our time."[9]

Cholera manifestations were not always deadly. Approximately 5–10 percent of previously healthy individuals develop severe symptoms. The percent is higher in populations where health has been compromised by poor nutrition, or in regions that include a high number of the elderly or the very young. In these instances, rapid loss of body fluids leads to dehydration, acute renal failure, severe electrolyte imbalance, shock, coma and death.

Symptoms of Cholera

- Profuse watery diarrhea, with a "fishy odor," or the appearance of "rice-water" stools
- Vomiting
- Tachycardia (rapid pulse)
- Loss of skin elasticity/dry skin
- Dry mucus membranes and mouth
- Excessive thirst
- Low blood pressure
- Muscle cramps
- Restlessness or irritability
- Lethargy/unusual sleepiness or tiredness
- Glassy or sunken eyes
- Dehydration/lack of tears
- Low urine output
- Sunken "soft spots" (fontanels) in infants[10]

Watery stools, characterized as having the appearance of "rice-water" (white grains mixed with fecal matter), result from flakes of mucus and epithelial cells containing huge amounts of vibrios.

Symptoms are typically seen within 2–3 days after ingestion of contaminated material, with a range of several hours to five days. Severe dehydration can occur 4–8 hours after the onset of diarrhea.[11] If loose stools are copious and the patient is left untreated, death can result between 18 hours and several days. In extreme cases, cholera is one of the most rapidly fatal illnesses known. A healthy individual may become hypotensive within an hour of the onset of symptoms and die within 2–3 hours. More often, shock occurs within 4–12 hours following the first bout of diarrhea, causing death in a window between 18 hours and several days. The loss of potassium in the liquid discharge also has the potential to cause serious cardiac complications and circulatory failure.[12] During epidemic outbreaks in underdeveloped countries where scant treatment or effective measures are not available mortality rates as high as 50–60 percent have been recorded.[13]

Treatment for cholera is basic and simple. Immediate replacement of fluids and electrolytes lost through diarrhea is achieved through an oral rehydration solution of sugars and salts mixed with water and consumed in large quantities. The World Health Organization supplies a prepackaged mix that is used throughout the world. With prompt treatment, less than 1 percent of patients die. Significantly, when administered with this or similar solutions, recovery is rapid. In the era before microscopes and bacteriology, this gave the appearance of a miraculous cure, lending credence to the effectiveness of numerous nostrums, quack techniques and divine intervention. In the present day, antibiotics (most notably tetracyclines) are occasionally prescribed to shorten the course of the disease and lessen its severity, but they are of secondary importance to prompt rehydration.

Simple Precautions to Avoid Cholera

1. Wash hands often with soap and water or an alcohol-based (60 percent) hand sanitizer.
2. Use only bottled or chemically treated water for drinking, washing, preparing food and ice and brushing teeth.
3. Eat prepackaged food or food that is thoroughly cooked and hot.
4. Do not eat raw or undercooked meat and seafood or unpeeled fruits and vegetables.
5. Dispose of feces in a sanitary manner to prevent contamination of water and food sources.

At present, there are two oral cholera vaccines available: Dukoral, a recombinant cholera toxin-B, killed-whole-cell vaccine (rBS-WC), manufactured by SBL Vaccines, licensed by WHO and used in over 60 countries (but not the United States), and ShanChol (manufactured by Shantha Biotec in India), licensed in India and pending WHO certification. The vaccine requires two doses, and weeks may elapse before offering protection. Neither vaccine is foolproof and prevention remains the best solution.[14]

2

What Is Cholera?
An Early Conundrum

Names are doubtless in some degree arbitrary, and a writer who has given a full enumeration of the symptoms of a disease, will be understood, whatever name he may give such disease: But it is much to be lamented that the negligence and confusion of authors, as to names and descriptions, have greatly increased the difficulties which necessarily attend the collecting histories, or forming the classes of diseases.[1]

Cholera is very much a disease of cities. Early humans were hunters, following the trail of game. Constant movement made it unlikely their excrements would contaminate the water supply. Later, as they became gatherers and remained in one place for long periods of time, the risk of polluting water became greater, but small settlements lessened the chances of drinking-water contaminations. It was only when large numbers of people gathered together in confined spaces that the danger of thousands of untreated privies leaking into ground water or rivers led to the spread of cholera on an unprecedented scale, striking the rich and the poor, the famous and the obscure with equal virulence.

The date of its first appearance is unknown, but clearly the disease has been endemic in certain parts of the world from at least the 5th century. Records of dehydrating diarrhea were kept by Hippocrates and appear in Sanskrit writings.

An interesting speculation on the early appearance of cholera in the British Isles came to light with the discovery of a letter preserved in the Scotch College. Written by the Bishop of Ross to the Archbishop of Glasgow, at Paris, it supplied details of the illness of Mary, Queen of Scots, while she was at Jedburgh in October 1566. In 1832, a researcher named Keith noted the similarity between the queen's symptoms and those of cholera victims of his day. The original letter was reproduced:

My Lord,—After maist hastie commendations, I wryt upon haist to zour Lorship with Sander's Bog, who was sent be Mons. de Croc, this last Weddensday to adverteis of the Queenis Majesty's Seykes quhilk at that time was wonderous gryt, for assuritlie her Myjestie was sa handleit with gryt vehemencie, that all that was with hir was disparit of hir convalescens. Nochtheles soone after the departing of Sanderis Bog, hir Majestie gat sume relief quhilk leslit quhill Frisday, at ten hourius at evin, at quhilk time hir Majestie swount agane, and failzet in her sicht, hir feit and hir neis was cauld, quhilkis war handleit be extreme rubbing, drawing, and others cureis, be the space of four houris, that na creature could indure gryter paine, and throch the vehemencie of this cure hir Majestie gat some relief, quhall about sax houris in the morning on Fryday that hir Majestie became deid, and all hir members cauld, eeyne closit, mouth fast and feit and arms stiff and cauld. Nochtheles Maister Naw quha is ane perfyt man of his craft wald nocht gif the mater owr in that maner, bot of new beyond to draw hir neis leggis, armis, feit, and the rest with sic vehement tormentis quhilkis lasted the space of three houris, quhill hir Majertie recovert agane hir sicht and speeche and gat ane gryt swyting quhilk was halding the relief of the seighnes, because it was in the nynt day quhilk commonly is called the creisis of the seykeis, and swae heir thocht the culeing of the fever. And sensyne continuallie thankis to God hir Majestie convalesces better and better; bot the vehement presse of vomiting and laxative with the gryt pain of rubbing and drawing of hir memberis, quhilkis hir Majestie hes sustenit, hes maid hir sae waik, that she is nocht abill haistile for traivel furth of thir partis.[2]

Roughly translated, the letter reads:

My Lord,—After most hasty commendations, I write upon haste to your Lordship with Sander's Boy, who was sent by Mons. de Croc, this last Wednesday to advise of the Queen Majesty's Sickness that at that time was wondrous great, for assuredly her Majesty was so [overcome] with great vehemence that all that was with her was despairing of her convalescence. Nonetheless soon after the departing of Sander's Boy, her Majesty got some relief which lasted until Thursday, at ten hours even [10:00 p.m.], at which time her Majesty swooned again, and failed in her sight, her feet and her knees was cold, which was [overcome] by extreme rubbing, drawing, and other cures, by the space of four hours, that no creature could endure greater pain, and through the vehemence of this cure her Majesty got some relief, until about six hours in the morning [6:00 a.m.] on Friday that her Majesty became dead, and all her members cold, eyes closed, mouth fast [rigid] and feet and arms stiff and cold. Nonetheless Master Naw who is one perfect man of his craft would not give the matter over in that manner, but of new beyond [knew] to draw her knees, legs, arms, feet, and the rest with such vehement torments which lasted the space of three hours, when her Majesty recovered again her sight and speech and got one great sweating which was heralding [?] the relief of the senses, because it was in the next day which commonly is called the crisis of the sickness, and saw her through the cooling of the fever. And since continually thanks to God her Majesty convalesces better and better; but the vehement press of vomiting and laxative with the great pain of rubbing and drawing of her members, which her Majesty has sustained, has made her so weak, that she is not able enough for travel forth of these parts.

Did Queen Mary suffer from cholera? Just as physicians in the 1830s could not positively differentiate between common diarrhea, vomiting and true cholera, it is impossible to make a definitive diagnosis, but the possibility is intriguing.

21st Century Disease Distinctions

It is apparent from the following definitions that practitioners working before the era of modern science were at a great disadvantage when it came to making a definitive diagnosis. The idea that miasma (poisoned air) caused many, if not all, of these diseases hindered effective preventative measures, while the similarity of symptoms complicated correct distinctions.[3]

Dysentery: Diarrhea containing blood and mucus, resulting from inflammation of the GI tract. It is caused by bacterial, viral, protozoan, or parasitic infections and is commonly seen in places with inadequate sanitation where food and water are contaminated with pathogens. Prevention is the major emphasis of health care providers.

Spotted fever: General and imprecise name for various eruptive fevers including typhus and tick fever.

Typhoid fever: A severe infectious disease marked by fever and septicemia. The disease is initially marked by a fever up to 104° F for about 7 days, followed by a flat, rose-colored, fleeting rash (which would have been the distinctive identifier for early doctors), abdominal pain, anorexia, and extreme exhaustion. About 14 days after infection begins, internal bleeding develops as the result of gastrointestinal ulcers. It is caused by *Salmonella typhi* (gram-negative bacteria, transmitted by water or food contaminated by human feces or by vomitus and oral secretions during the acute stage.

Typhus: An infection transmitted by lice, fleas or mites. Mild cases are marked by a flat rash that spreads out from the trunk or by flu-like symptoms. In more severe cases, fever, skin necrosis and gangrene on the tips of fingers, toes, earlobes and the penis is seen. Mortality is high except when treated early enough by broad-spectrum antibiotics.

Yellow fever: An acute, infectious disease caused by a flavivirus and transmitted by the *Aedes* mosquito. Symptoms include high fever, headache, muscle aches, nausea and vomiting and GI disturbances such as diarrhea or constipation. After a 1–2 day remission, 20 percent of patients experience abdominal pain, severe diarrhea, GI bleeding (producing a characteristic "black vomit") and jaundice, from which the nicknames "yellow fever" and "yellow jack" are derived. No antiviral agents are effective and prognosis is grave.

In 1563, Garcia del Huerto, a Portuguese physician, described epidemic cholera that had been present in India for hundreds of years.[4] By the mid– to late 1700s, reports of the incidence of cholera appeared more and more frequently in the newspapers. While the disease had not yet become widespread, death statistics at the end of the 18th century indicate that its dire effects were already being felt, although the first accredited epidemic did not begin until 1817. Anton van Leeuwenhoek had developed the first truly effective microscope in the 1660s, bringing the invisible world of bacteria into focus, but practitioners were slow to embrace the new technology, and for nearly 200 years, doctors predicated their diagnoses solely on the basis of symptoms.

Due to the fact a number of diseases produced similar effects, the diagnosis of "Cholera morbus," as it was called, was frequently confused or counted with statistics generically referred to as "Disorders of the Bowels." Being classified as an autumnal disease in accordance with the 18th and 19th century penchant for correlating changes in temperature and wind velocity with the prevalence of certain illnesses, cholera fell into a very broad category.

Autumnal Diseases (circa 1765)

- Cholera morbus
- Dysentery
- Bilious cholic* (*Colica Billosa*): colic from an excess of bile
- Dry gripes: pain in the loins
- Cholic Poictou: likely an inflammatory colic
- Hysteric cholic: brought on by a violent or emotional state; the word "hysteria" was used exclusively for females
- Gravel: (*Calculus*) small, sand-like concretions, or stones, which pass from the kidneys through the ureters in a few days
- Gallstones
- Wandering gout: rheumatism[5]

*"Cholic" was the British spelling; Americans dropped the "h." Colic is described by *Taber's Cyclopedic Medical Dictionary* (20th edition, 2001, p. 445) as being a spasm in any hollow or tubular soft organ accompanied by pain, particularly pertaining to the colon. Biliary colic causes right upper quadrant pain resulting from obstruction of a bile duct by a gallstone; intestinal, or abdominal colic is associated with intestinal obstruction; infantile colic in infants may be brought about by cow's milk or increased stimulation; renal colic causes pain in one of the flanks, radiating toward the lower abdomen and may be associated with passage of kidney stones.

In 1746, Dr. Charles Ayton Douglas noted, "the frequency of the Cholera, or Cholick, its various and terrible Effects, and often Fatality, especially among the poorer Sort ... can hardly have escaped the Notice of any one...." Describing cholera as "a violent Vomiting and Purging of Bile, and other acrid Humours; being a Disease so acute and deadly, as frequently to destroy a Man in 24 Hours," he made his patients drink "of warm Water, 3 or 4 Times; which they always throw up." He followed this with a Decoction of "Oat-Bread, baked without Leven, or Yeast, carefully toasted, as brown as the Colour of Coffee, but not burnt." If the patient convulsed, he added a strong dose of "Laudanum, 25 drops in an Ounce of strong Cinnamon Water and afterwards a Draught of Wine."[6]

As described by Andrew Wilson, M.D., Fellow of the Royal College of Physicians at Edinburgh, in his work, *Short Remarks Upon Autumnal Disorders of the Bowels, and on the Nature of Some Sudden Deaths, Observed to Happen at the Same Season of the Year* (1765), these illnesses "are ascribed to cramps or spasms, into which the state of the fluids is apt to throw the nerves of the bowels at these times: hence these grievous diseases are both translated and extended to the most extreme parts of the body, so as to produce cramps, fixed pains, numbness, and even palsies, themselves."

Dysentery was distinguished from "a Diarrhea" "by the remarkable inactivity of the peristaltic motion of the bowels, and *consequentially* by the hardened state of the excrements so commonly discharged in that disease."

Symptoms leading to death from any of the above-mentioned diseases were described as "an uneasy (and sometimes at the very first an acute) pain as in the upper part of the stomach between the breast and belly, or in the anticardium, commonly called the pit of the stomach." As the pain grew worse, the patient experienced trouble breathing, the heart either fluttered or did "its office faintly," the pulse weakened, and a ghastly cold sweat arose on the face. The sufferer was finally forced into an erect posture, "and soon after the circulation is totally suppressed. The patient all the while continues sensible." Wilson concluded: "These symptoms sufficiently indicate a violent spasmodic affection of the whole nervous system, by which the vital functions are almost instantly arrested." Criticized for its style ("perfect elegance is not necessary in a medical writer; but there is great merit in conciseness, simplicity, and propriety"), the work appeared in eight volumes and cost 1s, 6d.[7]

Style of a different sort was showcased in a letter written home by an Englishman in Paris. Aside from its humorous visualization, the missive clearly indicated that cholera, albeit in a mild form, had become engrained in the European consciousness: "You are misinformed, that Veneration, if ever it existed, is extinguished; the other Night, in a Company where Politicks had their Turn, I was seized with the Cholera Morbus, but was instantly relieved by the following Evacuation."[8]

As the medical profession inched along in its ability to diagnose and understand disease, Donald Monro, M.D., published *An Account of the Diseases Which Were Most Frequent in the British Military Hospitals in Germany, from January 1761, to the Return of the Troops to England in March 1763* (1766). Chapter 2 contained a discussion of dysentery, of which the author stated, "nothing contributed more to the cure, than keeping the patients clean, and in large airy wards." If the illness were attended with fever and pain, he suggested the "lancet to be freely used, notwithstanding the low pulse, which frequently rose as the blood flowed from the vein." Emetics were then prescribed, repeated as necessary. The following day, *sal catharticum amarum* (medicinal bitters), mixed with manna and oil was given. After four days, a moderate opiate was prescribed, alternating with minderi or saline draughts to which were added four drops of the Thebaic tincture, made with Egyptian poppies. When symptoms abated, rhubarb was preferred to the above cathartics. After several weeks of recovery, the intestines were braced and restored by gentle astringent medicines mixed with opiates. Mild purges were given at intervals.

The following entry in Monro's text was *cholera morbus*, "or a sudden and violent vomiting and purging; it is of the bilious kind, and the cure principally depends upon the free use of warm, mild liquors, in the beginning, to dilute and blunt the acrimony of the bile and other fluids, and to promote their discharge." Afterwards, gentle cordials to "support the strength" were given, along with warm formentations and mild opiates. Monro concluded: "If the sickness or gripping remains next day, after the cholera is stopt," give a dose of physic (cathartic) and an opiate in the evening.[9] The text, in 8 volumes, sold for 5s.

While Dr. Wilson took "pains" to describe the types of physical distress associated with autumnal diseases, Monro's emphasis was on the treatment for these pains. In neither case did the physicians prescribe immediate rehydration, and while the former described symptoms leading to death, the latter's casual summary presumed cholera would be cured within a day or two, indicating either his lack of experience or a serious misdiagnosis. As indicated at the beginning of this chapter, there was little, if any, regulation or agreement regarding nomenclature, leading to public and professional confusion.

Elements of the Practice of Physic, Part II, Containing the History and Methods of Treating Fevers and Internal Inflammations, by George Fordyce, M.D. (member of the Royal College of Physicians, and Reader on the Practice of Physic), 1768, did not make the subject any clearer. Under the subheading "Inflammations of the mucous membrane," Fordyce grouped together "the catarrh; the erisipelatous sore throat, or sore throat attended with ulcers; the cholera morbus, diarrhea and dysentery; the venereal disease; the gonorhaea benigna."

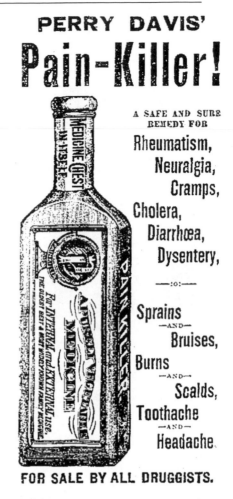

PERRY DAVIS'
Pain-Killer!

A SAFE AND SURE REMEDY FOR

**Rheumatism,
Neuralgia,
Cramps,
Cholera,
Diarrhœa,
Dysentery,**

—:o:—

Sprains
—AND—
**Bruises,
Burns**
—AND—
**Scalds,
Toothache**
—AND—
Headache.

FOR SALE BY ALL DRUGGISTS.

It was not uncommon to see a patent medicine advertised as a cure for a multitude of diseases. Perry Davis' Vegetable Medicine could be used either internally or externally for a wide variety of afflictions ranging from cholera to sprains and bruises. Attractively packaged, it could contain anything from colored branch water to ether, alcohol, cooling mint or other inexpensive spices to give it a "kick" and a pleasing taste (*Weekly Wisconsin*, August 1, 1883).

3

The Immortal Sydenham

Thus the observations of the immortal Sydenham in regard to the influence of the reigning epidemic on the other contemporary diseases, and the importance of keeping in view this fact in their medical treatments, received in every succeeding season, additional confirmation.[1]

The above quotation from 1799, referencing the symptoms and treatment of cholera morbus, diarrhea, dysentery and continued fevers (typhus) under the theory of *Vis medicatrix naturae*, harkened directly to Thomas Sydenham (September 10, 1624–December 29, 1689) and before that worthy physician to Hippocrates.

Known as the "Father of Medicine," the Greek physician Hippocrates (circa 460–375BC) was the first healer to attempt to record medical experiences for future generations, thus establishing the foundation for the scientific basis of medical practice.[2] Among his theories was the belief that an organism was not passive to disease, but made every attempt to correct imbalances. This led to the practice of allowing the living organism to heal itself by providing treatments that removed obstacles preventing self- recovery.

Born at Wynford Eagle, Dorset, England, Thomas Sydenham entered Magdalen Hall, Oxford, at the age of 18 years. After serving in the Parliamentarian Army during the English Civil War, he graduated from Oxford in 1648, with the degree of bachelor of medicine. His first book, *Methodus curandi febres* [The Method of Curing Fevers], was published in 1666; a second edition contained a chapter on the plague and a third edition under the title, *Observationes medicinae* [Observations on Medicine], appeared in 1676. Sydenham, known as the "Father of English Medicine," contributed to the study of fevers, fluxes and other acute maladies by studying them over a period of years, describing and comparing symptoms, similarities and outcomes. In his work, he expressed the belief that seasons and weather dictated the type and variety of disease and correct treatments could not be initiated until these were known. These observations constituted the doctrine of the "Epidemic Constitution of the Year or Season," which depended on "inscrutable telluric causes."

Sydenham's method of classification slotted diseases into "evident" and "conjunct." Fevers and inflammations (the "evident" symptoms), he believed, were the body's response to outside influences. Conversely, he considered "conjunct," or remote, causes of secondary importance and likely impossible to determine. Stressing that conformity of symptoms and the course of the illness resulted from unity of the cause (meaning that specific diseases ran a predictable course), he attributed acute diseases to the reaction of the body to combat outside influences. As with Hipprocratic teaching, he advocated the practice of observation and intervention of the natural crisis. He considered chronic diseases as a "deprived state of the humours," primarily caused by improper diet and lifestyle.[3]

Sydenham's influence on the practice of medicine was far-reaching and persuasive, and his belief that atmospheric conditions influenced the presence and course of diseases directly affected how cholera was perceived and treated.

Bad Winds and Good Winds

John Stedman, M.D., fellow of the Royal College of Physicians in Edinburgh, was clearly influenced by Thomas Sydenham when he wrote in his text, *Physiological Essays and Observations* (1769):

> The ancients universally ascribe a baneful quality to south winds.... With us, the good or bad effects of north winds seem to depend on the period of the year in which they blow; for about the end of the spring, or the beginning of summer, when pinching north winds follow a warm state of the air, these winds which are productive of rheums, coughs and inflammations, affecting chiefly the pleura and lungs. But from the summer solstice to the autumnal equinox, or some time after it, northerly winds are observed to correct that state of the air which promotes putrefaction, the causes of which in the air are heat, humidity, and continued calms, or warm south winds. The air when in this state, seems frequently to be impregnated with a sulphureous *gas*, which, at times, manifests itself by meteors, coruscations, thunders, and luminous appearances on swampy grounds.

Lamenting that scientific journals omit "the degree of winds," he argued that winds, independent of their source and direction, "have been found to acquire particular qualities, according to the nature of the tracts of land over which they pass." Citing Dr. Huxham, he stated that great storms frequently gave check to epidemic fevers. In the seven months of the two most sickly years (June-December 1732 and 1735), there were only four hurricanes, or winds of the fourth degree.

To determine the effects of air on the human body, he examined case histories during the latter part of these months and the period following, indicating that "unless the air be noxious to an uncommon degree," its effects did not appear until sometime after the cause. Beginning in August 1732, his study revealed that until the end of October, "low" fevers prevailed chiefly among "the inferior rank of people, and soon became mortal." These fevers were attended with headaches, ravings and sometimes diarrhea. In the two latter months, the disease took on a deadly cast, creating stupor and lethargic listlessness, eventually turning fatal about the 8th or 9th day. Many of the diseased voided worms of different kinds, which, in fevers, "generally proceed from bilious or acrimonious humours lodged in the intestines."

From the beginning of November to the end of December, "aguish complaints, cholera, quincies, rheumatisms, diarrheas, besides slow fevers," were common. About the middle of December, influenza broke out and soon became so general few escaped the disease. Interestingly, the author added that before influenza infected humans, the disease manifested itself in horses. Symptoms included coughs and a copious discharge of acrid mucus from the nostrils.

During the period beginning June 1735, measles broke out, becoming more frequent in the country toward December. Measles were followed by dangerous and intractable coughs, peripheumonies and diarrheas. Those with previous cases of measles were "taken with a fever similar to that of the measles." In July, slow fevers with low pulse (bradycardia) and diarrhea were most common. In the latter month, dysentery spread, while after the New Year until February, low fevers said to be of the pleuritic kind prevailed, of the species that proceeded "from a resolved state of the blood, and which is frequently produced by that constitution of the air, which generates putrefaction."

To further prove his theory that weather affected disease patterns, Dr. Stedman stated that the great plague at Messina in 1743 was thought to have been brought to England by a Genoese tartana, a small fishing boat, but the rapid propagation "of the disease seems to have been more owing to the state of the air some time before the arrival of that vessel, and to a pre-disposition in the bodies to receive the infection, than to any other cause." He concluded by remarking that the probability "of neglecting the degrees of winds" was grave and possibly gave erroneous conclusions.[4]

Dr. John Ruddy's work, *A Chronological History of the Weather and Seasons, and of the Prevailing Diseases in Dublin* (1770) covers the period 1725–1761. He concluded that in the spring season more than any other, coughs and defluxions were most common, "and undoubt-edly the N. and E. winds, usually then predominant, have a principal share in this." Quoting a poet, he added this:

> Each season doth its poisons bring,
> Rheums chill the winter, agues blast the Spring.

His tables included the following:

Diseases by Season

Disease	Spring	Summer	Autumn	Winter
Diarrhea	1	0	9	5
Dysenteries	2	5	10	4
Cholera morbus	0	2	3	0

Correlating statistics published in the *Memoirs of the Royal Academy*, Paris, he argued there was a great similarity between diseases and winds in both France and England, summarized as follows:

1. Agues and intermittent fevers are found chiefly in the spring.
2. The cholera morbus mostly in summer.
3. Inflammations in the bowels mostly in summer.
4. Dysenteries mostly in summer and autumn.
5. Diarrheas mostly in autumn.
6. Asthmas mostly in winter.
7. Military fevers equally in spring, summer and autumn.
8. Rheumatism and rheumatic fevers mostly in winter.[5]

William Grant, M.D., in his work, *Observations on the Nature and Cure of Fevers* (1773, revised from 1771) followed this well-established path, dividing fevers into vernal and autumnal. From the month of July onward, he stated, fevers commonly called "Putrid morbid lentor" reigned. In this category he included "cholera morbus, the new fever of Sydenham, bilious fever of Tiffot; the ague, dysentery, miliaria and erysipelas of the harvest season." His medical experience indicated that these fevers "easily yielded to the same, or a similar method of cure to that which agreed with the catarrh; excepting only some slight alteration according to the pressing symptoms, and variety of the temperatures of the sick."[6]

Diarrhea, Dysentery and Cholera

By the end of the 18th century, confusion still existed among practitioners attempting to differentiate various bowel diseases and fevers on the basis of symptoms. "Bills of Mortality" were commenced in the reign of Queen Elizabeth I, and beginning in 1603, were published by authority in London. A sampling of statistics reveals:

Diseases and Casualties in London
June 1–6, 1748

Convulsion	118
Consumption	104
Fever	67
Age	39
Smallpox	31
Teeth	21
Dropsy	15
Found dead	4
Suddenly	2
Drowned	2
Thrush	1
Killed by a blow	1

There were 245 christened and 452 buried.[7]

Diseases and Casualties in London
For the Year December 14, 1762–December 13, 1763

Convulsions	6,338
Smallpox	5,582
Consumption	4,892
Fever, malignant, scarlet, spotted, and purple	3,414

For the year there were 15,133 christened and 26,143 buried.[8]

Partial Account of Diseases in London,
August 20–September 20, 1798

Acute Diseases	Number of Cases
Diarrhea	26
Chronic Rheumatism	12
Scrophula	7
Dysentery	7
Cholera	4
Smallpox	3

Accompanying these numbers, text described the state of the city's health, remarking that disorders of the stomach and bowels had been very frequent, with diarrhea, dysentery and cholera prevailing in an uncommon degree. Concerning diarrhea, it was noted that most cases were so mild as not to require medical attention, proving "to be nothing more than a salutary effort of the constitution to throw off some offending matter." Cases in which the disease became troublesome and obstinate were attributed to the hasty attempt to check discharges by the use of astringents and opiates.

Dysentery was of a more alarming nature. Although it resembled the diarrhea in some symptoms, it "is sufficiently distinguished by others, and is to be traced to a very different cause." For this disease, writers for the *Monthly Magazine* described it as eliciting frequent stools, generally in small quantity and containing mucus sometimes mixed with blood. This was accompanied with severe gripings followed by tenesmus. Dysentery was sometimes preceded, and generally accompanied, by febrile symptoms and often proved contagious, particularly in military camps.

One instance of this was mentioned in a letter written by a British army officer, dated "camp at Long Island, about two leagues from the Bar of Charles-Town, South Carolina, July 7," 1776, during the American Revolution. After supplying details of some naval encounters, he added the following: "Some of the troops have been seized with the Cholera Morbus, but in general they are very healthy, though obliged to live on salt provisions."[9]

Distressed at the general lack of cleanliness at his camps, George Washington recommended the Mosaic code of Deuteronomy (which required latrine placement a certain distance outside camp), while Baron von Steuben, who trained the Continental Army at Valley Forge, issued specific regulations for latrine placement, emphasizing that health and cleanliness were matters of military discipline.[10]

Sir John Pringle, in his treatise, *Diseases of the Army*, described dysentery as a contagion arising from dead bodies unburied in the field of battle, or sometimes from the effluvia of marshes, and at other times from crowded jails and hospitals. Dissections proved that the seat of the disease lay in the larger intestines, while pathologists referred its proximate cause to a spasmodic stricture of the colon and a detention of hardened feces. The cure, therefore, consisted in the removal of the stricture and the evacuation of stool. Fomentations of the abdomen and the application of the blister sometimes succeeded in the removal of spasms.

Pringle stressed that if opiates were administered, they should be followed by cathartic remedies. If the stomach rejected oral medicines, the use of clysters became particularly necessary. Numbers reflected in the monthly statistics did not represent any dysentery in its worst form.

Most cases of cholera morbus listed above were mild, "which have yielded to the diluting and demulcent plan of treatment; though, in some instances, there has been occasion for the use of opiates."[11]

Partial List of Diseases in London
September 20–October 20, 1799

Acute Diseases	Number of Cases
Cough	14
Diarrhea	13
Dyspepsia	7
Dysenteria	6
Cholera morbus	4

Partial List of Death in London
August–October 1799

Disease	Number of Deaths
Consumption	972
Convulsions	785
Fever	334
Smallpox	161
Inflammation	99

Other causes of death and their numbers included "Suddenly, 31 [qm] and "Evil, 2."

Text accompanying the mortality list noted that disorders of the bowels were frequent and were, at times, obstinate. In most cases they constituted the principal disease but in some they "blend themselves with other diseases of the system." Cholera morbus tended to affect persons living in the same house, which made it appear contagious. During this period, symptoms were mild and "recovery was soon obtained."[12]

4

"The Cause of
Pestilential Distempers"

Relative Causes which affect the Health of Man: An inordinate use of impure water, often charged with earthly particles, animalcula both living and dead, noxious vegetable substances, mineral and poisonous impregnations, &c.[1]

An interesting case concerning the cause of yellow fever in America elicited some startling references to miasmas in general and dysentery and cholera in particular. During the summer of 1799, the New York State Legislature was called upon to answer and act upon the question as to whether yellow fever was of domestic origin or was imported from foreign ships and merchandise. Prevailing opinions settled the dispute by declaring the city had enough causes for the production of that distemper without any need for external sources.

In an effort to reduce the plague, lawmakers at Albany passed a bill prohibiting certain trades and manufactures within city limits. Among other things, the act forbade the manufacture of soap and candles under heavy penalty. Those directly involved with these businesses engaged Dr. Mitchell as their counsel to manage the business of procuring terms of mitigation. Dr. Mitchell presented his "Theory of Pestilential Fluids" to the seat of government, arguing that substances composed of "carbone and hydrogene," such as fat, grease and oil, "were incapable of yielding pestilential air; and that the substances containing septon, to wit, the skinny, lean, muscular and membranous parts of animals, together with the blood and alimentary faeces, were the substances whence unhealthy and noxious exhalations proceeded." Thus, persons engaged in business working with the "ashes, soap and fat" were protected from pestilential diseases.

Mitchell cited the work of Count Berchtold and Consul Baldwin, confirming the beneficial effects of oil in keeping off and relieving the symptoms of plague in Asia, while stressing the remarkable exemption of Nantucket whalemen from malignant fevers on long voyages. He also introduced the work of Citizen Guyton, stating that "the chief difference between common air and pestilential are consisted merely in this; that in the former, the septon with caloric formed azotic air, and the oxygene constituted vital air, each distinct from the other; whereas in the latter case the septon and oxygene are chemically blended with each other, base with base." He then stated that several cases of severe disorders in the alimentary canal, terminating in dysentery, came from the accidental drinking of diluted aquafortis, a weak and impure nitric acid. (Authorities in 1832 would also blame the existence of cholera on the admixture of aquafortis in whiskey.)[2]

Mitchell then expounded on the idea that privies and collections of human ordure (excrement) had long been observed to contain septic (nitric) acid, and the effluvia of privies had been known to excite dangerous sicknesses. Additionally, many articles of diet contained septon; and oxygen, in some form, always excited in the alimentary canal. It was therefore probable, he concluded, that septic acid might be formed in the cavities of these abdominal viscera, and that "irritation and inversion of the motions of the stomach, in some forms of *yellow fever*, as well as spasms of the colon, griping pains and tenesmus in some of the cases of *dysentery*, PROCEEDED FROM THE SAME EXCITING CAUSE."

From the operation of neutral salts in these kinds of illnesses, Mitchell derived the theory that these salts had the most efficacious and salutary effects upon septic acids, and "possessed a power, derived from their *alkaline bases*, to neutralize that mischievous and tormenting liquid. From this principle Dr. Mitchell investigated a theory of the *modus operandi* of these numerous and important articles of the MATERIA MEDICA."

Drawing from cases in a New York hospital as well as his private practice, the physician found watery solutions of the carbonates of potash and soda to be a most excellent antidysenteric remedy and valuable prescriptions in the cholera infantum. The acid/base relationship was used to explain yellow fever and to elucidate dysentery. Concluding, he said, "A general inference from all the phenomena was, that these maismata, or contagions, in all their forms herein contemplated, were violent STIMULANTS."

Taking his theory one step further, Mitchell believed that alkalies and lime neutralized the septic acid of animal excrements. Abandoning the common belief that lime was serviceable by its septic or putrefying quality, he became convinced its principal effect was to combine with septic acid into calcareous nitre, one of the richest manures, thus serving the added benefit of stimulating and feeding the plants which grow on such treated soil. When its use was applied to animals, he argued, dews and fogs impregnated with septic acid were the probable cause of mortal disorders in cattle, sheep and horses, as the aquafortis was taken into their bodies during the night. Rust and mildew in wheat was ascribed to the same cause.

Wrapping up the case for his clients, Mitchell stated that sweat, perspiration and excreted matter, all of which contained septon, rendered bedding, clothing and houses foul; in the heat of the human body, septic acid was produced, exciting morbid affections [*sic*] of the skin and engendering the worst forms of fever. Therefore, those in the business of producing alkalies actually provided a useful service to the community.[3]

Colonel Tatham, in his essay, "Remarks on the various Causes, which seem to affect the CLIMATE OF NORTH AMERICA, in those level Countries, which are less influenced by Frost, than the more mountainous Parts," had his own interpretation of conditions in the southern United States. After a lengthy discussion of how warm weather affected the constitution of this region's citizens, he delved into the subject of water. In an early discussion on the evils of drinking cold water—a prevailing attitude that persisted for over a century—he categorically stated that such a practice was often fatal in America. In an effort to explain the phenomenon, Tatham stated that even those seasoned to the country, and thus accustomed to the practice, were frequently "carried off with a *cholera morbus*, and the poorer class of emigrants from Ireland and other parts of Europe are still greater sufferers by it."

Without the benefit of microscopic science and bacteriology, he, like so many others, appeared to identify the source of contagion but missed the larger issue, perpetuating the mysticism of disease. Citing his experiences in Philadelphia in 1794, where wells were deep and the pumps stationary, he related several instances where individuals died in the streets near water pumps and was told that on one particularly hot day, not less than fifty expired from the imprudence of drinking cold water.

Closer to the point, Tatham advocated water filtration as a means of preventing sickness.

Referencing Staunton's *Chinese Embassy*, volume 2, p. 68, he reported that the Chinese put a small piece of alum in the hollow tube of a cane that was perforated with several holes. "With this instrument the muddy water is stirred a few minutes; and the earthly particles being speedily precipitated, leave the water above them pure and clear."

He added that Mr. Peacock at Guildhall had lately invented a more effectual method for purifying water by filtration *per ascensum*:

Water by Filtration—1800

The medium made use of is approximate to that by which nature operates; and the capacity of a machine of twenty guineas price is certified by a committee of captains, to whom Admiral Sir Peter Parker has lately referred the subject, to have proved capable, upon experiment, of clarifying at the rate of seven hundred gallons of turbid water in twenty-four hours.

Tatham added that further causes of ill health in the Southern states were directly attributable to a diet consisting of "salted meat, chiefly bacon, *hot* bread, and drink much cold spring water; those who assume a style of dissipation make equally free with ardent spirits and Madeira wine." Exposure to heat by the construction of homes using board planks or clapboards (of a thin kind split by malling) and nailed upon the outside of the frame, caused the inhabitants, particularly children, "to die (by inches as it were) from the moment in which he is born."[4]

Nostrums and Notions: The 18th Century Cure for Cholera

If Dr. Tatham, in his 1800 essay, deplored the use of cold water, hucksters of the same century were not as quick to dismiss its benefits, albeit with stipulations. In a lengthy dissertation on the benefits of "Baume d'Arquebusade Concentre, or Thompson's Concentrated Balsam of Arquebusade," the unnamed London author and former army surgeon noted that in Spain and other warm climates, when struck with cholera morbus, "or violent and copious discharges of green bile both by vomit and stool," natives had frequent recourse to plentiful draughts of cold water, "from which they often obtain relief." He stressed, however, with an eye toward selling his product, "it is not however meant to recommend such practice in this country." In his pitch to obtain a patent for Thompson's Balsam, he rightly noted that although "it is not customary with the Gentlemen of the Faculty, to act publicly the use of nostrums, yet he truths, that the well-informed and generous part of the profession will not withhold their countenance from this, without a fair and impartial trial of its virtues."

Made from the "concentrated juices of the most salutiferous, aromatic, saponaceous roots, plants &c.," Thompson's Balsam went speedily into the system. When rubbed on the surface of the body, it opened obstructed capillary vessels and passed through the whole course of circulation. Internally, it acted as a diuretic, mild astringent and a most powerful solvent of stony concentrations in the kidneys, urinary and gall bladders, strengthened the stomach and bowels and promoted digestion.

For those wishing to try this miracle cure, the balsam was sold only by the patentee at his warehouse, No. 415, Strand, nearly opposite the Adelphi. For the benefit of the poor, bottles cost 1s, 10d, while larger sizes sold for 4s, 6d, 6s, 10d and 12s, 6d. Each bottle was lettered with the title of the Balsam and sealed with the Patentee's Arms.[5]

Persons living in the year 1794, who wished to "cure the present very common complaint of the Stomach and Bowels" and prevent "the dangerous and fatal Consequences of the Cholera Morbus," needed to look no further than Dr. Molesworth's Anodyne Medicine," if his advertisement was correct. Scarcely ever failing to remove complaints from the above illnesses, it was promoted as being "perfectly innocent, and may be taken with the utmost safety." Sold only by the proprietor, E. Newbery, located at the corner of St. Paul's Church yard, it cost 2s, 9d. Duty was included.[6]

E. Sibly, M.D., went one step further in his 1799 advertising, using the testimony of the clergyman R. Thompson to promote "Dr. Sibly's Re-Animating Solar Tincture; or Pabulum of Life." Thompson wrote that as there was no medical gentleman near his parish, he was called upon to treat a female laboring under the violence of a Cholera Morbus. His patient "appeared indeed in a dying state, with a pulse scarcely perceptible, except when urged by frequent convulsions, every paroxysm returning with increased vehemence."

With little time to lose, he administered a tablespoon of Sibly's Tincture, diluted with water, despite the fact the mixture had not been promoted in Sibly's Medical Mirror as serviceable in complaints of this nature. After repeated doses, the convulsions ceased and in time the complaint was entirely removed, leaving the woman in better health than she had experienced for years. The advertisement concluded by stating a pamphlet extolling the virtues of the tincture could be had *gratis*; those wishing to purchase a bottle could do so for the hefty price of 7s, 6d.[7]

In 1804, "An Old Lady" wrote to the *Adams (PA) Centinel*, offering her "speedy and certain cure" for the flux and cholera: "Oil of Pennyroyal, two drops to a tablespoonful of molasses, syrup or honey; after being well stirred up, let one teaspoonful be administered every hour until it has the desired effect. For a grown person, the dose may be doubled."[8] A home remedy from 1811 promised "the bark of spruce pine boiled in milk, half-pint tumbler full taken at a time, and repeated at short intervals, as the stomach may be able to bear" never failed in curing bowel complaints.[9]

If that remedy did not "have the desired effect," Dr. Robertson's "Celebrated Stomach Elixir of Health" (price $1.50), offered to Philadelphians in 1812, purported to be "one of the most efficacious medicines, ever offered to the public, for coughs, colds, consumptions, the speedy relief and cure of obstinate hooping cough, asthmas, pains and wind in the stomach ... dysenteries, cholera morbus, severe grippings ... &c. &c."[10]

Gleaning from a New York paper, the London-published *Monthly Magazine* (November 1, 1819) offered this cure of cholera morbus:

> Take a soft cork, and burn it thoroughly in the fire; when it ceases to blaze, mix it up in a plate, with a little milk and water, or anything more agreeable to the palate, and repeat the dose till the disorder ceases, which it commonly does in the second or third administration of the remedy; the acidity of the stomach is immediately corrected, and the effect is instantaneous.

Unfortunately for professional hucksters and lay healers, Richard Reece, M.D., Fellow of the Royal College of Surgeons, London, in his tome, *The Domestic Medical Guide, in Two Parts*, third edition (1805), had harsh words on the "numerous nostrums, suggested by quacks, which they too successfully impose on the credulous public," justly observing the dangers presented "too often to the irreparable injury of those, who are induced to take their antibilious trash," and exposing "the mischiefs done by illiterate empiric(s)." Singling out "William Barclay's *patent* Antibilious Pills," Reece quoted from the advert that asserted bile to be "the fruitful parent of the complicated bodily miseries to which human nature is heir, (seen as gout, rheumatism, nervous affections, &c. &c.) that we bring into the world with us; that the *first pang* the infant suffers, proceeds from it! and that it *haunts* us more or less during our continuance in it."

Reece affirmed "a more absurd doctrine, blended with impiety, could scarcely be attended; nor could the reverend empiric have given a greater proof of his total ignorance of anatomy and physic, than in the passage just quoted." He added that the only disease produced by a vitiated secretion of the bile is the cholera morbus. In such cases, he had no hesitation in asserting that one dose of Antibilious Pills would "destroy the life of the patient, by producing inflammation of the bowels."

Significantly, in Reece's chapter on cancers, he quotes Dr. Lamb's study of common water, where he discovered not only a portion of lead (from the use of leaden cisterns, pumps and pipes) but also a mineral salt that he considered extremely prejudicial to the human frame. Lamb suggested his patients drink only water divested of these obnoxious combinations by the process of distillation.[11]

For those still accustomed to be their own physicians, Mr. Pouteau, a distinguished surgeon of the Hotel Dieu at Lyons (the second hospital in France), in his medical text, *Euvres Posthumes de M. Pouteau* (1783), noted that the explorer Belloin, in a voyage to the East Indies in 1686, mentioned that natives cured the cholera morbus by the application of a hot iron to the heel.[12]

Cholera by Degrees

The practice of "Medical Nosology" was first begun by Francis Boissier de Sauvages (born 1706, at Alais, in Lower Languedoc), who attempted to arrange diseases according to the plan suggested by Sydenham. Dr. William Cullen (born 1712, at Lanark, Scotland), among others, followed Sauvages with his own scheme of arrangement without entering into disease history or cures. The text, *The Edinburgh Practice of Physic and Surgery* (1800), attempted to clarify the situation with enumerations of the above authors' work:

GENUS LX. CHOLERA, THE CHOLERA MORBUS

Cholera, *Saxu*
Diarrhoea Cholerica
    The Spontaneous Cholera (no manifest cause)
    Cholera Indica
The Accidental Cholera (from acrid matters taken internally)
    Cholera crapulofa
    Cholera a venenis

Description:

The disease showed itself by excessive vomiting and purging of bilious matter, violent pain, inflation and distention of the belly. Patients sometimes suffered universal convulsions, great thirst, small and unequal pulse, cold sweats, fainting, coldness of the extremities, and hiccough. Death frequently ensued in twenty-four hours.

The weak and those rendered irritable by a long hot summer, or individuals living in a warm climate or in putrid vapours are peculiarly liable to this disease. It is produced by cold, or putrid vapours, arises as a partial result of fevers, from continual purging for any reason, or from inflammation of the intestines.

Care:

The first object is to counteract the accumulation of bile in the alimentary canal, particularly the stomach and to promote an early discharge of it. It is next necessary to restrain the increased secretion of bile, and lastly, to restore a sound condition to the alimentary canal, much weakened by the violence of the disease.

This ad was placed in *Allen's Indian Mail* (London, May 31, 1854) with the intent of catching the eye of those with any connection to the British possession. Readers of this newspaper were likely soldiers, their families, or, more important, those with investments in India. Well aware that cholera was rampant, everyone with interests in the colony was extremely concerned about preventing the sickness from affecting their commerce. Opium was a common ingredient of anti-cholera medicines at the time, considered essential for the treatment of diarrhea.

> The cure is effected by giving the patient a large quantity of warm water or weak broth in order to cleanse the stomach of the irritating matter, and injecting the same by way of clyster until pain abates. After this, a large dose of opium is administered. If the case is much advanced before the physician arrives, immediate recourse must be had to the laudanum because the patient is too weak to bear any further evacuations. If the laudanum is thrown up, a decoction of oat-bread, toasted as brown as coffee and mixed with water or weak gruel ought to be given; or, the simple administration of mint water is said to be efficacious.
>
> After the violence of the disease is overcome, vegetable bitters, particularly colombo root, strengthens the stomach and allays a disposition to vomiting, which often remains for a considerable time after the cholera may be said to be overcome.[13]

No one authoritative text ascended to prominence, and indicative of continuing confusion over the exact characterization of similar diseases, writers noted the following: "Indeed the cholera, diarrhea and dysentery are very nearly allied, and pass into each other by insensible gradations; the two latter especially, are so much alike, that except in a certain number of marked cases, which point out the peculiar circumstances of their distinction, it is doubtful whether we ought to affix to the disease the one name or the other." Eventually, the classifications *Spontaneous* and *Accidental Cholera* were eliminated, but it would be decades before more accurate and definitive terms were agreed upon.

Regardless of nomenclature, treatment remained similar. One generic approach consisted of administering 12–15 grains of rhubarb taken every morning for a few days to remove the complaint. A pill containing 1 grain of opium and 1 of ipecacuanha might also be taken at bedtime. It was recommended the diet should consist of nourishing emollient liquids, such as weak broth and rice gruel. In cases more purely dysenteric, a solution of neutral salts every morning proved more effective than rhubarb. In cases where diarrhea was prematurely checked by opiates (constipation was a side effect of opium), severe headache often resulted, indicating that in all cases, but especially when it prevailed epidemically, "the means of stopping it should be used with great caution." A diet consisting of nourishing emollient liquids such as weak broth or rice gruel was suggested.[14]

Partial List of Diseases in London
August 20–September 20, 1800

Acute Diseases	Number of Cases
Continued fever	54
Diarrhea and Dysentery	62
Asthenia	21
Rheumatism	12
Cholera	8

Cholera, which had been unusually prevalent during the latter end of July and the greater part of August, was in decline by October, while diarrhea and dysentery were spread in equal proportion. Most cases, however, were considered "mild," and the only recorded death from cholera was an 18-year-old woman who expired less than 24 hours after severe diarrhea and vomiting commenced.

The violence of cholera during the summer of 1800 was compared to data collected by Sydenham in the summer of 1669, affording some idea "of the severity of this disease in the tropical regions." Modern authorities add that "the symptoms of cholera afford a very good example of what Physicians call the *Vis medicatrix naturae* [the recognition by Hippocratic physicians that life is self-healing][15]; and its medical treatment was founded on this principle," advocated by Sydenham. Treatment had also advanced to the point where large quantities of mild liquids were administered, "in order to dilute the acrid bile and to render its discharge the more easy." Although this was a false premise (practitioners classified cholera as a disease of bile because of the patient's excessive thirst and the yellowish tinge to the eyes),[16] it did serve to provide appropriate care.

Again, without understanding the correlation between cholera and weather, writers for *Monthly Magazine* observed that the disease generally occurred in the warmest period of summer, "and its frequency and violence correspond, for the most part, with the intensity and duration of the atmospherical heat. As a hot summer immediately *excites* the cholera, so it *predisposes* to diarrhea and dysentery, which usually make their appearance on the accession of the chilling damps of Autumn." They added that the immoderate use of fruit, "to which these maladies are commonly attributed," may actually produce them, but minute inquiry revealed that matter taken into the stomach was not the cause. (Arguments on this subject would continue for decades.) Going further, these medical authors dismissed the "vulgar notion" that a quantity of damaged foreign wheat, mixed into bread and sold in London, had any share in promoting cholera, diarrhea or dysentery.

During the same 30-day period, the "continued fever, or typhus" had become milder as the "furious delirium" accompanying it during the heat of summer (given the name *brain fever*) had subsided.[17]

Partial Account of Diseases in London
September 20–October 20, 1800

Disease	Number of Cases
Continued fever	60
Dysentery	29
Diarrhea	13
Cholera	6
Small-Pox	1

By the fall of 1800, cholera had nearly disappeared, while diarrhea and dysentery were less frequent, although dysentery was more severe and had assumed "a more decided character." Its symptomatic fever, by which it was generally accompanied, was "very slight, and in some instances scarcely perceptible." Dysentery, however, remained "singularly obstinate." It did not terminate in death but left victims in an extreme state of debility and emaciation. Only by a strict attention to diet and regimen could they gradually recover a tolerable share of health and strength.[18]

Partial Account of Diseases in London
November 20–December 1801

Disease	Number of Cases
Rheumatismus	36
Amenorrhea	29
Scarlatina	18
Cholera	13
Dysenteria	6
Typhus	5

Partial Account of Diseases in London
July 20–August 20, 1802

Disease	Number of Cases
Rheumatismus	36
Amenorrhea	32
Typhus	28
Scarlatina	21
Cholera	11
Dysenteria	9

Interestingly, J. Reid, a reporter for the *Monthly Magazine*, commented:

The fact is, that inflammatory diseases are almost become *obsolete*. The bold and energetic practice of Sydenham, which, at his time, was, perhaps wise and judicious, cannot be followed, at the present moment, and in the existing state and habits of society, without producing consequences the most deleterious and destructive. That sacred reverence for the blood, the vital fluid of the human frame, which has been inculcated by the dictates of ancient and holy writ, and sanctioned by the fatal results of modern medical experience, is as yet not sufficiently attended to, in the ordinary treatment of disease.[19]

The Predominant Distemper of the Season

As predicted, cholera dominated medical news during the summer of 1803. Still lacking a positive cause, doctors' speculation centered on fruit as a causative agent, although too many cases existed where no such consumption ensued to make a positive correlation.

Practitioners were warned that cholera was one of the diseases of the human frame "which impresses strongly the folly and imminent danger of medical procrastination." In perilous or acute disorders, no more than a few hours were allotted for the effectual exercise of the physician's skill: too late a detection "of the actual *essence* of the case" often led to death within twelve to twenty-four hours. To healers, the warning was implicit: "A more than ordinary *quickness* of mental sight is the distinguishing and radical constituent in the character of a preeminently qualified physician."

Partial Account of the Diseases of London
August 20–September 20, 1803

Disease	Number of Cases
Cholera	39
Catarrhus	21
Rheumatismus	18
Typhus	14
Dysenteria	11[20]

Numbers for the year 1807 reflected a change in causes of mortality, with an emphasis on "semi-insanity," with the notation there was no radical distinction between the furor of madness and the gloominess of melancholy.

Partial Account of the Diseases of London
July 20–August 20, 1807

Disease	Number of Cases
Asthenia	14
Diarrhea	13
Amenorrhea	12
Hypochondriasis	11
Cholera	7
Dysenteria	1[21]

Confusion over exactly what constituted cholera persisted. In 1809, W. White, of the Royal College of Surgeons, published *A Treatise on Inflammation, and Other Diseases of the Liver*. His arrangement of diseases of the liver included "Hepatitis, or Sthenic Inflammation. Hepatitis Chronicus. Synochus Billiosa. Cholera Morbus. Periodical Cholera. Remarks on the indiscriminate use of Purgatives. Torpor, or Paralysis. Schirrous. Biliary Calculi."

A review of the book questioned under what genus in nosology came "Remarks on the Indiscriminate use of Purgatives," while considering *schirrous* an error of the press. Under the heading *Synochus biliosa*, the author described it as "a distinct genus of fever," and afterwards, as differing "only in degree from cholera." A third definition categorized it as "a diminutive species of the bilious, or yellow fever, which occurs in hot climates." In the opinion of the reviewer, the book presented "only a rude heap of uninteresting facts."[22]

5

Cholera Reaches the Pandemic Stage

The disease denominated cholera, has been observed by physicians to mark the decline of the hot season as faithfully as the appearance of swallows announces the spring.[1]

Temperatures in the summer of 1812 ranged from a low of 32°F to a high of 79°F, with scant rain and considerable dryness in the atmosphere, seeming to confirm the idea that weather played a role in the prevalence of such diseases as cholera and diarrhea.

Partial Report of Diseases, London, June 20–July 20, 1812

Disease	Number of Cases
Dyspepsia	6
Psora	5
Rheumatismus	5
Cholera	2
Diarrhea	2[2]

The idea of arranging diseases into categories continued into the second decade of the 1800s. Sir Gilbert Blane's paper, "Observations on the Comparative Prevalence, Mortality, and Treatment of Different Diseases" (1815) chose four distinct headings:

1st: Those that have appeared and then disappeared in England, including leprosy and sweating sickness.

2nd: Those that have arisen but not yet disappeared, depending on specific contagions.

3rd: Those that have occasionally raged with peculiar violence, and after having abated for some time again became prevalent, including plague, dysentery, typhus, scurvy and rickets.

4th: Those that are more common at present (1815) than in former ages.

Blane wrote that in general, the violence of the third class was much diminished, partly due to the attention of greater cleanliness in modern modes of life, while the increased luxury of the present, and some circumstances connected with trades and manufactures, had been favorable to the prevalence of scarlet fever, consumption, gout, dropsy, palsy, apoplexy, lunacy and all diseases of the brain and nerves. In conclusion, his view was that "the present generation may congratulate itself on its improved condition with regard to those great sources of human misery, epidemic and endemic disorders."[3] It would not be long before Sir Blane had reason to rue those words.

The First Known Cholera Pandemic, 1817–1823

The first known cholera pandemic originated in the Ganges River delta in India. The disease broke out near Calcutta and quickly spread throughout the country.[4] An early report from England dated April 1817 noted frequent cases of the disease, "very rarely met with in numbers at this season." Believing it to be a part of the epidemic constitution of autumn, physicians were quick to ascribe its occurrence to the excessive use of fruit. J. Want, late surgeon to the Northern Dispensary, remarked this was "clearly a mistaken notion," as the last epidemic occurred "in persons who had not eaten it." He further disputed the supposition, remarking that cholera "seems to be an effort of Nature to dislodge from the stomach offensive accumulations, from whatever source they may arise; hence we find solitary instances do occasionally present themselves without any seeming connexion with atmospheric influence." Want advised the safest practice in curing the disease was to "administer copious draughts of chamomile tea, or even warm water, until the offensive matter is freely evacuated, which may be known by the fluid which is taken being rejected unmixed."[5]

The incidence of cholera in India was also of particular importance to the British, who were engaged in extensive hostilities in that country. The whole of the army in the field consisted of ten divisions, each with approximately 10,000 men. Camp followers in the governor-general's division alone numbered 13,000 and for the transportation of luggage, 40 elephants and 400 camels were employed. On December 17, 1817, the forces of the rajah of Nagpore were defeated and on the 30th, the city of Nagpore was deposed, with the most productive portions of his state transferred to the British.

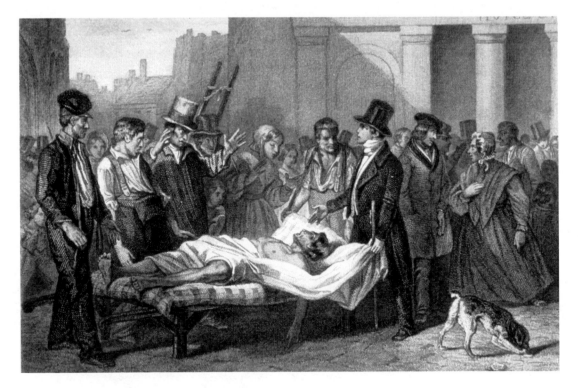

A man dying in the blue stage of cholera, J. Roze, engraver. It was commonly written about cholera that a man could be healthy at breakfast and dead by dinner (U.S. National Library of Medicine).

While the marquis of Hastings was receiving tribute from 36 rajahs and independent chieftains, cholera morbus was making severe ravages in the upper providence of Hindostan. In the district of Gorruckpoor alone, 30,000 deaths were reported. The disease appeared in Bengal and then crossed the peninsula "with rapid strides," quickly approaching Jualuah. Reports of "alarming sickness" in Hastings' camp were confirmed, but as it dissipated among them, camp followers suffered terribly. The report of one officer stated the following:

> This epidemic had all the characters of a decided pestilence. It had been gradually making its way along the banks of the Ganges and the Jumna, and suddenly broke out in the British camp. In the first day upon which it was distinctly recognised, 97 deaths were reported; on the next, above 500 died in the camp. Never, it is said, was a scene so dreadful witnessed. The dead and dying strewed every road. On all sides were heard the wailings of those who were seized, and gave themselves up to despair. At the time the malady was chiefly confined to the camp followers. Among the troops, European as well as native, who live well, the mortality was much less than among other classes; the loss even among them was severe. In the governor-general's establishment alone (who had himself been slightly affected) 17 native servants died. The remedy which was commonly administered upon the first appearance of the complaint was a tea-spoonful of laudanum in a glass of brandy. This in general retarded the progress of the disorder, and afforded time for further cure; but in many cases the malady was so rapid as to leave no opportunity for administering medicine. Natives were seen to fall suddenly without any previous sensation of illness, and die in a few minutes.[6]

A further report dated April 1, 1818, expressed grave concern over the spread of an epidemic disease assuming the form of cholera morbus, "which has fallen with fatal severity on the central division of the British army." While noting that native troops were the principal victims, "Europeans also have suffered from it." The article continued:

> Its ravages are nearly proportioned to the scanty sustenance to which those who are seized with it have been habituated. Laudanum, brandy, and calomel, are the medicines most successfully prescribed. The following statement of mortality from this disease, many years ago, is said to rest on high medical authority: At one of the greatest *Mallahs* held at Hurdwar every twelfth year, in the month of April, a sudden blast of cold air from the hills, which came down the course of the Ganges, produced so fatal and violent a *cholera morbis* [sic], that twenty thousand persons perished in the course of three or four days. Great as this number is, it will not appear incredible, when it is known, that nearly a million of people are supposed to be collected. In common years the number at the fair is estimated at 300,000.[7]

With concern over the war and the future of British interests in India running high, newspapers were eager to sate the public interest by publishing civilian reports from travelers and residents. News, always months behind the fact, reached Edinburgh in March 1819, concerning outbreaks of cholera in Calcutta and Decca, where it was stated the epidemic was of such formidable appearance that it carried off a number of natives, where in Bombay, obituaries listed a number of Europeans who perished from the distemper. Further reports indicated "that upwards of two millions of our fellow creatures have fallen victim to it within the last 18 months."[8]

During times of crisis, it is not unusual for people to seek redress for their miseries by appealing to a higher power. Eyewitnesses were often confounded and occasionally appalled at the desperation, and in some cases, the violence of these proceedings. Around the same time as the above, a gentleman residing in Calcutta reported that "upwards of 500 persons a day, for several days in succession" were carried off by the cholera morbus. The disease was supposed to be occasioned by the consumption of bad rice and by eating a species of "fat fish," taken in abundance in the spring.

Believing the sickness was sent upon them by *Oli Bibi*, the "Goddess of the Sickly Season," natives willingly followed an old woman pretending to be that incarnation. Her prescription for a cure was to go down to *Salempore* and eat of the fat fish. "In consequence, all the palanquin bearers and others of the lower classes deserted the city; and to their following her direction is attributed the alarming increase in the disorder." After several failed attempts by the government to seize her ("the people believing her not to be subject to the power of mortals"), she was finally apprehended and put in prison. That, the observer noted, restored order and "in some degree health, to the city."[9]

A letter by the Reverend C. Traveller, Vepery, Madras, India, dated October 12, 1819, brought home a more awful picture. Observing that the "heathen are both alarmed and sensibly concerned" about the epidemic of "Spasmodic Cholera," they made "great efforts to appease their deities, offering the most extravagant of almost every kind" of present. Hundreds of men, women and children poured forth "their libations of blood before their hideous idols, and vainly attempting to assuage the wrath of an unknown God, by services in which neither the judgment is informed, nor the heart affected."

During a trip to Pulicat, 30 miles from the Dutch possession of Madras, Traveller witnessed what he described as a mania affecting an entire village. At the instigation of their priest, the natives armed themselves with swords and other instruments of destruction, and paraded through every part of it, "brandishing their weapons in the air, beating their drums, and shouting with the vehemence of madmen, with a view to expel this disease from the borders." In addition, small branches of a peculiar tree were tied together and placed across doors to protect them from the plague.[10]

In a letter dated May 15, 1819, from Bombay, Mr. Horner, a Wesleyan missionary, described his own observations, beginning his missive by writing, "It appears as though God had a controversy with the people of India. War has slain its thousands, and pestilence its tens of thousands." He added that cholera, which had raged so dreadfully in 1818, had made a reappearance, sweeping away a great number of natives, as well as some Europeans. Describing the howling and lamentations heard during the night from families bewailing the loss of loved ones, Horner related how dead bodies were carried along in the streets, "while attendants loudly invoked Ramu or Narayau, or some other of their gods." Entire families were often seized with the disease, being carried away within a few hours of one another. Corpses were taken to great bonfires and consigned to the flames, "till the ground is strewed with the dead!"

In one remote village on the southern extremity, where the disorder had been very prevalent for several days, inhabitants forsook their homes and fled, leaving behind only a few priests to take care of their gods. The missionary added, in typical European style; "One circumstance makes it remarkable, namely, that the village is generally considered, by the Hindoos, as the most sacred place in Bombay, and where the Hindoo religion is observed in the greatest purity. Strange! that they should retain an attachment to the worship of gods who cannot protect them, and whom they are obliged to desert to save their lives!"[11]

The disease known as cholera morbus traveled quickly. Spread by increased exploration and trade in the early 1820s, it quickly left its devastating mark in Southeast and Central Asia, the Middle East, eastern Africa, India, China and the Mediterranean coast. Reports from the Philippines in 1820 presented a dire picture of how death from a mysterious and unknown cause wreaked havoc on a population. On October 9, 1820, a massacre broke out at Manilla (Manila was commonly spelled this way by 19th century writers), precipitated from an epidemic of cholera morbus. The banks of Lake Babia had overflowed by unusually heavy September rains, spreading water into the neighboring city of Manilla. After subsiding, a great quantity of filth and vegetable matter was left. Exposure to the hot sun, as it was believed, produced epidemic cholera, "which daily carries off hundreds of the natives." Local belief held that the disease was imported by strangers and rage was turned upon them. A number were murdered by a mob, their bodies horribly mutilated; an attack on a hotel frequented by foreigners soon followed.

According to contemporary reports, the governor pleaded with, but did not threaten, his people, leading to the suspicion that the authorities were aware of the danger to outsiders but did nothing to prevent it. The following morning, "the mob commenced plundering and murdering the Chinese" living outside the city walls. Colonel San Martin, commanding the Spanish troops, threatened to place himself at the head of his regiment and "for the honor of Spain," put down the mob without His Excellency's consent. San Martin's order to the natives to put down their arms and return peacefully home or be hanged on the spot had the desired effect and order was finally restored. Death counts included an American midshipman, an English captain and 10 seamen, and above 60 Chinese.[12]

Accounts from the year 1821 also indicated that cholera morbus raged dreadfully in Constantinople, Persia and throughout the Ottoman territory, especially in Schiraz. "More than 7,000 persons have fallen victims in a few days to this pestilential disorder. Among them were the mother, several children, and many other relations, servants, and slaves of the Schansade, Mahomet Ali Mirza."[13]

An officer from the United States Frigate *Congress*, off the coast of "Rio Janeiro," in a report dated March 17, 1821, informed readers that the ship had just reached port, being 91 days from Manilla, having sailed from Canton November 24 and Manilla on the 5th of December. The crew had left their business (the massacre) on the island "unsettled," having been driven off "by the distressing disease which was raging with great fury through the Island; it found its way on board our ship, and on the 7th we lost the boatswain, & on each five days succeeding, four or five hands were committed to the deep, having survived the attack but a few hours. Thirty-three died before we cleared Java Head, of cholera morbus; sixty-five of our crew have departed this life since we left the United States."[14]

His Majesty's ship *Termagant*, leaving Madras and Trincomalee on February 11, 1823, reported both areas healthy when they left, but off the south end of Ceylon, a "pestilential blast" assailed the ship, "and a very few days afterwards, eight of her scanty crew were buried, and two-thirds of the remainder were confined to their hammocks with Cholera Morbus. The blast continued a fortnight: it began in 3.25 N. and left the ship in 10 S.—the weather was very hot, very fine, and a clear atmosphere."[15]

In response to the increased awareness and spread of disease, it is not surprising that the *Gazette of Health* had reached its 72nd number in December 1821. For the price of 1s, citizens of England could read about recommendations of the Lettuce Lozenge for winter coughs, cases of gout and rheumatism cured by Colchicum Seed Tincture, "Successful Treatment of Hydrophobia in Russia, by Dr. Muller, of Paris," a "Fatal Case of Angina Pectoris and Lock-Jaw under Mr. Cline," and, of particular interest, "A Peculiar Disease of the Stomach, &c. in India, improperly termed Cholera Morbus."[16]

Although not considered a major health threat in the United States during the first pandemic, cholera was present to some extent in alarming numbers. A report from Baltimore, covering the period January 1, 1819, to January 1, 1820, indicated 2,287 deaths, the greatest number coming in September (474). Of these, 272 died of consumption, 258 from cholera morbus, 350 from malignant fever, 116 from measles and 77 of old age.[17]

Accurate numbers of fatalities are unknown, but based on the 10,000 recorded deaths among British troops in India, authorities place the death toll from cholera across that country in the hundreds of thousands. In 1820, alone, 100,000 individuals on the Indonesian island of Java succumbed to the disease. By 1823, cholera seems to have run its course around the globe, with the exception of the territory around the Bay of Bengal.[18]

Five Years Between Pandemics

Although the first known cholera pandemic ended in 1823, the intervening years of 1824–1828 before the next recognized pandemic were hardly free of the disease. Reports in this period typically followed a format similar to that reprinted from the *Nottingham Journal* in the *Courier* (London), September 11, 1824: "Nor has there been any sickness, beyond what is common to large towns: it is true there have been a few cases of the typhus kind, occasioned probably by the heat of the weather, and the *cholera morbus*, has prevailed in a partial degree, but we can safely aver, that not a dozen persons have fallen victim to either of these complaints within the last month."

In the United States, those wishing to stave off its appearance were encouraged to purchase "Dr. Vought's Valuable Medicines," or "Chemical Anti-Dysenteric Medicine," esteemed by all who used it for curing "Dysentery, (or Bloody Flux,) Diarrhea, (or Summer Complaint,) Cholera Morbus, Acidity, Vomiting, Sickness and Pain in the Stomach, Dyspepsia, Colic, Worms &c.—Prepared with directions. Price 62 1–2 cents per phial."[19]

In 1824, fearing that cholera might make an appearance in England, the Lords of the Privy Council sent data garnered from resident authorities abroad to the Royal College of Physicians. Their summary contained the following data:

> In 1817 [the Indian cholera] first assumed a pestilential character, and in the space of two or three weeks it traveled 100 miles, and exhibited itself in Calcutta, even amongst the European population; in two months of the following year, at Benares 15,000 persons perished, and on both sides of the Ganges a mortality equally great prevailed. In the Bengal army it appeared in the same year, and in a fortnight 9,000 soldiers fell victims, and soon afterwards spread among all classes. The disease traveled with a rapidity equal to 20 miles a day, and in one year traversed the whole of the Indian peninsula. Finally, it spread to Ceylon, the Mauritius, the Isle of Bourbon, Java, Cochin China, Arabia, where 60,000 persons died. In the city of Sheraz 16,000 died. It then traveled along the Mediterranean, and ultimately found its way to Astracan in Russia.

In 1826, cholera had reached the frontiers of Siberia, showing that cold could not arrest its progress.[20]

Underscoring the lack of public concern that cholera might make a deadly visitation to Great Britain, under the heading "Miscellaneous" the *English Gentlemen* (London) of August 21, 1825, informed readers that due to the late extremely hot weather and sudden changes in temperature, cholera morbus has appeared "in some of the more healthy quarters of London." Expressing the common notion that persons who had long resided in tropical climates were considered to be more at risk from this disease than others, the article mentioned that Mr. Buckingham, of the Regent's Park, who lived so long in India, was slowly recovering from one of the severest attacks ever experienced in England. The particular predisposing causes were said to be "bodily fatigue, mental anxiety, and a disregard of sudden checks of perspiration." To counter the latter, persons newly arrived from hot countries eager to enjoy the refreshing breezes were advised to adjust their dress according to health rather than taste.

A less encouraging notice appeared two months later when it was reported that typhus fever and cholera morbus, "a disease, the ravages of which are equal only to its severity, also prevails, especially among the working classes." The best preventative against the approach of these disorders was "cleanliness and sobriety in the former case, and a strict attention to proper food in the latter."[21]

As usual, war presented a calling card for cholera. During the First Anglo-Burmese War (1824–1826), European regiments of the British Army were so decimated by cholera that within 11 months of landing at Rangoon, nearly 50 percent had died. Chief causes included amoebic dysentery, malaria, scurvy and, later, cholera. Hospital admissions during the war amounted to 3,540. Out of a total strength of 2,716, disease-related deaths contributed 1,215, with only 96 deaths attributed to battle.[22]

In another indication that cholera was not destined to disappear quietly, a report on the slave trade (abolished in England in 1807) provided details of its presence on the small African island of Mauritius (then a sugar-growing British colony) situated near Madagascar. In calling for stricter measures to prevent slave trading, Sir R. Farquhar's statement that the practice of smuggling slaves into the colony had existed for an extended period was brought into evidence. He stated that between 1819 and 1825, from 7,000 to 10,000 slaves had perished from cholera morbus. Despite this diminution, the slave population remained steady. While the political discussion brought before Parliament by Mr. F. Buxton dealt with a total absolution of the slave trade, the incidental fact of epidemic (and likely endemic) cholera should have raised a red flag and elicited questions about quarantine. Unfortunately, with so little actually known about the cause and spread of this deadly disease and the fact that England had not suffered huge casualties, the subject was disregarded.[23]

In China, fever, ague, dysentery, cholera and bilious colic prevailed as the principal diseases, usually appearing around the month of October. Particularly affecting seamen at Whampoa, this oddity was accounted for by the fact that immense tracts of marsh—covered with rice and paddy—bound the river, extending back several miles. As the banks overflowed nearly every high tide, damp air and rotting vegetation were believed to account for the appearance and continuance of disease.[24]

Nor did evidence of cholera lessen in India, where Calcutta papers were filled with news of the disease. The years 1827–1828 proved to be devastating, spreading into districts nearer to the eastern provinces. Letters from Jubulpore indicated that the whole tract from Rewa had been equally afflicted, and that from Sagor to Jubulpore large villages were wholly deserted, "the inhabitants having fled from the pestilence, which had left but few to escape." One letter continued: "According to native superstition, the severity of this malady of late years has originated in the necessity to which the goddess Kali has been subjected to obtain human victims through disease, since she has been deprived of those sources of supply which civil war and Pindaree inroad have afforded."[25]

June 1828 continued extremely hot with little chance of rain, and cholera morbus continued its ravages, the Calcutta papers noting that "several Europeans had fallen victims to it."[26] By August, Bombay papers indicated cholera was "very prevalent," and that "the Europeans have suffered severely."[27]

The Second Cholera Pandemic
The Polish Insurrection, 1830–1831

We give, under the head of, "Hamburgh Papers," the last news from Poland, and in another column a curious circular of the Polish Government respecting the cholera, of which Russia made a fatal present to a nation which she has long oppressed.[1]

During the five years between the First and Second Cholera Pandemic, the unchecked disease spread steadily. According to a report made to the French Institute in 1830, by M. de Humboldt (based on his travels through Asiatic Russia), cholera first made its appearance in the Bombay army in 1818. By 1819, it had spread to the Isle of France and Madagascar. In 1821, it appeared at Basora before spreading along the Euphrates into Syria. Cholera then diminished for three years, but it continued to creep along the northern coast of Africa. By 1823, it appeared on the borders of the Caspian Sea, making dreadful ravages at Astracan before moving into Central Asia. Although Humboldt doubted the verity of conventional wisdom, he indicated that local authorities believed the disease had been spread by caravans consisting of 3,000–4,000 men and camels.

In 1829, cholera broke out on the Persian frontiers of the Russian Empire, marking the start of the Second Cholera Pandemic (1829–1849). The disease appeared at Tera in autumn 1829, disappeared during the winter, but returned with renewed vigor in the spring along the coasts of the Caspian Sea. On July 31, 1830, cholera again appeared at Astracan, where 21,000 persons died. By the 8th of August, the disease reappeared at Tiflis (Georgia) but was not correctly identified until the 13th. A report by M. Gamba, the French Consul at Tiflis, stated that during this time nearly "all the inhabitants of the town went in procession to the churches, in order to appease, as they hoped, the Divine anger, and from that moment, the malady became general: its ravages reduced the inhabitants of the town from 30,000 to 8,000.[2] From there, cholera extended into the heart of Russia, reaching Moscow by September 1830, having spread over 46,500 square miles of countryside.[3] This was the first significant penetration into the European continent and its presence attracted worldwide interest and concern.

Discovering the true nature and spread of the disease would prove vexing. On September 30, 1830, Prince Galatzin, governor of Moscow, reported that the health of the city had never been more favorable, stating that the average number of deaths per day was 30, but at present it was no more than fifteen, while at Penza, only 1–2 deaths were daily reported. However, the official bulletin published at Moscow stated that between September 28 (the first day on which it was observed), until the 11th of October, the number of sick was 216 (138 men, 78 women), of whom 18 were cured (11 men and 2 women), 76 dead (50 men, 26 women) and 122 still sick (77 men, 45 women). The contradiction was explained by stating that cholera had not appeared in any part of the government of Moscow except the city, nor in the areas of Taur and Novogorod.[4] The bulletin also stated that cholera had recently appeared at Constantinople: it was at Odessa on October 8, from where it was feared cholera would gain entrance into Greece, Italy and the southern parts of France, although it was hoped its effects would be suspended by winter weather.[5]

The Cholera Prizes

By November 1, 1830, cholera reports appeared in English newspapers on a daily basis. The *London Christian Advocate* of that date advised readers that the cholera morbus had reached Moscow, where it was making frightful ravages. The Russian government, it said, was making all possible efforts to stop its inroads, offering a prize of 25,000 roubles (about £1,000) for the best treatise on cholera morbus, to be written in Russian, Latin, German, English or Italian. Entries were to be addressed to the Council of Medicine at St. Petersburgh (the 19th century spelling typically added an "h" to the end of the word) by the 1st of September 1831. A year later, it was reported that the government had received 125 essays. Unluckily, almost all were "discovered in the closet of the writers, and never tried in a sick chamber."[6]

This was not the first attempt to discover a cure for cholera by offering a reward. In 1819, the challenge was issued for anyone to find an "absolute and reliable preventative." By 1854, the unclaimed sum had reached £148,000 and was to be presented by Napoleon III subject to the decision of the Royal Academy of Medicine, Paris. In December 1854, the New York Academy of Medicine also offered $100 for the best essay on "The Nature and Treatment of Cholera Infantum."

In 1849, Mons. Breant bequeathed the sum of 100,000 francs for the discovery of a "certain remedy in cases of Asiatic cholera." Conditions for gaining the prize included a medical prescription which would cure Asiatic cholera in the majority of cases, or to point out the causes of Asiatic cholera so that, "by leading to their suppression, the epidemic shall cease, or to discover some sure method of protection, such as the vaccination for smallpox." (Not surprisingly, Breant's heirs contested the bequest, but the courts subsequently validated it.) By 1885, Breant's gift, then equivalent to $20,000, remained unrewarded.[7]

Lord Heytesbury, British ambassador to Russia, reported to his government on the dangers of cholera spreading. Mr. Butler, clerk of the Privy Council, pursued the matter, addressing the commissioner of customs and "recommending them to call the attention of the quarantine officers to this subject, and to require them to use the utmost care and vigilance in regard to vessels arriving from places where the disease exists." Peculiarly, the matter was treated with humor in some quarters. After an incident at the Lord Mayor's residence, wild attention was placed on fisheries, which habitually placed plugs between the claws of lobsters to prevent their tearing each other. Poking fun at the Common Council, a piece in the *Age* (London, November 28, 1830) observed that Mr. Hobler, of that body, stated that lobsters thus treated brought on the cholera morbus, "for the substance contained within became mortified." Tongue in cheek, the article concluded: "Many an acquaintance of his, who complained in the morning of cholera morbus, or other internal complaints, could trace the disorders to nothing but lobsters on the preceding night."

News from Russia seemed to bear out this unconcern as reports from St. Petersburgh dated October 15 indicated that cholera in Moscow had been brought under control: the number of deaths had diminished and the precautions taken were so excellent "there was but little interruption to business, and the alarm created by the disease appeared to be subsiding."[8] Dispatches from Lord Heytesbury dated October 20 presented a far different picture, however. He stated that cholera still raged in Moscow and of 367 persons attacked, 72 died and many more were in a hopeless state. Despite advising that every precaution should be taken to prevent the progress of the disease to St. Petersburgh, cholera had already reached Tichwin, a place at which there was a large depot for merchandise to be conveyed by water to St. Petersburgh.[9] Reports from Paris indicated that on October 22, the number of sick in Moscow was 1,357, among whom 368 were considered likely to recover. The entire number of persons attacked by cholera up to that time was 3,542, of which 1,771 died.[10] Concurrently, it was observed, "its nature, and the nature of the proper remedies, seem to have hitherto defied the best skill which the medical men in the service of Russia have been able to apply to it. This infliction is now pronounced to be a different disease from the cholera of India."[11]

The November Uprising

As cholera continued to spread along the Russian frontier with Poland, the political situation between those two countries deteriorated. In 1815, the Congress of Vienna had solidified the long-term division of Poland between Prussia and the Habsburg Empire, with Russia assuming hegemony over the "Congress Kingdom," or the Kingdom of Poland, allowing it to maintain its own constitution and courts, elect its own parliament (the Sejm), maintain an army and control its treasury. This semiautonomy did not last long. In 1815, Alexander I of Russia appointed Grand Duke Constantine Pavlovich as de facto viceroy of Poland in opposition to the Polish constitution. Four years later, Alexander I revoked freedom of the press and after 1825, the Sejm was forced to meet in secret.

Amid rumors that the Russians planned to use Polish troops to suppress the July Revolution in France and the Belgium Revolution, in clear violation of the Polish constitution, on November 29, 1830, cadets from the Warsaw officers' academy led by Piotr Wysocki, attacked Belweder Palace, seat of the grand duke. The following day, armed civilians drove Russian soldiers north of Warsaw.

While negotiations between Poland and Russia were in progress, other martial activities came to the forefront. Reports in England, dated November 13, indicated a movement of troops continued in Germany, "but still Austria and Russia formally deny any idea of forcible intervention in Belgian affairs. The cholera morbus still rages with more or less violence in Russia. Some fear that it is the plague. The alarm throughout the empire is excessive."[12] Fearing contagion as much as war, the French Institute deprecated Russia for marching large bodies of troops from countries infected to those free of the disease, "more especially as it is historically known that it first appeared and was propagated in India by Lord Hastings' army."[13] How seriously this was taken by one French citizen was summed up by this comment: "Eu attendant la guerre, les Russes ont *le cholera morbus!*"[14] (While waiting for war, the Russians have the cholera morbus!)

At a time when communication was slow and official reports scant and unreliable, information in newspapers often came from civilians abroad. Writing from Frankfort to London, one writer observed that the progress of cholera in Russia was diminishing, "as the letters received from that country are no longer pierced or steeped in vinegar" to prevent contagion. Other letters from St. Petersburgh, however, belied that supposition, noting that mortality lists published in the journals of the city were incorrect, as the number of deaths in Moscow and the interior were far higher.[15] Accounts from Moscow by other sources supported the former's assumption.

Cholera Mortality Statement, Moscow
November 13, 1830

The number of sick, which on the 2^d, in the morning, was 1,399, increased for three days, being 1,447 on the 5th: it then decreased, and on the 9th, was 1342, of whom 427 were expected to recover. From the commencement of the disorder there had been 4,500 attacked, of whom 2,340 died; 818 had recovered. At Casan the disorder had rather abated, and on the 30th of October there were 54 sick remaining in that city. In the whole government of Casan, including the city, the number of patients from the commencement was 1,403, of whom 808 died, 474 recovered: 291 remain sick.

The cholera has also appeared in five villages of the district of Lascheff, and has also again manifested itself among the Calmachs and Kirghis of the government of Astrachan."[16]

On November 17, reports from St. Petersburgh indicated that the state of health in the provinces was "becoming satisfactory, and the precautions taken to preserve this capital from the effects of the cholera morbus will be more successful." It added that in the government of Novogorod only 3 deaths occurred between October 31 and November 5th.[17]

The Polish Insurrection, 1831

Toward the end of 1830, amid reports the disease spreading in Russia actually represented plague, as opposed to cholera, communication between St. Petersburgh and Moscow deteriorated to the point of virtual nonexistence. Anticipating the close of trade routes, inhabitants in the former city laid in provisions for six months, while the emperor, at his imperial palace in Zarskozeli, 25 miles from St. Petersburgh, cut off all intercourse with his subjects for fear of contagion.[18] In Moscow, as the disease raged, business was completely destroyed; merchants no longer paid anyone and even banks suspended payments.[19] This had repercussions as far away as England, where it was noted that the tallow districts in Russia had all but ceased production, eliciting fears that the supply for next season would be severely limited.[20]

By December 1830, reports from Odessa on the Black Sea stated that cholera, which had broken out with great fury several months ago at Taganrock (Taganrog), had subsided, while in Odessa itself no traces remained. In consequence, supplies of wheat to the Mediterranean ports of Italy had been "so copious as to leave the Odessa market almost bare of the article." The wheat crop, however, had not been abundant.[21]

On January 4, 1831, the two chambers of the Warsaw Sejm issued a manifesto, insisting on the reunion of all provinces of Poland. The concluding paragraph stated, "Persuaded that our liberty and our independence, have not been hostile to other nations, that, on the contrary, they produced a political equilibrium, and formed a rampart for the people of Europe, which may be peculiarly useful to them at this moment, we appear before the Powers and the people with the conviction that policy and humanity will equally declare for the defense of our scared cause." Any delay in answering from St. Petersburgh would be considered a declaration of war. On January 7, Poland's Count Drucki-Lubecki returned from Russia with no agreement, prompting the Sejm, on January 25, 1831, to pass the "Act of Dethronization of Nicholas I," the equivalent of war.

The Russian army continued to suffer from cholera, as a division of cavalry spread the disease among soldiers at Schewniserz.[22] Better news for Russia came from the opening of communications between Moscow and the governments of Wladimir, Kasan, Tola, Kaluga and Smolensk. Following necessary precautions, stations were established to inspect travelers there for any trace of disease.

Cholera at Moscow, 1831

(From the Prussian *State Gazette*)

January	New Cases	Recovered	Died
1	8	7	4
2	18	1	10
3	39	6	19
4	29	8	29

Since the beginning of the epidemic, 6,387 were attacked; 3,586 died; 2,707 recovered and, as of January 5th, 94 cases remained. At this point, the government of Saraloff also announced it was free of cholera and open communication had been restored. Simultaneously, *Le Courrier* reported that cholera had appeared in St. Petersburgh.[23]

Historians disagree on whether Russian troops introduced cholera into Poland or if the disease had already begun to spread well before the Russian campaign to suppress the revolution took shape.[24] Likely both are true, as news from Frankfort (published February 1, 1831, and probably 2–3 weeks old) brought intelligence that cholera morbus had broken out in Poland, while letters "From the Frontier of Hungary," dated January 13, indicated that a species of dysentery similar to that of cholera and equally contagious raged in the Hungarian counties of Maarinaros and Bihar.[25]

Within days of the declaration of war, Field Marshal Hans Karl von Diebitsch crossed into Poland. The first major battle took place on February 14 near the village of Stoczek near Lukow. Polish cavalry under Brigadier General Jozef Dwernicki won the battle but could not prevent Diebitsch from advancing toward Warsaw. On February 25, east of Warsaw, 40,000 Poles faced a Russian force of 60,000 in the Battle of Olszynka Grochowska. After two days of heavy fighting that claimed the lives of over 7,000 soldiers on each side, Diebitsch was forced to retreat to Siedlce, temporarily saving the city.[26]

Amid reports that cholera had broken out among Polish troops, the *Warsaw State Gazette*, dated Jamnow, April 22, contained a report from the commander in chief, providing an account of the defeat of General Scerawski. He reported, "Siedlec might have been taken, but the crowded hospitals and the contagious disorders in them, deterred me. This care was also in vain, the disease had communicated itself to our troops, on our meeting with the enemy on the 10th. We had some hundreds ill of the cholera, the precautions instantly taken will prevent the disorder from spreading, and from assuming too dangerous a character."[27]

Letters published in the *Journal des Debats* dated April 17 repeated the news that Russian prisoners captured on the 11th had communicated cholera to one of the Polish divisions of General Slaznecki. French physicians who went from Warsaw on hearing this information confirmed the statement. However, on April 19, the Municipal Council of Warsaw publicly contradicted the report that cholera was found among Russian prisoners taken near Siedlec.[28]

After a Russian victory on April 10, no serious engagements were undertaken by the Russians; in a letter from Warsaw dated April 28, the writer supposed one reason might have been that "the mortality in the Russian army is fearful. The cholera morbus, I am sorry to say, has certainly broken out here; but we are all in hopes that it will not be found so destructive as it has been elsewhere. The zeal of our medical men is exemplary, and, on the first appearance of infection, they hasten to afford every possible assistance. Cleanliness is most particularly enjoined as a preventative."[29]

On the medical side, at a sitting of the Royal Academy of Sciences at Paris, M. Moreau de Jonnes elaborated on a new phenomenon relative to cholera. In India, he stated, the cold of winter arrested, or at least suspended, the progress of the disorder, but such was not the case in Russia. He attributed the fact to housing and clothing. In India, poorly constructed homes left interiors as cold as exteriors, but well-closed apartments in Russia heated by large stoves, along with the fact inhabitants wore heavy furs, created a hot artificial temperature, allowing the malady to thrive.[30]

Cholera at Warsaw

The following is an abstract from a letter written by Mr. Searle, dated Warsaw, July 4, 1831. It brings home, as in no other way, the acute suffering brought on by the dreaded disease cholera, "The King of Terrors":

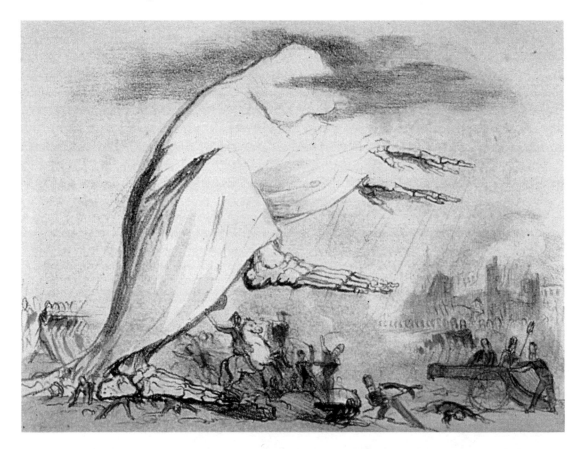

"Cholera 'Tramples the Victors and the Vanquished Both,'" by Robert Seymour, *McLean's Monthly Sheet of Caricatures,* London, October 1, 1831. In this sketch, cholera is depicted as a large shrouded specter with skeletal hands and feet, indiscriminately crushing soldiers on both sides of the Polish Insurrection (U.S. National Library of Medicine).

I am placed in charge of an hospital for the reception of the poor, a mile and a half from the city. The first difficulty I have to cope with is, that few patients are admitted till their extremities are livid, the pulse lost at the wrist, and the evacuations have spontaneously ceased: this comes of the Medical Board of this place having circulated advice that every person should be bled on becoming the subject of the disease, and drink plentifully of hot water; this treatment is consequently considered specific, and it is not, therefore, till every individual has proved the error that they think of coming to the hospital: to say nothing of the expense and trouble they are subjected to in coming so far. The next thing is, that, when admitted, there is nobody but a few Russian prisoners to see the remedies administered, or to attend upon the sick, except a couple of dressers, who invariably leave the hospital the moment my back is turned; that, in short, nothing is done for them but what is done by myself in person.

I have represented the thing to the heads of the department over and over again, promise has been made me upon promise, and in this way have I been fooled up to the present time. Yesterday I made a strong and pressing communication to the Government on the subject; what the result will be I know not. The true state of the case is this—that the Council de Medicine, consisting of a dozen private practitioners of the place, and a junto (for the most part) of ignorant men, and extremely jealous of us foreigners, both English and French, and I believe, do their utmost to thwart us in every way.

I say us, as, although they make great professions of respect and good feelings towards me, yet they do nothing that I require, but only promise. This may be well denominated the land of promise, for these they make in profusion; and it is the same yesterday, today, and for ever. Never, in any situation that I have filled through life, did I feel so truly humbled and disgusted.

I feel resources within myself, and burn to exercise them towards the poor and suffering creatures; but no, I am constrained to stand little better than an idle spectator of misery and death, which it is in my power to alleviate, but I am not permitted to do so.

The disease here, which is precisely the same in character with that in India, is unquestionably, as I have represented, of the febrile class, and dependent upon the same causes as the typhoidal orders of fever usually are—marshy and pestiferous exhalations, arising in low, damp, filthy, unventilated situations. To the development of the disease, or to render the individual susceptible of its attack, it would, however, appear that a certain condition of system or predisposition must exist, or it would be of more general influence where filth of every kind so much abounds as it does here. This condition I believe to consist simply, or principally in debility: hence the indifferently fed, the badly clothed, and comfortless poor, or those exposed to the inclemencies of the weather and vicissitudes of temperature, and particularly under exhaustion from want of food and bodily fatigue, are the most frequent subjects of its attack.

The treatment I find most successful, corresponds with the advice given in my work; evacuating the stomach, in the first instance, with a solution of *salt,* in the proportion of a large table-spoon in a tumbler of hot water. This operates almost instantly as an emetic; or where, from atony of stomach, it does not so, a second is administered. The patient then, for cleanliness sake, is sponged all over with one pint of nitric acid, diluted with two of hot water, and hot flannels being in readiness, he is well rubbed with them for half an hour; when, being placed in a warm bed, in an airy room, five grains of calomel are administered every half hour, with a spoonful of brandy added to two of hot water.

As excitement becomes developed, the spirit is diminished in quantity, and the intervals between each dose of calomel prolonged, but continued till bilious stools and urine are obtained. Should the breathing be much oppressed, or the fulness of the praecordia, or oppression of the brain considerable, bleeding is required, but not in too large a quantity.

The fever which generally follows being of the typhoidal character, requires a great deal of nice management, and they almost invariably here die from neglect; it is always attended with some organic inflammation, which is not to be cured by evacuents. This fever is, however, to be prevented, I am of the opinion, by carrying on the calomel to the production of a tender state of the gums, or gentle ptyalism; but my views are, instead of persevering with the calomel to this extent, to follow up the treatment, on the appearance of bilious evacuations and urine (or the restoration of secretion), by the quinine, or bark and wine.

I have just completed an apparatus for the inhalation of chlorine, which I intend giving a trial to. The nitrous oxide, or oxygen gas, I should have preferred, but there are difficulties attending these which I fear are insurmountable.

I think it by no means improbable that you will have the disease, or something of the kind, in England, as I cannot help connecting its appearance in Europe with some peculiar epidemic influence of atmosphere, seeing that when I passed through Berlin there was an epidemic fever prevailing there, with which 40,000 persons were attacked out of a population of 200,000, and hearing since that an influenza, or something of the sort, is prevailing in Paris.

The connexion between cholera and fever has been remarkably exemplified here; at least I have been told that intermittent fever was prevailing to some extent before the cholera; on this appearing the former vanished and re-appeared on the cessation of cholera. The weather here is the most unpleasant I have ever experienced; for a few days it was so hot that I never felt it so oppressive that I remember of, all the time I was in India; this has been followed by constant rain; and with the few comforts the country affords us it is truly wretched.[31]

The Spread of Cholera—Quarantine Regulations

Reports dated February 2 indicated "the spasmodic cholera has been raging with great virulence in Persia, and particularly at Tiflis, and the route between that town and Tabrez. The plague, which has existed for some time in Persia, has undergone no abatement, but seemed rather to gain ground, and it was computed that within a circle of twenty miles around Tabrez, 30,000 people had died since the month of June," 1830. These reports also observed that reports from Lemberg concerning the spread of cholera were very alarming.[32] On June 1, 1831, extracts from German papers announced the appearance of the cholera in two circles of Gallicia, inducing the government to adopt strict measures to prevent the spread of the disorder into the interior of the monarchy. "There is the more reason to hope," the paper continued, "that this measure will be effectual, as the mortality seems already to abate in the Jews' quarter at Lemberg, where eighteen persons fell victims to it in a few days."

Reports from Berlin, June 8, announced that by official proclamation, bills of health granted in Russia, Poland, or Austrian Gallicia "will not exclude travelers and merchants from the quarantine regulations." This measure was considered necessary in light of the fact that ships from Riga "provided with the regular documents generally granted to vessels leaving a perfectly healthy place" were heavily infested with the disease.[33]

On June 1, the Royal Board of Trade at Stockholm issued an ordinance through the Royal Swedish and Norwegian General Consulate stating that, independent of the quarantine station at Kanso, two other quarantine places at Hasselo (about four miles within Sandhamm) and in the harbor of Slito (in the island of Gothland) were to be established. The ordinance likewise decreed that the town of Polangen was considered infected with cholera morbus, as were all intermediate places on the coast between the mouth of the River Vistula and the extreme eastern boundary of Estonia, including the coastal islands. Every vessel arriving from an infected or suspected place was required to proceed to one of the above-named places, there to undergo quarantine.[34]

Further sanctions were issued on July 2, 1831, when the Royal Marine Department of the kingdom of Norway declared Archangel (contaminated by vessels coming by the Dwina from Vologda and Wialka), Lieban, Riga and Dantsic as infected with cholera. Those places suspected of being infected included all Russian ports in the White Sea and Artic Icy Ocean and all Russian and Prussian ports in the Baltic.[35] This was followed, on July 8, by an ordinance from the king of Holland containing a strict injunction to enforce regulations against the introduction of cholera, and particularly to prevent all persons from touching any dead bodies or effects thrown onshore by the tide. Anyone coming in contact with the dead or their effects was to be placed in quarantine and afterwards punished according to law.[36]

Quarantine regulations were not always appreciated. In a letter from Lubeck dated July 6, 1831, it was reported "the *Nicholas I* steamer arrived from St. Petersburgh, this morning, and brings afflicting intelligence that the cholera morbus has now extended its ravages to that capital likewise.... As the steamer was leaving the roads she saw two vessels driving out to sea with the quarantine flag half-mast high as a signal there were sick on board.... Among the passengers on board the steamer is the Duc de Montemart, the French Ambassador to the Russian Court. His Excellency is said to be very much annoyed and surprised at the delay to which our measures of precaution are like to subject him."[37]

The State of Cholera
Warsaw, April 23–May 5, 1831

Total infected	2,580
Died	1,110
Recovered	192
Remain sick	1,278

The number of those who died after contracting cholera was 1:20, but percentages for survival were greater for those with private houses and presumably better health care.[38] Interestingly, a letter written from Warsaw May 16 advised, "The cholera morbus is no longer a subject of alarm; it has wonderfully decreased within the last week; it is now fatal to very few, and not many new cases. The Prussian government has, however, established a rigorous quarantine of 21 days, which, as the disease here is not infectious, is considered as a political one, calculated to impede communications with foreign countries rather than to circumscribe the complaint."[39]

From the first appearance of the cholera epidemic at Riga to the morning of June 21, there were 4,117 cases; 1,918 cures; 1,750 deaths.

The State of Cholera
Riga (Reported June 25, 1831)

IN HOSPITALS

	Cases	Cures	Deaths
From June 21 to 22	23	26	9
22 to 23	33	51	5
23 to 24	28	33	6
24 to 25	28	19	10

IN PRIVATE HOUSES

From June 21 to 22	26	19	5
22 to 23	16	30	6
23 to 24	26	39	6
25 to 25	23	29	5

After giving the death statistics, the article noted that it was a fixed opinion among the natives that goods and merchandise were not liable to spread contagion; "and, in fact, comparatively few of the labouring people in the hemp ambars, or of those employed in dressing flax, have been attacked by the cholera."[40] It is interesting that oil of cameline, also known as "wild flax," was occasionally used as a preventative of cholera (see chapter 5).

To alleviate suffering at Riga, the emperor granted a sum of money to the orphans of cholera victims, as it was noted that, "as the cholera seldom attacks children, the number that are left fatherless in a place where the malady has raged is always great."[41]

Rybensk (100 miles from St. Petersburgh)

Total infected	80
Died	60[42]

Dantsic June 23, 1831

Total infected	15
Died	13
Recovered	2[43]

Accounts received June 28 at Stutgard from Jassy, the capital of Moldavia, stated that cholera existed in the two principalities of Mondavia and Wallachia and especially at Jassy. Between June 2 and June 19, no fewer than 800 persons fell victim; on the 11th, out of 280 infected, 155 died and deaths gradually increased to 200 a day. In consequence, the government directed all citizens to retire from the city and disperse themselves in the open country.[44] Munich was also under a cholera alarm, where a commission was appointed to inquire into the situation, although it had not yet been deemed necessary to establish a sanitary cordon.

Death from cholera was not limited to the common man. In the early morning of May 28 (other reports give June 9), Field Marshal Diebitsch fell ill and was tended to by M. Schegel, physician in ordinary to the emperor. Witnessing severe attacks attributed to cholera, the doctor ordered the patient bled, leeches applied and very strong friction employed. By 7:00 a.m., the patient felt easier, but within the hour he fell into alternate fits of shivering and burning heat. As his vital powers diminished, Diebitsch fell into a lethargy, his eyesight failed and by 11:15 a.m., he expired. On June 28, the Prussian *State Gazette* confirmed that when Dr. Koch "opened the body" (performed an autopsy), he indicated the cause of death as cholera.[45] It is curious to note that before the autopsy report was published, so great was the fear of cholera that early reports indicated Diebitsch had either died of apoplexy or taken his own life.[46]

The State of Cholera in Gallicia
from the first appearance until the end of June 1831

Number of Cases	37,000
Died	13,356
Recovered	19,655
Still ill as of July 7	3,989[47]

In an interesting political comment on the situation in Poland, *Bell's Life in London, and Sporting Chronicle* of July 24, 1831, reported that a treaty had been concluded between France and England to interfere on behalf of the Poles. The newspaper added that the concern of the Great Powers had less to do with Poland than with the fear that despotism and cholera should both be introduced into the west of Europe, "and therefore they wish to stop the progress of the Russian arms."

In fact, although the Polish uprising elicited great sympathy in Europe and the United States, there was little chance of a united cooperation on their behalf. Louis-Philippe of France was more worried about being recognized by European governments, while Lord Palmerston of England did not desire to weaken Russia, fearing that as Poland was a natural ally of France the two countries might form a powerful union against England. Austria and Prussia adopted a position "of benevolent neutrality towards Russia," closing the Polish frontiers to prevent the transportation of munitions and foodstuffs.[48]

On July 25, the *London Courier* supplied information that at St. Petersburgh, since the first manifestation of cholera to July 7, the number of persons attacked reached 1,230, with 558 deaths. The report added that the "number of persons recovered was very small, there being on the 8th, in the morning, 665 sick remaining."

According to accounts from Vienna (July 17), cholera was no more than 44 miles from the capital. Pesth was already surrounded by a cordon, as cholera continued to spread on both sides of the Theiss, with some cases reported at Szelnok, Heves and Erlau. In consequence, it was felt more serious precautionary measures would be needed at Vienna. A sanitary cordon composed of 36,000 chosen troops were ordered to protect the capital against cholera; in order to prevent the scarcity of provisions which might ensue from this form of seclusion, bakers were ordered to lay in corn sufficient for the consumption of the inhabitants for three months.

To raise spirits, the emperor resolved that "whatever may happen" he was to remain in residence, and he "intimated to the members of the Imperial family to do the same." Taking a firmer stance with public functionaries, none were allowed to leave their posts, request a passport or take a leave of absence. The establishments Josephinum and Theresianum were converted into hospitals, while no Jews ("known for their want of cleanliness and their mode of life," being "peculiarly susceptible of contagion,") coming from Poland were permitted to pass through Brunn, in Moravia. They were also to be expelled from their closely built quarters at Prague, Pesth and probably Vienna while the police "purified" their habitats.

While German newspapers chiefly related news of cholera, "which has been for some time a prominent feature in all the Journals of the North of Europe," foreign ministers at Vienna, dreading the disease, all removed to Baden, a city not known to be infected by any epidemic disease.[49]

In mid–August, a private letter from Vienna painted a melancholy picture. "The approach of the cholera has filled every mind with alarm. The public has given itself up so entirely to dread, that already several persons have died with fright or become mad." The writer indicated that all communication with Hungary, from whence almost all provisions arrived, had been severed, greatly augmenting prices.

Precautions in Vienna included dividing the city and suburbs into 50 districts, each with four physicians under the supervision of a doctor who had been practicing at Warsaw. Because people did not know how cholera was contracted and thus presumed it was contagious, a commissary was appointed to every four houses, bound to visit them daily in order to prevent more than three persons from sleeping in the same room. Every house was furnished with a quantity of chlorate of lime and fumigated every day with vinegar. It was also recommended that the mouth be washed every morning with vinegar and that a drop of the essence of chamomile on a piece of sugar should be taken while fasting. Houses were also required to be supplied with a quantity of vinegar, herbs, tea, flannel and heated sand.

The emperor gave 2,000,000 florins toward the establishment of hospitals, for which the most extensive houses and the theatre were appropriated. No one was allowed to go three leagues from the capital without a certificate of health, but at the same time, numerous carriages set off "in crowds" for Switzerland and the Tyrol. By August 16, all theatres were to be closed and all unemployed foreigners were ordered to leave within eight days. The emperor went with his court to Schoenbrunn, where the outside walls and windows were closed with planks. The young king of Hungary, Prince Metternich, and the foreign ambassadors joined him there.[50]

Notices from the German newspapers up to September 1 indicated that the sicknesses in

Vienna "were to be classed, according to the medical report, not under the head of oriental, but of sporadic, cholera."[51] Cholera continued to rage at Lemberg, where 50–60 daily deaths were recorded. At Frankfurt, preemptive measures included a house of quarantine for strangers coming from suspected places and a hospital to care for those attacked by the disorder. A separate report indicated that greater exertions were being made at Stockholm to prepare hospitals for cholera patients.[52]

In what may be viewed as germ warfare, a correspondent for the *London Courier* wrote the following in a letter dated July 18: "One of the feats of the Russians must be observed. In Sienpic, they broke open the church, robbed it, and left the cholera in the place." He added, "The cholera here is treated as a *tangible* article: something to be laid hold of—and yet we are completely in the dark as to the precise situation, in the church of Sienpic where the alarming personage was secreted—whether in the reading desk, in the folds of the parson's surplice, or in the belfry." He added the disease was making great ravages in St. Petersburgh: on June 29, the total number of cases was 3,418, with 1,479 deaths.[53]

Adding to the confusion, a letter from Pesth, dated July 21, noted, "We know nothing of the cholera here, except some cases of sudden death, which at another time would not have been regarded, but which many persons immediately took to be the destructive Indian disorder. The cases of death in other parts of Hungary appear also, as many assert, not to be caused by the Indian cholera, but by a kind of dysentery, not uncommon in these parts. However, the

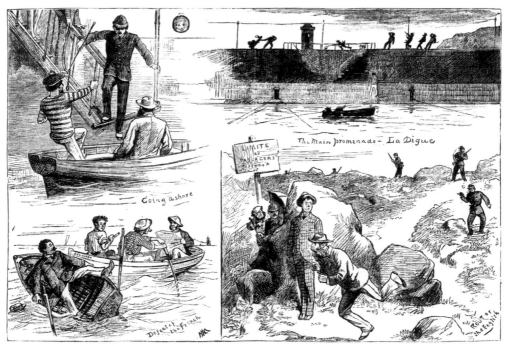

THE CHOLERA IN EGYPT—IN QUARANTINE AT MARSEILLES

"The Cholera in Egypt—In Quarantine at Marseilles." Quarantine was a subject of continuing debate throughout the cholera era, extending from the 1800s to the present day. Health authorities used quarantine to prevent contaminated immigrants from entering a country; businesses complained it hurt commerce. Taxpayers railed against the cost and occasionally took to arms to prevent a quarantine station from being constructed on or near their property. Governments used it as a political tactic against other nations (*London Graphic*, August 4, 1883).

question must soon be decided, and, at all events, the precautions adopted by the government deserve to be gratefully acknowledged."

Precautions included placing placards on street corners announcing that quarantine was reestablished, "but that the pontoon bridge is not to be taken down again." Doors of all private houses were to be closed at 9:00 p.m. and all coffee-houses and hotels shut at 10:00 p.m. In case of disturbances during hours of darkness, nightlights were to be put in all windows facing the street. Due to the fact that several cases of "incendiarism" had occurred, city magistrates of Pesth were authorized to sentence persons convicted of this crime to a rapid execution. The final order warned all citizens that in case of public disturbances they were to keep their distance from the rioters, "lest they should suffer with them for their disobedience of the lawful authority."[54]

Diseased Properties of the Blood

Contradictions in the type and symptoms of the disease continued to perplex both the civilian population and the medical community. Dr. David Barry, writing from St. Petersburgh on July 20, 1831, stated that in contrast to the typical symptoms he expected to encounter, vomiting and purging were among the least important in the present epidemic. His concern lay in the sudden paralysis and rapidly diminishing action of the heart, in conjunction with the "shrivelling of the fingers and toes, the colour of the skin, the shrinking of the features, the coldness of the tongue, the feebleness or extinction of the pulse and voice, the rice-water evacuations when there are any, are the true marks of the disease, not to be mistaken."

To the modern practitioner, these symptoms are indicative of severe dehydration and kidney failure. Barry found magisterium bismuthi and cordials serviceable, assisted by synapisms (blisters) covering the whole belly, and friotions (frictions, or rubbing). He noted that neither warm nor vapor baths were appropriate, as they warmed the body, "as a dead animal would be," but failed to restore native heat, adding that opium appeared contraindicated. Two German physicians of Barry's acquaintance, Ysenbeck and Brailow, recommended bleeding, followed by two tablespoons of common salt in six ounces of hot water, repeated as a cold mixture every hour. Using this treatment at the Customs-House Hospital, St. Petersburgh, they claimed success with 30 cholera patients.[55]

A follow-up to this story noted that the two physicians first learned of using salt from "the talk of the town," but paid it no heed until one witnessed an old woman dying of cholera consume large quantities of salted herrings. This remedy, suggested to her by the "common people," brought about an astonishing recovery, inducing the doctor to administer the above stated salt and water mixture to two other patients dying from the disease. After witnessing them return to health in 48 hours, he prescribed the mixture on 16 successive hospital admissions. They all "got rid of the disease by that remedy, but died with the typhus fever, in consequence of the severeness of it."[56] This salt mixture used in 1831 came very close to approximating the modern treatment for cholera. In order to prevent death by dehydration, an oral solution of water, sodium chloride and bicarbonate is administered. *Taber's Cyclopedic Medical Dictionary* (page 405) advises use of an oral rehydration solution made of 1 level teaspoon of salt and 1 heaping teaspoon of sugar added to 1 liter of water, used to replace 5–7 percent of body weight.

Interestingly, Dr. William Stevens published "Observations on the Healthy and Diseased Properties of the Blood" and "On the Employment of the Alkaline and Neutral Salts in Cholera," London, 1832. He claimed that Ysenbeck and Brailow copied his theory and cited

Sir William Crichton as saying the team lost 3 of the 30 patients thus treated, as had Mr. Searle in Warsaw.

From the preternatural thickness and dark color of the blood seen in cholera patients, Stevens deduced that the method he had used successfully in the West Indies and the United States on violent fevers would be useful in cholera patients. With permission from Mr. Wakefield, surgeon at the Cold Bath Fields Prison, he applied his treatment in April after several cholera cases were reported.

DR. STEVENS TREATMENT FOR CHOLERA

1. Seidlitz power was administered with a view of allaying gastric irritation.
2. A large sinapism was applied to the epigastric region and rubbed with hot flannel to alleviate stomach irritation.
3. A powder of half a drachm of carbonate of soda, one scruple of muriate of soda and 7 grains of chlorate of potass was dissolved in half a tumbler of water and administered every 15 minutes to every hour until circulation was freely restored.
4. If the stomach was very irritable, a common effervescing mixture of small doses of common soda powders, with excess of carbonates, was used, after which carbonate of soda with larger doses of chlorate of potass was given without muriate of soda.
5. A solution of muriate of soda at as a high a temperature as could be borne was injected into the intestines.
6. In two cases, patients were immersed in a hot saline bath, as suggested by Mr. Marsden, a surgeon at the Free Hospital, Greville St.
7. Seltzer water was swallowed *ad libitum* when the patient desired to drink. A strong infusion of green tea was also supplied.
8. A fire was to be kept going at all times as external cold acted as an exciting cause of cholera.
9. Patients were not to be considered cured until 7 days out of danger.
10. No solid or indigestible food until 5 days after recovery.
11. The saline treatment was to be trusted entirely and exclusively: no calomel, brandy or opium, although 25–30 drops of laudanum was allowed, diffused in tepid water. Milk with carbonate of soda was also recommended.
12. As a last resort, injection of saline into the veins was to be tried.
13. All contaminated material was to be removed, wards fumigated with gunpowder twice a day and clothing boiled for half an hour in a strong solution of common soda.

When cholera subsequently appeared at Sunderland (see chapter 7), Stevens urged local physicians to try his method but was ignored. (See a further discussion of Stevens' method in chapter 22.[57]) As noted in number 6 above, Dr. Marsden, physician to the Cholera Hospital, was an early proponent of effervescing saline draughts, "containing the salts common to the blood in a healthy state," and recommended them even in the last stages of cholera.[58]

Drs. David Barry and William Russell presented their findings in a letter from Calais, dated November 6, 1831. Writing on the epidemic in St. Petersburgh, they concluded the following:

1. Cholera germs were brought to the city by boats and barks (small water craft) from the interior, prior to June 26, 1831.
2. The germs were diffused and the disease propagated in two ways: the first was called

"personal," meaning they were spread by passengers and boatmen who came from infected places. The second was called "atmospheric," meaning emanations from the barks and their contents carried by currents of air to susceptible persons, independently of direct communication.

3. Germs of the same disease were carried to Cromstadt and propagated there from the barks already mentioned and by persons who had contact with them or who had been in the immediate neighborhood.

4. The cholera was introduced into all the villages around the city by persons from the city or other infected places.

5. Neither the near approach nor the immediate contact with infected individuals was indispensable to the infection of a healthy person if he were susceptible at the moment.

6. The epidemic in St. Petersburgh did not possess the absolute communicable qualities of plague and smallpox, and the risk of infection to persons who approached the sick was in direct proportion to the want of ventilation, cleanliness and space around the latter.

7. In a generally infected atmosphere the additional danger of infection by approaching the sick was not greater than if they approached a typhus patient under similar circumstances.

8. Under favourable conditions of body and mind, personal seclusion did afford protection from cholera, especially if the shelter kept out currents of air passing through sources of infection.

9. Those who avoided communication with infected persons and who resided windward of infection were likely to remain exempt from the disease. Next in point of immunity were those in favorable health, with strength and cheerfulness and who lived temperately.[59]

Unfortunately, while this theory of using salt was correct (which the authors did not mention in their letter), they propagated the belief that cholera was transmitted by miasmic air and personal contact. This idea would prevail for another two decades.

On a slightly different track, it was observed that in Prussia and Russia cholera spared all persons employed in the manufactories of tobacco (or snuff), the tanyards, and medical laboratories: "The smoke of tobacco seems to neutralize most animal miasmata; and it is generally considered as a preservative against the cholera; accordingly the Prussian, Austrian and Russian magistrates have given permission to smoke in the streets."[60] In Upper and Lower Egypt and along the Barbary Coast, a similar belief held that not a single oilman or dealer in oil ever suffered from the plague or cholera.[61]

The *Messager des Chambres,* France, published a different summary of the disease on August 14, 1831:

> The cholera of the ancients, the Chinese *holouan,* the Indian *maudechin,* the Persian *ouebb,* the Arabian *houwa,* the *trousse-galant* of France, and the cholera morbus which spreads its ravages over the North of Europe, are all one and the same disease.
>
> Modified by the difference of climate and change of seasons, the cholera loses much of its violence in winter, and increases in summer. It may also exist in conjunction with other epidemic diseases, and occasionally render them so complicated, that the real character of the affliction cannot be discovered. as has occurred in Warsaw, where the cholera commits less ravage than the typhus in our army. We have grounds for hoping that the severe discipline of our army, the exertions of the police in our large cities, especially the excellent practice in our hospitals, both civil and military, will preserve us from this dreadful scourge.
>
> The cholera morbus is not contagious, but so rapid in its effects that the slightest delay in checking its progress may lead to the most fatal consequences. L. LABAT, M.D.[62]

The Deadly Swath

A letter from Warsaw, dated July 27, indicated "the fatality of the cholera has not been more extensive in Warsaw than at the present time; 130 Jews have been known to fall victim to this dreadful malady in the course of 36 hours. That class of society feels its effects more severely than any other, though all do so in a more or less degree. The disease is said to have extended itself in Prussia, in the direction of Posen." From Berlin, private correspondence dated August 6, depicted an even more frightening description.

> The cholera advances more and more, and precautions continue to be taken; but as we learn from the events at Petersburg, Pesth, and Konigsberg, a rigorous shutting up of the infected houses, and a barricading of the sick streets, will not do much good in large towns, if it be at all possible. The rabble believe it is a measure only intended for the comfort of the rich. Loudly, they say, "It is better that thousands perish from the cholera than that 50,000 should starve, while they have nothing to do or to eat." At Pesth the history of old Galileo has been revived. A physician and a professor of the University have been forced by the rabble and by the students (scarcely one can believe it) publicly to declare that he had erroneously before declared the sickness of some individuals to be cholera! At Konigsberg, the town where the great Kant was born, ignorance and credulity have so prevailed amongst the rabble, that they do not hesitate to say the physicians were hired to poison the poor people. From that opinion may spring a revolution stained with blood. Indeed, it seems already to have begun, but we shall find that opinions and sicknesses are not so powerful to rule and control as soldiers and imposts. We hope, if the cholera comes to us, no such strong measures will be adopted as shutting up and barricading. Our King, now at the baths of Toplits, has declared, upon the first appearance of cholera in Berlin he will return to share all dangers with his beloved and loyal subjects.[63]

On July 30, as the Russian army moved on Warsaw, cholera continued its own crusade, raging at Cracow (Krakow) and its environs with unabated violence. From Pesth, it rapidly approached the frontiers of Germany, while prevailing to a considerable degree at Kran and reaching into Raab.[64]

Cholera had not finished its deathly swath. In the first two weeks of August, 2,000–3,000 persons were attacked in Constantinople, although with less severity than other places. The disease was also reported at Stettin (present day Szczecin, Poland) and at Sweaborg, on the south coast of Finland. One interesting statistic came from Posen, where the disease was observed to make more havoc on Tuesdays and Wednesdays, "on account of the excesses in which the people indulge on the Sundays and Mondays."[65]

Mortality by Cholera in St. Petersburgh
From its first appearance until August 8, 1831

Number of Cases	8,699
Died	4,438
Remained ill	226

By this point, Russian physicians were almost unanimous in the opinion that cholera was not contagions, citing the fact that at the great cholera hospital on Wasslli Osbrow, none of the doctors were taken ill and of the 90 nurses and servants, only 2 died. A hopeful, if not inaccurate addendum to this came from *Bell's Life in London*, September 11, 1831, where it was noted, "If the cholera be really contagious, its progress will probably be arrested by the sea, and, consequently, it will not appear in this country."

September losses in the Polish army were severe and outlying cities of Warsaw fell to the Russians. On October 5, 1831, the remainder of the Polish army crossed the Prussian frontier and surrendered at Brodnica. In summary, at the height of the cholera epidemic in 1831, the monthly count of cholera cases in Russian military hospitals both in Poland and in Russia grew from less than 700 in March to over 8,700 in April, resulting in over 2,800 deaths. In September, as defeat was inevitable, Warsaw recorded 22,700 cases of cholera, with 13,000 fatalities.[66]

The war may have been over, but cholera was hardly defeated. In May 1831 cholera broke out at Mecca and the viceroy issued the necessary precautions. "Unfortunately, however, in consequence of the ideas which the Turks entertain respecting predestination, these precautions were almost useless." Travelers leaving the city introduced the disease into Cairo and at Suez. Between July 30 and August 1, a total of 120 (of 400) inhabitants perished, including the governor. A general terror spread through Cairo and inhabitants fled, filling the Nile. Business was suspended and diplomatic offices closed. Foreign vessels refused to put into port, and a great part of the squadron of the Pasha was infected.

From this period, the scourge made rapid progress through Cairo and Alexandria, with dead bodies abandoned in the street. The prince departed for Upper Egypt after forty women from the harem of the Ibraham Pasha were lost. "The cholera, according to custom, followed beaten tracks, and the courses of canals and rivers. It manifested itself with violence at Fouah, at the entrance of the canal Mahmoudich, where there were a great many pilgrims fugitives, and at Rosetta and Damietta."[67]

Despite official reports, by September, eyewitnesses indicated that the continuing epidemic in Mecca had claimed the lives of 5,500 people in 30 days, while of the 50,000 pilgrims who visited the Prophet's shrine since January, 20,000 were said to have perished of cholera.[68] A November 1831 edition of the *Augsburg Gazette* gave "a most frightful account of the late ravages of the severe Asiatic cholera at Cairo and Alexandria. In 24 days, it carried off 30,000 Egyptians: of the 60,000 inhabitants of Alexandria, 10,000 had died."[69]

Dispatches from Vienna dated November 3 indicated that within the prior three days, the number of cholera patients had increased from 18 to 24, but there were no new deaths to report. Statistics from the Austrian *Observer*, November 3, presented complete data:

Vienna, November 3, 1831
Numbers Since the Commencement of Cholera

	Cases	Recoveries	Deaths
In the city	1,042	614	404
In the suburbs	2,262	872	1,183
	3,304	1,486	1,587[70]

By December, reports from both Vienna and Berlin indicated cholera had been nearly extinguished in both cities.[71] Rounding out the year, the *New York Estats Unis* carried a story from St. Petersburgh, where six healthy criminals condemned to death were held in a hospital set aside for cholera victims. Three weeks later, when none had contracted the disease, they were offered a pardon if they would willingly expose themselves to the contagion. They agreed and were moved into an *uninfected* hospital and placed in clean beds. "In a few days they were all *frightened into* the Cholera, and four of the six died of it!"[72]

The Second Cholera Pandemic
England and France, 1831

To the philanthropist, the statesman, and the philosopher—to the sagacious enquirer into abstruse and distant causes, and the acute observer of present and practical effects—the new and fatal disease by which this country is now afflicted, is a subject for careful observation and deep and serious reflection. The origin, the former course, and the probable future progress of the malady—the means of prevention, and the mode of cure—the effect that has been, and will hereafter be, produced upon commercial intercourse and political combinations—these are objects which demand the profound consideration of the most powerful intellects. They afford abundant matter for the searching eye of speculative inquiry in the present day, and will in future times be the subject of the curious and minute investigation of the historian, who shall record the occurrences of this eventful period.[1]

The *London Medical Gazette* issued a report on June 4, 1831, denying rumors that cholera of the same character that prevailed in the north of Europe had appeared in the metropolis nearest the port of London. The paper conjectured that a severe fever, then common in various districts in the neighborhood of the river, was the true cause. This had little effect on those who believed the city to be infected. On the same day, a notice appeared in the *Courier*, remarking that the government "had acted very properly" in taking the precaution of quarantining ships recently arrived from places of contagion. It cited the Hamburg steamboat then isolated at Stangate Creek, where letters and papers were being fumigated. The *Christian Advocate* of the 6th echoed this sentiment, but had cause to complain that the commissioners of customs were "daily allowing large parcels of dried calf-skins in the hair to be imported without interruption of any kind." In defense, officials stated only hides were mentioned on the manifest, to which the newspaper responded, "but surely skins are equally calculated to carry the infection; and thus, taking advantage of a quibble, the interests and welfare of the public are sacrificed to the profits of the few individuals concerned in those vessels."

With the topic of cholera on the minds of citizens, Sir Anthony Carlisle addressed a letter to Lord Brougham, alluding to the conflicting evidence respecting the contagious character of cholera. His opinion was that the disease assumed different features according to place or climate, "thus being contagious in one spot and not in another."

In view of the confusion, the Lords of the Privy Council transmitted to the Royal College of Physicians a mass of statistical returns furnished to the government by the British authorities resident abroad. To allay public fears, it was noted this was a common practice, not indicative of any apprehension that cholera would appear in England. On June 15, the Royal College of Physicians issued their unanimous opinion, stating, "That the Cholera Morbus may be communicated by infected persons to those in health; but that no information which has reached the Committee justifies the supposition that it is communicable by merchandize. As a measure of safety, however, the Committee approve of the establishment of quarantine."[2]

The British College of Health, New Road, King's Cross, London, had its own solution to cholera by promoting its concoction, "MORISON'S VEGETABLE UNIVERSAL MEDICINES," that might be had at the college, and where "advice is daily given, gratis." Mr. Morison, a hygienist who had published "Address to the Hon. Court of Directors of the East India Company" in 1825, republished the work in 1831, entitling it "Morisoniana." In it, he "clearly laid down the inefficiency of the past medical practices for the eradication, or even stoppage of the ravages" of cholera, while promoting his own nostrum.

Interestingly, in 1841, an inquest was held over the body of Mary Cracknell. Her father deposed that she was poisoned by "quack medicines," administered by her husband, whose father was one of Morison's agents. The physician attending the woman testified that she died of peritoneal inflammation of the bowels, "and the administration of drastic purgatives, such as Morison's Pills, was exceedingly improper, and tended to aggravate the disease." The jury returned a verdict of "natural death."[3]

Such advertisements, in the form of news articles like the one above, typically included testimonials from distinguished persons. In a July 11, 1831, notice, Michael Gardner, general agent for the College of the County of Durham, avowed that before sailing, the ship *Halcyon* (of which Gardner was part owner) put in a plentiful supply of Morison's Universal Medicines. Despite putting in at Riga, where cholera was "raging at its highest," the infection was kept away from the crew. The advertisement cleverly added, "Surely this ought to induce all Commanders of vessels to take them to sea every voyage, not only as a certain preventative to all diseases, but a sure investment of trade, the Medicine being now in high request in all parts of the Baltic."

On July 26, the president and members of the British College of Health announced that, in the Baltic, "none have died who took the Medicines." After adding more information on the *Halcyon* voyage, a letter of praise from John Carr was published as "proof that the Cholera Morbus is not unknown in that densely populated manufacturing district" in London. Mr. Carr suffered a loss of strength, his sight nearly left him, his body was convulsed all over and he was tormented by a violent purging; but after taking "Morrison's [*sic*] Vegetable Universal Medicines" under the guidance of Mr. Poole, agent, he obtained immediate relief from his symptoms.[4]

An advertisement for "MOXON'S EFFERVESCENT MAGNESIAN APERIENT" noted, "The influence of heat, combined with too free indulgence in acid fruits and vegetable diet, during the summer and autumnal months, generally disorders the digestive functions. The bile becomes acrid—acidity predominates in the fist passages—the stomach loses its tone and energy—the intestinal canal is subject to unnatural irritation; hence arise acid eructations, sickness and purging, and those painful and dangerous diseases, Cholera Morbus and Dysentery." Moxon's Aperient, obtained in Bottles at 2s, 94, was clearly the answer. The ad boasted of an international clientele and indicated the mixture could be obtained from "all respectable Druggists and Medicine Venders" in London, Hamburg, Quebec, New York and Calcutta.[5]

A common over-the-counter preventative consisted of wearing camphor in a silken bag around the neck and placing it against the chest. If the disease was contracted, a teaspoonful of mustard (ground white mustard seed) in a pint of warm water, repeated every hour until vomiting occurred, was prescribed; afterwards a small teaspoonful of carbonate of soda with 5 drops of laudanum and a little warm brandy and water repeated every 3rd or 4th hour was recommended. Injections (enemas) made from a tablespoon of oil of turpentine and a pint of warm water was then to be administered every two hours until reaction was produced. After an "untoward outcome," it was recommended interment take place as quickly as possible. All clothes that could not be boiled were to be burned and the room in which the patient expired was to be fumigated and ventilated speedily and completely.[6]

One of the great newspaper responses to such advertising came from the *London Times*, July 4, 1831. Under the heading "To Correspondents," it warned, "We receive, by almost every post, letters from physicians, and surgeons, and apothecaries, on the subject of cholera morbus, each recommending his own peculiar mode of treatment, and most of them containing very precise descriptions of the places of residence of the writers. This is a very ingenious mode of advertising, but it won't do. *Quaere peregrinum.*"

Physicians, generally eschewing nostrums, had their own ideas of treatment. Dr. Ainslie considered the sudden sinking of strength and the disordered state of the blood as the most urgent manifestations of cholera. He advised the immediate trial of "inhaling a super-oxigenated air, for the purpose of revivifying the blood, until other remedies, such as ammonia, shall have time to act upon the morbid materials in the alimentary passages." He relied on the immediate and often-repeated doses of ammonia "because of the attending spasms in the limbs, an occurrence which is generally connected with alimentary acidity." He added, "So that, in addition to the cordial effects of ammonia, it may probably act as an antidote."[7]

Dr. Hope, an eminent surgeon with 30 years' practice, provided a remedy for cholera consisting of "one drachm of nitrous acid (not nitric, that has foiled me), one ounce of peppermint-water or camphor mixture, and 40 drops of tincture of opium. A fourth part every three or four hours in a cupful of thin gruel. The belly should be covered with a succession of hot cloths dry; bottles of hot water to the feet, if they can be obtained; constant and small sippings of finely strained gruel, or sago, or tapioca; no spirit—no wine—no fermented liquors till quite restored."[8]

M. Anthony Kraus sent Prince Lobkowitz, governor of Gallicia, two preservatives against cholera: oil of cameline and a stomach plaster. The prince subsequently responded that since the 22nd of May when cholera first appeared in Limburg, he and his family made use of them with good effect; he also gave the them to Professor Berres, who tried them on the sick of the Jews' hospital and those employed in burying the dead, "all of whom, as well as every other person who used these preservatives, escaped the disorder."[9]

The Board of Health and Economic Conditions in Britain

In June 1831, King William IV took a huge step forward in promoting public welfare by announcing that he "has been pleased to establish a board of health, to prepare and digest rules and regulations for the most speedy and effectual mode of guarding against the introduction and spreading of *infection,* and for *purifying any ship or house in case any contagious disorder* should unhappily manifest itself in any part of the United Kingdom, *notwithstanding the precautions taken* to guard against the *introduction* thereof; and to communicate the same to all *magistrates, medical persons,* and others, his Majesty's subjects, who may be *desirous,* and may *apply* to be made acquainted therewith" (italics in the original).

The Privy Council appointed Sir Henry Halford, president of the Royal College of Physicians, to serve as president of the board. His selection of board members elicited immediate howls of discontent. A letter to the editor of the *Courier* (June 27, 1831) protested that these individuals "never were in India, or indeed ever had an opportunity of witnessing this disease

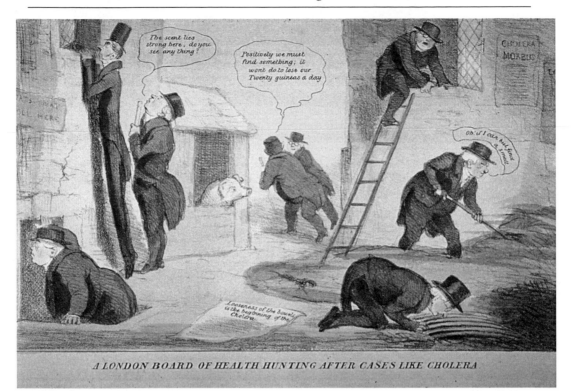

A LONDON BOARD OF HEALTH HUNTING AFTER CASES LIKE CHOLERA

McLean's Monthly Sheet of Caricatures, **London, published this farcical scene March 1, 1832. Created by Robert Seymour, it depicts a group of London physicians "sniffing" about a courtyard for signs of cholera. Seeking the smell of cholera is a clear reference to the belief that poisonous air caused the disease, while the clear incompetence of doctors was a recurring theme among the press and many in government (U.S. National Library of Medicine).**

in all its activity." On June 29, the *Albion* reprinted an article copied from the *London Royal Gazette,* noting that the board consisted of "seven FELLOWS of the Royal College of Physicians, and a few OFFICIALS with snug places at home under government" to enforce and fortify quarantine regulations. The writer added that among the first class, only those educated at "our *two* Universities" were included.

He also asked a question: "Is it not strange that among the numerous surgeons and assistants who have been where cholera raged, and have obtained experience in those formidable diseases against which the quarantine regulations are made, *not one* is mentioned as a coadjutor in the Board?" He went on to answer his own question by writing, "To those who are not aware of the internal workings of the college, their jealousy of the licentiates, of surgeons, and of the army and navy medical officers in general, and of the effects of the President's favour and patronage, the omission must appear strange.... Do Oxford and Cambridge confer superior excellence in medicine, as they exclude the members of all other colleges from an equal share with the fellows of Pall-mall East in the patronage of their exclusive grade? The fact is, that 'the green-eyed monster' resides in the college, and, backed by high aristocratic influence of church and state when anything is to be got, or anything to be done in which medical interest is concerned, it is grasped by the College of Physicians, who effect to despise the neophites of other colleges, and to consider the *ungraduated* as excluded from all pretension to judge of medical subjects." Asking whether the College of Physicians was justified in prejudging the nature of a disease "about which at present they know nothing from experience," the editorial called for them to seek further information "before we are convinced of [cholera's] *infectious* and *contagious* properties, and even of the disease being anything resembling cholera at all."

The appearance of cholera and the validity of quarantine continued to vex the public. One report stated that the master of a vessel from Riga landed a boat on a retired part of the coast and discharged a passenger suffering from cholera in order to avoid being detained in port. Another described how a case of influenza at Birmingham had initially been diagnosed as cholera, causing great alarm.[10] Of even greater concern, however, at least to men of commerce, was the state of the economy. One editorial began, "We never (except in periods of commercial convulsion) recollect the state of business, in the City of London, being in a more stagnant and unsatisfactory condition than it is at this moment. The freshest, and the most prominent, of the causes which have conduced to this effect, is the Cholera Morbus, and its consequences, on the Continent."

From a business perspective, the presence, or supposed presence of cholera, presented three different scenarios. In the first, it was assumed to materially affect present commercial interests by influencing the value of almost all articles imported from the north of Europe. "Of these there must be a cessation in part of the supply, as the owners will cease to send them on when certain to encounter the inconvenience of strict quarantine regulations, and in doubt, perhaps, whether they will ever reach their place of destination." This created a good deal of mercantile speculation, "as the truth may be exaggerated, or suppressed, to serve the object which the speculator may have in view." The example was given that in Stettin, one report affirmed that cholera was committing great ravages, while another claimed that the place was wholly free from it.

While acknowledging that cholera had a great potential to affect commerce, a second interpretation suggested that English business had not yet suffered in consequence of the contagion. It being only June, the largest quantities of corn, timber, wool, tallow, hemp and flax imported from the northern states of Europe, including Prussia and Austria, were not due until the months of October, November and December and none of which were purchased later than May, that being "the particular time for freighting Ships from this country, to bring home such commodities as arrive here in the three last months of the year; and in preventing such ships from being engaged in the trade, the Cholera will produce an injurious effect upon the shipping interest; but its effect on imports from the Continent will not be felt in our markets until about three or four months."

Consequently, the third, immediate, problem lay in the fact that alarm was very prevalent throughout the principal parts of the Continent, preventing circulation in all channels and diminishing consumption. Merchants and traders had already quit their desks and counters, repairing to the country, thus checking and impeding trade. In summary it was felt that markets for colonial produce and English manufacturing had begun to suffer, but not the market for the sale of goods brought from the Continent for sale in England. In fact, it was believed that the anticipated stoppage of supplies during the autumn and winter would drive prices up. This state of affairs, along with the uncertainty of ships being chartered at Hamburg and the Baltic due to the waxing and waning of the cholera epidemic, made for unfavorable speculation.

In summary, all three fears had succeeded in creating a "very stagnant state in Mincing-lane and merchants connected with it are extremely gloomy; and the principal of the minor causes is the effect of the cholera upon traffic, in Germany, Prussia, &c." Making matters worse, there was no great abundance of bills or money in the Money Market and London bankers were changing the discount upon bills to 5 percent instead of 4. As a point of interest, the price of gold bars was £3:17:10½ per ounce and silver was 4s. 10d per ounce.[11]

Matters would grow worse with new regulations concerning quarantine. While opinions varied on whether cholera was imported from areas of contagion, the government took immediate steps to protect against the possibility. Quarantine was established on all vessels from Hamburgh and those originating from the north of Denmark and Rotterdam. Similar to the spread of smallpox, a standing belief held that cholera germs were to be found in rags, and by mid–October the importation of rags was prohibited.[12]

Who, if Anyone, Brought the Cholera Morbus to England?

While mortality lists and horror stories of death and destruction from Russia, Poland and Northern Europe filled British newspapers, the final months of 1831 also saw their fair share of humor, directed at those who believed the disease, if not already wreaking havoc, was soon to become epidemic. Not atypically, the *Age* (November 20, 1831) poked fun at these doomsayers by writing of the "astounding intelligence that, a sailor named Crawford, 'kicked the bucket,' after having been drunk regularly for a fortnight—died of the Cholera Morbus! An old woman of sixty-two, who had led a drunken life for years, 'popped off the hooks'— died of the Cholera Morbus! Again, a fisherwoman, who had for years been afflicted with the dropsy ... was immediately cured of that disease, and made her die of the Cholera Morbus!" Nor were politicians free from ridicule. The *Age* questioned whether it did "not seem exceedingly probable that they *have* introduced the bugbear, in order to avert as much as possible that indigestion which the people of England must feel at their perfidy?"

Another article presented a fictitious dialogue from the House of Commons ridiculing medical treatments and politicians' penchant for kickbacks by imagining Alderman Wen say that he "thought their time would be well spared by referring the investigation [of cholera] to the City Reform Committee, who had a natural predilection for dirty jobs." Alderman Thompson suggested the general adoption of iron bedsteads as the best public safeguard, and he would "contract to furnish the *materiel* at little more than cost price." Alderman Wood suggested *Quassia* and *Coculus Indicus* "might be given in considerable quantities, and he knew where a large supply could easily be procured on the most moderate terms." Alderman Waithman suggested wrapping patients up in flannels and stout shawls, such as could be procured at very reasonable rates at the corner of Fleet-street. Mr. Mayhew thought decoctions of sloe-juice an infallible remedy; Mr. Tennyson declared an ordinance should be issued for fumigating the metropolis by keeping fires blazing in all streets, but Alderman Atkins "extinguished the honourable gentleman's motion, which would after all be only a *fire-escape* from the malady."[13]

If nothing else, the satiric *Age* suggested, the cholera scare would, at least, have "the effect of causing a few waggon-loads of filth—which is alone sufficient to generate a plague—to be taken from the city and its vicinity; and that, together with a good supply of food, flannel, and chlorate of lime, *will* be of *some* service to poor families."[14]

As politicians did not actually introduce cholera and physicians did not have it within their power to control it, the faithful turned to religion for explanations and redress. The *Christian Advocate* (September 5, 1831) began an editorial by warning princes who sacrificed their subjects on the shrine of policy or passion that there was One mightier than "the king of terrors." The author opined, "We are not surprised that so many persons, of various countries and opinions, regard this scourge as a visitation,—a *judicial* visitation from heaven" against

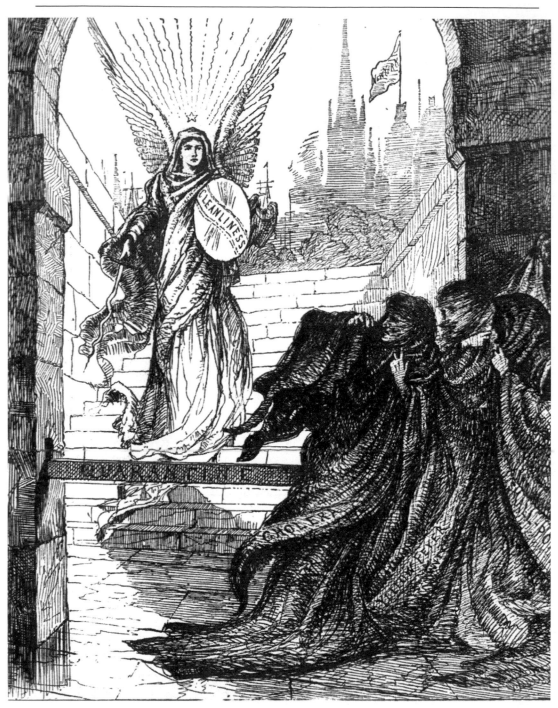

"At the Gates: Our safety depends upon official vigilance." First published in *Harper's Weekly,* September 5, 1885, this winged angel carries the shield of "Cleanliness," warning terrified women, on whom the cloak of darkness has already descended, that the only true preventative of cholera, the "disease of filth," was to keep their domiciles free from contamination (U.S. National Library of Medicine).

Russian ambition. In a bit of politicking of his own, he continued that while it was a duty to pray that "in the midst of deserved wrath" God would remember mercy, no one should be surprised that his anger should "wax hot" against imperial robbery, and that God should come "out of his place" to judge and afflict those who aim at the extermination of a whole people.

On October 31, in a letter to the editor of the same newspaper, a writer suggested that the best defense against contagion lay in "spiritual remedies." He suggested a day be set apart for a solemn fast, where prayer was to be made at all the churches and chapels throughout Great Britain. "Who can tell," he asked, "but that God looking down from heaven, and seeing this highly favoured (but deeply depraved) land, imploring forgiveness with fasting and with tears, may exclaim as he did of old, 'It repenteth me of the evil that I said I would bring upon it—I will not do it.'" This remedy, the author concluded, "was tried by the Ninevites, *and it succeeded.*"

A "Considerable Excitement" at Sunderland

The only hope England had of escaping cholera was its "insular position, and the neutralizing powers of the sea air on the miasma."[15] That sentiment offered little comfort to those who realized their country was only a 36-hour steam voyage across the German Ocean (North Sea) from Hamburg, where the disease had proved itself a known killer. Reacting to the growing fear, the *Courier* (October 29, 1831) informed its readers "a considerable 'excitement' (as the fashionable word now used on all occasions) existed in the city."

That fear stemmed from reports out of Sunderland (on the northeastern coast), dated November 4, that cholera was supposed to have been brought in by a seaman late of Riga or by a seaman who had died of cholera at Riga and spread to the locals through his wife, who contracted the disease on opening his sea chest. During the next several weeks, London newspapers were filled with contradictory information. While businessmen in Sunderland were unwilling to admit the disease was cholera, considering the injury that would be done to the port by subjecting its ships to quarantine, physicians failed to agree on everything from the number of deaths to the specific type of cholera, or even if the contagion were cholera.

A medical board was formed at Newcastle (12 miles distant) as the number of fatalities increased. As a preventative, commissioners ordered streets, lanes and alleys cleaned of nuisances; the plan was also adopted on the opposite coast, where Liverpool authorities began cleaning and white-washing all dwellings of the poor.[16] In London (300 miles distant), complaints arose about the negligence of scavengers employed by city authorities to keep streets clean. It was believed these hirelings had hitherto escaped punishment by confusing the dates of the days on which they were to take their turns cleaning the streets.

Resorting to traditional measures, large quantities of chloride of lime were sent to places where purification was most needed. The commissioner of sewers became actively engaged in affording facilities for passing off all sorts of rubbish "which may tend injuriously to impregnate the air," while the New River Company offered to supply a greater abundance of water to sluice the streets, particularly the narrow lanes and alleys. In conjunction with the hoses of parish engines, it was expected the water would carry off all the offensive matter "after every day's occupation."[17] The following year, the New River Company raised rates charged to the London House of Corrections from 40l. to 60l. in order to deal with requirements for a new influx of inmates (making a total population of 930 males, 30 females and 29 children), some of whom were suffering from cholera.[18]

Water suppliers were in the news again in July, as the prevailing theory on the "unknown subject of cholera" centered on the belief it was produced and propagated by local malaria. Anyone passing the gratings of the common sewers could "perceive that there is much in the way of malaria there, which a little liberality and attention on the part of the Water Companies might remove."[19]

In order to alert the public of this and other dangers, 20,000 copies of new rules were ordered printed and circulated throughout London.

REGULATIONS FOR THE CITY OF LONDON
TO WARD OFF CHOLERA—NOVEMBER 1831

1. Chloride of lime was to be used to purify receptacles; refuse matter in drains, cesspools, dustbins and dirt heaps was to be cleaned and prevented from accumulating.

2. All reservoirs, cisterns and sinks were to be cleaned; running water was to be used to carry away impurities.

3. Apartments were to be kept clean by frequent washing and ventilated by fire and fresh air.

4. Windows were to be kept closed at night to prevent currents of air from exposing sleepers to disease.

5. Bed linen and furniture were to be changed regularly.

6. Personal cleanliness was encouraged—washing and a change of clothing.

7. To guard against sudden changes in temperature, flannel was to be worn around the bowels, while feet were to be protected by woollen stockings.

8. Excessive fatigue was to be avoided and wet or sweaty clothes removed at night.

9. The diet should consist of plain meats, bread and well-boiled vegetables; salads, fruits, nuts, rich pastry or any articles found to create acidity, flatulence and indigestion were to be avoided.

10. Undiluted spirits, acid drinks, stale soups and sugar were to be avoided.

11. Regular habits pertaining to moderate exercise were encouraged.

12. Citizens were encouraged to maintain a cheerful disposition while keeping a full reliance that the government was taking all appropriate measures, best calculated, with divine assistance, to meet the exigencies of the occasion.

One unintentional consequence of the last admonition was pointed out in a letter to the editor. Remarking that if cheerfulness were to be one anti-cholera remedy, the writer found that directive nearly impossible to obey if a quotation from Mr. Ritson of Sunderland were to be taken on face value. (Ritson had reported, "There is not one body lies unburied in this town.") The writer lamented this sad fact by wryly commenting, "Surely he does not mean to say that that devastating disease, the Cholera, has taken off the whole population of the town of Sunderland, and that he himself is the only melancholy exception, having performed the duty of consigning his fellow townsfolk to their mother earth." The editor was obliged to add a postscript, "We presume Mr. Ritson alluded only to *dead bodies,* but those alarmists should be guarded in their expressions in these times of terror."[20]

The government sent medical expert Dr. Robert Daun to Sunderland but his presence did little to clarify the nature of the malady. On November 7, he publicly stated his belief it was Asiatic cholera, while his private letters continued to insist the disease was "malignant cholera," "Indian cholera," "spasmodic cholera," or no more than "common bilious cholera," lamenting, "the medical men are greatly blamed." The same day, six new cases of cholera were identified; other doctors immediately brought the diagnosis into question, offering lengthy discussions on alternate explanations.

By November 9, nineteen persons were reported dead at neighboring Newcastle; authorities denied this, calling the state of health there "excellent," which prompted the national Council Office to issue its own report.

Daily Reports of Diarrhea and Cholera Cases
Sunderland, November 11, 1831

	Diarrhea	Cholera Morbus	
		Common	Malignant
Remained at last report	2	3	3
New cases	12	4	1
Total	14	7	4
Recovered	–	1	1
Died	–	–	2
Remaining at this date (10 P.M.)[21]	14	6	1

By November 12, there were 11 new cases of diarrhea (for a total of 20), 2 new cases of common cholera (for a total of 8) and 3 new cases of malignant cholera (for a total of 3).[22] The same day, a report of two cholera cases, both fatal, was reported at Sheffield.[23]

News from Paris

In early June, a letter written by an Englishman from St. Omer warned his countrymen that cholera had just made its appearance there among the English, who consisted of upwards of 400 families. The symptoms, he wrote, "are the same which invariably accompany the plague; and confirm me in the opinion that the Russian cholera morbus is neither more nor less than the plague itself." Singularly, only the English were afflicted with cholera, measles and smallpox.[24]

Similar to other countries, a conclusive diagnosis proved elusive. By June, "alarmists" declared that cholera had reached the capital, while others declared it to be no more than influenza, arguing that the febrile infection attacking the poorer classes was no more than was "usual at the same season of the year." In the same newspaper, a physician was quoted as saying that the disease was "a catarrhal affection ... arising solely from the variable state of the atmosphere."[25]

In July 1831, the *Messager des Chambres* felt obliged to print an article respecting the contagion of cholera. Stating it was "a positive fact" that persons who led a "regular life, and live in healthy places" were likely to be spared its ravages, the article went on to say cholera would strike "without pity every man worn out by excess, and weakened by dissipation"; more specifically, 90 out of 100 persons who contracted the disease were in the habit of drinking ardent spirits to excess. The writer added the following: "This scourge must find an ample harvest among the Russians, who never cease drenching themselves with brandy. Field Marshal Diebitsch used frequently brandy and punch." Women, according to the report, "rarely addict themselves to strong liquors, and accordingly few of them are attacked with the cholera."[26] Unfortunately, while a common belief throughout the 1800s, the idea that temperance protected men and women from cholera or other diseases was based on selective interpretation of data rather than impartial scientific studies.

Similar to the actions of the British, by July the French minister of marine ordered those in charge of the ports to follow the strictest observance for preventing the introduction of cholera into the country. Vessels were to "cruise incessantly along the coast, to watch the smaller landing-places" so that passengers and merchandise could not be smuggled in without passing through quarantine.[27] Later that month, French papers reported that cholera had made an appearance in Italy, where it had been brought through the Austrian frontier. It was also suggested that the disease had reached the north of France, but telegraphic communications contradicted the rumor.[28]

Fear continued to mount. Despite conflicting reports from England about the nature and severity of the disease, the Commission Sanitaire (Board of Health) decreed that no vessel coming from Scotland or any part of the North of England, including Yarmouth, would be admitted into the harbor at Calais. All packet and commerce boats from London and Dover were required to carry bills of health, delivered by the magistrate at the place of their departure or by the French consul, or suffer quarantine.

The French took their preventative measures so seriously that when a vessel from Hamburgh (typically spelled then with an "h") attempted to force her way into Boulogne, she was fired upon twice as a signal to prevent her coming in. When the captain refused to withdraw, the boat was surrounded by armed vessels and driven off. Equally alarmed, the British consul at Boulogne communicated with the collector of customs at Dover, warning him not to allow the renegade craft to enter port. The matter was settled by having the steam packet *Britannia* tow the ship into quarantine near Havre. Their fears proved groundless when it was subsequently learned the captain ignored the warning shots because his boat was not seaworthy, having sprung a leak and carrying four feet of water in the hold.[29]

One ray of hope, if indeed it had been true, came from Dr. Guilot, of St. Etienne (Department of the Loire), who published a letter in the *Segusian Mercury*, purporting that in towns where coals were used for fuel, residents were secure against pestilential contagion.[30] Beliefs such as this were based on the premise that smoke from bonfires or the discharge of cannon rid the air of miasma.

8

Sunderland

The Continuing Saga, 1831

"Burking Versus Burning"

The surgeons have it (it has been said)
A private interest lurking;
They pay high prices for the dead,
And thus encourage Burking.

With equal truth, we may avow
To Burking they conspire;
A patient's cured of Cholera now
By setting him on fire.

What shocking men the doctors are,
How little they must feel—
If iron's so successful,—rare!
Why next—they'll take to steel.

By fire the Cholera is cured.
Thanks to the surgeons' learning.
Our bodies now must be insured,
Since they encourage Burking.[1]

In point of fact, "burking" was a dangerous occupation in the 1830s. During January 1832 in Edinburgh, the home of body snatching, two resurrectionists went into a churchyard for the purpose of procuring "something." The mother of one of the men had died of cholera on the previous day and had been interred by the side of a plump "subject" on whose grave they intended to operate. Unfortunately for them, they opened the wrong grave and lifted out the body snatcher's mother. The men quickly replaced it and retreated. The following morning, both were seized with the disease and died that evening. A day later they were buried alongside the corpse they had so lately exhumed![2]

Less than a month later, "Crouck, the notorious resurrectionist-man," and his fellow body snatchers "got wind" that a female cholera victim had been recently interred. Knowing they could get a good price for the "article," they snuck into the churchyard, but a grave watcher overheard them and gave the alarm. Crouck's cohorts escaped but the authorities arrived in time to apprehend Crouck in the grave, surrounded with implements of the trade. On the way to the office, police had much difficulty in preventing a mob from attacking the "snatcher." The offender was held to answer the charges at the sessions.[3]

Several days later a riot took place at Paisley, Scotland, in consequence of a false report that six graves containing cholera victims had been opened and the bodies carried away.[4] "Choleraphobia" apparently ran rampant at Paisley, as they requested physicians treating cholera victims to stay away from coffeehouses, while "self-afflicters" resorted to muffling their faces in order to avoid breathing "air charged with infection."[5] Similar riots also broke out in Ireland when locals concluded that doctors treated cholera patients "merely to try experiments on them!"[6]

When statistics of cholera deaths were collected, the death rates of individual towns were published in order for civilians and authorities to track the progress of the disease. While not a specific place, "Afloat in the River" became a fixed residence in these tables, as a significant number of seamen who contracted cholera either fell off their ships and drowned or were placed there in lieu of burial. Resurrectionists quickly discovered that collecting these specimens was easier than disinterring bodies and gathered them in for the purpose of selling them. These atrocities finally prompted Mr. Hume to present petitions from the Glasgow students of medicine and London Surgical Institution, praying that some legislation might be immediately passed to regulate the mode of procuring bodies for dissection.[7]

Determining the exact moment of death—or even an accurate determination that death had actually taken place—occasionally led to what Edgar Allan Poe so graphically immortalized as "premature burial." Stethoscopes were rarely used and a patient, while under the influence of "the indiscriminate use of opium, may remain for twelve or sixteen hours without a symptom or evidence of life." Victims, presumed to be dead, often shocked friends and family by exhibiting signs of life while the coffin lid was being nailed down or kicking the coffin lid at the graveside. One unfortunate, after bleeding failed to restore animation, was discovered the following morning to have rolled off the table, dead in pools of her own blood.[8] Three children of a poor workman living in Chelsea, subsisting on potatoes and "broken victuals" (refuse of a baker's or pastry-cook's shop) and drinking *water out of a tub*, were found to have been buried alive when the bodies were exhumed for a coroner's inquest. In this case, the jury reached a conclusion of death by "the visitation of God."[9]

Sites selected for interment were no less controversial. Fearing that the usual kirkyards were too close to thoroughfares and might be the means of propagating cholera, local aldermen suggested bodies be buried in secluded areas at the water's edge. The board of health offered no objection but raised the question of whether the ground was to be consecrated. Predetermining that the bishop of London would refuse to perform the requisite service, the officers ultimately decided "they should be able to get over that difficulty" somehow.[10]

In taking up the subject of burial, the House of Commons supported local authorities by determining that on no account should the bodies of those supposed to have died of cholera be carried into churches. "Such bodies should, without being washed, be wrapt in the clothes in which *they may have died*, and deposited, as soon as possible, in a well-fastened coffin, carefully pitched within." Pitch and tar were used to seal coffins in suspected cases of contagion.[11]

Perhaps the best way to state the continuing saga at Sunderland (and consequently the metropolis) is to quote from an editorial printed in the *Courier*, November 14, 1831:

> It is really amusing, notwithstanding the gravity of the subject, to read the medical and non-medical communications from Sunderland relative to cholera. They are all exceeding curious, but the medical statements are more so in a high degree. One physician has doubts, another wonders how any medical man with common knowledge of his profession could have any doubt at all. Dr. Daun, in his reports, extracts of which only find their way to the public, is stated to have said one day, "I have doubts of it being the Asiatic cholera"—another day, "I have strong hopes that it is not the true cholera"—on

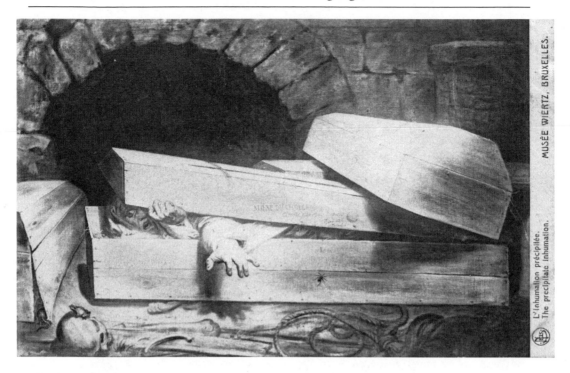

This fascinatingly gruesome Victorian postcard from Musee Wiertz, Bruxelles, depicts the fate of many cholera victims: premature burial (Authors' collection).

a third, "My hopes of the disease not being the Asiatic cholera are growing hourly less and less"—on a fourth, "My hopes revive that this is not the true cholera, or at least that, if we have been visited by that pestilent disorder, it is now disappearing.... [T]o non-medical people it must appear strange that with all the boasted skill of medical men in this country, there should be any doubt. The cholera at Sunderland is stated to have attacked in the same way as on the Continent; to have killed in the same way, and to have left the same traces behind. How then can pathologists mistake the character of the disease?

The article goes on to say the following: "It is almost certain that the disease has not been imported, but that the same extraordinary change of atmosphere which induced it elsewhere has been in operation here. That the effect has been so slight is to be attributed to our ever-varying climate, which is, in fact, a better security against the extension of the disease than all the decrees of the Board of Health.... It is some satisfaction to an Englishman, that, bad as his climate is, it will kill an enemy." For its "zealous" crusade in promoting the presence of cholera, the *Sunderland Herald* accused the *Courier* of perversely influencing all of London, when, in fact, the city was experiencing "excellent health."

By mid–November, under the growing penalties of quarantine, shipowners and merchants of Sunderland, situated in northeast England, issued a statement avowing that the present disease was "not Asiatic or foreign cholera imported, but aggravated cases of English cholera, and were not contagious or infectious." The last was based on the fact that "no seaman or custom-house officer belonging to the port, has been attacked by any complaint resembling it." The statement further complained that, while Sunderland continued in a state of proscription, cholera, if it really existed, was "allowed to be conveyed by the daily traffic inland between that town and the metropolis!"

Denial that a fatal disease, by whatever name, existed in their city was standard practice by businessmen. The presence of smallpox throughout the 19th century was similarly dismissed on the grounds that even a rumor would destroy commerce.[12] Merchants in Sunderland lamented the fact the ports in the Mediterranean and other parts of the world would be closed to them, throwing manufacturers out of employ, "at the very season of the year when they stand most in need of it. There can be little or no doubt, that many of the alarming reports have been propagated by interested persons, by speculators in coals, or gamblers in the drug game."

Considering the source, the last statement was ingenuous but nevertheless true. As proof of the flourishing state of the drug swindle, the *Morning Herald* published a report that camphor (sold as a curative), which had been selling in the 80s two or three months previously, now went for £17 and that cajeput oil rose from 9d an ounce to 15s. The newspaper also reported that the government obliged coal "to perform quarantine," but allowed cotton from Alexandria, where cholera has been raging most virulently, to be brought up the river in lighters: "Now, if there be any one thing more calculated than another to propagate a pestilential disease, it is cotton; and, on the contrary, nothing can be less likely than coals!!"[13]

A less provocative article in the *Christian Advocate*, November 14, 1831, informed readers that "The speculative demand for drugs administered in cases of cholera has been very brisk": camphor sold as high as 16 guineas per cwt, cajeput oil at 9s. 3d per ounce; oil of peppermint advanced from 36s to 60s per pound; American oil of peppermint ("which a short time since was a 'complete drug'") rose from 9s to 30s per pound. However, quotations on laudanum and ether had not proportionally risen and continued to be readily obtained. By December 16, however, reports on the Markets stated that anti-cholera drugs were on the decline.[14]

Nearly as insidious as drug speculation was the news out of Sunderland concerning a "system of concealment," whereby local physicians did not submit cholera reports to Dr. Daun, thus keeping new cases and deaths out of the statistics.[15] Newspapers, too, were not without their critics. The *Patriot*, March 7, 1832 (citing the *Medical Gazette* of March 3), fearful that

BEWARE OF CHOLERA!

| SAMMIS' ESS. JAMAICA GINGER. A few Drops In the Water you Drink. | DON'T | SAMMIS' CHOLERA DROPS! |

Be without them in the House.

To be had only at

62 BROADWAY.　THE BROADWAY DRUG STORE,　62 BROADWAY

FARQUHAR & SAMMIS.

1y26

Large typeface and bold lettering was sure to catch the eye of prospective clients. Apparently this was all the proprietors felt was needed as they failed to list any other diseases Sammis' Cholera Drops cured, offered no exotic ingredients (although they were also promoting Jamaica ginger drops) and included no testimonials (*Logansport (IN) Weekly Journal*, July 5, 1873).

the full truth was not being published, wondered, "How far a meretricious press, interested in concealment, may prostitute itself for lucre, and how far a credulous public, ready for persuasion where it is anxious to believe, would be misled" by false predictions that cholera "would not show itself in the 'happy climate' of England."

Charges that physicians and newspapers willfully withheld information on deadly diseases, whether from ignorance, to alleviate panic, to protect their "boasted prognostications," or to preserve commerce in infected cities, frequently appeared throughout the 19th century when epidemics such as cholera and smallpox were present.

Based on the observations of Dr. David Barry, who had extensive contact with the disease on the Continent and who was sent to Sunderland to ascertain the true nature of the disease, the malady was confirmed as Indian or spasmodic cholera. In consequence, the classifications originally called diarrhea, common and malignant cholera were discontinued.[16]

Daily Reports of Cholera from the Commencement of the Disease at Sunderland on October 26, 1831

December	Cases	Deaths
6	369	119
10	422	141
15	449	155
16	456	157
17	464	159
21	507	184
22	509	186
25	511	188
26	525	196
28	528	197
29	529	198
31	541	207[17]

On December 20, 1831, the *Kent and Essex Mercury* commented on the state of cholera, adding that it was "not pleasant to see six places now set forth in the daily medical reports," indicating the spread of the disease. The date of the commencement of the disease at Newcastle was December 7; at North Shields, December 11; at Seghill Colliery, December 12; at Walker, near Newcastle, December 14.

Official Report of Cholera Issued from the Council Office For the Month of December, 1831

City	Date	Cases	Died
Newcastle	14	46	13
	15	61	23
	19	112	41
	20	123	48
	22	164	59
	26	226	83
	28	285	99
	29	307	107
	31	492	122
North Shields &	14	3	2
Tynemouth	15	3	2
	20	7	5
	22	11	9

City	Date	Cases	Died
	26	13	9
	28	16	9
	29	16	9
	31	19	11
Seghill Colliery	14	4	2
	15	4	2
	19	12	6
Walker	14	2	0
	15	2	1
Seaham	15	3	1
Houghton-le-Spring	19	8	3
& Penshaw	20	8	3
	28	29	14
	31	29	14
Gateshead	26	41	12
	28	143	55
	29	172	63
	31	234	74
South Shields	28	2	1
& Westow	29	2	0
	31	2	0
Haddington	27	6	4
	28	10	4
	31	13	4[18]

As indicated by the table, cholera spread quickly. Prior to December 26 there had been no reported cases at Gateshead, but the morning report indicated 39 cases and 9 deaths; by afternoon, 15 new cases had been added and 6 more deaths. By December 31, the disease at Gateshead was described as "fully equalling in virulence" any Dr. Kennedy had seen in India. In four days, he reported 271 cases and 63 deaths. Although the city had only one-third the population of Newcastle, the marked contrast was explained by the fact the former comprised vagrants, adding to the wretchedness of the disease. (Newcastle authorities solved that problem by moving most of their vagrant tribes out of town.) Unfortunately, as disease there continued to spread into the higher parts of town the cause was blamed on atypically warm weather and Christmas imbibing. Reports of "ghost stories" (false deaths) continued to be used against the official reports. Complicating matters, warm clothes and flannel issued to the poor were often pledged for drink money.[19]

The unprecedented violence of cholera caught parish authorities by surprise. At Gateshead in particular, proper medical aid could not be provided for one-tenth of the diseased, as the number of medical men was extremely small. Coffins could not be procured fast enough to permit interments being performed within a short time of death and a new chapel-yard set apart for cholera victims "presented a pitiable sight." A long trench, capable of holding 12 coffins, two abreast, had been dug, while clergy read the service as more and more corpses arrived. One coffin was much deeper than the others and upon investigation it was revealed that the man had been doubled up by cramps and his body was unable to be straightened. "The burial service was finished by the dim glare of a lamp, and the whole scene was certainly calculated to leave a lasting impression on the mind of the observer."[20]

Significantly, a November 9 report of the common council observed that in a town as large as North Shields it was "somewhat reprehensible that there are no public water-founts, at which the poor might procure that necessary article free of expense." Plans to address the matter were to be discussed by the local parish. The subject was one of paramount importance, but unfortunately, without a firm awareness that cholera was waterborne, the source of water being pumped through the fountains was not a consideration. Consideration continued to center around removing rubbish that "may tend injuriously to impregnate the air."[21]

Cholera: Caution

Seeking preventatives and cures understandably became a driving passion. As the Russian government discovered, however, when their effort to solicit a cure failed, suggestions were varied and ineffectual. Claims were wild and unsubstantiated; lacking any government control, proofs were left to the eye of the beholder, often leading the credulous down a path of unintended self-destruction.

In 1831, one fad was the steam-bath. Its origins were attributed to Dr. Ucelli, a medical officer in the Russian service who used it in the Crimea. During the course of his career he treated over 2,000 patients for cholera and lost only 8–9 out of 100. In 1828, a treatise written by Captain Jekyll of the Royal Navy promoted the use of the vapor bath. This method was used by a surgeon of the East India Company, who claimed the application of steam cured seamen on a voyage to India and China. Later, a London medical practitioner invented a "Spirit-air Bath," which he claimed to be efficacious in cases of derangement of the bowels and the English cholera of ordinary seasons, "its effects being a ready determination of blood to the skin and the production of speedy and copious perspiration."[22]

No less a publication than the *London Medical Gazette* (December 3, 1831) recommended the "Bath for Hot Air or Vapour," stating that it fit into an extremely small compass (space), and was equally efficient and much cheaper than any similar devices. Created by I.J. Rippon, the device was constructed "upon a principle which renders it unnecessary to Remove the Patient from the bed; is remarkably portable, and, at the expense of twopence, will produce in four minutes sufficient heat to cause perspiration." Price for the machine with spirit lamp was 10s; frame for the bed 10s; packed for the country at 1s. 6d extra. S. Jones' "Portable Hot Air and Steam Bath" promised a "cure of cholera morbus" and sold for 1 guinea.[23]

Not everyone agreed with these bold pronouncements. Dr. Schleiden felt that bathing of all descriptions was successful only in the beginning of the malady, but never in its progress. He recommended frictions, poultices and blisters on the stomach and grimly added that, if the disease was well advanced, "generally, every assistance will be useless."[24] In fact, steam baths and all methods used to promote sweating were actually detrimental to cholera patients, for they exacerbated dehydration by the very perspirations advocated.

Surgeon Silas Blandford, Royal Navy, advertised that his experience in India enabled him to "ascertain the precise cause of the complaint," and he avowed his medicines would cure 99 out of every 100 cases, if "taken in anything like reasonable time." A more ingenuous advertisement stated that Sir Henry Halford and the boards of health recommended "PRICE and GOSNELL'S CAMPHOR SOAP," which combined "the greatest possible quantity of camphor with cajeput and other anti-contagious ingredients." Packaged with full directions, prices ranged from 10s. 6d to 30s. depending on the amount required.[25] While it was true Halford and numerous boards of health recommended soap for personal cleanliness, no specific brand was ever mentioned.

Camphor continued to be promoted as a preventative against miasmic contagion and even Rigge, Brockbank and Rigge, perfumers to the Royal Family, got into the business, selling camphorated *eau de cologne*, lavender, smelling salts, cold cream, soap, pastilles and *eau a bruler*, camphorated tooth powder and paste, sachets and powder and Adelaide bouquets.[26] Samuel Gray promoted his newly invented "Lavement Syringe" for a healthy and regular action of the bowels[27] and Dr. George Rees was called upon to communicate his ideas with respect to "Carbon, Oxygen, and Vitality," calculated to "throw some light on the nature of Asiatic Cholera."[28]

Harkening back to a method used in 1686 (see chapter 3), Dr. Lange, chief physician at Cronstadt, applied a heated iron (*ferrum condens*) to each side of the spine in the region of the lumbar vertebrae. He claimed this immediately stopped spasms brought on by cholera, the pulse grew stronger, heat of the extremities returned and vomiting and diarrhea ceased. Of 14 patients treated in this way, 12 were cured and two died the same day.[29]

Dr. McKechnie, who learned the technique in India, advocated a similar procedure. After declaring a decided preference for the use of actual cautery, he explained the less formidable application of moxa over the spine of the precordia in the cholera stage of collapse. Moxa (*Artemisia Chinesis*) was a Japanese word describing a fine powder made from the leaves of young mugwort trees. The substance, in the shape of a cone, was placed on moistened skin and set on fire. After burning down, a dark colored spot remained, the ulceration of which was promoted by applying a little garlic. This treatment was believed to prevent or cure many diseases.[30] Dr. McKechnie's method of "moxa" (in his case the use of the word referenced "burning") consisted of saturating a small quantity of cotton wool in oil of turpentine or spirit of wine and then rolling it into the thickness of a finger. This was placed at the nape of the neck and extended 9 inches down the spine. After setting it on fire, a vesication appeared and the application was removed. He stated this method had "been attended with very great success in the most hopeless cases."[31]

In 1832, the *Caledonian Mercury* reported that Haddington medical practitioners used a galvanic battery on several persons suffering from cholera, finding "great efficacy,"[32] and in Ireland, a Dr. Ferguson suggested people have themselves "galvenised" so "you may be a man again." The theory was in the experimental stage but the newspaper carrying the story thought it amusing enough to speculate that it was a better alternative than boiling or baking in hot and vapor baths and humorously suggesting galvanic batteries be set up on every street corner to defy cholera, "the foul fiend."[33] On a different order, troops stationed in Ireland were ordered to cease washing out their barracks rooms as a precautionary measure against cholera. Instead, the rooms were to be left perfectly dry and cleaned with large scrubbing brushes.[34]

If such techniques did not appeal to the sufferer, Mr. G.H. Bell suggested the application of dry heat to the body of cholera victims. His method, "within the reach of every family," consisted of filling a sufficient number of large pans with dry salt or clean sand and setting them on the fire or a hot table until the contents were as hot as the skin could bear. The contents were then to be poured into pillowcases or shirts tied at the ends and put in immediate contact with the body. By a succession of these, the heat could be kept up for as long as necessary.[35] One "grave correspondent" recommended with "great fervor," that champagne be used as a remedy for cholera. The newspaper dryly noted, "'Pleasant but wrong,' we suspect will be the answer of the medical practitioners."[36]

9

Trials and Tribulations

Whilst we cannot go along with those who utterly deny that the genuine *Cholera has yet actually existed in England, much less London, we are strongly of the opinion that the nature and extent of the disease have been greatly exaggerated, partly by the professional ardour of our medical men, and partly by the natural feats and apprehensions of humanity.*[1]

From a detached perspective, one of the more interesting aspects associated with cholera had to do with the similarity of its symptoms with poisoning. Because a definitive diagnosis was often difficult to make in the early 1800s, defendants in murder trials occasionally used the disease as a means of protesting their innocence.

A case in April 1817 involved Robert Saul Donnald, a man of 26 years, who carried on the business of a surgeon and apothecary. He was accused of murdering his mother-in-law, Mrs. Elizabeth Downing, on November 3, 1816, by administering arsenic in a cup of cocoa, upon bread and butter, or in some other undiscovered manner. He pleaded not guilty.

In July 1816, Donnald began borrowing heavily, promising his debts would be repaid upon his marriage, as his wife was worth £3,000 and her mother, Mrs. Downing, was worth £14,000. After representing his practice as in a "flourishing state," the couple married in July. Witnesses testified that, soon after, he was often heard to proclaim his mother-in-law "would not live long." On October 19, Mrs. Downing took tea with her son-in-law, became ill, vomited and complained of cramps in her legs. After a second party where she drank tea, the woman sickened and died. The coroner's jury returned a verdict of murder by poison and Donnald was brought to trial.

In his defense, Donnald stated that Mrs. Downing died from an attack of cholera morbus, having recently suffered from that disease. A physician then testified that "he had never met with a case of cholera morbus that had produced death in a shorter time than three or four days" and was of the opinion she had not died from that disorder. An autopsy revealed the stomach to have been in a state of "stellated inflammation, and both the coats of the stomach were softened, as if by the action of some corrosive substance," most certainly arsenic. On cross-examination, the doctor stated that cholera was produced generally in hot seasons by the overflowing of bile. A second physician deposed cholera often killed a patient within 24 hours and "might be considered the most acute disease known in Great Britain." He attributed the autopsy findings "to nothing but the cholera morbus, though they did not indicate that disorder exclusively," and tests made on the victim's stomach contents indicating the presence of arsenic as "by no means infallible." Several other doctors also presented conflicting testimony, after which the jury consulted for a quarter of an hour, returning a verdict of not guilty.[2]

On May 22, 1818, a coroner's inquest was held on the death of Elizabeth Danvers. A medical practitioner called to treat her in the last few moments of life diagnosed an acute case of

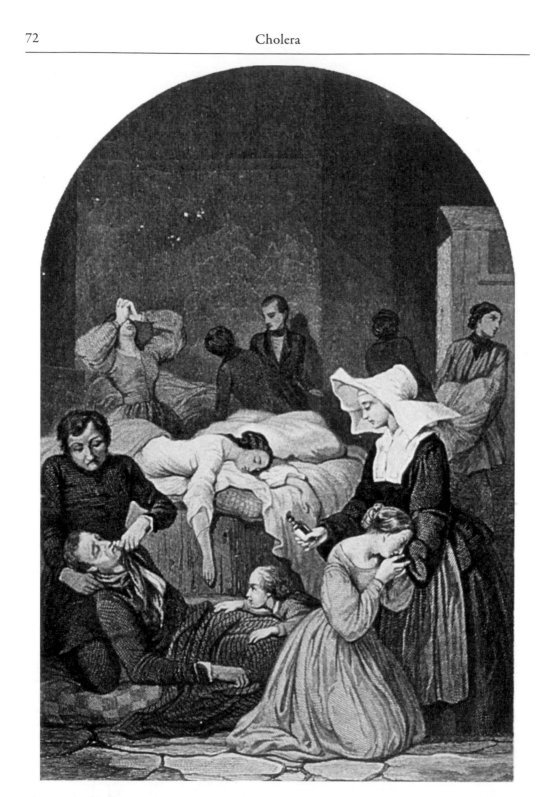

This engraving of lament in a sick room vividly captures both the agony and the terror of "King Cholera" during the 1832 epidemic in London. Viewed through an open doorway, aid is being rendered to a victim who appears to have just been struck down. The chances of survival were grim (U.S. National Library of Medicine).

cholera morbus, and testified that would have been the verdict had there not been a supposition that she had "drunk something improper." At autopsy, the stomach contents were removed and sent for analysis, revealing the presence of arsenic. The jury concluded the woman, "from disappointment in love and a consequent state of despondency, had put an end to her existence by means of arsenic."[3]

A case of a different sort occurred the same year when a young gentleman applied to the lord mayor, stating his father had been poisoned and directly charging his uncle with the crime. Application was made to have the body disinterred but the coroner refused on the grounds too much time had passed for a fair conclusion to be drawn. In order to satisfy all parties, however, an inquest was held, whereby the attending physician swore on his oath that the gentleman died of cholera morbus. The lord mayor expressed satisfaction with the termination of the matter and it was intimated that the young gentleman who preferred the complaint "was actually insane."[4]

Not even the dead were allowed to have their final wishes respected. In the year 1815, a man named Dickson effected insurance on his life for a period of 7 years through the Hope Insurance Office, London. A medical man (who subsequently died) made the usual certification of health. In 1818, Dickson died of cholera and his executor claimed the money. The insurance company refused to pay on the grounds that in 1813, the policyholder had suffered an attack of palsy, the knowledge of which had been withheld at the time of issuance, making the policy fraudulent. The case was brought before a special jury and testimony for both sides was reviewed. A physician for the plaintiff stated Dickson had been in good health for years and described the supposed palsy as rheumatism. A physician for the defendant testified that a shock of paralysis in conjunction with cholera undoubtedly shortened Dickson's life. Verdict was for the plaintiff, with damages set at 2000*l*.[5]

A rather spectacular insurance case was brought to trial in 1831, when Mrs. Evans, executrix of Ann Elsworthy's estate, put in a claim for her life insurance amounting to £2,500 after the latter died of "cholera morbus acute inflammation of the liver." The defendants were three directors of the British Commercial Insurance Company, who refused to pay on the grounds that Mrs. Evans had no interest in the life insured, the law being such that unless a person effecting insurance on the life of another had a pecuniary interest in that life he should not be allowed to recover in a court of law. They also claimed that a codicil stipulated Miss Elsworthy was to continue to lead a temperate life and she had not.

Attorneys for the plaintiff stated that Mrs. Evans had loaned Miss Elsworthy the sum of £2,500 to set her up in business and the insurance policy was a bond to protect Evans' interests. Legal representatives for British Commercial attempted to prove that the deceased had operated a dressmaking shop and later a toy store, but her combined assets were less than £30, making it difficult to believe she had ever received a large sum from the plaintiff. Furthermore, they argued that a second life insurance policy had been taken out by Mrs. Evans on Miss Elsworthy's life in the amount of £700, and that seemed suspicious, especially since the deceased had also taken out a third policy from the economic office for £3,000 (paid for by Mrs. Evans) that had lately been paid to the estate.

Sir James Scarlett, in speaking for the defendants, stated that suspicion had been aroused when the insurance company discovered Mrs. Evans had previously taken out two life insurance policies on her sister, one for £2,700 and the second for £2,500. Her sister died three months later of cholera. She also insured her mother's life and "actually endeavoured to insure in six other offices, the Asylum, the Economic, the Pelican, the European, the Globe, and the Albion," to no less a sum than £18,700. Both her sister and mother also died of cholera morbus. This indicated the lady was "trafficking in insurances on the lives of different members of her family, and of her dependents; and that they all died a few months after the insurances were effected." Since all the policyholders died of the same disease, this implied murder by cholera, creating a crime "even worse than that of Burke and Hare, for their victims were strangers." After lengthy and contradictory testimony was given on Miss Elsworthy's temperate or intemperate life, the jury conferred for about five minutes and returned a verdict for the plaintiff, with damages set at £2,500.[6]

In 1832, directors of the Asylum Life Insurance Company determined that "henceforth all domestic policies for terms less than the whole duration of life, shall contain a clause excluding death by Cholera, unless an increased rate of premium be paid to cover that disease—the present restriction to continue during the prevalence of the epidemic within the United Kingdoms."

Life Insurance Premiums, Per Annum, 1832

Age	Seven Years Excluding Cholera	Seven Years (Covering All) Risks within the UK	Whole Life
20	£0 17 1	£1 2 5	£1 11 9
30	1 2 10	1 9 10	2 2 0
40	1 10 8	2 0 2	2 17 1
50	2 1 7	2 15 3	4 2 0
60	4 1 0	5 2 10	6 10 9
70	8 8 10	10 5 3	10 18 6

Interestingly, the rates of insurance on the lives of persons residing in or voyaging to foreign parts were not affected by the new modifications.[7]

Misunderstandings about cholera continued to appear in the newspapers. In 1824, an impoverished couple named Wilson arrived at the Isle of Ely from St. Ives. After obtaining lodging, and with no money to buy food, Mrs. Wilson prepared a stew from mushrooms that she called "champignons." Although warned by the landlord that she was cooking "toad-stools," the couple, another lodger and the landlord's daughter ate the meal. By morning, the couple were in a deplorable state and died within several days, soon followed by the girl. The coroner's jury returned a verdict of death "of cholera morbus, occasioned by eating poisonous fungi, which they mistook for mushrooms."[8]

Another case in 1825 centered around 24 students of the Royal Polytechnic School who experienced violent cholic and every effect usually produced by the cholera morbus. They were attended to by physicians who later diagnosed the condition as having been brought on by a breakfast of "cold meats, jelly &c."[9]

Murder by Cholera

The connection between murder and cholera persisted. In the midst of political unrest in France, suspicion ran as rampant as contagion. In April 1831, it was commonly believed that both government and health care providers were on a mission to murder civilians. The ministerial journal, *France Nouvelle*, published an account of a workman who averred that cholera victims who had died within the past year were poisoned. He stated, "The governments understand one another. They will not make war, and thus by poisoning they attempt to get rid of the excess population." After offering several other examples to the same effect, the newspaper

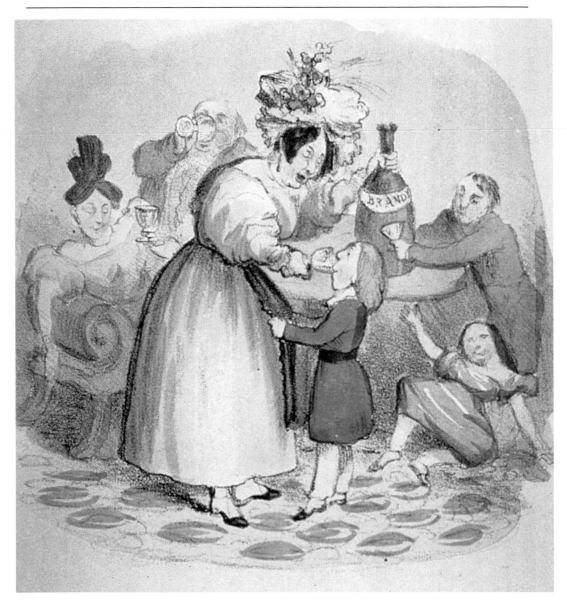

"Fortifying Against the Cholera," by Robert Seymour, *McLean's Monthly Sheet,* London, August 1, 1831. Nostrums and notions for the treatment of cholera were heavily marketed. Many contained alcohol as their prime ingredient, along with bitters or sweet herbs for taste and color. In some fairness to these hucksters, alcohol (in this case brandy) was long believed to ward off or cure cholera. This illustration takes that concept to the extreme with a clearly intoxicated, wealthy family offering brandy to children (U.S. National Library of Medicine).

noted that even the most respectable who exposed their lives and health for the benefit of the sick and dying "were publicly hissed and hooted as poisoners, and were publicly upbraided by the populace as guilty of poisoning their brethren."[10]

Interestingly, in September 1831, similar occurrences were reported from Stettin, where the "common people" formed a mob, believing that all cholera patients in the hospitals were being poisoned to prevent the spread of the disease. Their "fatal error" was based "on the circumstance that not one of the cholera patients has yet been cured. The Crown Prince has just left for Stettin, to tranquilize the populace." The newspaper added that a somewhat similar idea had taken hold in Hungary when the peasants took hold of the idea that the nobility had poisoned all the springs to destroy them. This led to a "complete war of extermination of the lower orders upon their superiors, but it has, happily, been put a stop to, and the chief leaders shot."[11]

Even the beginnings of the cholera outbreak at Sunderland were attributed to poison. As early as November 7, 1831, the *Courier* carried a story that the deaths in that town were believed by some to have been caused by poison rather than Asiatic cholera. Acknowledging there was nothing in the government reports to justify such suspicions, it was noted that the symptoms of poison so closely resembled that of cholera as to be nearly indistinguishable. Several months previous, a man in London had all the symptoms of Indo-European cholera and physicians were called out in the middle of the night to witness "a real case of Indian cholera." The man died the next morning and on his dissection there were found marks "of violent inflammation in the stomach and bowels." Evidence at the inquest brought out that the victim had purchased poison a day or two before.

Readers were warned that in all works on medical jurisprudence, the symptoms of poisoning and cholera were so similar that "in times like these, every sudden illness or death, with symptoms at all resembling cholera, will be placed to the account of that disease, and thus excite or augment alarm." The newspaper then mentioned an instance of sudden death by cholera in 1829 at a school at Clapham. The fatal cases were caused by emanations from the accidental opening of a drain at the bottom of a garden belonging to the school. More than 20 pupils became alarmingly ill and two died. The paragraph concluded: "Had such an occurrence happened a week ago, the panic in London would have been dreadful."

Perpetuating the misunderstanding of cholera, Dr. Brown, an eminent physician of Sunderland, published a text in 1829, writing that "the most decisive proof of cholera being the effect of malaria is to be found in the fact, that many of the most obstinate cases of remittent fever which have occurred in this district (Sunderland) commenced with that disease. During the autumn of 1827 I treated a case which commenced with cholera and passed into a remittent fever; but, during the two preceding years, the number of cases in which *remittent fever* commenced with *cholera* was very great." In fact, most medical men believed fatal epidemic cholera was what might be called "the first or cold state of a malignant fever, from which state, if the patient emerges, he is nearly safe, the succeeding re-action being a salutary effort of nature."[12]

On January 19, 1832, a coroner's inquest to determine cause of death was held over the body of John Potts, a seaman who died after a few hours' illness. Potts apparently entered a bar, called for a glass of purl, drank it and began vomiting. Complaining of being unable to walk, having "trouble in his mind," and suffering "stitching" pains in his heart, he was considered drunk and carried to the workhouse. A physician was called the following morning; after ruling out intoxication and poison, he made the diagnosis of cholera. The patient cried for a drink of cold water but was refused on the grounds warm tea was the better remedy. The patient subsequently died and, on post mortem, metallic poison was ruled out, as the internal coats of the stomach and intestines were not eroded. Jurors were of two minds: one felt it was highly desirable not to reach a conclusion as the public would be greatly alarmed if they became aware cholera had arrived in the metropolis. Another argued that if cholera were indeed present in London, a positive verdict would put them on guard. After deliberation, the beadle was ordered to bury the body "as deep as possible, clothes and all."[13]

A second case the same month was held over the body of a seaman off the *Mould* collier brig. Three of four physicians argued for a verdict of death by cholera; the fourth declared death to have been caused by "a case of rapid inflammation, and consequent mortification." The Government Board of Health was appealed to, declaring the fatal disease "was not that of cholera.... After much animated discussion among the medical men as to the real cause of death, without any satisfactory result, the Jury returned a verdict, 'That the deceased died by the visitation of God, from natural causes, but not from cholera morbus, nor from the effects of any poison or external violence.'" [14]

The appropriateness of coroners' juries in such cases became a matter of public concern; opinions divided over the same issues brought by jurors in the Potts and the seaman's inquests. The coroner of the London borough of Southwark was unmoved by the argument that open discussion was necessary, stating his opinion that it was not his province to inquire into death from natural causes, and that a certificate from a medical man was enough to permit the body to be buried. He furthermore opted to ignore the law calling for an inquest over the deaths of prison inmates, particularly those attributed to cholera, by "deeming it improper to subject twelve persons to the possible danger from immediate contact with an infected person and place." [15] More specifically, another authority argued that post mortems on cholera victims threw no light on the nature or the treatment of the malady, while dissections were injurious to family and friends of the deceased. [16]

The connection between cholera and poisoning persisted throughout the century. In 1876, one London physician aptly summed up the problem by stating that he feared cholera outbreaks because sudden deaths were taken as a matter of course, leading to a frightful increase of secret poisonings. [17]

One fatal case that did not require formal investigation occurred to Mr. Kyme, a 61-year-old farmer from Wyberton. After being attacked by a bowel complaint, he swallowed a bottle of strong patent medicine. His bowels being previously inflamed, the "drug" proved too much for him, death being the consequence. [18]

As late as 1886, Dr. W.S. Janney, former coroner of Philadelphia, expressed his opinion that "under the innocent guise of medical certificates of death from cholera morbus," there were enough murders from arsenic poisoning to keep the sheriff busy for the whole of his term. [19]

A bizarre death in Japan in 1906 created another international "murder by cholera" sensation. According to news reports, Kiota Nga fell in love with the wife of his best friend, Murta Toya. Nga, a member of the nobility, decided murder was his best option and infected a white spaniel with the disease. After he presented it to Toya, Toya contracted cholera and died. A Japanese detective with a grudge against Nga secured the dog that he suspected to be the medium. Proving his theory after two beggars slept in the same room with the animal and died, he made a formal accusation. Nga, failing to swear his innocence, was convicted and sentenced to die. American newspapers concluded it was strange that a man who killed for love was put to death while the detective who caught him by literally murdering innocent men to test a theory was honored. [20]

Another astonishing case involved Dr. Pantchenko of Russia, who was accused of operating a murder-for-hire scheme by injecting his victims with cholera bacilli. In April 1910, he received $10,000 to kill Count Bouturlin and successfully committed the crime. He was subsequently caught and at trial it was revealed he had enough cholera germs to infect 100,000 persons. Similarly, Dr. Bennett Clarke Hyde of Missouri and Dr. Randall Williams of England were implicated in murder by germs, the latter having collected enough deadly germs to depopulate England. Such atrocities brought to public attention the fact that any doctor or scientist could purchase disease germs in sufficient quantity to cause thousands of deaths without giving any adequate explanation for what purpose he required them. The *London Lancet* called for a law regulating the sale and distribution of disease germs whereby only certain laboratories would be authorized to distribute such germs and no cultures would be dispensed in unusually large quantities.[21]

Oddities such as the following instances also occurred regarding cholera. In lieu of legal recourse to settle their differences, two Berlin students decided to duel to the death with cholera. The participants each embraced a person so afflicted but after 24 hours, neither contracted the disease. Their seconds declared "honour satisfied," and the affair "terminated."[22] If this was not strange enough, a "non-contagious" physician intent on proving that cholera was not spread by contact, undressed and lay beside the corpse of a person who had just expired from the disease. He remained there for 2½ hours before leaving. His medical brethren were so convinced he would fall victim that numerous inquiries were made at the hospital next day asking the hour in which he died. Fortunately for the doctor, he remained in excellent physical health.[23]

10

England, 1832

"Who shall decide when doctors disagree?"

Prophetic Almanac for 1832 January 1st. New Year begins—expected to last till the 31st of December, twelve p.m., unless previously put an end to by the cholera or a comet.[1]

An article from *Bell's New Weekly Messenger* (London, February 26, 1832) entitled, "Pro and Con; or Cholera, or No Cholera," cleverly offered seven points of disagreement on the subject.

    I.   As to the symptoms by which English and Asiatic cholera may be distinguished from one another—"Violent spasms, rice-coloured evacuations, and blueness of skin, are symptomatic of Asiatic cholera," cries Dr. A. "Violent spasms, rice-coloured evacuations, and blueness of skin," are symptoms of the English cholera," cries Dr. B.

    II.   As to the existence of the disease in England, "The disease is undoubtedly in London, and undoubtedly will spread," say one party. "The disease is not in London, and will not spread," reply the other.

    III.   The pathological signs observed in the several cases—"There was a great deal of blueness," says one doctor. "There was no blueness at all," says another.

    IV.   The causes—"Exposure to cold," "Eating too much," Eating too little," "Having nothing to eat."

    V.   The cure—"Cleanse the streets—feed the poor," "Swallow plenty of mustard and salt," "Rarify the air, get up bonfires, burn and tar-barrels," "Inundate the streets with water," "Damp is more favourable than dirt."

    VI.   How was the disease brought to London?—"It was brought by a vessel from Sunderland," says one. "That is impossible," cries another. "It came by water," "It came by land."

    VII.   In Parliament, one hon. member remarks, "It will run like wildfire," and another, "It will not run." "It is contagious," says a third. "It is not contagious; it is a mere epidemic," says a fourth. "The best way is to make everything public," says a fifth. "I would not allow people to speak about it," says a sixth. "It is a mere alarm of the anti-reformers," says a member of the Political Union. "It has been spread through interested motives," says a newspaper correspondent. "It is the last blow given to the commerce of London, already declining under the competition of Liverpool, and the other northern ports," thunders the "leading journal."—"The trade of London is not declining on account of any competition of the northern ports," retorts the editor of a Sunday paper.

While written in a humorous style, the article accurately and succinctly summed up what dozens of newspapers, numerous medical conferences and hundreds of letters argued to the

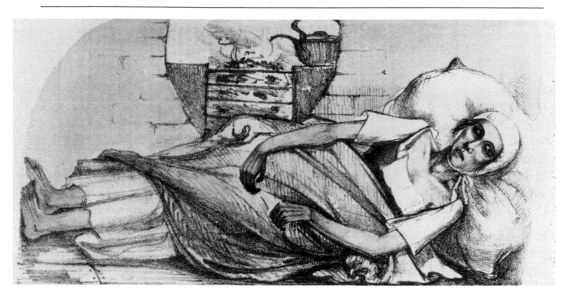

"Blue stage of spasmodic cholera." Sketch of a young woman who died of cholera at Sunderland, England, November 1831. First published in the *Lancet* (U.S. National Library of Medicine).

point of near hysteria. Nor were the authorities and physicians any closer to a definitive answer than they had been in 1831. No consensus seemed possible. On the "anti-cholera side," the disease was a "hobgoblin" and a "bugbear"; these people believed newspaper columns alone were "enough to infect the whole land with Cholera," and espoused the sentiment "Certain cure for Cholera: Hang the Board of Health," found on "a *dead* wall (an appropriate spot) in the Albany Road." On the "cholera side," statistics appeared to speak for themselves.[2]

Cholera Morbus in London and the Country: January–February, 1832
Total Cases from Commencement of Disease

Date	Cases	Deaths
January 23	2,350	791
January 26	2,639	874
February 1	3,247	1,026
February 7	3,967	1,204
February 9	4,273	1,281
February 10	4,146	1,250
February 16	4,519	1,358
February 23	5,106	1,511
February 28	5,460	1,609

During January, Sunderland dropped off the list; Newcastle registered the highest numbers, with Gateshead second. In February, Newcastle maintained the highest; Gateshead dropped off the list and was replaced by Hetton, followed by Musselburgh, Scotland. The *Glasgow Chronicle* reported that every case of cholera in Kirkintilloch was traced to a boy who contracted the disease on a vessel laden with hoofs and horns from Newcastle, adding, "So rapid is the effect of the pestilential effluvia that persons predisposed for the disease are infected by *merely entering* the room where the patient lies." Ireland reported rare, isolated cases.[3]

Were these steadily increasing numbers truly representative of an epidemic, or were they, in fact, no more than seasonal fluctuations in the mortality tables? Were they actually greater than common? Was cholera the dreaded disease some medical men made it out to be, or were the publications of official and daily reports merely creating an alarm of pestilence? Would similar official and daily returns of inflammation, fever, consumption, asthma and apoplexy create in peoples' minds a Miltonian "land of death?" Which physicians were better qualified to identify cholera—those who were *not* paid for their opinions, or the "20 guineas-a-day gentlemen" hired by government ministers? Was cholera contagious? Was it simply a species of typhus or putrid fever? Was the disease mitigated by the different climates through which it passed? Was mortality modified by different degrees of medical skill and treatment? Did quarantine protect countries or did it simply depress commerce? These were questions not easily answered, but they were vigorously argued in 1832. On the lighter side, a poem published February 28, 1832, expressed the contemporary English view of cholera as an over-diagnosed disease used by physicians and apothecaries to fill their purses.

The Lament of the Stomach Ache

If now old women make a face
Through swilling too profusely swipes,
'Tis entered, "a new Cholera case,"
Forget the stomach ache or gripes.
If wind creates a bowel row,
As Cholera straight 'tis understood,
It fills your purse—I've heard ere now,
"An ill wind 'tis blows no one good."

What twists, what turns, can Cholera bring,
What draughts demand—what rubs and scrubs,
Which came not erst to Clown and King,
From good old English mulligrubs?
I cramped you well, if truth is told,
I chilled you by the warmest stove,
And made you look, to say I'm bold,
As blue as bilberries, by Jove!

Then, Chieftains of the Pulse and Pill,
At length give up your Cholera prank;
Let patients, as of yore, be ill,
And let me hold my ancient rank;
Let men respire from wild alarm,
Dismiss the source of needless grief!
O let my prayer your ire disarm!
A humbugged nation claims relief![4]

Adding to the confusion was the juxtaposition of terms. Cabinet ministers used the words "spasmodic cholera" and "new Asiatic cholera" as synonymous; the single word "cholera" meant "English" or "common cholera" (an endemic rather than an epidemic disease); "Indian cholera," "Hamburgh cholera" and "Russian" or "St. Petersburgh cholera" referenced a disease specific to those areas. Most symptoms were common to all "choleras." For example, the *Encyclopaedia Britannica* used in 1832 described the disease generically: "Sometimes the patients fall into universal convulsions; and sometimes they are affected with violent spasms in different parts of the body. There is a great thirst, a small unequal pulse, cold sweats, fainting, coldness of the extremities, hiccough: and death frequently ensues in twenty-four hours."[5] Dr. Majendie offered a more distinct definition of Indian cholera by describing it as "a disease beginning where other diseases end, with death."[6] "Plague" might refer to any contagious disease causing fever.

In a vain attempt to avoid confusion, the British Medical Board published a description so that the word "cholera" might be understood as a disease characterized by the following symptoms:

CHOLERA

A purging and vomiting of fluids, neither feculent nor bilious, with cramps and prostration—to which, in extreme cases, are added, a coldness and shrinking and lividity of the surface, particularly of the extremities; with suspended pulsation at the wrist, and suppression of urine.

It must, not, however, be supposed that the whole of these symptoms will be found in each, even of the most extreme cases; for one or two of them are sometimes altogether absent, or so feebly marked as not to attract particular notice. This is more especially the case with respect to young children, in whom, for instance, cramps have hitherto been but seldom observed in this country as a well-marked symptom of cholera according to experience.[7]

There were three points upon which most authorities agreed: first, that the disease almost invariably followed the banks of rivers and the low and flat lands that adjoined them. Dr. Daun suggested cholera was generalized *de novo* along the banks of a river liable to inundation, citing that provinces on the banks of the lower Danube, Moldavia and Wallachia were annually visited by both plague and cholera.[8] Second, that cholera traveled in a northwest progression:

If we draw a straight line on the map of Europe from Gratz, near Vienna, to Ayr or Irvine, it will be about 1,000 miles in length, and while the Cholera has been raging at a thousand points on the north side of that line for nearly twelve months, it has never got a footing at a single spot on the south side, though the intercourse *across* this boundary is as great and constant as in any other direction. And hence, we have the singular spectacle of a disease which has migrated from the east of Europe, committing ravages on the shores of Britain, while Bavaria, Italy, France, Switzerland, Rheinish Germany, and the Netherlands are still untouched by it.[9]

Concerning the direction of disease, it was also pointed out that the Great Plague of 1348 began in Tartary in 1345, and after desolating Asia and part of Africa, it extended its ravages to the west and was supposed to have swept away one third of the population of Europe.[10]

Finally, the greatest fear was indifference. *Bell's New Weekly Messenger,* February 19, 1832, aptly stated, "Danger and habit render us familiar with death in its most frightful appearance; and the progress of the particular plague being probably slower than fancy had pictured, the impression grows fainter every hour." In arguing that the people must be saved in spite of themselves, *Bell's* tragically concluded, "Does our contemporary know *why* the 'lower orders' are so obstinate and rash in these affairs of death? They are not bound to life by so many captivating ties as the rich are; and to but too many of them, death is the best comfort which the earth can afford."

In an observation that applies as much to modern politics, the *Spectator,* February 19, 1832, questioned a motion made by Mr. Briscoe in the House of Commons to resolve that cholera was "an infliction of God" by asking whether that body was a proper place to discuss religion. "Nothing can be more unjust," the article continued, "than the attempt to hold up those who object to the idle, unauthorized use of the Divine's name, as irreligious persons.... The practice must be put down.... If longer permitted, it will soon occupy the House to the exclusion of every thing else."

The Cholera Morbus Prevention Bill

The House of Lords took up the Cholera Morbus Prevention Bill on February 16, 1832. Early debate centered around legality and it was proposed that any orders issued by three of the lords of the Privy Council for preventing the spread of contagious diseases should be legal and binding. The second subject concerned finances: it was proposed that expenses for new regulations were to come first from the poor-rates in the parishes, but ultimately the county treasurer would pay them from the county purse. Sir Robert Peel countered that, as cholera was not a parochial disorder but had started at Sunderland, travelled to Edinburgh and was then in London, the entire country had an interest in the subject and poorer parishes would be taxed out of proportion. The chancellor of the exchequer objected, fearing that if expenses were paid out of the public funds, it would lead to great extravagance. That discussion led to the concern that quarantine was a greater threat than disease and might lead to famine. On a wider scale, it was noted that, as cholera had ravaged India for 14 years, there was every reason to believe it would be permanently fixed as an addition to the diseases of England.

On February 17, discussions focused on the lack of receptacles (coaches) with which to transport cholera victims and the fact that cases of malignant cholera were being turned away

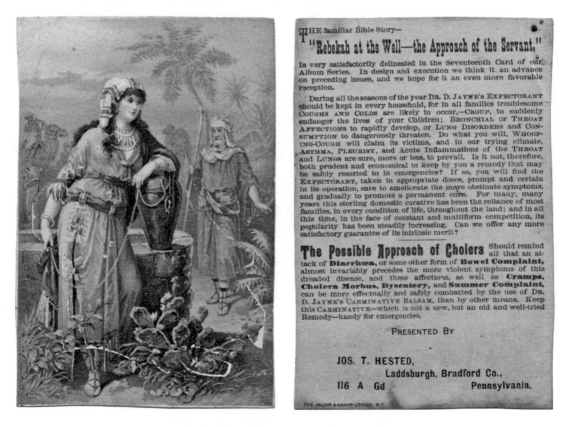

Left: This attractive color postcard, entitled, "Rebekah at the Well—Approach of the Servant" (number 17 in a set) is actually an advertisement for Dr. D. Jayne's Carminative Balsam. The preprinted text on the back urges people that with "The Possible Approach of Cholera" they should be reminded that any diarrhea or bowel complaint "almost invariably precedes the more violent symptoms of this dreaded disease," for which the tonic was "an old and well-tried Remedy." The religious theme added to a sense of trust and by being issued as a numbered set encouraged people to collect and possibly even display them, the promoters thus cleverly keeping a reminder of the product visible in homes. The postcards were probably given to druggists free of charge as a means of encouraging them to stock the item. There is even a blank space at the bottom for the druggist to stamp the name of his business. On this card, the text reads, "Jos. T. Hested, Laddsburgh, Bradford Co., Pennsylvania." *Right:* Back side of the postcard.

from St. Bartholomew's Hospital. Dispensaries were available to the poor but these offered no more than advice and medicines rather than in-door treatment. It was agreed that an establishment of receptacles for cholera patients be created in each district of the metropolis and that public hackneys were not to be used.

One disgruntled citizen gave his opinion of the cholera bill by posting a placard warning that the people ought not to be "imposed upon by the villanously false report that the Asiatic Cholera has reached London. A set of half-starved doctors, apothecaries' clerks, and jobbers in parish funds, have endeavoured to frighten the nation into lavish expenditure; with the Government they have succeeded in carrying a Bill which will afford fine pickings. A ruinous system of taxation, starvation, and intemperance has been long carried on; it has now arrived at its acme, and disease is the natural result."

Cholera also played a role in the reform movement then preoccupying England. One of the more outspoken Tories, Sir John Malcolm, suggested a "cholera prescription" by recommending that "the people should not be permitted to *speak* of it; and acquainted the House that he had pursued that plan of interdict "with admirable effect in *India*." Those on the opposite side lamented this military suppression by crying, "O, merry—once merry, merry England! to what dismal Hades is your glorious spirit descending?" adding that "the working classes, lower classes, labouring classes, &c. &c." were acquiring "the new and most miserable distinction of being the cholera-morbus class."[11]

Looked at in a humorous light was the anecdote of two Bristol women who had just returned from the committee for the prevention of cholera: "I soy, Martha, what hast thee got?" "Why, I got five yards of flannel. What hast thee?" "Why, I have got seven; and dang me if I don't think, after all, the cholera's better than reform."[12]

Cholera Morbus in London and the Country: March–May, 1832
Total Cases from Commencement of Disease

Date	Cases	Deaths
March 2	5,559	1,652
March 3	5,717	1,738
March 5	5,825	1,757
March 7	5,891	1,768
March 8	5,949	1,791
March 10	6,006	1,829
March 12	6,087	1,857
March 13	6,121	1,877
March 14	6,144	1,892
March 15	6,176	1,904
March 16	6,223	1,927
March 17	6,237	1,938
March 18	6,478	2,025
March 22	6,642	2,100
March 23	6,689	2,127
March 24	6,784	2,169
March 27	6,927	2,232
March 28	6,995	2,258
March 29	7,042	2,279
March 30	7,089	2,305
March 31	7,119	2,321
April 2	7,260	2,381
April 3	7,289	2,465

Date	Cases	Deaths
April 4	7,331	2,429
April 6	7,416	2,470
April 7	7,455	2,489
April 9	7,581	2,547
April 12	7,738	2,626
April 13	7,980	2,747
April 17	8,064	2,782
April 18	8,144	2,834
April 21	8,364	2,944
April 23	8,503	3,019
April 25	8,623	3,064
April 27	8,796	3,195
April 28	8,879	3,229
April 30	8,976	3,280
May 1	9,019	3,302
May 2	9,112	3,336
May 3	9,198	3,371
May 5	9,271	3,427
May 7	9,393	3,485
May 8	9,485	3,528
May 9	9,529	3,551
May 10	9,576	3,565
May 11	9,630	3,583
May 12	9,691	3,608
May 14	9,776	3,656
May 15	9,867	3,689
May 16	9,913	3,715
May 18	9,994	3,753
May 19	10,024	3,784
May 22	10,093	3,786
May 23	10,149	3,808
May 24	10,191	3,821
May 25	10,218	3,830[13]

On May 15, 1832, the council office declared it would not publish any further reports for the metropolitan districts, under orders of the Central Board of Health, which "declared the cessation of cholera in London as an epidemic."[14] On May 24, the *Courier* noted that cholera was "fast approaching its total extinction." This elicited the lament that dire government predictions had been overblown. Although Hungary and Galicia contained perhaps 10,000,000 inhabitants, of which 400,000 perished of cholera, in London, with a population of 1,500,000, fewer than 4,000 persons died. A second newspaper drew this conclusion: "The alarm does seem exaggerated, and the quarantine not merely useless, but highly reprehensible."[15]

Cholera in Ireland

In 1826, upwards of 70,000 persons died of typhus; of that number, the deaths in the metropolis of London amounted to 20,000. Great apprehension was therefore felt when cholera appeared on March 22, 1832. On April 25, the board of health had registered only 147 cases of cholera, which would have been comparatively insignificant. But due to the prevailing sentiment against cholera hospitals, authorities believed the propagation of the disease had been facilitated, and their numbers were low estimates.[16]

Fresh statistics from the council office, Dublin Castle, April 26, indicated that Dublin had a total of 462 cases with 188 deaths and Cork had a total of 471 cases with 143 deaths. Among nine cities reporting, there were 1,002 cases with 380 deaths.[17] On May 5, Dublin reported 100 new cases, 269 patients in the hospital, 131 being treated at home, 40 recoveries and 35 deaths.[18]

A letter dated May 4 from George D'Aguilar, deputy master, Royal Hospital, Dublin, to the General Board of Health indicated that upon inspection of a burial ground, he discovered that within the previous 10 days upwards of 500 bodies (mostly cholera subjects) were brought for interment. "I found the whole place so *occupied and encumbered with the dead,* that it is impossible to open a fresh grave without encountering at every stroke of the spade some remnant of mortality." He begged the board of health "to reconcile the lower orders of the metropolis to other places of interment."[19]

As a consequence of the cholera epidemic, in early March 1832, Dr. James Yorke Bramston, the Catholic bishop of London, issued orders that for the future, none of the Irish Catholics should hold any wakes over their departed family. On March 26, under Bramston's name, the Catholic bishops of Ireland issued a circular through the central board of health, urging the faithful not to remain with the dead and to have victims interred 12 hours after death. After concurring with the order to eliminate wakes, they added, "all persons who assist at such wakes act most unwarrantably and wickedly, by unreasonably putting their lives in danger."[20] The orders were not well received; and to complicate matters, numerous riots were reported among the Irish when authorities attempted to take victims to the hospital. The people fearing the victims would either die there or doctors would perform dissection, blood was often spilled and numerous arrests made. Expressing a not-uncommon prejudice of the day, a Mr. Halls of the London police implied that some good might come of the cholera by making it a matter of necessity "to cause the Irish to be removed entirely from the Metropolis."[21]

In May 1832, epidemic cholera raged through Limerick, preceded by a "most unwholesome thick fog, which covered the city almost to suffocation, and in 24 hours after, the disorder began in earnest, stalking with gigantic strides through our streets and alleys, aggravated by poverty, uncleanness, and want of common necessities of life." Slack lime was spread over the flagstones and channel ways, giving the strange appearance of snowfall in June, while the official report showed "a dreadful increase in mortality." Within a fortnight, business became totally stagnant and the city was forsaken by most of the respectable families.[22]

On June 14, Southern "anti-cholera fanatics" entered Monaghan and Cavan counties, carrying bits of burned turf, hot stones and wood as specifics against cholera. In their "enthusiasm," they burned half a dozen towns but refused to serve the "blessed turf" to any Protestant homes on the ground as "they are not of our creed." It was said the "holy turf and straw carriers" met with no encouragement from the locals. English papers, determined that the idea of disseminating the "blessed turf" originated with "Romish priests," noted that such "blessed turf" had been, on former occasions, used to staunch the plague and bring about a Protestant massacre.[23]

The *London Times* feared that the above transactions, far from being a "Roman Catholic superstition," actually represented some political movement. "All accounts concurred in stating that the proceedings in question, however farcical it appeared at first sight, had excited the population to a degree which was hardly to be credited. The house must be aware that he was alluding to the burning of what was called holy straws as a pretended charm against cholera," which took place on the same day in several counties, implying conspiracy.[24] Complicating matters as far as the Irish were concerned, reports from Dublin stated that Lord Anglesey, the chief governor, abandoned his post in consequence of the death of one of his grooms from cholera, and went "yacht sailing" away to his seat, Plass Newydd, Isle of Anglesey.[25]

Another act of violence occurred when the country people between Tullamore and Ballinasloe cut down the banks of the Grand Canal running to the latter town on the belief that "it was the communication by water that cholera was carried throughout the interior of the country with such rapidity."[26] Less incendiary news from an Irish newspaper reported that in the Cork jail, where cholera was raging, musicians were engaged to play for the prisoners, "which has been attended with beneficial effects."[27]

"If ducks and doctors both quack, are we not justified in classing them both as birds of a feather?"[28]

By March 6, 1832, the intense speculation in drugs related to the treatment of cholera had wholly subsided. The Essential Oil of Cajeput, a once-reputed anti-cholera specific, fell from a high of 10–12s. per ounce to 1s. and was considered quite unsellable. Camphor, still being used in cholera cases, maintained its value at £12–15 per cwt, according to quality, but for the essential oil, the demand was very bad.[29]

The idea of self-medicating, whether to treat an actual illness or to ward away cholera, occasionally had tragic consequences. On March 31, an inquest was held over the death of Nicholas Robert Bruin, aged 28. Apparently, the victim had been in the habit of taking laudanum mixed in Cognac brandy as an antidote because he had a "touch of cholera." On his way to purchase an emetic, he became dizzy and complained of pain that he ascribed to cholera. A watchman found him and returned him home. The following morning Bruin was found dead; the attending physician ascribed the cause of death to be "from the effects of poison." The newspaper titled the article, "Death from Taking Cholera Medicine." More sensational than accurate, it is just as likely the man had become addicted to opium and used cholera as an excuse. The jury returned a verdict somewhere in the middle by declaring death from "temporary insanity."[30]

On the lighter side, a man attired in a blue jacket and trousers, with a belt round his body in which were a brace of pistols and a cutlass, was brought before the magistrate on a charge of quackery. The accused had made the rounds of public thoroughfares with a printed bill on his hat upon which was inscribed, "*Preventative Service*," selling a cure for cholera. Upon inspection, the weapons turned out to be pieces of wood similar to children's toys that the "quack doctor" used to gull the public. The magistrate told him to go home, give the toys away and never return, for which the man thanked him and retired. Less amusing to "royal watchers," King William IV came to London on April 4 for a levee, then immediately returned to Windsor Castle, announcing he would not return until after the departure of the cholera morbus.[31] Cholera did not prevent him from celebrating his birthday with a drawing room party at St. James's Palace on May 29. Two days later, while he was holding court, the Privy Council agreed that the archbishop of Canterbury should prepare a prayer to return thanks to Almighty God for the abatement of the cholera.[32]

Consumption of contaminated fish was one way to contract cholera but there were few who made the direct connection. In June 1832, a small article (picked up by numerous newspapers) appeared, stating that a medical gentleman named N. Canstall alerted the sitting magistrate that he had seen a quantity of fish, "in an absolute state of putrescence," for sale as food.

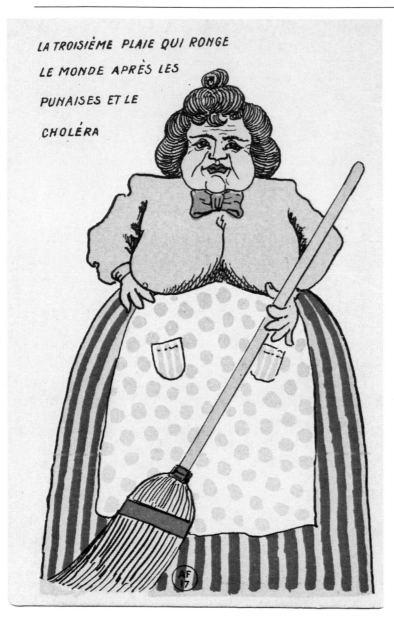

LA TROISIÈME PLAIE QUI RONGE LE MONDE APRÈS LES PUNAISES ET LE CHOLÉRA

This humorous 1910 French postcard depicts the matron ready to sweep away the dreaded cholera (Authors' collection).

He stated that in his practice he had recently attended two cases of cholera that he distinctly traced to the use of unwholesome fish such as he had seen in the market. He hoped the magistrates would interpose and destroy it.[33] Undoubtedly, spoiled fish would cause sickness, but the actual point Canstall missed was that the fish were likely carriers of the disease whether or not they were unfit to eat.

After the appearance of cholera in Bohemia, reports indicated that the animal kingdom also suffered great mortality from the disease. Prevalent among them were fish and hares, leading to a banishment of these foods. Similar stories followed from various parts of the world. The English Agricultural Report for April 1832 indicated that ewes, lambs and horses were suffering from a disease resembling cholera morbus. A similar phenomenon was seen in Montreal when horses employed in drawing sick carts were taken with the staggers and soon died. An officer who had seen service in the East Indies predicted this, noting that after cholera abated there, many dogs would "go mad." In Dublin, a large mastiff found in the vicinity of the cholera hospital was observed to suffer from violent spasms and a frothy tongue. Two medical men diagnosed the case as cholera. The dog died within half an hour after being attacked and its body was declared to be "capable of imparting greater infection than the dead bodies of twenty human beings." It was instantly interred.[34]

11

"From Our Correspondent—
Foreign News"

Great News for France

The cholera morbus, it is said, has reached Edinburgh: On learning this news, Charles X. demanded his passport for France.[1]

Private correspondence from Paris to London dated January 21, 1832, included this sentence: "From the Departments, it is not possible, even by telegraph, to learn the news, as Paris has for two days been covered with a dense fog, which the citizens suppose to be the forerunner of the cholera morbus."[2] It did not take long for panic to spread and within the month the French government ordered quarantine against all places on the eastern coast of England between Yarmouth and Ramsgate, and Glasgow and all ports of the Clyde. Quarantine was to last between 3 and 10 days, depending on the ship's origin. Although vessels coming from other English ports were exempt, all dispatches and papers coming from London were to be submitted to purification "and shall be pierced and passed through vinegar, or an aromatic fumigation."[3]

Precautions proved ineffectual and, although the government endeavored to deny the presence of cholera, newspapers continued to report a growing number of casualties. By March 26, seven deaths were reported and the Hotel Dieu (the chief hospital in Paris) was making preparations for the reception of many more. Two days later, the *Gazette de France* indicated 38 cases of cholera.[4] Reports on March 30 indicated 178 persons had contracted cholera, of whom 118 were male and 60 female. Proven deaths were 60: 41 males and 19 females.[5]

By April 1, amid lingering doubts that the disease actually existed in Paris, reports of an epidemic were "confirmed by better evidence than hearsay," as 9 persons were brought to the Hotel Dieu with symptoms of cholera. Four died the same day and after performing autopsies, physicians declared "all the symptoms of this horrible epidemic were detected." In consequence, a meeting of the board of health was held, attended by the minister of trade, the prefect of the Seine and the secretary of the prefecture. Surprise was elicited at the fact the disease appeared at the capital, away from all communication from strangers, instead of along the coast, where it might have been introduced by contagion from abroad.

Extract from the Popular Instructions
as to the Cholera Morbus
Issued by the Minister of Commerce and Public Works

1. Observe the strictest cleanliness both in person and dwellings.
2. Avoid all chances of being chilled.
3. Abstain from sleeping with the windows open.

4. Sobriety cannot be too strongly recommended.

5. Eat as little as possible of *charcuterie* and salt meats; abstain entirely of heavy pastry.

6. Abstain from undressed food of every description.

7. All cold drinks taken when a person is heated are dangerous; Water used as a beverage ought to be clear; filtered water is better than any other. Instead of drinking it pure, mix in two teaspoonfuls of brandy or wine.

8. All persons affected with dull pains in the limbs, heaviness or giddiness in the head, a feeling of oppression, uneasiness about the chest, heartburn or cholic should apply to a physician.

9. Persons thus affected should go to bed and take, quite hot, an infusion of peppermint and flowers of the lime tree.[6]

Numbers continued to escalate and all doubt was erased when the sanitary bulletin was published.

Cholera Report, Paris, April 1, 1832

Location	Admitted	Men	Women	Deaths
La Pitie	6	4	2	1
Beaujon	3	2	1	1
La Charite	5	3	2	0
St. Antoine	4	2	2	3
Necker	2	0	0	0
Hotel Dieu	33	0	0	20

Immediately afterward, 53 new cases were reported. Thus, between March 30 and March 31, a total of 281 cases were confirmed, with 100 deaths. Of these, 66 were men and 34 were women.[7] The medical men of the Hotel Dieu considered cholera to be noninflammatory and recommended it be treated with stimulating medicines. They also agreed that the disease was not contagious, "though by all accounts, the Paris epidemic is the same as the English, the Indian, and the continental, which goes under the same name."[8]

Eminent physicians may have agreed on the state of cholera, but political unrest in France continued. On April 6, Premiere M. Casimer Perier came down with symptoms of cholera. His lingering illness disarranged the administration, allowing cabinet members to draw up new lists of ministers, while disturbances broke out at Nantz in consequence of an article in a royalist journal tracing the cholera "to the avenging wrath of heaven against the authors of the late revolution." Furthering French ire was the offer of 12,000 francs (nearly £500) by Madame Du Barry to aid cholera victims in Paris. Editorials against her noted that her generosity was "an evident intrigue ... to turn the cholera against the revolution of July, 1830."[9]

Adding to the political unrest was the belief that the government (or those against the government) had initiated a "preconcerted plan" to poison the poor by adding arsenic to drinking water and wine. Beginning around April 1, 1832, windows of druggist shops where anticholera medicines were sold were broken and street lamps smashed. A correspondent from Paris wrote, "It is remarkable that all the riots that have taken place since the beginning of the year seem arranged in such a manner as to suit certain bears of the Exchange, who wish to make a profit on the settling-days in the beginning of each month."

Joining the riots (the *Revolte des Chiffonniers*) were the *chiffonniers* (rag-gatherers), or the *boueurs* (mud-men), who complained that a new government contract for cleaning the streets would hurt their occupation. The Carlists were also said to have joined the riots "with the hope of proving that no tranquility can be expected in France until the return of Henry V." In consequence, the newly contracted parties were afraid to perform their work, resulting in a massive accumulation of filth.[10]

Understandably, the situation in Paris deteriorated quickly. One writer among many encapsulated the gloomy mood with particular sensitivity:

Alarm has superseded presumptive security and incredulity. The Boulevards, public walks, and gardens are comparatively deserted—the theatres literally empty. Every third person you meet holds his (or her) handkerchief to the mouth, impressed with the belief that the disease is in the atmosphere, and that to respire is death. No man laughs, or appears amused: even the street minstrels—that unwearied class of the industrious—have become silent or have fled the city. I verily believe that the only pleasurable sensation experienced in Paris at this moment arises from the exercise of benevolence; and to their honour be it spoken, that virtue is practiced to an extraordinary extent by the Parisians.[11]

Among those participating in charity events was Niccolo Paganini (1782–1840, Italian violinist and composer), who gave a concert in Paris producing 9,750 francs.[12] On the subject of music, an auction of the splendid collection of "Ancient Pictures" owned by Sebastian Erard (1752–1831, the genius who specialized in the production of pianos and harps) that had been delayed in April 1832 due to the cholera outbreak was finally listed for sale in August 1832.[13]

Mortality numbers fluctuated wildly based on official numbers, personal observation and guesswork. By April 9, one letter noted the death toll as 11,300, "and since that day, nearly as many more have perished." Grave diggers could not dig fast enough, sextons had no time to arrange bodies "that were continually arriving in all sorts of vehicles, even in the military hospital waggons," and the authorities were obliged to employ artillery horses "to relieve those employed in the hearses and hackney-coaches, which are no longer able to convey the dead." Funerals took place at night. "In vain do our Journals assure us that the virulence of the disease has diminished, whilst we see such a frightful succession of funerals, and the layers of carcasses, which the grave-diggers have not time to cover, but as they are in measuring the intervals between the full-grown bodies, in order to fill them up with children and women."[14]

Grim responses to the epidemic came from the caricaturists of Paris. One effort represented cholera as a female of terrible aspect, "with one foot upon Hindustan, and the other on Europe. From a large box which she carries before her she ever and anon takes a handful of pestilential vapours, which, as she stalks along, she drops over the cities and towns of the earth. In one corner of the picture the Hotel Dieu at Paris is represented, on the roof of which stands old Baron Larrey, the celebrated surgeon, looking up at the Lady Cholera, and exclaiming, 'What a stride!'—Whilst Dupuytren, another eminent surgeon, is mounted on the Baron's shoulders, discharging the contents of a tiny syringe at the monster."[15] More humorously (to the English), *Figaro in London* had this to say: "In England the Cholera attacked only the poor—in Paris it extends its ravages to all classes. There is no wonder in this, for in this country, the *plague is* an Aristocrat, while in France the *plague is* a Republican."[16]

The Quality of Water and Sewers

An important article connecting cholera to water appeared in the January 9, 1832, edition of the *London Courier*, although it took the form of an advertisement:

Water by Filtration—1832

A novel theory has been started by some of the most eminent members of the French faculty, that this modern plague is engendered by the use of impure water. If such be the case, it is to be feared that it will not be long ere it reaches our shores, for nothing can be more fearfully unwholesome than the fetid and disgusting liquid daily poured into the domestic cisterns. The Parisian *savans* recommend a general course of filtration; and the most eminent medical authorities of this country have written

RANSOME'S PATENT ARTIFICIAL
POROUS STONE FILTERS,

For Purifying Water, manufactured in the Patent Stone which has obtained the Medal of the Society of Civil Engineers, the Medal of the Great Exhibition of 1851, the approval of the most distinguished men of Science, as Faraday, De la Beche, Buckland, Cubitt, Ansted, Phillips, &c. &c., of the most distinguished men in the medical profession, and of the leading journalists.

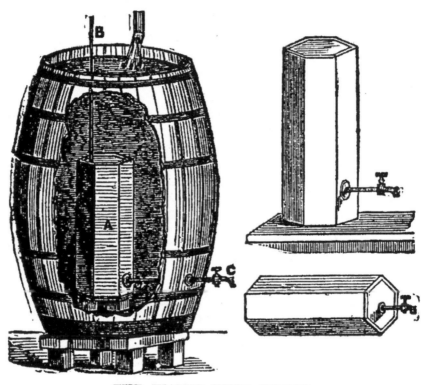

THE WATER-BUTT FILTER.

On October 11, 1853, the following quote appeared in the *London Times*: "People owe it to themselves, and the establishments over which they have control, to secure an ample supply of water which has been filtered chymically as well as mechanically, having passed through charcoal (animal charcoal is the best), as well as through porous stone or gravel." Ransome's Patent Artificial Porous Stone Filters, along with the Model Sanitary Tank for supplying filtered water for the working classes, were on display at the manufacturer's depot. This ad appeared less than a year before Dr. John Snow proved his theory that cholera was transmitted through water coming from the Broad Street pump, Golden Square, Soho, England (*Allen's Indian Mail* (London), November 14, 1853).

and spoken in terms of the warmest eulogium of the great and *exclusive* advantages of Robins' Royal Portable Filters; and to all our readers who feel the slightest wish to preserve their health, we would suggest an early visit to the Royal Filter, 69, Strand, (opposite the Adelphi Theatre.)

The cost for a 2-gallon size capable of purifying 12 gallons per day was £1, 5s; a 12-gallon size capable of purifying 90 gallons per day ran as high as £3, 10s. It is unlikely anyone would have purchased the water filter if they read an article dated March 25, 1832:

THE CAUSE OF CHOLERA: Some clever fellow, in a morning paper, tries to prove that a peculiar state of the water is the cause of cholera. He talks confusedly of its chemical and mineral properties being the remote spring of the epidemic, and hints that the purity of the Thames is one reason of the disease being so mild in London. Poor gentleman! he must have been bit by a mad dog. He may be sure that no water has any thing to do with cholera, except it be water in the head![17]

Notwithstanding, Mr. Baron Gurney, presiding in the Crown Court, England, August 13, 1832, observed that in the city of London, the healthy state of water was attributed to its being well supplied with sewers. The subject, however, was not universally agreed upon. Inhabitants of Bennett's Hill asserted that the common sewer that had recently been made between the end of Watling Street and the Thames presented a terrible nuisance, giving the town a stench "so intolerable by the effluvia which arises through the different gratings" that they could not sleep at night. In consequence of several corpses lying immediately contiguous, parish authorities resolved to indict the sewer. The money expended in its completion was immense, "and now there is likely to be a serious dispute respecting it."[18]

A private correspondent from Paris, April 3, 1832, offered some relevant comments concerning the French water supply. After noting "the mortality of the cholera morbus is proportionate to the degree of knowledge and civilization of the people among whom it appears," he suggested that a national policy of widening the streets, the formation of a common sewer system and the introduction of an adequate supply of water for domestic and sanitary purposes would have prevented the extent of the disease. While some improvement had been made in the English quarter of Paris, the form for common sewers and the materials of which they were composed were "unsuitable and expensive." As described, the "section is nearly semi-circular, the bottom being broad and flat, and covered with a composition consisting partly of clay and plaster of Paris. The arch is built of a very rough sandstone, extremely porous, requiring a very large proportion of mortar and incapable of holding together, except in considerable masses. The weight of matter employed must be at least three times that of brick, the quantity of mortar must be doubled, and, as the current is not continued to a straight line, as when the section of the sewer is an oval, the stream, in dry weather, meanders in all directions through the flat bottom, the solid substances which find their way through the gratings are not carried off, but get time to consolidate, and already the new sewers have been obstructed in several quarters."

An abundant water supply would have corrected the problem, but the water-carriers who made a considerable living selling water to customers by the week or month made formidable opponents. As they were chiefly Savoyards of respectable character, an attempt to deprive them of their livelihood would have made them "a more formidable race of malcontents" than the chiffonniers.

A greater obstacle to creating a domestic water supply by means of cast-iron pumps based on the English system was the huge expense, not less than the 30,000,000 francs expended in bringing the waters of the Oureq to Paris. This had been achieved by means of an open canal; but by passing through mineral strata, the water had become unfit for most purposes for which it was designed. The municipal council had attempted to find a company that would contract for the introduction of the requisite supply of filtered waters of the Seine, to be taken from the river before being contaminated with the impurities of the town, but it imposed two conditions. The first stipulation was the payment of 300,000 francs per annum that the city received from the water-carriers for permission to draw their supplies from public fountains and the second that the company should assume the burden of maintaining the canal of the Oureq and the pipes employed in its distribution to the monumental fountains. Only one company made an offer and ultimately withdrew it in consequence of the conditions.[19]

Work on the sewers progressed "with great activity," however, and when considering the question of whether emanations from animal and vegetable matter had an injurious influence in epidemic cholera, the French Academy of Medicine decided in the negative. Their rationale stemmed from the fact that workers exposed to soil removed from sewers were no more liable to the disease than other classes of laborers. They added that the quarter of the Place Vendôme, though traversed by a vast sewer, suffered very little from cholera, while at the Faubourg St. Germain, where there were no works of the kind, cholera appeared in its most virulent form.[20]

A notice in the *Gardeners' Gazette* (December 2, 1837) stated that an English and French company had finally succeeded in obtaining permission to begin work on a new water system for Paris "at a trifling expense per annum, as the river Seine will give an ample supply of good and salubrious water, as the current always runs one way (there being no tide), emptying itself into the sea at Havre de Grace." Pipes and tunnels were to be laid down for the leading streets only, so as not to injure the water-carriers who made their living selling water drawn from the fountains at a penny per bucket. The same company also offered to cut sewers so the night soil might be emptied into the river, thus preventing a recurrence of the cholera as it was in 1831–32 when it was "proved by the faculty of medicine" that deaths were produced "from the miasma arising in the closely inhabited streets, in consequence of the filth allowed to accumulate, and no means to carry it off."

Debate on sewers would carry on throughout the century. In 1887, when the county commissioners of Reno, Nevada, considered rebuilding their sewer system, they called in General Irish to explain their options. Warning the city was building for generations to come, Irish advocated cast iron as the best material, but it was cost prohibitive. Other alternatives were salt-glazed vitrified pipe, followed by brick and wood. Advocating the salt-glazed pipe, the entire project cost then revolved around size and grade. Estimating the quantity of water used per person to be 32–212 gallons per day averaged to 56 gallons. In cities where sewers were designed to carry off storm water as well as sewage, large pipes were needed; smaller cities with an estimated 80 persons per acre required smaller ones. A complete system dictated manholes for the purpose of examining pipes, with water and grease traps and ventilation pipes. If the sewer were properly constructed, Irish assured the commissioners, pestilential diseases could not spread in their midst.[21]

"Latest from Europe"

By early February 1832, an epidemic called "scarlatina or cholera morbus" had appeared in Chili with so much violence that "people die in the streets in a few minutes after leaving their houses." At Valparaiso, letters indicated that 363 persons died of the disease in 8 days, and during one week, 591 perished in this capital. In the same month, cholera had reached the Swan River settlement in New South Wales.[22]

Reports from Berlin during 1832 indicated that the number of new cholera cases continued to decline, although sporadic cases were reported in the German provinces besides in the town of Magdeburg. On January 10, nine cholera patients remained at Hamburgh and two in Berlin. By May 22, as the incidence of disease diminished in England, the Senate of Hamburgh relieved her ships of quarantine. At Brunn, no new cases were reported by January 13, but several appeared in Moravian villages. Gallicia was nearly free.[23]

Reports from Moscow, St. Petersburgh and Lisle in April 1832 indicated that "an innumerable quantity of midges or gnats obscured the atmosphere upon the arrival of cholera."

Calls to light fires in the streets, a measure taken by the ancients to rid the air of contagion, was offered as a preventative to further disease. In England, the publication "Inquiry into the Remote Cause of Cholera" attempted to prove that cholera could be traced to an insect, possessing either in itself or its eggs or its larvae poisonous qualities, based upon the Biblical reference in Isaiah 7:17–19.

In a new twist, residents of Liege, Belgium, were able to purchase cholera insurance for 25 francs. If they contracted the disease, they were afforded comfortable quarters and treatment. If they left the institution alive, they were asked for 100 more. If they died, no further payment was extracted![24]

The *Nuremberg Correspondent* reported in April that the medical men of Vienna were persuaded that cholera had been naturalized in their country as cases continued to appear. At Prague, from January 14 to January 16, there were 112 new cases, 58 recoveries and 33 deaths.

**Total Cases of Cholera in Vienna
Since the Commencement (18 weeks)**

	Cases	Recoveries	Deaths
City	1,101	690	411
Suburbs	3,000	1,451	1,547[25]

By July, the number of cholera victims reached 15–20 a day, with attacks considered quite violent. To explain the visitations, scientists reverted to Sydenham's theory of the 1670s, that cholera was of telluric origin, created by mephitic vapours in the earth and first communicated to the water. In consequence, many persons drank only boiled water. Being right, but for the wrong reason, Sydenham's hypothesis would account for the track of the epidemic along the course of rivers, "and for other phenomena, such as the death of fish, ducks, &c."[26]

As an indication of how cholera affected commerce and public transportation in particular, an advertisement ran in June advising passengers that the "Switzerland, Cologne, &c." line was the only conveyance to Italy that avoided all places suffering from cholera. The route left London and went via Rotterdam up the Rhine.[27] On the same subject, on March 10, the Lisbon Board of Health prohibited all vessels from England and the north of Scotland from entering any ports in the kingdom. As a preventative measure in Madrid, theatres were closed and a board of health was appointed for determining what further steps were needed.[28] Brussels papers from June 23 indicated 67 new cases of cholera at Ghent on the 20th and 60 on the 21st; deaths were at 23 and 20. The whole number of cases to that date was 583, with 195 deaths.[29]

Letters received in England as of May 1 indicated "many thousand lives" were lost by dysentery and cholera in the suburbs of Calcutta, commencing from Diamond Harbor, while another stated that the disease had made an awful appearance at Faltah and other adjoining villages, where victims perished in the course of a few hours. He attributed the cause to a new type of rice, obtained at a cheap rate, that obstructed the viscera from its turgid propensities. Other correspondents mentioned that the plague and cholera had "hardly begun to subside" in Persia. In some provinces more than two-thirds of the population expired, with Ghillan among the greatest sufferers. Out of 300,000, citizens only 60,000 men and 44,000 women and children remained. Through neglect, the eggs of the silkworms were completely destroyed, and it was calculated it would take seven years to produce the same quantity as before.[30]

Shocking news in May revealed that cholera had appeared on his majesty's ship *Racehorse,* on the St. Kitt's station. West Indian proprietors worried that mortality "amongst the (N)egro population" would further depress their already ruinously depreciated property. On a far wider scale, it was feared "neither distance of voyage, temperature of climate, nor lapse of time" afforded any security against the extension of the disease and that cholera would spread through the Western Archipelago and the American continent.[31] Tragically, they were correct.

12

Cholera in North America
"Imported by Immigrants"

ENGLAND—The Cholera fast diminishing—not the population, but its extent of ravage. Emigration the order of the day, in all parts of the united kingdom. Peers and parishes shipping off in scores their pauper dependants to America, and the paupers themselves going off in a merry cue.[1]

The observation above was intended to be humorous, but in 1832, immigration was the order of the day, with many poor, particularly the Irish, leaving their homes for better opportunities in the New World. Unfortunately, they took cholera with them, leaving scores dead before ever reaching their destination.

Although passengers and crew underwent requisite health examinations before departing, many passengers soon contracted cholera, either from previous exposure or more likely contamination by onboard drinking water. On May 18, 1832, the *Brutus*, under Captain Neilson, sailed from Liverpool for Quebec with 330 passengers and 19 crewmen. On the 27th, a 30-year-old man came down with the disease. The following day, a 60-year-old woman died within 10 hours and thereafter numbers rapidly increased, until reaching a high-water mark of 24 deaths in one day. The captain had no intention of returning to port until his crew fell ill on June 3, which forced him to change plans. By the time he reached the Mersey on the 13th, there had been 117 cases, with 83 deaths and 36 recoveries. Survivors were immediately placed aboard the Newcastle lazaretto ship. Although the *Brutus* had been at sea only 26 days, provisions were nearly exhausted (not an untypical occurrence aboard immigrant ships) and the laudanum was completely depleted.

Other immigrants suffered similar fates. After cholera was discovered aboard the *Lord Wellington,* Captain Culleton was forced to return to the passage of Waterford where he landed several infected families. These unfortunates were shunned by the locals until persuaded to offer assistance by a clergyman. The vessel then sailed for the quarantine station at Milford where physicians discovered dead bodies lying on deck.[2]

For those reaching the Promised Land, their fate was often just as tragic. By June 9, 1832, no fewer than 25,700 immigrants had arrived at Quebec from Great Britain. One of the earliest "plague ships" was the *Carricks,* out of Dublin. During the passage, 42 persons perished and within two days of landing, 80 fresh cases were reported, of which 60 died. Cholera spread quickly, crossing Lake Champlain into New York, "with results fully as fatal as in any part of Europe.[3] Other cholera ships arriving at Quebec included the *Robert* (sailed from Cork May 14; 10 deaths); the *Constantia* (from Limerick on April 28; 29 deaths) and the *Elizabeth* (from Dublin, 17 deaths). The ships were placed in quarantine at Grosse Isle, a few miles below Quebec.

On June 7, the St. Lawrence steamer *Voyageur* conveyed a load of immigrants to Quebec; on June 8, cholera broke out in emigrant boardinghouses and by the following day, 15 cases were reported, with 7 deaths resulting. The pest steamboat continued to Montreal; along the route, a man and woman picked up a mattress thrown from the *Voyageur*, contracted cholera and died. Another man was asked to bury a passenger who had died aboard ship; soon after, he, his wife and nephew perished; six Indians who were also asked to bury a passenger suffered the same fate. The remaining passengers were discharged at Montreal on the 10th. The 200-mile trip required fewer than 30 hours, but in this short span, many passengers had either died or were dying.[4]

Immigrants became easy targets for blame, but six weeks before the shipping season opened (around late April), "many cases of Cholera" appeared in Montreal. The cause was imputed to be easterly winds blowing constantly for 40 days toward Canada, bringing with it the tainted atmosphere of Europe. The epidemic quickly subsided, however, and no new reports were received until June 10 when the *Voyageur* arrived. The malady was then described as appearing "like a shower of hail," reaching rapidly across the suburbs.[5] As further proof that immigrants were not wholly to blame for the influx of cholera, the Montreal *Canadian* reported cholera among Native Americans residing 100 leagues from the sea. Suffering from cramps, diarrhea and vomiting, they were said to have cured themselves with a decoction of barks.

The Montreal Board of Health registered 431 cholera cases, with 82 deaths as of June 16; by the following day, the number had risen to 475 cases, with 102 deaths. Most fatalities occurred among the French Irish Catholics and immigrant population, the blame being placed on their drinking impure, unfiltered water from the St. Lawrence.[6] The rapid expansion of the disease was attributed to a delay in the organization of the board of health—which prevented a complete purification of the city—the careless treatment of the disease and the too free use of nostrums. Eventually, the artillery went through the streets discharging cannon "with a view, if possible, of disinfecting the atmosphere." The same evening, fires of rosin and other bituminous matter were set in every part of town. Business was almost entirely suspended, with the Bank of Montreal open only 2–3 hours each day.

Statistics from Quebec, "the very seat and throne of Cholera,"[7] on June 20 indicated 60

To Americans, sarsaparilla is a nonalcoholic drink most identified with being served to youths in Wild West bars on episodic television. In these cases, the drink was a beverage flavored with sassafras and an oil from a birch. In a wider context, sarsaparilla had been used as a medicine since the 16th century to cure venereal diseases. In the 1800s, sarsaparilla was sold as a tonic to invigorate the body after mercury poisoning or an attack of cholera. Although this ad states Wilkinson's Essence was an extract of Jamaican sarsaparilla, Jamaica was merely a channel of exportation to Europe. The extract was probably derived originally from plants grown in Honduras (*London Atlas, February 14, 1868*).

patients admitted to hospitals, 20 discharged cured, 44 convalescent, 40 deceased, and 189 remaining, for a total since the commencement of 572 cases and 329 deaths. Reports indicated cholera prevailed to an alarming extent in Caughnewaga, a small Indian village on the south side of the St. Lawrence and at Prescott, U.C., where 15 out of 30 stricken died. At Kingston, 14 cases resulted in 8 deaths: 6 residents and 2 immigrants. At Three Rivers (midway between Quebec and Montreal), cholera was alleged to have been interrupted by burning 200 pounds of brimstone with a quantity of rum.[8]

Dr. Ayres, Cholera Physician

One interesting story concerned the appearance of a stranger named Stephen Ayres. Wearing a long beard and attired in rags, he attracted numerous followers by reputedly being able to cure cholera by a prescription of two spoonfuls each of charcoal pulverized, maple sugar and hogslard, later followed by drinking spruce beer and eating chocolate on dry bread. He was looked upon as a saint, with people bowing down to touch the hem of his coat. Ayres charged nothing for his services and was said to have been a graduate of a medical college in New Jersey, although he had not practiced "in this century."[9] Two months later, the *Frederick Herald* (September 1, 1832) stated, "Dr. Ayres, the Cholera physician, who has made such a noise in Canada, made a triumphant entry into Montreal, accompanied by the Indians among whom he has been and who have christened him Dr. Cure-all. The Indians cut his garments, and take the pieces, which they believe will keep off the disease."

A further follow-up in the *Sandusky Clarion* (September 19, 1832) remarked that more than 200 citizens of Quebec addressed a letter to Dr. Ayres, thanking him in the warmest manner for his humane and efficient exertions in "saving the lives of so many of them." Ayres replied, "My arrival and continuance here, in the deplorable and forlorn situation of the place so ably and feelingly depicted by you, seems to me as it does to you, a special interposition of Divine Providence, for which I cannot be too thankful; for independently of the practical knowledge gained by attending the many cases of different ages and sexes sick with this most dreadful disease, with what success your address testifies, it has enlarged my views of medicine and its sister sciences. It appears probable to me that this disease is one of those so often mentioned in the Old Testament by the name of pestilence, as its appalling terrors in the present day fully coincide with those described in Scripture. If I am correct in the opinion that it has troubled the inhabitants of this earth before, it must have been two, three, or four thousand years ago; and it will be truly fortunate for the world, if its future periodical returns, like those of the planets, are thus far distant. I sincerely reciprocate my best wishes for your health and prosperity in this world, and your eternal happiness in the next. Stephen Ayres."

By February 1834, the "eccentric Stephen Ayres" turned up in Boston, offering his professional services for the cure of "obstinate coughs, consumption, and the natural disorders of the climate."[10] A similar savior appeared in Italy around 1886. Luigi Grazziotin, called "il re del cholera" (the king of cholera) because of his unselfish devotion to his patients, reportedly traveled from Egypt to Spain to Italy dispensing his mysterious "elixir." After his arrival in Rome late in 1887, he submitted to the king and the Venetian deputies his remedy, which he hoped would interest the scientific community.[11]

Cholera Reports from Montreal, 1832

Date	New Cases	Deaths
June 19	165	88
June 20	274	149
June 22	113	41

A private letter placed the total as of June 20 at 3,112 cases and 990 deaths.[12] Published reports as of July 10 indicated that 1,000 had died in a population of 25,000 within a 10-day span, and that the Protestant dead were left unburied in the churchyards. Worse, regulations aboard the steamboat *John Molson* directed that all patients dying from cholera be thrown overboard immediately.[13] Purification fires continued to burn in the streets, while a great part of the community wore bags of camphor around their necks. Commenting about this phenomenon during a trip to Montreal, Dr. Bronson, of Plattsburg, warned that "the effluvium of camphor is powerful and penetrating, which cannot but do harm when constantly in contact with the sensible olfactories." He also warned against the too-frequent and indiscriminate use of nostrums, "carried to a most absurd and dangerous extreme in Montreal." He continued:

> Every man had his phial, or his pill box, or his powders of different kinds, in his pockets. Literally, he carried about him an apothecaries' shop. Whenever he perceived a bad odour, or felt a disagreeable sensation, at the stomach, or imagined he did so, he suddenly stopped, felt his pulse, pulled out his medicine, swallowed a dose, smelled his camphor, felt his pulse again, and hastened on.

Dr. Bronson believed that apothecaries "did an immense deal of injury by advertising and recommending their nostrums as preventatives of cholera, and as specifics in its cure. A hundred different preparations, some of them inert, some of them powerful, were in this way distributed among the community." Equally obvious to everyone who read the newspapers, editors "scraped together and published all the Recipes which could be had," leaving it up to the individual which, whether singly or in combination, offered protection. He concluded that cities should pass regulations preventing such evils.[14]

As proof of how rapidly news of "preventatives" spread, a letter appeared in the August 18 edition of the *Frederick Herald,* citing the effectiveness of a Prussian plaster placed on the pit of the stomach. The device was called the "Burgundy Pitch," commonly called strengthening plaster. An ad for "Alcoholic Camphour" and "Burgundy Pitch Plasters," followed almost immediately.

Similar to reactions in Europe, authorities could not agree on the identity of the pestilence, calling it Asiatic, malignant, spasmodic, congestive or epidemic cholera, or "Endemic or Domestic Cholera of the United States and of the Canadas." Debates raged as to whether it was contagious, on what preventative measures to take, and how best to cure the disease once contracted. Relying on the experience of Great Britain, newspapers were filled with rules and regulations from Edinburgh and London, sanitary measures and "sure cures," many printed verbatim.

Saline Injections

New cases of cholera in Montreal on July 31 totaled 38, with 14 deaths; by August 1, 28 cases were reported, with 27 deaths. Amid such alarming numbers a new method of saline injections into the veins (as opposed to enemas) was used with success in North America. The *Montreal Gazette*, August 2, 1832, referenced the work of Drs. Stephenson and Holmes, who practiced the technique on a patient considered mortally ill from cholera. After a second infusion, the woman appeared in a favorable state. The newspaper added, "We trust that this will prove a permanent cure, as it is of much importance to the medical world, & to the community in general, that a cure should be discovered for a class of patients, whose case is so hopeless, under any other treatment."

On July 22, a patient named Mehan was brought to the Crosby Street Hospital, New York, in a collapsed state with no pulse, cold skin, sunken eyes and lividness over the body. She was administered 14 ounces of "Mur-soda 2 drachms, sub carbo. soda, 1 drachm, aqua hiej." into the vein at the bend of the arm. This was followed by a slight increase in the volume and force of the pulse, an improvement in respiration and deeper inhalations. An hour and a half later, a second infusion of 40 ounces of the same fluid was injected into another vein, followed by a decided improvement of all bad symptoms. Several days later she was discharged, perfectly cured.

Dr. Cox of Philadelphia, who had been visiting New York, performed the injections, considered to be "very simple" and performed with "great ease." Dr. Depeyre, the assistant physician, had performed two other cases with equal success. Dr. Rhinelander, another assistant, declared that the operation was performed by every doctor at the hospital, and was "done with as much facility as cupping or bleeding."[15]

The History of Intravenous Injection

The origins of intravenous therapy probably originated with Sir Christopher Wren in the early 1650s, when he injected wine and ales into the venous circulation of dogs. Although unsuccessful, they led to later attempts at blood transfusions.[16] In 1830, reports circulated of Russian soldiers being treated for tetanus with intravenous opium,[17] while Dr. T.J. Murphy, Liverpool, claimed to have been the first to use the therapy by recounting several cases and collaborations,[18] but this was subsequently dismissed.[19]

Credit was ultimately bestowed on William Brooke O'Shaughnessy, born in Limerick in 1808 or 1809, who was the first to present the idea of intravenous injection. As a youth, he studied medicine, chemistry and forensic toxicology at the University of Edinburgh with Sir Robert Christison and anatomy professor Robert Knox, dissecting cadavers supplied by the infamous grave robbers Burke and Hare. After receiving his medical degree in 1829, he relocated to London but was unable to obtain a license to practice. In consequence, he established his own forensic toxicology laboratory, performing chemical analyses of blood, feces, urine and tissue for private physicians, hospitals and the courts.

On December 3, 1831, he delivered a lecture to the Westminster Society on the "blue cholera." From his study of the blood of cholera victims, he reported that "universal stagnation of the venous system, and rapid cessation of the arterialisation of the blood, are the earliest, as well as the most characteristic effects." Most physicians of the time promoted the idea of venesection (blood-letting) or the inhalation of oxygen gas, a mixture of oxygen and atmospheric air or the protoxide of azote (laughing gas) to achieve artificial arterialization. O'Shaughnessy concluded that venesection might have its merits but was not an adequate solution and he saw no evidence to favor oxygenation. He suggested the idea of an intravenous injection of nitrate or chlorate of potash, "salts which contain the greatest quantity of oxygen." The method employed consisted of a small tube, "which should be of gold or ivory" into the external jugular vein because of its proximity to the super vena cava and the reduced risk of air embolism.

His article, "Proposal of a new method of treating the Blue Epidemic Cholera by the injection of highly-oxygenised salts into the venous system,"[20] appeared in the *Lancet*, followed by a second work, "Experiment on the blood in cholera."[21] Of major significance, his research proved that there were only 860 parts water in 1,000 parts serum, from which he concluded "the copious diarrhoea of cholera leads to dehydration, electrolytic depletion, acidosis and nitrogen retention": "treatment must depend on intravenous replacement of the deficient salt and water." The following year, W.R. Clanny, a researcher from Sunderland, confirmed that blood from one of his cholera patients had only 644 parts per 1,000, with an increased proportion of "colouring matter."[22]

In 1832, the central board of health published O'Shaughnessy's book, *Report on the Chemical Pathology of Malignant Cholera*. A review in the *Lancet* observed, "The author recommends the injection into the veins of tepid water, holding a solution of the normal salts of the blood; his experiments having, we presume, led him to abandon his former ideas respecting the superiority of highly oxygenated salts for this purpose."[23]

Inspired by O'Shaughnessy's work, Dr. Thomas Latta, of Leith, abandoned his attempt to correct blood deficiencies via injections into the rectum (the common practice) and performed intravenous therapy by inserting a tube into the basilic vein. His first patient was an elderly woman on the verge of death from cholera. Fearful of the consequences, he began by infusing one ounce of liquid; when he saw no change, more was added, until "she began to breath less laboriously, soon the sharpened features and sunken eye and fallen jaw, pale and cold, bearing the manifest impress of death's signet, began to glow with returning animation.... [I]n the short space of half an hour, when six pints had been injected she expressed in a firm voice that she was free from all uneasiness...." Unfortunately, the patient relapsed and died several hours later. Latta remarked, "I have no doubt the case would have issued in complete retraction, had the remedy, which already had produced such effect been repeated."[24]

The apparatus Latte used was "a Read's patent syringe, having a small silver tube attached to the extremity of the flexible injecting tube. The syringe must be quite perfect, so as to avoid the risk of injecting air; the saline fluid should never be injected oftener than once in the same orifice, and the vein should be treated with much delicacy to avoid phlebitis." Causes for failure included not enough fluid, underlying disease and late application of the remedy. In the same issue of the *Lancet*, letters from Drs. Robert Lewins, Thomas Craigie and J. Macintosh described similar methods.[25]

Dr. O'Shaughnessy responded with enthusiasm: "The results of the practice described by Drs Latta and Lewins exceed my most sanguine anticipations. When we consider that no practitioner would dare to try so novel an experiment, except in cases beyond hope of relief by any ordinary mode of treatment, and, consequently, desperate to the last degree, even a solitary instance of recovery affords matter for congratulation."[26]

Mr. Read quickly saw the advantage of promoting his apparatus, mentioned by Dr. Latte. Under the prestigious heading "Central Board of Health," he ran the following advertisement. Although the comment supplied by Dr. Barry (a prominent and well-known physician who had extensively studied cholera on the Continent and who had been selected by the government to investigate the outbreak at Sunderland, England, in 1831) fell short of a testimonial, it provided a strong selling point:

CENTRAL BOARD OF HEALTH
COPY OF SIR DAVID BARRY'S TESTIMONIAL.
Council Office, 21st June, 1832
Without adverting to the efficacy of saline injections into the veins as a remedy for Spasmodic

Cholera, I feel pleasure in declaring as my opinion that Mr. Read's Apparatus is admirably well calculated for effecting that operation.

     (Signed)   D. Barry, M.D.

J. READ most respectfully begs to inform the Profession and the Public, that the Instrument thus approved by the Board is his PATENT STOMACH PUMP and ENEMA SYRINGE, which he now fits up with additional Pipes for Saline Injections. He also begs to caution them against spurious Instruments, which continue to be circulated throughout the kingdom in his name, and which are daily sent to him, with complaints, to be repaired. None are genuine except stamped with the Royal Arms and the Patentee's name, to imitate which is Felony!!

Manufactured and sold by J. Read, 35 Regent Circus, Piccadilly. Sold by Mr. Pepys, 22 Poultry; and Mr. Stodart, 401 Strand.

N.B. Venous Pipes fitted to Read's Brass or German Silver Instruments, if sent to him for that purpose.[27]

A follow-up advertisement included a quotation from Sir Henry Halford, dated July 9: "Mr. Read's instrument seems to me to be very ingeniously and effectually adapted to the purpose intended." Dr. Charles Scudamore, M.D., F.R.S. added, "From a careful examination of Mr. Read's apparatus, I have no hesitation in declaring my conviction, that it is perfectly and admirably adapted to the purpose of injecting into the venous circulation."[28] For all the method's seeming promise, however, an editorial in the *Courier*, July 13, 1832, made the following observations:

> The necessity of precaution is the more evident as we become convinced that the disease is, when in its confirmed state, really beyond the reach of medicine. We hear a great deal indeed of cures having been effected by this or that mode of treatment; but how do we know that where recovery takes place it is not the spontaneous work of nature? At one time the Carbonate of Soda, freely administered, was said to effect cure—at another Saline Injections into the veins of the patients, on the ingenious supposition that such a process would restore to the blood the peculiar property of which it is deprived by cholera. But who now places any dependence on Saline Injections or the use of Soda?
>
> The apparent result of a few cases, treated by injections of this kind, did, indeed, seem to promise a mode of treatment as successful as it was ingenious; but it should not be concealed that of the patients who appeared to have recovered, some relapsed, and others died of a new disease—inflammation of the veins, caused by the process, which is at all times a dangerous one, from the great liability of the veins to inflammation, and the probability of admitting atmospheric air, which, even in the minutest quantity, is fatal to the patient.

Tragically, the technique of intravenous injection fell into disuse and it would take decades for acceptance to follow. Ironically, Dr. O'Shaughnessy would be knighted by Queen Victoria in 1856 for his telegraphic work in India. He died in obscurity in January 1889.[29]

"Will the Cholera arrive in America?"

As early as January 14, 1832, before the influx of immigrants reached Canada, those in the United States were concerned that the European epidemic would reach their shores. In answer to the above question, Dr. Paul F. Eve answered, "I *think* it will, inasmuch as other epidemics have generally made the tour of the world, and this one follows, as has been observed, the general law of all epidemics."[30] The same month, the New York Board of Aldermen (acting as the board of health) sent a memorial (request) to Congress, recommending that experienced persons be sent to England to ascertain the nature of cholera, and that some general laws should be passed for the protection of the citizens of the country.[31] By mid–February, the Medical

Society of Massachusetts had appointed a committee of physicians to investigate spasmodic cholera.[32]

A startling confirmation seemed to confirm their worry when it was reported by the *New Orleans Argus* that on February 20, the brig *Jesse* out of Liverpool brought nine infected persons into Mobile, of which five died within the space of 20 hours. Doctors declared them to be suffering from cholera.[33] On April 3, a 12-year-old girl at Topsham, Maine (a small seaport 136 miles from Boston), was reported to have contracted cholera from handling her brother's clothes. He had recently returned from Hamburg where he had suffered from the disease. Further information disclosed that another English vessel had lost the greater part of its crew, but in returning to New York, the captain had neglected to inform authorities and thus escaped quarantine.[34]

While a "new disease," strikingly similar to cholera was breaking out at Niagara, New York, a memorial of the Philadelphia Board of Health was presented to the United States Senate, praying for the establishment of quarantine jurisdiction in Delaware Bay for the purpose of preventing the introduction of cholera. It was voted down, 30–8.[35] And to prove "murder by cholera" was not solely the province of Europeans, the celebrated case of Mr. and Mrs. Mina made headline news. Trial summaries from Buck's County, Pennsylvania, revealed that the former Mrs. Chapman engaged in an illicit affair with Mina; they poisoned her husband with arsenic and blamed his death on cholera. Once Mr. Chapman died, the two married and attempted to escape but were caught and brought before justice. After disinterring the body, the cause of death was determined to be arsenic and Mr. Mina was convicted. On the gallows, he was alleged to have said, "If my life is ended by hanging, I shall certainly escape the cholera."[36]

Headlines of May 9 indicated the presence of cholera at New London, Connecticut, with 160 cases and upwards of 30 deaths. Although the classification of cholera was argued, victims suffered chills and pains in the head and back. If they survived for 12 hours, they were thought likely to recover.[37] By August, however, "very respectable physicians" of Connecticut determined the epidemic was not cholera but *typhus syncopalis* (sinking typhus), improperly called "spotted fever." This disease had been present in the state since 1806 and identified in New London during the winter of 1831–1832. Dr. Minor of Middletown differentiated cholera from spotted fever by indicating the former attacked greater numbers and extended over a vastly larger territory. In his mind, cholera was no more dangerous than sinking typhus and treatment was the same except for a variation of medication.[38]

By June 22, cholera had been reported in Burlington, Vermont, and Plattsburg, Whitehall, Fort Ann, Fort Miller, Mechanicsville, Troy and Albany, New York. In response, the *Adams (PA) Sentinel* (June 26, 1832), observed the following:

> Afflicting Intelligence!
> The Destroying Angel Has Reached America!
>
> It is with feelings of no ordinary nature, that we announce to our readers the alarming fact that the India CHOLERA, that dreadful scourge of Asia & Europe, which has swept off, it is thought, at least *fifty millions* of human beings, has reached the shores of America, and is already carrying death and desolation before it.

Adding that "the alarm felt in Albany and New York is beyond description," the paper noted that authorities of the Empire State had placed $25,000 at the disposal of the board of health for the purpose of having the poorer classes attended to and other precautions taken against cholera. The Episcopal bishop of New York and the governor of Maryland called for renewed spiritual endeavors; on June 29, Senator Henry Clay suggested a voluntary "General Day of

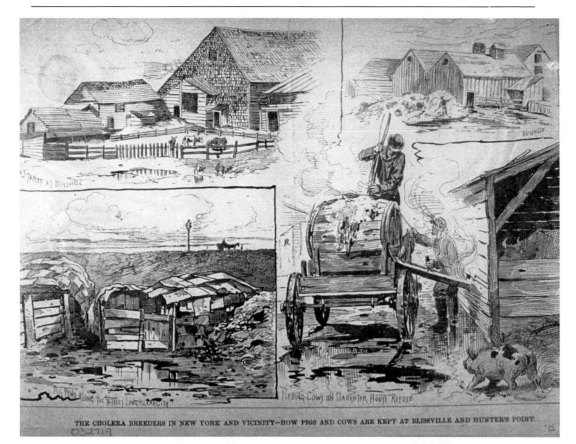

"The Cholera Breeders in New York and Vicinity—How Pigs and Cows Are Kept at Blissville and Hunter's Point," from *Pictures of Life and Character in New York*, circa 1875. Poisoned air and filth: these were a sure prescription for cholera. These images portray the deplorable condition of cow stables at Blissville, pig pens along the street in Long Island and feeding cows on slaughterhouse refuse (U.S. National Library of Medicine).

Humiliation and Prayer" to avert the "Asiatic Scourge" (the resolution passed). The price of camphor rose from $1 to $2.50/pound; calls were made to Boston's in Wall Street for their 120 percent stronger chlorine of soda; and persons were advised to carry a phial of laudanum and one of peppermint to be resorted to upon being attacked by the malady. Mixtures such as sulphuric ether and aromatic spirit of hartshorn, each half an ounce, combined with compound tincture of cinnamon, one ounce, were to be kept on hand in the home, along with a concoction of 24 grains opium, camphor, one drachm; spirit of wine and conserve of roses, enough to make a mass of proper consistency divided into 24 pills.[39]

The special medical council of New York assured the board of health that cholera in the city involved only "the imprudent, the intemperate, and those who injure themselves by taking improper medicines."[40] Harlem and "Five Points," a depressed area in the city where five streets met (500 yards from Broadway, the principal street in the city and close to Central Park and city hall), was particularly hard hit. Described as one of the greatest regions of "vice and iniquity, of distress, and misery, of any in the United States; where the abandoned of all ages, sexes and colours, congregate in small rooms, and even in cellars," no one was surprised to find disease there. Descriptions given matched those of "classic" cholera: disordered stomach, looseness of the bowels, the discharge becoming thin with a rice water appearance, dizziness, nausea, retching, vomiting and "oppression."[41]

Not surprisingly, along with prostitutes and drunkards, immigrants were particularly hard hit. Upward of 7,000 arrived in the city per month, living in cramped houses, destitute of the ordinary comforts of life and unable to find work due to the stoppage of business. Cholera victims of this class were often found lying dead among the living.[42]

Cholera in New York City, July 1832

Date	New Cases	Deaths	Total Cases	Total Deaths Since July 3
4	7	4	–	–
5	20	11	–	–
6	37	19	–	–
7	42	12	–	–
8	42	21	–	–
9	105	28	–	–
10	120	44	–	–
11	129	55	495	116
12	119	57	614	237
13	101	42	715	286
14	115	66	830	352
15	133	84	963	436
16	163	94	1,126	530
17	145	60	1,265	590
18	131	72	1,503	656
19	90	32	–	–
20	126	100	–	–
21	310	103	–	–
22	239	90	–	–
23	231	93	–	–
24	296	96	–	–
25	157	61	–	–
26	141	73	–	–
28	145	68	–	–
29	122	39	–	–
30	103	39	–	–
31	121	48	–	–
Aug 1	92	41	–	–
2	81	34	–	–
8	85	21	–	–
9	73	28	–	–
10	97	26	–	–
11	76	33	–	–
12	67	23	–	–
13	106	23	–	–
14	42	15	–	–
15	75	26	–	–
16	79	26	–	–
17	63	21	–	–
18	76	19	–	–
19	56	18	–	–
20	58	13	–	–

Date	New Cases	Deaths	Total Cases	Total Deaths Since July 3
21	52	18	–	–
22	48	22	–	–
23	72	31	–	–
24	45	30	–	–
25	37	16	–	–
26	50	24	–	–
27	40	13	–	–
28	41	15	–	–
29	21	16	–	–

Cholera in Albany, July 1832

Date	New Cases	Deaths	Total Cases	Total Deaths Since July 3
16	29	7	–	–
24	19	10	–	–
25	29	7	–	–
26	32	7	–	–
27	40	13	–	–
28	28	18	–	–
29	36	17	–	–
31	26	10[43]	–	–

If there were any good to come from cholera, the *Boston Transcript* reported that after chloride of lime was used to purify and disinfect drains, thousands of rats, repulsed by the smell, deserted the city. The same also occurred in Providence, Rhode Island, where rats, mice and small deer were chased away by the score.[44]

The Black Hawk War

Known contemporaneously as the "Border War," the "Frontier War," or the "Indian War," the "Indian question" came to the attention of Americans when the Sauk and Fox tribes murdered 28 Menominee Indians at Prairie du Chien. In April 1832, the 6th Regiment of United States Infantry left Jefferson Barracks (10 miles below St. Louis) with the intention of capturing the renegades who had perpetrated the slaughter. Black Hawk, leader of the warriors, defeated a contingent of militia at Stillman's Run, prompting Governor John Reynolds of Illinois to call for volunteers to defend their country.[45] On June 2, the Missouri *Intelligencer* reported that Governor Miller had received expresses that the Indians were stealing hogs and cattle from settlers on the western frontier, while in the southern part of the state Black Hawk was recruiting other tribes to join his efforts to drive off the invaders. Under the overall command of Generals Atkinson and Dodge, pitched skirmishes took place at Rock River and along the four Lakes, about 80 miles from Galena.

Colonel Twiggs, commanding three companies of artillery and two of infantry, landed below Fort Gratiot by the steamer *Henry Clay*, a boat known to have carried cholera victims. With the disease already rampant, a dispatch from Fort Gratiot, dated July 10, indicated that 13–14 cases of cholera remained, of which it was hoped two-thirds would recover. The detachment of 400 had dwindled to 150 by pestilence and desertion from an "overwhelming dread of the disease." Bodies of deserters were "literally strewed along the road" between the fort and Detroit, with no one offering relief. Reports of bodies being devoured by wolves and hogs were common. A letter of July 12 indicated that the condition of troops there was "disastrous,"

**SIR WILLIAM BURNETT'S PATENT DIS-
INFECTING FLUID,**

For the Prevention of CHOLERA and CONTAGIOUS DIS-
EASES, DISINFECTION OF SICK-ROOMS, CLOTHING,
LINEN, &c., PURIFICATION OF BILGEWATER, CESS-
POOLS, DRAINS, WATERCLOSETS, &c.

As a DEODORIZING and PURIFYING AGENT, it is the
Best, the Cheapest, and the Most Healthful.

It is INODOROUS, and it does not stain the most delicate
fabrics—advantages possessed by no other preparation offered
to the public for similar purposes.

At mid–19th century, health authorities were desperate to
find a means of preventing the contagion of cholera. Chloride
(sold under many brand names) was usually the agent of
choice for disinfecting sickrooms and treating water. Sir
William Burnett's Patent Disinfecting Fluid had an advantage
over similar products by promoting the namesake's title (*Nautical Standard and Steam Navigation Gazette*, London, October 27, 1849).

GREAT REDUCTION IN PRICE
OF
SIR WM. BURNETT'S DISINFECTING FLUID.
Gallons, 6s. ; Quarts, 2s. ; Pints, 1s. ; Half-pints, 6d.

THIS valuable DEODORISER and DISIN-
FECTANT instantaneously destroys all BAD SMELLS
without producing any itself.

Its free use, as directed, Prevents CHOLERA and all CON-
TAGIOUS DISEASES.

Sold by all Chemists and Druggists, and at the Office, 18,
Cannon-street, London-bridge.

N.B.—Beware of a spurious imitation.

Still in business five years after his earlier ad in 1849, Sir
William Burnett tried a different tactic for attracting customers in 1854: the tried-and-true "Reduction in Price."
There is little doubt the tactic appealed to customers among
the poorer classes. The same day this notice ran, the registrar-
general released his report stating that 2,050 persons had been
stricken with cholera the previous week. Mortality was confined, for the most part, to squalid districts, low grounds
along the river and Liverpool (*London Patriot*, September 14, 1854).

the soldiers being "swept off by disease, and nearly all the others had deserted." Twiggs and surgeon Everett (who subsequently died) were also afflicted. Reinforcements departing Detroit for the front aboard the steamboat *William Penn* under Colonel Cummins were also attacked by cholera and lost 17 or 18 on the voyage to Fort Gratiot.

Although bloody success was reported against the marauders (Gen. Dodge's troops annihilated a band of 12 "savages," scalping 11 of them, and Capt. Stephenson's men killed 6–7), General Atkinson was blamed for his slow movements and reinforcements were called for. To combat the Indian uprising, U.S. troops were congregated at Detroit before transport to the theatre of war. One factor that had not been anticipated by the army was the spread of cholera. During the Canadian outbreak earlier in 1832, the Emigrant Society forwarded newcomers away as soon as they arrived and the disease was sown at each stopping place. The infection reached Toronto, Kingston and Niagara, while spreading with fatal rapidity along the waterways of the northern frontier and across the Great Lakes.

The garrison from Fort Niagara was transported to Detroit, reaching there on June 30 without sickness. By July 6, however, the first case of cholera appeared; by July 12, there were 39 cases reported, with 18 deaths. The situation worsened and by July 20, out of 78 soldiers, 47 had been attacked. The sudden appearance of cholera in Detroit, which, up to that point had been relatively unaffected, was believed to have originated from an infected steamboat on which troops were conveyed from Buffalo to Detroit, as the vessel had recently been employed in transporting "crowds of filthy foreign emigrants westward from Montreal and Quebec."[46]

Fort Dearborn, near Chicago, was temporarily reoccupied during the Black Hawk campaign. In June, the War Department issued orders that 1,000 men of the regular army from garrisons upon the seaboard and Great Lakes were to concentrate there under the command of General Scott. That officer and advance companies of the army arrived aboard the steamboat

Sheldon Thompson on July 10.[47] It was feared, however, that "one half of the detachment under Gen. Scott will never reach him, from the two causes of disease and desertion." That concern proved accurate: out of 1,000 troops, over 200 were admitted into hospitals over a 7–8 day period. Surgeon DeCamp attributed the sickness to the contagious nature of the epidemic, stating there had been no disease before the arrival of the soldiers by steamboat.

The United States Army Report for 1832 indicated the entire force being sent by the Great Lakes suffered from cholera to such a degree that they were incapable of taking the field. Some were landed but the main body was rerouted to Chicago "in a most deplorable condition." Six companies of artillery left Fortress Monroe, Virginia, in perfect health, contracted cholera at Detroit and reached Chicago with a loss of one out of every three men. The schooner *Napoleon*, chartered to transport supplies for the army at Chicago, left Detroit. But Captain Hinckley, her commander, died before she reached Lake Huron. Fear of contagion caused a panic among the civilian population and even the Indian agent left with his family for St. Louis. Upon their leaving Mackinac, cholera broke out in these six companies; by the 12th, twenty-five soldiers had died of the disease and 60 more were sick. By the time they reached the Mississippi, the disease was as bad as it had been at Fort Dearborn.[48]

Colonel Twiggs returned from the front on August 11 in a state of convalescence, giving an account of cholera among the troops and the subsequent dispersion of General Scott's command as "lamentable." From their original point of debarkation at Norfolk, the command traveled through Baltimore and Detroit, the trail of cholera in their midst.

Before the friendly Winnebagoes captured Black Hawk and his warriors, effectively putting an end to the war, cholera had appeared at Fort Crawford on the Mississippi, two miles above the mouth of the Wisconsin; Fort Leavenworth, on the Missouri River, about 500 miles above its confluence with the Mississippi; Jefferson Barracks and Fort Gibson, on the Neosho (Grand) river, Arkansas. Cholera was more devastating than war, and the U.S. Army Report for 1832 observed, "Our troops handed the disease over to the Indians."[49]

As true as this statement was, cholera had not abandoned the U.S. troops. When Black Hawk and his warriors arrived at Jefferson Barracks on September 7, cholera had claimed three officers and a number of privates at Rock Island and Galena. A dispatch from General Scott on the 15th stated that the disease had "entirely disappeared" from Rock Island, but attrition had been horrific. Of the 6 companies of artillery that left Fortress Monroe in June to oppose the Indians, only 180 remained on November 7 when they returned to Norfolk.[50]

By November 24, cholera raged among the Sacs and Foxes around Rock Island. Among the dead was Ke-o-kuck, the great orator of the Sacs who had participated in the "Great Talk" between the Northwest Indians and the victorious U.S. troops. Prior to this, Col. John Brandt, the celebrated Indian chief of the Six Nations and member of the Upper Canada parliament, had died of cholera in Brantford, U.C.

Matters would only get worse for the displaced Native Americans. On November 21, Arkansas's *Gazette* reported that cholera continued to prevail among emigrating Indians and had carried off at least 50–60. On December 6, Major Pool, assistant agent in the forced emigration of Indians, wrote from camp 30 miles west of St. Charles, Missouri, that cholera was ravaging the Ohio Indians lately removed from that state. War-tesh-ne-wa, principal chief of the Ottowas, had died that day and others were not expected to live until morning.[51]

13

The Scourge of God

It is right, nay, it is a duty, to make use of all natural means for protection from the power of the plague. Religion does not discourage the use of such means, but urges men to resort to them in all cases where they are at hand. The cholera, though we have reason to look upon it as a special visitation from God, is nevertheless, as we have seen, subject to the established laws of nature in its action; and if these laws can be ascertained, so as to enable us to avoid the evil in any measure, we are as much bound by religion itself to attend to them for this purpose as we are to attend to any other conditions on which our comfort and happiness are known to depend.[1]

The above, extracted from a sermon preached at the First Presbyterian Church, Pittsburgh, July 6, 1832, noted of cholera, "Its natural history has never yet been elucidated. The laws of its action are hidden even from the wise.... Whatever theory we construct in order to account for the disease in this instance, the fact continues unchanged, that the cholera, before which other nations have been made to tremble, is on our borders." In his thoughtful lecture, Reverend Nevin added that he had no doubt cholera was governed by general and fixed principles established in nature, "as is the lightning in its mazy track, or the planet circling in dread amazement around the sun." In calling out a day of fasting, humiliation and prayer (officially proclaimed by Governor George Wolf for August 9), Nevin attempted to place the scourge in proper context with humanity and his God. "Be not afraid," he said. But America was afraid.

In reference to Canada, Dr. Rhinelander, the New York surgeon, remarked, "You cannot conceive the panic in every part of the country—the absorbing theme of all thoughts appears to be centered in this disease."[2] The *Philadelphia Inquirer* of July 17 announced 5 new cases of malignant cholera, adding, "This was to be expected. A few deaths will certainly occur here.... Treated properly and in time, there is no danger." It would not be long before their confidence was put to the test. Before the month was out, mortality tables began to appear.

Cholera at Philadelphia

Date	New Cases	Deaths
July 27	2	3
28	6	5
29	6	1
30	15	8
31	19	9
Aug 1	21	8
2	40	15
3	35	14
7	136	73
8	114	46
9	154	58

Date	New Cases	Deaths
10	142	41
11	126	33
12	110	31
13	130	49
14	111	37
15	73	23
16	94	30
17	90	26
18	74	18
19	49	11
20	54	18
21	51	9
22	49	9
23	33	10
24	48	10
25	24	10
26	30	6
27	21	7
28	16	2
29	20	4
30	20	3[3]

The *Saturday Courier*, August 11, reported that the ravages in Philadelphia had far exceeded all anticipation: "This immense augmentation excited serious apprehensions, and the public mind was greatly and properly agitated." At the city prison, cholera attacked so suddenly and violently, men "alternately begged and prayed for a release, or abandoned themselves to the most furious rage and defiance." The rapid progression of disease among the "scum and refuse of the population" was attributed to "long continued excesses in the vilest debaucheries."[4]

Philadelphia was not alone. At the state prison, Westchester County, New York, the final week of July registered 97 new cases and 30 deaths among inmates, while at Sing Sing Prison, between July 27 and July 30, forty-one cholera cases were reported, with 16 deaths. Among those who died was the notorious Englishman John Stephens, who committed some of the most extensive and daring forgeries ever heard of in the U.S.[5]

Not unlike citizens of other cities, the people of Philadelphia charged physicians with forcing patients into hospitals. Doctors denied the charges but the resultant anger prompted them to threaten to "wash our hands in innocency, and retire from the charge of our hospitals." The situation deteriorated to the point the sanitary committee was forced to beg the mayor to punish all persons who molested any medical practitioner.[6]

Cholera Among African Americans

While "the whole fashionable world" had abandoned New York and the last new novel was "laying on the work table unread,"[7] cholera continued its insidious march. By late July, reports from Portsmouth, Virginia, indicated a "strange disease" had carried off 11 blacks and one white man, while at Norfolk, two blacks also perished. (The cause of death for the African Americans was in question because a physician had not treated them.) The distinction between black and white victims was an interesting one, illustrated by a letter from Quebec that stated "no colored people had been attacked there by the cholera," causing instant speculation "in different parts of the country." These concerns were allayed, however, when Messrs. Gates & Co. from Montreal assured the people there were not "two dozen blacks in Quebec and here."

That the Grim Reaper had not singled out Caucasians, interested parties were further reassured by the *Commercial*, which quickly published the fact there were 14,000 "colored" persons in New York and that they were "as liable to cholera as whites, and that as many die in proportion to their number." From July 24 to July 29, however, 18 more black men had died, compared to three whites. The report was followed by this observation: "If the cholera shall get among the slave population of the south—careless of themselves and badly provided for, we apprehend very awful accounts of its doing." By August 4, twenty-three cases (no distinction given) were reported at Portsmouth. By August 9, Elizabeth City, North Carolina, reported cholera progressing at a very rapid rate, principally among the blacks.

Cholera in Norfolk, Virginia

August	New Cases	Deaths
9	48 (38 colored)	11
10	43	11
11	38	12[8]

Cholera among the "poor Negroes" continued to worry the slave-owning population. A letter published in the *Charleston Patriot* detailed their condition in Norfolk, observing that "they would not, and they will not nurse each other—you cannot compel them, unless you are with them constantly. They looked aghast at you if you offered to hire, or persuade them to attend a sick brother." The writer added that the slaves were "so perverse," although daily admonished and entreated," to inform their owners if they have any symptoms, until it was too late to save them. He attributed the high rate of cholera to their penchant for putting up food "all day long, and eating enormously very late at night." In the hot weather, the food fermented, and as "*they live to eat*," they fell on the ground and died. He estimated that three-fourths "have gone off in that way," as their whole manner of living ("with which you are as well acquainted as I") was the reason of "greater fatality among them than the whites."[9]

As the disease traveled down the great western waterways, African Americans held in bondage suffered terribly. In a letter written August 2 from Natchez, one plantation holder indicated that the genuine Asiatic cholera had appeared among "our blacks," attended with violent spasms. On one of his "places," disease struck 49 out of 69 souls. They were treated with calomel in a pill (20 grains) and the application of a poultice of peach leaves, made by stewing them in whiskey and then placing over the abdomen. In 700 cases, the writer heard of only 5–6 deaths.[10]

Spirituous Liquors Predispose to Cholera!

The mayor of Troy, New York, Nathan S.S. Beman, called for "efficient means to suppress *nocturnal dissipations*" and "regulations in relation to *the retailing of ardent spirits*." Defending his position that cholera was "a disease principally dependant for its existence and malignancy on the use of ardent spirits," he cited numerous contemporary experts: Dr. Ricche's observation that in China the disease was due to filth and intemperance; Ramohun Fingee, the Indian doctor, who stated those who abstained from spirits or opium did not catch the disorder; Dr. Joenichin of Moscow, who declared "drunkenness, debauchery, bad food, and personal indiscretions" were "indubitably" the predisposing cause; Monsieur Huber, who saw 2,160 persons perish in Moscow in 25 days, noting "every drunkard has fallen!" Dr. Becker recorded the caution "above all things, avoid intemperance," which at Berlin (and everywhere else) rendered its votaries the first victims. The *London Medical Gazette* remarked "intemperance gives a claim to the pestilence which it never overlooks." The *London Morning Herald* added, "The same preference for the intemperate and uncleanly has characterized the Cholera every where," while the Edinburgh Board of Health concluded "the most essential precaution for escaping the disease is sobriety."

Other cited authorities were Dr. Thomas Sewall of Washington, D.C., who warned, "The epicure and the intemperate have no safety but in a speedy and thorough reformation." Dr. Bronson, of Montreal pleaded, "The habitual use of ardent spirits *in the smallest quantity*, seldom fails to invite the cholera." He remarked that five-sixths of all who fell to the disease in England were "from the ranks of the intemperate and dissolute." When asked who were the victims of cholera, Dr. Rheinelander, of New York, answered, "The *intemperate*—it invariably cuts them off." He added that physicians who prescribed brandy as a preventative or treatment were "unaccountable."

In further defense of his position, Beman quoted the July 5 edition of the *Journal of Humanity*: "Of what avail is it to remove external filth, or to pave the streets with chloride of lime, while rum, twin brother to the cholera, is sold by hogsheads at every corner? Ought not the sale of intoxicating drink be forbidden by law?" The mayor concluded his July 1832 editorial by stating, "The profit of *vending*, or the pleasure of drinking is not, for a moment, to be regarded when the lives of thousands are at stake."[11]

Hoping to avoid the fate of gardeners and fruit growers who saw their businesses nearly destroyed by physicians who charged that eating such foods brought on cholera,[12] those in the brewing business made a rapid counterattack. Members of the fraternity from Philadelphia, New York City, Poughkeepsie and Baltimore were surveyed as to the effects of malt liquor on their employees and customers. In defense of their product, a series of letters signed "Brewers" noted that in Europe, where malt liquor was not the common beverage, cholera made its greatest ravages, while in England, where people were more accustomed to the drink, of all those engaged in the occupation, "not one person had died of the cholera." Conversely, at Quebec and Montreal, where malt liquor was little known, the disease raged.

At Philadelphia, home of "the greatest consumers of malt liquors in this country," many eminent physicians recommended the use of porter and ale and introduced it into hospitals. No brewers in that city or county died of cholera, although they made free use of these drinks. The same held true at Poughkeepsie, where "*eminent physicians* advocate our articles as being the best and most *wholesome* beverage for the common purposes of *life*, and during the existence of the epidemic." Spokesman J.N. Vassar added that of the 30–40 families in the vicinity, all of whom used malt beverages instead of coffee or tea, none were attacked by cholera. Of the 13 breweries in New York City and one in Brooklyn, no deaths were reported among employees, which spokesman Samuel Milbank considered "conclusive" as to its safety.

The "Brewers" could not account for the fact some physicians took an opposing stance, "for surely we might as well nay soon exclude sugar from our table as the saccrihine of malt from drink, and surely nothing is more healthy than the hops, for its fragrance is grateful to a sick man, laboring under any disease; these extracted by water, united by fermentation, are the component parts of malt liquor." They concluded by remarking the subject was well worth consideration, "believing that the good morals and health of society will be preserved in proportion to the consumption of malt liquors."[13]

In England, Bennett and Company's "Syrup of Malt," added to porter or ale, was promised to counteract "the influence of all deleterious matter that too frequently bespeaks the bad qualities of such liquors, and which have consigned many thousands of our fellow-creatures to a predisposition for Cholera and other Bilious Diseases."[14]

"For the week ending..."

Rhode Island "surrounded herself with quarantine laws and bayonets against the cholera! Panic never reasons," the *Frederick Herald* of August 4, 1832, proclaimed. Perhaps she had reasons. For the week ending July 28, Buffalo reported 41 new cases and 14 deaths, while Princeton, New Jersey, had four cases, two of which terminated fatally. Buffalo had 15 new cases and four deaths on July 27, and Brooklyn registered 35 new cases and seven deaths on August 1. Among the more noted deaths was the "Ourang Outang," the "Pungo" of Africa. Soon after reaching New York, it contracted cholera and after passing through the regular stages of the malady it perished, "to the amusement of spectators."[15] On a wider scale, hundreds of pike and perch were found dead on the shores of the north of Oneida Lake, reputedly killed by cholera.[16]

Doctors were of unanimous agreement that "never was there less disease in Baltimore ... at this season of the year, than at present."[17] Barely a week later, however, newspapers reported, "Baltimore is now passing through her season of trial." For the week ending August 20, fifty-four deaths were recorded.

Cholera in Baltimore, 1832

Month	Deaths
Aug 21	13
22	15
23	29
24	10
25	14
29	15 (4 whites, 11 colored)
30	13
31	30
Sept 1	29[18]

For the week ending September 10, there were 226 cholera deaths were reported. From that high point, numbers slowly decreased. For the week ending September 17, there were 135, and for the week ending on the 24th, there were only 40.[19]

Saturday, September 1, the *Washington National Intelligencer* reported, "The Cholera is amongst us at last, beyond doubt," with 18 new cases reported by the Central Hospital. By the end of the year, cholera had "at length" reached Nashville.[20]

While Henry Potter, professor of the practice of physic in the Medical College, Maryland, lectured that cholera was "an atmospherical epidemic" affecting everyone differently depending on their susceptibility to such stimulation weakening the nervous system. Another author was opining on cholera and comets. He wrote, "The most probable hypothesis in relation to comets, is that they are the agents for distributing electricity through the planetary surface. The prevalence of malignant diseases may be attributed to the want of excess of electricity in the atmosphere." Supposing the revolution of the earth from west to east might explain the progress of cholera from east to west, he expected that the visit of two comets in 1832 would be the means of restoring a healthy medium to the atmosphere, "particularly as one of them will cross the orbit of the earth."[21]

From June 13 to September 18, there were 1,832 Catholics and 1,165 Protestants who died of cholera in Quebec, the numbers in general reflecting the religious proportions. A letter from Montreal indicated that since June 12, in a population of 30,000, nearly 3,000 deaths were recorded, more than two-thirds from cholera. By October, it was estimated one out of every nine of the population had succumbed to the disease; Quebec was said to have suffered even greater casualties. At York, estimates ranged between 500 and 600 out of a population of 4,400, equating to the loss of one out of every eight persons. Despite these staggering numbers that were well chronicled in the United Kingdom, immigration to Canada remained heavy. As of July 31, a total of 14,375 persons had arrived in Montreal from England, 23,242 from Ireland and 3,823 from Scotland.[22]

If cholera took a devastating toll on human life, it also extracted a considerable cost in treasure. In New York, a special medical committee consisting of eight physicians was appointed. The president of the board received $25 per day and earned $1,525 during the epidemic. Other members received $15 per day, with the aggregate of their compensation reaching $7,000. Attendant doctors at the several hospitals and their assistants (who actually risked their lives by exposure) received sums between $350 and $600. The whole expenditure of the city from cholera was $110,000, not including private contributions.[23]

Cholera Along the Waterways

Reports from Wheeling, Virginia, dated September 1, 1832, indicated that the current rate of emigration had never been equaled: within the prior 3–4 months, wagonloads of Germans passed through the area, some crossing the river but most descending it for Cincinnati, Indiana and Illinois. The first notes of cholera came 12 days later, when cases were identified at Boonsboro and Sharpsburg, a small village six miles from the canal. As this strain proved particularly fatal, contractors dismissed canal hands and fled. It was observed that many foreigners (but not the Germans) showed no pity on their sick comrades but left them for dead.

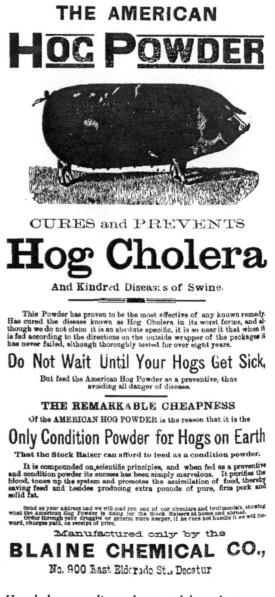

Hog cholera was a disease that spread throughout the Midwestern United States beginning around the middle of the 19th century. Symptoms in the animals resembled cholera in humans but the two diseases were not related (*Saturday Herald,* Decatur, Illinois, October 23, 1886).

While the disease prevailed at Richmond, it made dreadful ravages along the eastern bank of the Potomac, 20 miles below Alexandria. By October 4, "Death's Doings" were said to have swept through Halltown, four miles from Charlestown, taking 16 of 100 souls.[24]

Cholera came with the same blast as "the equinoctial storm" to Cleveland, showing little diminution between July and October. Cincinnati registered 19 deaths on October 25; 17 on the 26th; 13 each on the 27th and 28th; 8 on the 29th; 9 on the 30th and 7 on the 31st. By mid–November, 400 had perished within a two-week span, with business entirely suspended. Cholera was acknowledged in St. Louis on October 21: in a population of 6,000, there were 100 deaths registered in one week; by mid–November, 22 were dying daily. The same month, Louisville registered eight deaths per day, while Pittsburg reported occasional cases.

It is no surprise that cholera followed the rivers: since Robert Fulton had proved the practicality of steam-operated boats, they literally opened the western waterways to national trade and transport. Goods and passengers traveled the Ohio and Mississippi rivers from the opening of the waters in spring to the close by ice in winter. Every stopping point along the line was exposed to the disease, with captains and immigrants coming in for their share of the blame. Nor was it uncommon to read brief notices, such as one from the *Adams Sentinel* (November 20, 1832): "Eleven persons died [from cholera] on board the steamboat Freedom, on her passage down the Ohio."

If Pittsburgh and Cincinnati were the starting point, St. Louis was the figurative middle ground, with Natchez and New Orleans the end. By late October, New Orleans was in "the utmost consternation and confusion" over the appearance of cholera. One hundred and ninety-two deaths had already been recorded, primarily attributed to the slave population and persons of intemperance and unclean habits. Coming on the heels of a yellow fever epidemic (which began in early September), it was not uncommon to see 100–200 bodies lying in graveyards awaiting burial. The *Emporium* of November 1 calculated that if the current rate of deaths from the "king of terrors" continued, New Orleans would be depopulated within one year. Reports on November 4 indicated deaths from both epidemics were taking off 300 a day, leaving the city "nearly deserted by its inhabitants," while a letter from November 12 claimed "about 3,000 have died in the last 15 days (ending on the 9th)."

The *New Orleans Bee* of November 8 carried a report from a committee summoned to investigate reports of ill treatment at a cholera hospital run by a Dr. McFarlane. They discovered the most disgusting filth, night vessels full and patients claiming they had received no succor. Seventeen bodies in a state of putrefaction were so long dead they had to be burned. In rebuttal, Dr. McFarlane stated he, too, had been suffering from cholera and excused the accumulation of bodies by stating that the secretary of state lay several days unburied because his wealthy friends would not intercede. The *Courier* added that the epidemic, "which by some is designated as the Cholera, by others the cold plague, and which many call *a compound of all the evils which hell may contain*," found no obstacle to check its destructive course. "The rich and the poor, the temperate and the intemperate equally fall victims to its baneful course." Only the appearance of frost later in the month significantly reduced the death toll.[25]

The Annual Bill of Mortality for New York City, 1832, revealed that the total number of deaths was 10,359, or 3,996 more than had occurred in any previous year. The extraordinary increase was attributed to malignant cholera, which carried off 3,515 souls, all in the months of July through October.

Mortality in New York City, 1832

Month	Deaths	From Cholera
January	564	–
February	735	–
March	545	–
April	478	–
May	515	–
June	410	–
July	2,467	1,797
August	2,206	1,202
September	1,064	451
October	586	63
November	400	–
December	389[26]	–

The *New York American* reported that the direct monetary cost of the cholera visitation amounted to $118,000, which did not include actual expenses for medical treatment, hospital stores or employment given to the laboring poor thrown out of work during the epidemic. Put in twisted context, the visit of the emperor of Russia to London cost more. Compared to larger cities, cholera expenses for Huron County, Ohio, for the fiscal year ending June 8, 1833, totaled $367.36.

For the year 1832, there were 3,572 deaths in Baltimore, of which 1,162 were colored persons. (The population in 1831 was 88,990, including 18,940 blacks—14,783 free and 4,124 slaves.) Of the 1,832 deaths, 853 were attributed to cholera: 502 white and 351 black; cholera infantum 322; cholera morbus 2; consumption 403; influenza 114; intemperance, 40; old age 164; stillborn 145; smallpox 79; childbed 33; hydrophobia 1.

The "chief outlets to human life" in Philadelphia for 1832 included deaths from malignant cholera, 945; consumption, 681; cholera infantum, 366; scarlet fever, 302; and cholera morbus, 73. For the year, there were 7,253 births and 6,699 deaths. For Boston, out of 1,761 deaths, 199 were ascribed to scarlet fever; 70 to measles and 78 to malignant cholera.[27]

Nullification

Of all the stories to emerge in 1832, one that readily draws attention was the rupture between the Northern and Southern states over the threatened separation of South Carolina from the union. This threat was not lost on contemporaries. The July 30, 1832, edition of the *New York Inquirer* put the problem succinctly: "Surrounded at all points by the ravages of a fearful pestilence, we cannot but feel a comparative insignificance of any or all plagues affecting individual life, when a danger rises up before our eyes, menacing the glory of a great people— the march of free principles—the safety and happiness of millions yet unborn." The *Pennsylvanian Inquirer* added, "The cholera has naturally monopolized the attention of all classes of the community; but while we attend to the preservation of life, the preservation of our liberties, through the integrity of the Union, should not be disregarded."[28]

The subject of nullification would not end in 1832. Like cholera, its dark cloud would hover over the United States for decades to come. Both would extract a horrific toll on the lives and spirituality of humanity, challenging North and South, white and black, Native Americans and immigrants to question why these calamities struck with such unremitting inhumanity.

believed doctors there had murdered and mutilated a small boy, presumably on the pretext of medical study or experimentation. Mobs forced the gates and removed patients, some of whom subsequently died. Dragging out pieces of furniture, they tore them to pieces and set them on fire. Order was not restored until the Hussars were called out.

An example of the fear people had of the medical profession was a similar riot that occurred at Wick, in Caithness-shire, Scotland, "originating in the unfounded supposition on the part of the mob, that Dr. Anderson, from Edinburgh, who had the charge of the hospital, was only sent from thence to procure subjects for Edinburgh College, and that he therefore poisoned the cholera patients under his care." Crying, "Murder him, off with the murderer, &c.," about 1,500 individuals forced Anderson to resign and he escaped with great difficulty back to Edinburgh.

Under the heading "The Cholera and Robbers," a case from Devonshire aptly demonstrated how fear influenced the law courts. After a number of strangers were caught stealing, they were brought before the magistrate. This justice, laboring under the "painful terror" of cholera, refused to have the thieves in his presence and ordered they be "conducted to the boundary of the parish and seen to pass into another! Thus did cholera triumph over justice." Leaving the door open for some humor, one wag noted the best mode of escaping cholera was to enter the army, as military personnel avowed there had not been a single case of cholera among soldiers, their wives or children. On a slightly more realistic note, an expedition to Africa was held up in Milford to obviate the risk of carrying cholera to that nation.[8]

The Stirrings of Homeopathic Medicine

Challenging times, when dread diseases plagued the world and answers were few, compelled adventurous individuals to summon forth creative methods of treatment. One of the more enduring was the idea put forth by Samuel Hahnemann (spelled with one "n" in some contemporary accounts), whose doctrine was based on the theory that one ten-thousandth of a grain of the mildest drug would cure the most acute disease (the "Law of Infinitesimals"). Although the basic premise dated to Hippocrates and was used by ancient civilizations and Native Americans, Hahnemann was the first to systemically test the theory of "homeopathy."

His first book, the *Organon of Homeopathic Medicine*, appeared in 1810, followed in 1811 by *Materia Medica Medicine*. Arguing that the body had its own healing power, he wrote that practitioners must test and administer only one remedy at a time, carefully tailored to fit individual needs.[9] Although ridiculed by members of the medical establishment, this discipline found believers across Europe. Dr. Belluomini, a disciple of Hahnemann, published the pamphlet "A Few Plain Directions on the Employment of Camphor in the Asiatic Cholera," purporting that "two drops of camphorated spirit placed upon the tongue every four or five minutes will effectually remove the worst symptoms in the most decided cases of cholera."

An editorialist in the *Courier* (July 21, 1832) was less than convinced, writing, "we would as soon think of putting out the conflagration of Covent Garden if it were in fire, with the contents of a watering pot, as of subduing so severe a disease as cholera by the administration of such almost imperceptible doses of camphor." He added that, while what was called the "bold practice" of administering large doses of medicine was carried a great deal too far, every man of science knew "that the only chance of arresting the progress of a rapid and violent disease is by grappling boldly with the enemy, and effecting that timely revulsion which gives nature an opportunity of reasserting her influence." He warned that "we cannot too strongly caution the public against placing reliance upon new schemes, which are as absurd in theory as they must be fatal in practice."

Dr. Belluomini went further by asserting "a thin piece of copper, two or three inches in circumference, and highly polished, worn at the pit of the stomach, will effectually preserve the wearer from an attack of the malady." To prove his point, the doctor avowed that the comparative immunity from disease at Vienna arose chiefly from the practice of wearing these amulets. Considering this a "species of quackery," the editorialist suggested credulous persons believed they owed their safety to these charms, but he feared they would diminish the observance of cleanliness, temperance and good air.

Homeopathy was introduced to the United States in the 1820s and became one of the first alternative medicines to seriously compete with conventional practitioners. Although bitterly fought by these physicians (who organized the American Medical Association [AMA] in 1844 to defeat doctors calling themselves homeopaths), homeopathy claimed many 19th century luminaries, including William James, Henry Wadsworth Longfellow, Nathaniel Hawthorne, Harriet Beecher Stowe, Daniel Webster, Louisa May Alcott, William Cullen Bryant and Abraham Lincoln's secretary of state, William Seward, as believers. During the three devastating cholera epidemics in the U.S. between the mid–1800s and the early 20th century, statistics revealed "homeopathically treated patients suffered fewer deaths than those treated in allopathic hospitals. Some life insurance companies even offered a 10 percent discount to homeopathic patients, in the belief that they lived longer"[10] (see Appendix I for more details).

THE PATENT CHOLERA PREVENTION BELT (recommended by the Board of Health) scientifically constructed to secure warmth, support, and ease, to protect the bowels from cold, and improve the figure. Sent in return for post order free, price 7s., with Elastic Hips 10s. 6d., small size 5s. Also the PATENT ANTI-CONSUMPTION CORSET; Elastic without Bones or Lacing, yet imparting fashion and elegance to the figure with perfect support and ease. This corset is admirably suited for Invalids and Married Ladies. Price 15s. and One Guinea. Childrens, 7s. Directions for measurement sent per post. E. and E. H. Martin, Surgical Bandage Makers, 3, Mabledon-place, New-road, near St. Pancras Church; of whom may be obtained every kind of Truss, Belt, Supporter, &c.

Temperature changes were considered a sure harbinger of cholera and, as this 1848 advertisement notes, protecting the bowels from cold was of paramount importance. In 1876, British soldiers in India were issued "cholera belts," as it was believed such girdles acted as a preventative against the disease in hot climates. By 1885, the name was considered to carry an unpleasant connotation and when issued to British soldiers in Africa, they were referred to as "flannel belts." During the fad that promoted the use of copper for protection, cholera belts were designed with thin sheets of metal wrapped in cloth. Such articles were still in use as late as 1906 (*London Church & State Gazette*, December 1, 1848).

The Visitations of Cholera

More temporal than universal cures was the not-unjustifiable dread of premature burial. To address such fears (although, in fact, excusing them), a French paper ran a lengthy article on the subject, detailing the mortal symptoms wrought by cholera. Among them was a state of lethargy that might easily be confounded with death: cold extremities; the livid circle of the eyes being more prominent; the pulse almost ceasing to beat; and falling into a state of immovability without breath. In the latter instance, the suddenness of change "should excite the greatest distrust among persons who would otherwise be inclined to imagine that all was over with the patient."[11]

According to official reports from Paris, cholera deaths did not exceed 80 per day for the month of July 1832, but correspondents typically ascribed numbers closer to 200 and, on one particularly bad day, nearly 500 new cases were identified, with 300 deaths. The new buoyancy was attributed to extremely hot weather reaching 92°F and the use of unripe fruit. Victims continued to be taken indiscriminately from all classes. The prevalence of cholera was worse in the country: the department of Aisne lost 3,584 souls and that of the Marne above 4,000.[12]

News out of Dresden, July 6, indicated cholera had been present at the watering place Toplitz for a fortnight, although carefully concealed until the discovery of 40 new graves offered incontrovertible proof of its existence. Reports from The Hague, July 26, indicated a small decrease in cholera patients, but at Scheveningen it was increasing, 37 new cases being reported over a two-day span. Locals believed cholera had entered Holland by this port when a deserted vessel laden with tallow and wool was discovered. Bodies of the dead crew were stripped and their clothing brought ashore, thereby contaminating the population. At Rotterdam, between July 25 and July 26, there were 46 new cases, 20 deaths and 4 recoveries reported. Concurrently, gardeners discovered the morning dew presented an oily appearance that adhered to the fingers, causing speculation whether this was a new quality in the dew itself or some unwholesome emanation from the plants somehow connected with an increase in cholera. By the end of the month, The Hague reported 28 cases remaining, Scheveningen, 120, and Rotterdam, 71.[13]

Reports from Vienna for the month of June indicated 654 cases of cholera and 384 deaths. The situation in July was no better; on the 17th alone, there were nearly 100 cases and 38 deaths. This was attributed to temperatures reaching 90.5°F and to the fact the Festival of St. Brigitta on July 15–16 brought many people to the city. The *British Quarterly Review* also reported that in Bassora in Asiatic Turkey, in the space of 14 days, cholera carried off between 15,000 and 18,000 inhabitants out of a population of 60,000. At Bagdad (the 19th century spelling), cholera was blamed for destroying one-third of the population.[14]

15

"I do not know who is dead
and who is alive"

The Cholera is raging in New Orleans, and is attended with more malignancy and fatality than it ever was, in any known part of the Globe, not even excepting the Jungles of India. No premonitory symptoms attend the disease. The first warning a man has, who may be in perfect health, is, that he is dying. A man a few days since, actually died standing up: He felt faint and unwell, reached a fence, which he grasped, and then died, his hands cramped to the rails, which held him up after death.[1]

The year 1833 did not start out well for the nation's capital. A case of cholera involving the family of President Andrew Jackson's stepson-in-law required two outside physicians to be called in to consult with the family physician. Unfortunately, doctors in Washington had arranged for a "tariff of charges" by which they bound themselves not to accept less than a certain rate of compensation. The consultants refused to advise the primary physician on account of his not having agreed to their compact and the patient subsequently died.[2]

The *Cincinnati Gazette* noted that during the autumn of 1832, the city lost one out of every 50 inhabitants to cholera, "a proportion greater than the *average.*" To pacify readers, the paper noted that in the higher parts of the temperate zone (a latitude of 32–34°), epidemics had not prevailed with a greater mortality a second time, making them comparatively exempt. More accurately, the Philadelphia Board of Health issued a warning to the community that cholera had a tendency to reappear in the warm season and urged them to be alert to places of possible contamination that not only included persons and clothing but also houses, yards, privies and streets. In order to avoid a recurrence of the "filth and wretchedness," they urged the destruction of all "nuisances."[3]

The major step forward in public sanitation was positive, but there was a long way to go. Already, by the opening of the western waterways, cholera had begun its insidious march. By early May, New Orleans had already reported 17 deaths over one weekend, while the steamboat *Tobacco Plant* arrived at Nashville from that city May 10 with the bodies of eight cholera victims.

Small villages in northern Virginia that, nearly three decades later, would become infamous as battlegrounds of the Civil War (and later incorporated into the new state of West Virginia), found themselves in the news as hotbeds of death and destruction from cholera. Between May 16 and May 24, twenty-nine cases of cholera were reported at Wheeling; a dispatch of May 24 from Romney indicated the disease at Wheeling (population 3,500) was so great that within 12 hours after the first case was identified, five people died. No one recovered nor did any survive more than half a day. Significantly, it was observed that cholera was "much more alarming than it was last season, because then all who had the Cholera in that place, had brought the disease with them from abroad; but now it has its origin in the place, and none of the cases can be traced to any other." By June 3, the number had risen to 127 with 67 deaths. A day later, 142 had contracted the disease.

Because medical authorities persisted in the belief cholera was a disease of bile, "recipes" for cures continued to favor treatments allaying gastric and intestinal irritation. The mayor of Wheeling advocated the anti-cholera decoction prescribed by Dr. Zollickoffer of Middleburg, Maryland. This contained 2 ounces each of cayenne pepper and laudanum and eight ounces of lime juice, taken in doses of 100 drops. Coffee, it was noted, was "incompatible with its execution."[4] If the nostrum did not work, at least residents received a good omen in early July when the martins and domestic pigeons, which had left town during the prevalence of cholera, began returning.[5]

Cholera's path along the great waterways soon became clear. Across the river, cholera struck Bridgeport with such malignity that the residents fled, prompting those from neighboring Wheeling to bury the dead. Reports later in May indicated cholera raged in St. Louis, Nashville, New Bedford, Cincinnati and St. Clairsville, while Vicksburg was "depopulated" by the disease. At Nashville, by May 28, cholera of "more than ordinary malignity" resulted in 20 cases, with 7–8 deaths. The first instance at Maysville, Kentucky, occurred on May 29 and prevailed to such an extent that by June 2 there had been 20 deaths. The city was nearly deserted and all business suspended. At Lexington, Kentucky, 37 deaths, chiefly among colored persons, were recorded between June 2 and June 6. Within a 12–day span, the death toll reached 150. By August 17, the total had reached 502: whites, 252; slaves, 184; free blacks, 48.[6]

"Painful Intelligence"

Transmission by water included more than inland rivers. The brig *Ajax* left New Orleans bound for Liberia with 150 emigrants but lost her mate and two blacks to cholera when only two days out. She was compelled to put in off Key West, where 30–40 more died. One hundred of the passengers were from Kentucky, of whom 96 were slaves who had been manumitted upon condition of their deportation to Monrovia. Forty were from Tennessee and the remainder from Ohio and Kentucky. After the *Ajax* left Key West on May 16, cholera appeared in town, nine cases proving fatal out of a population of 200.[7]

Bad news from New Orleans continued to fill national newspapers. As the disease progressed, authorities copied the supposed success at Edinburgh by discharging cannon in hopes of "agitating the air and decomposing the poisonous *miasma*." The experiment, "however doubtful," was "cheap," with the only harm stemming from carelessness and want of skill in managing the guns. During May, 435 deaths were attributed to cholera, and from June 1 to June 13, an additional 617. By June 25, there were 764 Catholics buried compared to 268 Protestants. Of these, many were from the respectable class, who were previously thought to be immune. The wealthy may indeed have lost their exempt status, but the heaviest toll continued to be "valuable negroes." Cholera spread from one plantation to another, often claiming 50–100 souls within short periods of time. As owners fled, slaves not indisposed escaped to the swamps, forced to abandon the dead and the dying, whose bodies became food for dogs and buzzards.[8]

On April 23, a correspondent from the *Portland Daily Advertiser* took a tour of two New Orleans graveyards, aptly observing that due to the high water table, those who could afford it were buried aboveground. He described one French Catholic cemetery, estimated at 5–10 acres, as having "elegant" tombs of the affluent, constructed chiefly of brick and occasionally plastered over. Measuring 2½–3 feet high, they contained an "oven hole," or front door, through which the body was slid. Weeping willows shaded some, while others had little palings for a guard; many had inscriptions.

Because the land was at ground level, during rainy days it was inundated with water, creating a swampy morass. The poor and the black population were buried in these areas, placed in graves excavated by hoe and spade to a depth not exceeding 2½ feet. The clay bottoms were of a mud-like consistency, with water reaching to within a foot of the top; when a coffin was placed into it, it floated level with the surface. The gravedigger held the casket down by standing on top while an assistant tossed in heavy clods. Rank weeds and broken boards, used as markers, littered the scene.

In the Protestant ("American") cemeteries, tombs were aboveground but badly plastered, with "little neatness, propriety or even decency. The whole is shameful." Prices were expensive, with ovens offered for sale at $60–$70. Ready-dug graves were also for sale but these were filled with water, the surrounding earth so wet mourners sank into the clay. Uncoffined bodies of cholera victims were piled in masses, around trenches or pits, awaiting mass burial as "draymen raced off [at] full gallop to the yard, so brisk was their business—and then boasted their profits."

The reporter added, "The exhalations from these ditches were insupportable. I turned from it to catch a breath of fresh air. The third ditch was filled only with water. Thank God, there was no call for it." After losing his breakfast over the sight, he left the revolting scene for his hotel, where patrons were gay, courteous and happy, "calculating on life many years yet, and large masses of wealth." Regretting that he had indulged his curiosity, he concluded: "Death loses its terrors in such a grave yard, and life its objects and allurements—for what is there worth living for—an oven—a hole of clay and dirty water! 'Bury your dead with decency. Have a fitting grave yard'—if I had the power, I would emblazon these words on every lamp post in New Orleans."[9]

Above New Orleans, the steamboat town of Natchez fared little better as cholera-infected travelers passed through on their way up and down the river. Reports dated June 21 indicated some days the disease appeared to have abated, only to return with renewed violence and fatality. During the week ending June 18, the deaths of eleven blacks and five whites were recorded. More dreaded than gamblers, "Mr. Cholera's" death spread across all the smaller intersecting rivers, laying his hand on crews as well as passengers. On June 11, the *Asinaboine* [*sic*] arrived at St. Louis from the mouth of the Yellow Stone River having lost three hands and a pilot on her upward voyage near the mouth of the Kansas. During August, the *Yellow Stone* was abandoned after eight crew members died during a voyage up the river of the same name. At the tiny river village of Galena, Illinois, 30–40 persons died of cholera between July 19 and August 18.

Nor were "estates" of the rich and powerful ignored, although attrition lay heavily on the blacks. During July, on the plantation of General Wade Hampton (located on the Mississippi a little above New Orleans), more than 700 out of 1,500 slaves perished from cholera. (This number was later amended to 700 sick and 40 deaths.) The *Natchez Journal* estimated 1,000 slaves died in Mississippi and 10,000 in Louisiana, or 8 percent of the slave population. Valuing each slave at $400, this placed the pecuniary loss of Louisiana at four million dollars.[10]

Across the Gulf of Mexico at Tampico, cholera made an unwelcome appearance. By early June, in places where the disease was described as being "very fatal, 19 vessels were unable to get pilots, several of whom had died and the rest fled. Outside the harbor, there were 10 vessels unable to get in, from the same cause." (Pilots were typically local men hired by captains to guide their ships into or out of harbors.) During a 3-day period, 275 inhabitants were said to have died out of a population of 4,000; after 17 days, the loss was estimated at 900.[11]

Fear of cholera at the "Bay" near Columbus, Georgia, prevented farmers from bringing their produce to market. In what was called a prospective panic, a near famine set in as flour reached $13/barrel and cornmeal sold at $1.25/bushel. Fear was more readily perceived in Mississippi with the death of Governor A.M. Scott from cholera and in Missouri, where Senator Alexander Buckner and his wife perished from the disease.[12]

While a somewhat humorous account of Davy Crockett stated that he "grinned" at the cholera in Nashville and the next day it abated (a play on the legend of Crockett's "killing stare"), the next line was less amusing: "It is supposed by this time that the colonel has grinned it out of Tennessee into Kentucky." Of the latter state it was written, "The present year will be long and awfully remembered ... for the 'scourge of the human race,' the mysterious and terrible cholera, has passed over most parts of the state, and, in some, decimated the people in ten or twelve days—and then retired, as if appeased with the sacrifice made!" Chickens at Frankfort, Kentucky, also displayed all the symptoms of cholera, but apparently they fared better than their human counterparts, many recovering after the administration of spirits of camphor.[13]

16

Mowed Down by Cholera

Malignantly the cholera took
Quick from him life, and healthful look;
Could Science stay this awful rod!
No! 'twas a judgment from our God![1]

Throughout the various pandemics of cholera, it was not unusual to read of deaths attributed not to physical symptoms but to mental agonies precipitated by fear. One particularly tragic fatality happened aboard the brig *Daddon*, of Swansea. When Captain William Bayley did not appear on deck, his mate went to take him tea. Receiving no response from his knock, the mate broke a pane of glass in the stateroom door and discovered the master's body a bloody corpse, he having shot himself in the head with a fowling piece. Witnesses testified that the deceased had been convinced he suffered from cholera although he would not see a doctor. The coroner's jury rendered a verdict stating death came to the victim "while in a state of temporary derangement of mind."[2]

Cholera deaths declined in Great Britain during 1833–1834, but the origin of the disease remained elusive. The Rev. W.R. Clarke, writing in the September 1833 issue of *London's Magazine of Natural History*, attributed cholera and influenza to "recent metoric phenomena, vicissitudes in the seasons, and the prevalent disorders contemporaneous, and in supposed connexion with volcanic emanations." The same argument was made in the German text *The Black Death*.[3] Further experiments in England ascertained that the weight of atmospheric air was considerably heavier during the prevalence of cholera, indicating that some heavy foreign body had been diffused through the lower regions of the atmosphere and was "in some way connected with that disease."[4]

The consumption of fish also continued to be a matter of debate. In January 1834, in the first prosecution of its kind at the Court of the King's Bench, the case of *The King v. Old the Younger* charged the defendant with selling fish in an unwholesome state and unfit for human food. Initiated by the Corporation of the City of London, the case was defended on the grounds that the offense had been committed "at a time when great alarm was excited in the public mind in consequence of the prevalence of the cholera morbus." After a guilty verdict, the defendant was charged a fine of £50.[5]

Drawing another correlation to cholera, at the January 17, 1833, meeting of the River Wandle and South Metropolitan Water Works Company, the discussion centered on a "matter of notoriety" that the parishes of Saint Savior, Saint George the Martyr, Saint Thomas, Saint John, the Borough of Southwark, Christchurch, Lambeth, Newington, Battersea, Wandsworth and others were supplied with water drawn direct from the Thames at sources between Chelsea and London Bridge and that between Chelsea and the River Lee. There were 139 common sewers in addition to "multifarious nuisances from dyehouses, gasworks, &c. which are discharged into the Thames." The report continued:

> That the odour, filth, and other impurities thus introduced each day are carried down the river by the tide and returned by the next for several days, undergoing by the operation of tides and the agitation caused by steam vessels, more minute dilution and dissemination through the waters of the river.
>
> That from evidence laid before a Committee of the House of Commons, reported 21st April, 1828, it appeared to be the opinion of medical men. derived from experiment, and of persons having the charge of numbers of the working classes, that the water taken from the Thames is highly deleterious and prejudicial to health, and that its impurity cannot by any process of filtration be so separated as to make the water a wholesome beverage.
>
> That the opinion appears to the meeting to have been strongly corroborated by the melancholy truth, that the ravages of the cholera were much more destructive in the districts above London, situate at the south side of the Thames, where Thames water alone is used, than in those on the north side, where the inhabitants have the benefit of other supplies: and likewise by the circumstances proved before the House of Commons, that salmon and other fish, which used to frequent the Thames in such abundance so as to afford a livelihood to upwards of 400 fishermen, are now very rarely seen in the river....

The meeting determined that the water of the river Wandle, which was surveyed, gauged and analyzed by chemists, proved to be a "pure unadulterated stream," more capable of affording a regular and abundant supply of "pure and soft water" to the borough of Southwark and its suburbs, inasmuch as the water was above the level of the Thames and could not be affected by tides. Members recommended a joint stock company be formed to make this water available, which they anticipated would be met with "general and increased demand."[6]

If discerning individuals preferred other beverages, the Great Wine Depot in Bath offered "Old Sherries and East India Madeiras" at auction, noting "the whole stock may confidently be stated to be Anti-Cholera."[7]

Although the Second Cholera Pandemic continued through 1849, a trend in England offered some hope for the beleaguered population.

Decline of Cholera Deaths in England, 1832–1834

1832

Month	Fatalities
July	1,006
August	777
September	607
Total	2,390

1833

Month	Fatalities
July	181
August	853
September	199
Total	1,233

1834

Month	Fatalities
July	37
August	247
September	241
Total	525

From these tables, the *Medical Gazette* concluded that cholera would continue to diminish in successive years. On an interesting side note, as Dr. Drake of Cincinnati was advocating that the bodies of persons supposed to have died of cholera be kept as long as possible for the fear they may merely have been in a state of "suspended animation" (he stating there was no danger of contagion before or after death[8]). Dr. Herisson introduced a new invention for measuring the pulse to the *Academie des Sciences*. Called the "Sphygmometre" (sphygmomanometer), it gave the numerical force of the pulse (arterial blood pressure). Dr. Herisson presented six years of research demonstrating its use in studying diseases of the heart and in determining the effects of blood-letting upon the strength of a patient. Its future use would help determine whether patients were actually dead or merely in an unresponsive state as seen in many cholera victims.[9]

In Paris, the number of cholera deaths in 1831 amounted to 18,602 but were in decline over the next three years, a circumstance attributed to "the great diminution in the consumption of different articles."[10]

Cholera in Cuba

Cholera reached Cuba toward the end of February 1833, with early reports citing 40 cases. While the "Board of Directors and Intendant" denied the disease was cholera, "they cannot deny there have been a number of sudden deaths."

Excitement over the disease quickly reached a fever pitch with mortality escalating to 100–150, primarily among the blacks. Soon, "deplorable accounts" from Havana indicated business was at a standstill and the number of fatalities had risen to 400–500. A week later, deaths among slaves were said to reach 100 per day. One editorialist sympathetically observed, "This is a great loss to their owners, but whether it is to be lamented on their own account, we know not. Perhaps, considering the wretchedness of their condition, with them 'to die is to gain.' The horrors of slavery under a tropical sun would be well exchanged even at the price of death."

Accounts received from the ship *Fan Fan* represented an appalling picture. From the 24th of February until March 24, five thousand deaths (1,000 whites and 4,000 blacks) were attributed to cholera. Nearly 500 victims were said to be buried daily. The captain general issued orders that artillery be fired at sunrise each day in hope of purifying the atmosphere, but the government kept close control over newspapers so that little official word reached the outside world.

The Cuban Board of Health at Havana prohibited the sale or distribution by apothecaries of any medicines specific for the cure of cholera, despite the offer to dispense them *gratis*, leaving the superintendents of hospitals to receive patients in the last stages of the disorder who were absolutely incurable.

A letter dated March 31 indicated deaths at Havana averaged 350–500 per day among a population estimated at 180,000, supposedly exceeding a total of 10,000, among whom was the American consul, Mr. Shaler. Because the public prints were forbidden to carry news of cholera, people in the U.S. relied on information from letters and ship captains. One report noted that, while the population of Havana within the walls was comparatively clean, the suburbs were intolerably filthy and here the mortality was greatest. Another letter dated March 31 placed cholera death tolls at 18,000.

Official Mortality List, Cuba, March 1833

March	Whites	Colored	Total
19	41	191	232
20	35	193	228
21	24	211	235
22	75	258	333
23	60	254	314
24	62	190	252
25	54	207	261

The above tally did not include five large cemeteries in which, up to March 27, as many as 3,000 had been interred. However, when the Cuban government reported cholera fatalities to Spain up to March 31, they indicated 13,435 deaths. Losses from that point until April 7 added 1,500 more, for a total of 14,935.

On April 11, the *Ariel* arrived in New York with news that cholera had spread to Matanzas (population between 10,000 and 16,000) and the brig was immediately ordered into quarantine. As of April 5, reports indicated between 200 and 250 died daily, indicating the disease, at first mild, had become extremely malignant. People died so quickly that there was no time to make coffins, and "as soon as the breath appears to be out of the body, they are thrown into a cart, prepared for the purpose, with whatever they may have on, and hurried away to 'Campo Santo'; and it has not infrequently happened that they have been buried before dead."

The governor suspended the labor of blacks in the boats and forbad the entrance of persons from the interior of the country. Further suffering was caused by the order that no launches were allowed to go up the Canimar River where most of the produce originated. A letter dated April 12 indicated two cargoes of slaves (slavery was legal in Cuba) were landed in the vicinity of Matanzas in perfect health and within days all had perished. Two months later, letters indicated that the "colored population" had literally been mowed down.

Not surprisingly, reports from Key West as of April 8 indicated cholera had been present there for about a week, prompting the removal of soldiers from the garrison to the mainland.[11]

News dated June 5 from Matanzas indicated that while cholera had nearly ceased in cities, in the country its path was "marked with desolation and ruin." On one "estate" (plantation), all 100 slaves died, while another slave ship with 400 aboard lost all but three.[12] The *Mail* (Maryland, August 9, 1833) gave official statistics from Havana and its suburbs: The total number of deaths from cholera was placed at 8,263, of whom 2,365 were white and 5,070 black. Broken down further, there were 1,450 white males and 1,029 white females; 215 male free mulattoes and 311 females; 983 male free Negroes and 1,198 females; 1,331 male Negro slaves and 909 females. Clearly, government tallies lagged behind those of eyewitnesses.

One point brought up in the hope it might lead to a useful discovery in the nature of cholera was the reported fact that although the disease occasioned great violence on sugar plantations over the Island, no cases were known to have occurred on *coffee* plantations, even when they were surrounded by sugar growers.[13]

Cholera in Mexico

After the termination of Mexico's successful war for independence against Spain in 1829, political turmoil followed. Antonio Lopez de Santa Anna was elected president on April 1, 1833, and appointed Valentin Gomez Farias as vice president. Santa Anna soon regretted his decision and forced Farias into exile. He dissolved the congress and assumed a military dictatorship. Several states, including Coahuila y Tejas (the northern part of which would later become the Republic of Texas), Yucatan, Durango and San Luis Potosi, rebelled, throwing the country into protracted war.

By the summer of 1833, cholera had reached such a height that "the whole country was but a vast field of battle," while in the state of Yucatan, "the whole population may be said to have been destroyed." While noting the accounts were "probably much exaggerated," there was great lament over "more human wretchedness and degradation than any other part of the globe."[14]

By September, cholera was so bad in Mexico City and St. Luis de Potosi that the 2,500 troops under Montezuma were obliged to relocate to safer locations. Notwithstanding, cholera depleted both the ranks of the rebels and those of the government, including Duran, the associate of Arista. Letters from the capital dated August 10 stated "nine men of a piquet of cavalry fell dead of cholera in descending from their horses." By August 27, news from Mexico City indicated cholera deaths had reached 14,000 out of a population of 180,000. At Vera Cruz up to August 30, cholera had devastated the poorer classes, although persons "in comfortable circumstances" were comparatively exempt. That would change, as 8 members of the congress, 2 judges of the supreme court and the collector of customs perished of the disease, although it was further claimed that four-fifths of the victims were female.

Statistics from a Mexican Mercantile House provided more detailed information.

Interments as a Result of Cholera in Mexico City, 1833

August	Deaths
15	533
16	611
17	1,219
18	954
19	1,165
20	1,460
21	1,100

Over the span of 35 days in September–October, cholera deaths were estimated at 22,000 in Mexico City, while at Vera Cruz, one-fourth of the population had succumbed. By November, the disease was considered less malignant, "yielding more readily to medical skill."[15]

Cholera would continue to plague Mexico, but religious rituals often sidelined medical practices. During 1846, "Our Lady of the Remedies" (a little alabaster doll purportedly given by the Virgin to Cortez to revive the valor of his soldiers after their Mexican defeat) was held by priests to stop "all contagious diseases," and was "remarkably active in times of cholera." At Mier in 1849, one ceremony to avert cholera consisted of a gaily dressed population bearing small flags marching in procession to the cathedral, where the organ was played and bells rung. Afterward, men, women and children carried candles and proceeded to the plaza, where they knelt and prayed for an exemption.[16]

Cholera Gleanings from Around the World

By the spring of 1834, great fear arose in the British Parliament over concern that Canada, its most important colony, might cast off its allegiance and seek admission into the American union. Since the opening of the shipping season, 13 vessels chiefly carrying Irish emigrants suffered a total of 600 deaths (and a loss of £3,000 in gold) from the dangers of cholera and navigating the St. Lawrence after a difficult Canadian winter. By mid–July, the malady prevailed in Quebec and Montreal, where "a considerable number of persons were dying daily." Newly arrived emigrants made up the greater number, in part because of their "free use of cold water." Newspapers soon reported, "It can no longer be doubted that this fearful scourge is now committing its ravages in various sections of the country." As the summer wore on, the *Montreal Herald* indicated that by August 15, cholera deaths numbered 816.

Between July 12 and August 5, there were 548 persons who died of cholera at Montreal; during the prior week, 222 perished. At a public meeting in October, the mayor of Quebec stated that 14,000–15,000 had perished of the disease. Mid-September news from Halifax noted that the disease continued to rage, with 440 new cases reported within the previous 10 days, causing 131 fatalities. Death, however, was not limited to those on land; the *Canadian Eagle*, carrying 300 passengers, reported 20 cases on board with 5 deaths. "The boat was in a most crowded state, and the spectacle of the dead and dying was truly shocking."[17]

In July 1833, Lisbon was reported to be suffering from cholera; carrying over into January 1834, the disease continued to rage. Many attempted to escape by boat to Abrantes, but the greater part died before they reached their destination.[18] Spain also suffered violent attacks in 1833. The citizens of Malaga were so alarmed guards were placed around the perimeter to prevent any communication with the country. In consequence, it was feared merchants would suffer a heavy financial burden as they had sent large advances for fruit that would not be permitted to enter. Despite precautions, cholera quickly made its appearance, spreading as well to Seville, Cordova, Estramadura and Grenada; in consequence, government officials quickly placed a quarantine three leagues outside Madrid, keeping travelers under quarantine for 12 days.

News continued to worsen. In Triana, the poorest suburb of Seville, deaths were reported at more than 100 per day and when the inhabitants endeavored to flee, they were driven back by bayonet, and cannons were planted to fire grape shot at them. By September 26, the number of cholera cases at Seville (with a population estimated as one-third that of New York City) reached 3,001, with new cases a day later reaching a high mark of 777. Mortality continued to climb, at times averaging as many as 300 per day.[19]

Cholera in Seville,
September 1–November 8, 1833

Ecclesiastics	67
Nuns	24
Military	157
Males	2,612
Females	3,755

From this point forward, the disease was said to have disappeared.[20] Not so in Madrid, where political unrest since the death of King Ferdinand had been usurped by news of cholera. A September report began with this: "Frightful excesses have been committed by the populace at Madrid on the bursting forth of cholera. As in Paris and elsewhere the ravages made by the disorder were believed to be the effect of poison, and it having been suggested that the monks had poisoned the wells, the mob broke into three convents, pillaged them, and massacred several of the monks."[21] In October 1834, a correspondent for the *New York Times* wrote that the number of cholera deaths had been immense: "For some days the carts loaded with the dead, piled up, without coffins, passed our house nearly all hours of the day, on their way to the burying ground outside the gate, where they were thrown into holes, hundreds together, and covered over. All was gloom."[22]

Between 8 and 16 September 1834, there were 360 new cases of cholera reported at Bilboa, Spain, with 240 deaths. On the 18th, the disease attained a lamentable intensity, reaching 90 deaths out of 105. The town was "left entirely to the undertakers and the priests," as the rich "hasten into France by land or water" and the poor sought asylum outside the city.[23]

News from Switzerland in late 1833 indicated that at Drameix, 82 cholera patients out of 157 perished, while at Christiana, 34 out of 78 perished. Late in the year at Nykoping, official accounts indicated 15 deaths for every 100 inhabitants.[24] Between July 26 and August 21 at Gottenburg, out of a population of 23,000, the dead were estimated between 2,000 and 9,000, many from the highest class. All business was suspended, leaving the few workers remaining to bury the dead. The great mortality among lower classes was attributed to unwholesome provisions and irregular modes of life. Among the entire Jewish population, only two were said to have perished. At Stockholm, the Prince Royal enacted the "ridiculous farce of walking through the wards of the hospital to encourage the sick!"[25]

17

"Times are no better, they are worse"

Guessing at Hard Words.

I am often reminded of the missionary who was ascending the Mississippi river with some religious tracts, and stepped on shore from a flat boat to accost an old lady who was knitting before a low shantee, under a tree near the river. It was in the Asiatic cholera time, and the epidemic was then in N. Orleans.

"My good woman," said the evangelist, as he offered her a tract, "have you got the GOSPEL *here?"*

"No, sir, we ha'nt," replied the old crone, "but they got it awfully down to New Orleans!" The question was a puzzle. Knickerbocker.[1]

Early 1834 reports from New Orleans indicated the disease had already appeared by February, and although the numbers were not very great, it was said to be extremely severe. On March 12, the *New Orleans Advertiser* acknowledged the continued presence of cholera, adding that it owed its origins "to the extreme filthiness of the streets." In Manchester, Mississippi, a letter dated April 20 stated that 116 cholera cases had occurred during one week on a nearby plantation, while in Louisiana, the great destruction of slaves induced the legislature to repeal their laws against their introduction from other states.

As early as March, alarming news of cholera aboard steamboats in the southern trade began appearing with regularity. By March 8, news of the disease's advancement on the Mississippi River cited the deaths of seven passengers on the steamboat *Hudson* on her passage from New Orleans to Louisville. The *Pittsburg Statesman* reported a boat left New Orleans with 60 passengers and lost 23 before arriving at Louisville. At Montgomery's Point, a detachment of U.S. troops aboard the *Philadelphia* landed with six cases among the soldiers and several among the passengers: two deaths were recorded.[2]

From Little Rock, Arkansas Territory (AT), news of April 22 indicated that over the past four weeks isolated cases of cholera had been spread by emigrants passing through the country. This was followed by news that the Cherokee, who were being transported by the U.S. Army up the river on the *Thomas Yeaman,* suffered from measles and cholera, which carried off "a good many victims." Less than a month later, soldiers at Fort Mitchell, AT, were almost totally annihilated, taking all but 15, and of those, seven were sick. Twenty-three out of 60 passengers on a steamboat also died as the disease "resumed its desolating march in the Western country."[3]

At Natchez during the first week in June, nine deaths from cholera were recorded while yellow fever raged to a considerable extent. By the third week, the *Randolph (TN) Record* wrote, "This desolating pestilence still traverses the lower part of the Mississippi. Several boats have lately passed up from Orleans, having buried from 6 to 15 passengers. The *Kentuckian* passed up last Tuesday [June 17], having buried 17, principally Dutch emigrants. The disease breaks out and confines itself most exclusively among crowded deck passengers, who neglect all necessary preparations of cleanliness, and against exposure to the burning sun and night air."[4]

In fairness to deck passengers, such "preparations" were virtually impossible. People were literally packed belowdecks and were supplied with few communal buckets meant to serve as drinking and washing water. Personal space was limited to no more than a foot or two, privacy was nonexistent, bodily waste accumulated in pails, insects were horrendous and the only food available was that which these wretched souls brought aboard. When trips lasted longer than anticipated, and most did, victuals spoiled in the heat or ran out, compelling people to beg from their fellows (as they were not permitted on the deck, where luscious banquets, gilded gaming halls and orchestras entertained the well-to-do) or purchase grossly overpriced supplies at landing sites or starve. Not only were they exposed to the fluctuations of outside temperatures, but tremendous heat from the boilers also made life intolerable, while the open end of the steamboat subjected them to killing sun, constant spray and waves, occasionally washing the unfortunates overboard. Proving no one was exempt, Captain Knowles of the steamboat *Eclipse* was attacked by cholera and died within 5 hours.

While the "real Asiatic cholera" prevailed on steam-, flat- and keelboats operating on the Mississippi and Ohio rivers, its first appearance in Cincinnati came in mid–July as it spread from Newport, opposite that city. At Fulton, located above Cincinnati, 35 deaths out of a population of 1,000 were reported in a single week. As noted by the *Baltimore Patriot*, "Times are no better, they are worse."

In normal years, the average weekly mortality in Cincinnati throughout the year was about 20. The presence of cholera raised those numbers dramatically.

Deaths in Cincinnati During the month of July

Year	Deaths
1830	74
1831	113
1832	116
1833	360
1834	300

Although 1833 was considered an epidemic year, death totals in 1834 came close to approximating it.[5]

At Beaver (outside Pittsburg), cholera was introduced by a traveler from Louisville. Unfortunately, an additional case that "went very far to prove the contagious character of Cholera" occurred when a woman observed a bundle floating in the river. Upon retrieving and opening it, she discovered bedding and a small board on which was written, "*Cholera—Beware!*" Notwithstanding, she kept the articles, contracted the disease and was a corpse within two days. Dr. Daniel Drake (a frequent newspaper contributor) warned citizens that "Malignant Cholera" could be "distinguished from the common cholera morbus and cholera infantum, with which we are familiar, by the watery discharges, the want of bile, and the absence of fever." In a succeeding edition he wrote that it was remarked on the river that cholera was constantly worse after a thunderstorm and warned persons to guard against the action of the air on the surface of their bodies in the latter part of the night.[6]

At St. Louis, cholera raged during the months of July and August 1832, but as the citizens and newspapers suppressed news of the disease to the point of "criminality," reports of fatalities could only be estimated at 5–15 per day. One visitor from Kentucky who did not anticipate the disease there visited a sick friend, became contaminated and died within a few hours: one reporter observed, "A little precaution might have saved him."[7]

By September, the presence of cholera was still felt in Ohio. Statistics included 10 cases at Newark; 67 in Cleveland (of whom all but 10 were emigrants or transients); Lower Sandusky, 15; Huron, 43; Massillon (on the canal), 12; Zoar, 15; Chester, 10. At Painesville (near Lake Erie), there were 16 deaths; New Carlisle, 24. Reports from Detroit for the summer gave a death count of 200 out of a population of 5,000. The same month, cholera prevailed on plantations along the Savannah River and was "making some progress on the Carolina side." At Randolph, Tennessee, a little town on the Mississippi a short distance from Memphis, 40 out of 350 people died within the space of several days, cholera having been introduced by a flatboat lying at the landing. The disease prevailed through December at Flemingsburg, Kentucky, which, in addition to the epidemic of 1833, carried off one-sixth of the population.

As a hint to sailors, an account was given of the frigate *Undaunted* that left Madras, India, in 1833. An epidemic of cholera broke out, quickly infecting 103 of the crew, with nine fatalities. So long as the ship was before the wind, the disease increased until the ship's surgeon recommended the captain change course and haul to the wind. This he did and the frigate was soon free from the complaint.

In an equally interesting story of how a cholera death revealed political corruption, a lawyer in Vermont named Charles Robinson died of the disease. In his effects were 40 sheets of blank paper and numerous political letters to him from various correspondents, all bearing the frank of the Hon. Mr. Plum, member of Congress from Mississippi. "Here we had a political emissary from Vermont, traveling through Ohio, with quires of letter paper franked by a member of Congress from Mississippi! This most profligate abuse of the franking privilege [free postage] deserves, and we doubt not, will receive the attention of Congress."[8]

Cholera in New York City

The board of health reported on August 9, 1834, that the first fatality from cholera that year occurred on July 23. Between that date and August 9, the total reached 14.

Deaths in NY City, August 1834

Date	Cases	Deaths
10	–	3
11	–	5
12	12	4
13	13	6
14	24	11
15	23	9
16	26	16
17	49	18
18	33	17
19	31	17
Total		**120**

Compared to the scourge of 1832 that resulted in a mortality of 1,450, these numbers were low. On July 21, 1832, there were 104 deaths reported, only 16 fewer than the entire number that died in the summer (up to August 19) of 1834. The final report from the board of health on September 17, 1834, indicated total cholera deaths for the year as 656; the city inspector gave a higher total—734. During the corresponding period of 1832, total cholera deaths numbered 3,513, or nearly five times as great, prompting the *New York Post* to comment: "This presents a view of the subject which ought to excite the most grateful feelings." The disease continued to linger, however, being responsible for 48 deaths for the second week of October.[9]

The Long Arm of Cholera

A report from the *New Orleans Bee,* May 9, 1835, stated that cholera had again made an appearance in the city, but most of the 150 deaths attributed to the disease within the past 16 days were confined to persons arriving onboard steamboats who had become intemperate and careless of diet: "many of them were but the progress of disease from dysentery to diarrhoea and death. But every fatal indisposition must now be termed cholera." Noting there was not much fear among the citizens, as cholera had proven to be noncontagious and "scarcely regarded any more than an endemic ... easily conquered by our medical practitioners,"[10] the *Bee* called for precautionary measures to be adapted to address problems associated with the levee where passengers congregated.[11] Isolated cases were reported throughout the rest of the decade but yellow fever remained the primary health concern.[12]

Cholera appeared in Memphis, Tennessee (population 2,000), in early May 1835, forcing the *Gazette* to publish only a half sheet on the 14th, as three of their journeymen were sick. The disease was considered "mild," however, yielding "so easily and readily to medicine." Four days later, however, attention turned to the explosion of the *Majestic.* Bound for St. Louis from New Orleans, the steamboat put in at Memphis. But owing to the fact so many passengers flocked to one side of the steamboat, it dangerously listed, producing a transfer of water from the starboard to the larboard boiler. Sixty persons were scalded, most of them fatally, although in this case deck passengers were believed to have entirely escaped. As an afterthought, one report indicated "thirty-four deaths by Cholera had already occurred in that ill-fated city ... and four transpired on the day of the accident."[13]

At Nashville, an interesting fact made many trade journals: of 25 deaths in the penitentiary, not one who suffered the disease two years earlier when cholera prevailed "had now been a subject of the disease." Cholera also affected the political news of the state when General Dunlap, the leading opponent of Governor Carroll, was struck down and forced to withdraw from the election. (This was supposed to ensure Carroll's reelection, but in a surprise conclusion, Col. Newton Cannon rode to victory on the grounds the former supported Van Buren for President.[14])

Reports from the *Lexington (KY) Gazette* of July 4, 1835, indicated cholera prevailed through most of the western country; at Russellville (population 600), 80 deaths were reported up to the 27th of July, indicating the town exhibited "a scene of desolation and distress, appalling to the beholder"; at Columbia, in Adair County, the disease raged "with great violence," with similar reports from Maysville. Near Bueyrus, Ohio, on the Sandusky River, 17 cases were reported, but Cleveland, St. Louis and Cincinnati were relatively free of the disease.[15]

Not insignificantly, cholera was reported at Madison, Indiana, during July. The cause was attributed "to the effluvia arising from the immense quantities of hogs which were killed there last winter, and which was permitted to remain in the yards and cellars of those who slaughtered them. We are informed that a similar neglect was practiced at Chicago, the stench arising from which is intolerable, and that the cholera was daily expected to break out there also."[16]

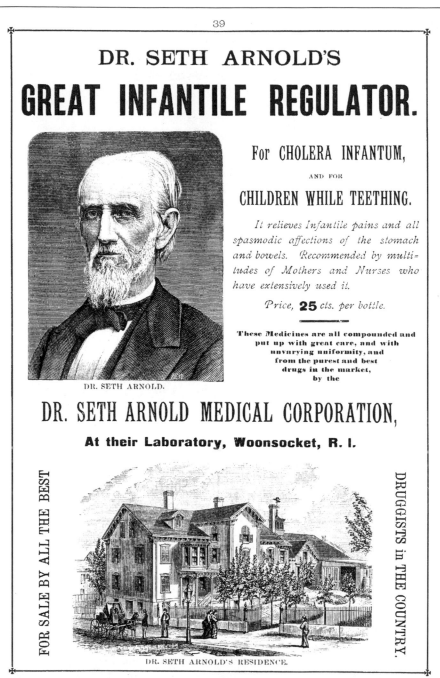

It is not surprising to see that Dr. Seth Arnold's "Regulator" combined cures for both cholera infantum and teething. Throughout most of the 1800s, both diseases were linked. Physicians believed teething brought on convulsions (mortality tables frequently listed both together), weakened the body and made young children susceptible to diarrhea and cholera. This 1881 ad featured Dr. Arnold as a stern, respectable father figure whom mothers of the era instinctively trusted. It even included an illustration of his well-kept, upper class home as proof of his success, implying the efficacy of his Regulator. Many doctors of his stature had an office in the rear or lower level of their private dwellings (from the authors' collection).

On August 1, 1835, H. Pratt, mayor of Buffalo, announced there was no cause for alarm over eight cases of cholera in the city; during the two weeks ending August 27, however, 41 deaths had been recorded. To reassure the citizens, the board of health asserted that "all these were entirely of local origin, and that the disease has not prevailed as an epidemic." Sporadic accounts for the rest of the decade occurred, but little general alarm was raised, and reports from New York City, such as the one for the third week of September 1839, listing 24 deaths from cholera infantum, were taken as the natural course of events.[17]

"No tongue could tell of the sufferings I have witnessed"

Cholera reached Charleston, South Carolina, on September 1, 1836. Between that time and the 11th, the number of deaths reached 62, of which 49 were black and 13 white. Of these it was said, "Negroes and intemperate people had been the only sufferers." During the week ending October 2, ninety-four deaths were recorded—80 blacks and 14 whites. A letter dated October 19 included the following:

> Since I have been here I have seen much misery, and much of human suffering. The loss of *property* has been immense, not only on South Santee, but also on the river. Mr. Shoolbred has lost, (according to the statement of the physician,) 46 negroes—the majority lost being the primest hands he had—bricklayers, carpenters, blacksmiths, and coopers. Mr. Wm. Mazyck has lost 35 negroes. Col. Thomas Pinckney, in the neighborhood of 40, and many other Planters, 10 to 20 on each plantation. Mrs. Elias Horry, adjoining the plantation of Mr. Lucas, has lost, up to date, 32 negroes—the best part of her primest negroes on that plantation.

Another letter placed the losses of William F. Capers of Daniel's Island at 31, noting the disease was spreading from place to place, with "bilious fever and measles" almost as destructive. The official report from the Charleston Board of Health stated that the cholera epidemic ran from August 24 through October 31, resulting in the deaths of 59 whites and 321 blacks, while on the Santee, deaths amounted to two whites and 247 blacks.

Of additional interest to slaveholders was the case of a Negro who had supposedly died of cholera. As he was being carried to the public burying ground, he displayed signs of life and by the use of "proper means" was restored to health. The man who first perceived signs of life in the slave, "and thus led to his preservation, claims the property as his own," and brought suit "for its recovery."[18]

An officer of the army, writing from Garey's Ferry, Florida, July 30, 1836, described the tragic state of affairs among the indigenous population. After remarking "the half is not known" about the prevailing sicknesses, he detailed that

> The measles broke out among them, and their insufficient shelter caused colds; death has raged among them most frightfully—80 or 90 have died within the last 5 or 6 weeks, and it is supposed that no less than 2000 are now sick with the measles, ague and fever, and the cholera morbus, the latter takes off adults as well as children.... I have today been in the huts of some 3000 to 4000 of the miserable creatures—my heart bleeds, and no tongue could tell of the sufferings I have witnessed, and the tales of woe I have heard.... The occupants of these beds were the most distressing objects I ever saw—some emaciated with the cholera morbus—some almost burning with fever—others again having taken cold with the measles, were swollen most frightfully.[19]

In another plaintive cry from Native Americans that touches on cholera, the displaced Wa-san-coo-sa band of Muncies made a claim to recover land near Rochester, New York, they had left in the care of a Quaker friend during the Revolution. Around 1836, they sent chiefs to Buffalo, but three took sick with cholera and died on the road; the others got discouraged and returned home. In 1842, poor, landless and few in number, the band appealed through Henry Harvey, superintendent of the Friends Mission among the Shawnees west of the Mississippi, to their friends the Quakers and David Evans, agent of the Holland Company, for help. The editors of the *Bangor Daily Whig & Courier* (October 4, 1843), which reprinted the plea, made no comment.

"Is This the NINETEENTH CENTURY?"

The above question was asked by the *New York Pleabian* under the opening of a brief introductory paragraph published by *Ohio's Independent Treasury*, July 20, 1842: "The *King* party in this ill-stared State [Rhode Island] are carrying on a horrible war of persecution against the suffrage party. It is horrible to reflect on—and all this, too, because the laboring people asked the right of voting at elections, and being a majority actually formed a Constitution and elected officers under it." The text from the *Pleabian* stated the following:

> The accounts of the cruelties practised by Algerines in Providence upon the suffrage men are really horrible. The Norwich News informs us, upon unquestionable authority, that fifteen of them are now confined in one cell in the Providence prison, the size of which is only 8 by 14 feet. For the want of proper food, and treatment, many of them are now sick; the cholera morbus has now broken out among them, and two inmates of the above room, Gen. Sprague and Mr. Smith, of Gloucester, died on Monday, the 4th inst. Neither of them had taken up arms against the King's Government.... Worse than the Black Hole of Calcutta! far worse than the Jersey prison ships of the revolution!

Compared to that very deliberate inhumanity, the state of medicine remained in flux. The celebrated physician, Dr. Roberts, was confident that a cure for cholera was effected by the external application of mercurial ointment and the inward administration of ice and opium, while in the chapter "Botanical or Vegetable Principles," from the text *American Practice of Medicine,* W. Beach, M.D., recommended the total abolition of metallic remedies and the rare use of blood-letting and surgical operations. A physician from Ohio warned against eating fruits, or pies made of them, and drinking freely of cold water, as these were likely to produce cholera.[20]

Into the decade of the 1840s, cholera infantum was said to be prevented by allowing children to eat as much boiled fat pork as they liked, while one apothecary promoted "Fosgate's Anodyne Cordial, a safe and efficacious remedy for *Diarrhea, Cholera Morbus, Grippings, Cholic, &c. &c.*" If that did not work, "Bour's Cordial" was recommended and if both failed, "why then, you may as well try the Doctors, for we can sell you any thing in this line."

In cases considered incurable, a new cure developed in France consisted of putting the sick person into a warm bath of very salty water. Over the course of three hours, discolored skin gradually changed every half an hour until it had resumed its former whiteness. Success was said to be achieved because warmth opened the pores, "and as the salt has the property of liquifying the coagulated blood, it causes the blood congealed in the veins to resume its ordinary course towards the heart, and thus prevents death." More tasty, the following recipe was "successful in more than one case of Cholera." The addendum said, "It may spoil practice, but it will save life":

Blackberry Cordial

To 2 quarts of juice of Blackberries, add
    1 pound of loaf sugar

½ oz. nutmegs, ½ oz. cinnamon, pulverized,
¼ oz. cloves, ¼ oz. allspice,   do [ditto].
Boil all together and when cold, add a pint of fourth proof brandy.

Dr. Bennett, professor of midwifery and the diseases of women at the Medical College of Lake Erie, stated that the tomato was a better agent than calomel, adding that "the free use of the Tomato would make a person much less liable to an attack of the Cholera, and that it would in the majority of cases prevent it." Inasmuch as a degree was not required to practice medicine and any man might call himself a doctor, the following provides an example of self-credentialing:

NOTICE
Dr. G.W. Chalmers,

From Baltimore, Maryland, offers his Professional Services to the inhabitants of Hunterstown, and the neighboring vicinity, in the

Practice of Medicine,

Surgery, and Obstetrics. Having regularly studied Medicine for 7 years—attended Lectures for 5, in the different Medical Schools—also, attended in the Infirmary, the Baltimore Hospital and the Dispensary, where from two to three thousand patients are treated annually—and having practiced on the Potomac River, contending successfully, as far as could reasonably be expected, with the Cholera, and all kinds of Bilious diseases—he thinks himself competent in his Profession, and has in possession ample testimony to witness the same.

Concerning sanitation in 1840, the idea was to "keep the air sweet," for "surely the impurities that enter the system through the respiratory organs are as pestilential as mere dirt that may adhere externally." People were advised to go into the cellar and hunt out decomposing vegetables and give the walls and ceiling a coat of white wash, as "nothing is a surer cause of cholera morbus, dysentery, and other summer complaints, than an impure cellar under the house you live in."[21]

18

Windows, Potatoes and Avatars

The King of Prussia loud doth holla—ah!
Monarchs twain, beware the cholera!
Werry glad to see you at Berlin,
But werry sorry to see you twirling
With the belly-ache, and other throes,
Which leads grim Death to tweak *your nose!*
Therefore, good kings—I say that, ergo,
'Tis right that both your visits forego.
When cholera's gone and left all Prussia,
Just then drop in and I'll make you lushy!

This rhyme, published in the always-witty *Age* (September 24, 1837), referenced the gesture by the king of Prussia towards the kings of Wirtemberg and Hanover, whom he warned not to visit him because cholera was present in his country. The gesture was surely appreciated, as the disease continued to make horrific inroads throughout the 1830s–1840s.

Italy was particularly hard hit, with epidemics breaking out across the country. Two sentences from November 1835 are enough to evoke an image of the tragedy: "The Cholera in Italy appears to be subsiding. The aggregate number of deaths at Genoa is stated at between 3000 and 4000, of which 1000 occurred in a single week."[1] Fourteen-day quarantines were established on the Roman frontier before a traveler was permitted access into Tuscany, while a similar restriction was placed on those passing from Rome to Naples. An interesting letter written by a Scottish physician in September detailed his interview with Pope Gregory XVI.

> I was next introduced as the writer of a medical work: and his Holiness said, "What, is it on cholera?" The Count [translator] answered that it was not. The Pope then said he had received about forty volumes on the cholera from different medical men; and that one was sent from Vienna the other day with a note earnestly recommending him to try the remedy it advocated, which consisted in washing the body over with oil and vinegar. His Holiness said it was not a bad receipt; but it only wanted a little salt to make a salad of him! There was no withstanding this sally; and we all became uproarious.

Carried over into 1836, by July 4, cholera invaded Austrian Lombardy, where the Pontifical Government imposed a 14-day quarantine, while the archbishop of Milan granted 100-day indulgences to those attending the sick. The same month, reports indicated Parma, Milan and Rome were affected. By November, deaths at Naples reached 140–160 per day and authorities threatened the bastinado (foot whipping) to any who exhibited fear of the disease. The *New York Evening Star* reported mortality had reached 6,000. The Festival of the Conception, December 8, was celebrated "with extraordinary solemnity" in December, as it was avowed the Virgin Mary had appeared to a clergyman of high rank, promising to see the ravages of cholera "brought to a happy termination on her fete."

The year 1837 proved no better: by April 13, the disease reappeared at Naples. From that date to June 1, there were 990 cases, with 560 deaths. On the night of June 24, Mount Vesuvius shot flames into the air, "but it had not affected the atmosphere so as to reduce the intensity of the cholera which carried off four hundred daily." Since April 13, the number of deaths was estimated at 10,000, with a malignity so great a "patient's fate was decided in 24 hours." Chaos led to uprisings and during the first week in August, a conspiracy was discovered in the Neapolitan regiments. As English ships had been reported off the coast of Sicily, "to their apparition are traced all the evils of cholera and insurrection. England is evidently the bug-bear of these poor people."

Letters from Rome to August 20 represented the inhabitants "as in the greatest terror," as the disease was within eight leagues of the city. It was written that great blame was attached to the government and the cardinals "for remaining inertly shut up during the crisis; and the common people, seeing that persons of high rank were amongst the deaths from cholera, loudly manifested their satisfaction at its impartiality."

By August 29, there were 366 new cases and 217 deaths reported in Rome. Schools and tribunals were closed but the disease invaded the Quirinal Palace and several convents, as physicians refused to treat the sick. At Palermo, 30,000 were said to have died of cholera, reducing the city of 120,000 to 90,000. So great was the mortality that bodies lay in the streets and during the 22-day period when cholera raged at its height, the town was prey to famine, pillage and assassination. Atrocities included some persons being buried alive, others being nailed up against church doors and still more being "buried in the earth up to the neck, and then pelted with stones."

At Catania, although abating in September, cholera deaths were still 80–100 per day and out of 30,000 inhabitants who remained in the city, between 6,000 and 10,000 had perished. The board of health in Rome issued new regulations displaying its belief that cholera was contagious, but German physicians, sent by the king of Bavaria and the Austrian and Prussian governments, expressed no fear, giving aid to others besides their own countrymen.

At Malta, British officers of the Fleet reported 2,025 new cases of cholera, 803 deaths and 616 recoveries for the week ending July 18, 1837, while at Palermo, cholera deaths were given as upwards of 100 per day.[2]

Advices from Pesth, Hungary, of August 10, 1836, mentioned that during the prior four months, "only from 400 to 500 persons had fallen victims" to cholera out of a population of 85,000. Cholera being considered endemic in Germany, August 1837 reports made light of the disease by observing that what few cases they had yielded to "judicious medical treatment." Cholera bulletins the next month told a different tale.

Cholera at Berlin, September 1837

Date	New Cases	Deaths
4–5	72	42
5–6	70	32
6–7	81	41

Citing statistics to November 20, the *Berlin Courant* reported cholera deaths for the previous 12 weeks totaled 1,972. By the second week in October, new cases were averaging seven per day with six deaths, and all but two cholera hospitals were closed. Unfortunately, melancholy accounts of premature burial persisted. At Hermannstadt, Trannsylvania [*sic*], one particularly gruesome story concerned Lieut. Col. Elasser, the auditor general. Upon his death from cholera he was placed in a tomb but afterward, it was ascertained an heirloom ring had been interred with him. Subsequent investigation revealed the unfortunate had turned in his coffin and devoured the flesh from his arms, through hunger, before he died a dreadful death.[3]

"Extracts from a letter, dated..."

Accounts from Algiers in mid–1835 indicated people fleeing from the scourge of cholera with the total of sick reaching 1,237 and deaths 800. All hospitals were crowded and that of Caration alone recorded 258 casualties. Official numbers placed total deaths up to September 2 as 1,200, while private letters estimated 1,800. Under the heading "Cholera in Arabia," news was given that the last caravan, "attacked by cholera at Mecca, worn down by fatigue and destitute of water, almost wholly perished. No less than 40,000 pilgrims were left behind in the desert. The dust of the desert surrounding Mecca is, in fact the dust of men."

Cholera persisted in India through the 1830s and 1840s, doing particular harm to British troops. In May 1842, two hundred men of Her Majesty's 22nd regiment stationed at Kurrache died, while in the 14 days ending May 22 in Bombay, 1,483 natives perished, for an average of 106 per day. At Koiapoor, casualties were said to reach 5,000. The following year, 130 of Her Majesty's 63rd foot soldiers and their families died within a few days. To protect his own people, the king of Delhi, "on advice of his spiritual adviser, sacrificed a buffalo, the flesh of which was exposed with vessels full of wine, sherbet and milk, on each of the towers at the three gates of the city." At Calcutta, cholera deaths for 1843 reached 4,686, while in the first four months of 1844, the total stood at 4,426.[4]

Cholera news from Central America broke on the scene in 1837, when a letter from St. Juan indicated the disease was raging on the west coast and that between May 4 and May 9, 600 persons died. Another letter dated June 25, from Guatemala, stated that in the city, 1,200 had fallen victim, while in the province, the number rose to 3,500 and at San Salvador, 4,600 died in that city and province. A correspondent from Grenada (Nicaragua) wrote on July 2, reporting cholera was committing great ravages in Leon. In St. Salvador, it destroyed 1,300 in 19 days and at Touganta, 1,200 perished within the span of 21 days.

In a sadly continuing theme, in two Indian villages near St. Salvador, the natives rose "*en masse*, and butchered many of the inhabitants, stating that the President of the Republic and others, had poisoned all the rivers to kill the poor people and deliver the country up to the English; and, as farther proof, they inquired why none of the rich died.... So general has been the idea that the waters are poisoned, that the people there (Grenada) will not drink the well water on any account." (In 19th century correspondence, "St." and "San" were frequently interchanged.)

When providing data from the West Indies, the *Journal of the London Statistical Society* (no. 7, 1838) offered the opinion that "the (N)egro race suffer to a much greater extent than white troops by epidemic cholera. When this disease made its appearance at the Bahamas, though none of the white troops died of it, there were 20 of the black troops cut off out of 62 attacked, and it ran very rapidly to a fatal termination. The same has been observed whenever the native troops in the East Indies have been attacked by this disease."

A report from 1842 indicated that at Java, in the Malay Archipelago, cholera affected not only humans but also animals: "Birds struck with it fall suddenly to the ground, and other creatures die as suddenly."[5]

The Window Tax—Excitement in Wales

In consequence of the new "Window Tax," the surveyor of assessed taxes appeared at Machynlleth, Wales, in 1840, to survey windows as suggested by the chancellor of the Exchequer in his budget. The surveyor was met with great anger, expressed at a town hall meeting. Among the resolutions proposed by Hugh Davies and H.J. Evans, Esquires, to be presented to Parliament was the following:

> That, during the fearful apprehensions of the infectious disease called the Cholera Morbus, a few years back, the public was recommended by, or in consequence of the orders in Council to avoid breathing the pestiferous atmosphere of ill-ventilated apartments; and in consequence, many persons opened windows—that on the faith of pledges given by the present, as well as past Governments, of a great reduction in taxation, rather than an increase thereof, such windows have been kept open, and are now about to be taxed.[6]

Interestingly, the same year, it was proposed to beautify Kensington Gardens by planting trees; arguments against the idea cited the 1832 report by Paris commissioners appointed to enquire into the causes of cholera, and they "reported earnestly upon the necessity of keeping extensive open spaces in populous towns."[7]

In 1850, deputations of the sanitary, philanthropical and architectural associations applied to the chancellor of the Exchequer for a repeal of the window duties on the grounds that they "operated as a direct premium for the encouragement of dirt, darkness, and defective ventilation," leading directly to the appearance and spread of cholera. Evidence was also presented on the beneficial influences of light on both plants and animals: "A tax on light could only have originated in the most profound ignorance of the physical laws."[8]

On the subject of medical insurance, the prospectus of "The Medical Invalid and General Life Insurance Company," 1843, found ready investors when they revealed the following statistic on cholera: "It has been ascertained that out of every 100 persons attacked in this country 38.5 have died; hence a company would be safe in insuring persons attacked with cholera at a premium of 45 per cent, and would reap a paying profit."[9]

"No cholera to be spoken of here!"

During one cholera epidemic a Parisian belle painted the above warning over her door.[10] As a tonic against hearing grim news it may have had its benefits, but unfortunately, the malady was usually the foremost topic in the mid–1830s. A letter from Toulon, France, dated July 6, 1835, indicated that "the violence of this dreadful scourge has been beyond all expression, and universal consternation prevails." The writer added that the roads have been crowded with fugitives driven by terror from the city, "most of whom have no means of subsistence. The disorder has already made many orphans…. The attacks of the cholera are so severe that a person who is seized in the streets falls down on the spot instantly."

Another letter, dated July 8, added that civilians were obliged to beg the military for coffins, and convicts were employed to dig the pits in the burying ground. During the day, large fires were burned, into which were thrown quantities of spices and aromatic herbs and during the night, gunpowder was exploded in hope of purifying the air. Adding to the chaos, "a species of society" formed of 200 "wretches" organized a system for plundering the houses of those who had taken their departure, while those escaping overcrowded neighboring villages brought contagion with them. Such an epidemic was not anticipated, however, as the burgeoning population of Toulon, having reached 40,000, forced intense crowding, "without the conveniences or even the necessities of life, in houses without any court yards or drains" and raised to an enormous height to accommodate the increasing numbers."[11]

Cholera also reached Versailles in July and within 24 hours there were 20 deaths, including a number of physicians. After many in Marseilles fell victim, a letter dated September 24 revealed "it will be a long time before Marseilles will be able to redeem what she has lost—the deaths some days from cholera amounted to 7[00] and 800—numbers of rich persons were buried without coffins, there not being mechanics to make them."[12]

Cold Hard Numbers

Cholera was a deadly plague destroying lives and, in some cases, wiping out entire cultures in distant lands, but in the mid–19th century, it was easy to consign this misery to cold statistics. A letter dated April 4, 1845, remarked that in Calcutta, from 500 to 600 died daily. Other statistics, from June and July, indicate the disease "had been for some time raging at Lahore, in its most terrific form. From 500 to 700 deaths occur daily, and between 20,000 and 30,000 persons had fallen." By September, "in the Punjaub it had made sad havoc, carrying off at Lahore from 500 to 600 daily." In 1846, while giving news of British troops, two bleak sentences read, "We regret to learn that cholera continues to rage with unabated violence betwix Mhow and Ahmedabad. The 22nd N.I. continues to suffer fearfully." Another supplied this: "At Kurrachee the cholera was raging with great fierceness. The number of deaths of Europeans alone on the 15th, 16th, and 17th of June, is stated to be 155, and upwards of 100 of these cases belong to Her Majesty's 86th Regiment. The natives were dying by hundreds."

Toward the end of summer, another letter reported: "The cholera is raging here—and no wonder! A hundred thousand people assembled twenty days ago for a grand native festival which only takes place once in twelve years." Many were too poor to buy food and were in a state of "dirt and filth.... The poor natives go on beating their tom-toms, or drums, all night, in hopes of driving it away; and the want of rest weakens them, and makes them still more liable to catch it." In the United States, readers were informed, "the British accounts from India, are painfully distressing. The cholera—that scourge of the human race—is sweeping all before it in Sinde. Hardy veterans, long inured to toil and fatigue, and to all 'the pride and circumstance of glorious war,' are being mowed down by thousands." After noting cholera had visited Ahmedabad since October, one correspondent's letter, dated May 1, 1837, offered his opinion that recent thunder and lightning storms had "conduced to the augmentation of cholera, which I regret to state is sweeping myriads away."[13]

Words such as "raging," "mowed down," and even "suffering fearfully," were vivid, but overuse and repetition rendered them dry and unemotional. What about the "poor natives," covered in "dirt and filth?" Who were these individual human beings whose lives were shattered? They were harder to find among the mortality tables and atmospheric conditions, but without them the soul of humanity was lost to a faceless, inscrutable destroyer.

On a voyage from Bombay to Sinde in August 1842, Captain Von Orlich accompanied Sir Charles Napier. Along the way, cholera broke out, which he described in his book, *Travels in India, Including Sinde and the Punjab*:

> One fine young woman, in the prime of life, with an infant at her breast, threw herself on the ground in an agony of pain; though already struggling with death, she would not resign her beloved babe, and before sunset the bereaved husband had committed both his treasures to the deep.... Most affect-

ing was the separation of a young woman from her husband and child only three years old; in the agonies of death she embraced both; neither would let go of the other till death had cast his dark shadow over the distorted countenance. Not less moving and painful was it to see the engineer, a fine young man, in his dying moments: he was married only two days before our departure, and implored God with tears to grant that he might expire in the arms of his beloved wife.[14]

The Avatars of Cholera

In his firsthand account of conditions in Bombay, *Notes on the Epidemic Cholera*, 1846, Hartley Kennedy, M.D., late physician-general and president of the medical board, Bombay, offered a graphic view of what doctors in the East India Company's service witnessed. Required to be a "surgeon physician, accoucheur, dentist, aurist, [and] occulist," all at the same time, these men also functioned as occasional soldiers, "cutting down some enemy with a sabre, now cutting off the hand of some friend with a penknife."

In the chapter "The Fear of Cholera," Kennedy deviated from more gruesome details of cholera to cast some amusement on the Europeans with whom he came in contact. One man had notes written to every medical officer within reach, to be delivered the instant he fancied symptoms of the disease. Another kept cauldrons boiling night and day that he might "ensure the advantage of an early recourse to the warm bath" if he became afflicted. Many others furnished themselves with medicines, keeping constantly about their person "*quantum suff.* of poison, after the old Roman fashion, only that in this case it was marked 'Cholera dose.'"

Among the natives, "superstition arrayed itself in its most disgusting and debasing attributes; religious ceremonies, rather as magical incantations than in the spirit of devotion, were every where resorted to.... The ostensible, unconcealed object of every magic rite, is to purchase for the sacrificer, not an actual release from danger, but to transfer it to some less liberal sinner,—the principle acted on being this, that the fiend of destruction needs a certain number of victims, and the supplicant cares little who suffers, so that he be permitted to escape." In the Mosaic institution of the scapegoat, a buffalo was dedicated to the spirit of the plague and turned loose in the woods. Whenever it was seen, villagers drove it away. The buffalo "was not only supposed to be accursed, and bearing the curse and punishment for the people, but the pestilence was expected wherever it was seen." The district was only relieved of the disease when the "devoted beast had been destroyed by tigers, or sank exhausted under the pitiless persecution which goaded it from village to village." Even more common were the Avatars of the fiend pestilence:

> Wretches of both sexes, who, affecting to be possessed by the demon of the plague, carried terror whithersoever they proceeded; and by their frantic gestures and language, had more the appearance of maniacs labouring under delusion, than imposters practising on the credulity of others; the more especially as avarice does not generally appear to have been the motive of their conduct, but rather the desire of notoriety, as it were, or that diseased state of mind which sometimes leads half-crazed individuals to extravagances of conduct, for no apparent object but to attract attention.

This was not to say profit was never a motive. At Severndroog, in the Southern Konkan, a band of imposters, through the love of novelty, bribery, threats or drugs, enticed a party of young girls to impersonate the demons of cholera. While they danced their way through crowds, "their brutal companions were levying contributions, as they prowled through the country." In the Island of Basseen, a poor unfortunate who was believed to be possessed by the demon of cholera was "most inhumanly butchered" by a mob and his body towed out to sea and sunk with heavy stones in deep water. Nearly 100 persons were charged and sentenced to death for the murder, "and were of course all pardoned after a short confinement."[15]

Missionaries in Ceylon reported similar rites during a frightful epidemic of cholera in 1846. The natives held a great festival in honor of the goddess of pestilence, "to propitiate her favor." The ceremonies were closed by "sending forth a scape-goat, bearing on his person the dreadful pestilence. By this means they expected to rid themselves of the terrible scourge. Some £100 has already been collected to defray the expense of this great sacrifice."[16]

The "Potato Cholera"

On October 15, 1845, the *London Nonconformist* ran a small article from Galway, mentioning a disease known as the "potato cholera." Although crops presented a healthy appearance, owing to apprehensions elsewhere prices were high for the season. There was, however, "not the slightest reason to dread a short supply."

Interestingly, a month later the *Huron Reflector* noted the new potato disease in Europe bore the name of "American potato cholera," possibly stemming from the fact that for several years the American crop suffered from rot. Another explanation, offered in May 1846, suggested that the disease was "generated from some peculiar state of the atmosphere, and of which cholera and endemical diseases in the animal system are analogous."

Optimistic reports notwithstanding, by April 1846, every part of Ireland revealed a general distress "attributed to the use of diseased potatoes." Fevers and typhus followed unemployment and a scarcity of food, quickly leading to cholera outbreaks and starvation. At Warwickshire, the entire crop failed, leading to one farmer's dire prediction: "Three months hence I doubt much if there will be a good potato in England." Roots were reduced to a pulpy mass and the smell emitting from them was "most offensive, and sufficient in low-lying marshy grounds to produce a pestilence." Rumors spread quickly that eating bad potatoes occasioned English cholera.

After replanting with seed from countries where the disease had not appeared and using different soils universally failed, attention was again turned to atmospheric conditions that destroyed the plant from the stem down. In his book, *The Preservation and Treatment of Diseases in the Potato and Other Crops*, John Parkin, M.D., argued that as the potato disease and cholera originated at the same time they sprang from the "emanation of subterranean gaseous or volcanic matters," both of which geologists proclaimed to be "yearly more and more circumscribed." Based upon his theory, Dr. Parkin recommended the use of charcoal or carbonic acid to treat humans and potato plants.[17]

On the Western Islands off Scotland, where residents were forced to eat diseased potatoes and small fish called "cuddies," near starvation led to seriously weakened health conditions. In November 1846, on South Uist, "cholera and inflammation of the intestines" became so serious the *Greenock Advertiser* called for "sympathy and aid," correcting assumptions that the destitution in the highlands and islands was "exaggerated."[18]

"I regret to say ..."

... that the cholera appears to be advancing with rapid strides" toward St. Petersburg, a letter writer penned on May 22, 1846. In what had, by this period, turned into a sad ritual, the following year the Swedish ambassador to St. Petersburg warned "the cholera is travelling on with such speed that it is now scarcely 18 miles distant from St. Petersburg, and will doubtless soon appear in the capital itself." Reports turned out to be all too true. The *Universal Russian Gazette* indicated that from November 29 to December 6, cholera attacked 231 persons in Moscow, of whom 112 died. That brought the number of cases since the beginning of the epidemic to 2,795, of whom 1,419 died.[19]

Cholera made its appearance at Aden (Arabia) in May 1846. During the few days it raged, four out of five persons attacked died, totaling 400. Mortality was also described as "fearful" along the territory of Yemen and at Mocca, Lidda, Jambo and all the coast of the Red Sea on the Arabian side; the Abyssinian coast was healthy.

By the first of August, the malady appeared at Tehran (also spelled Teheran), claiming 40 deaths per day. After one of the shah's sons died, the shah and his ministers abandoned the city for the mountains. At Bagdad, information indicated that 1,400 persons had perished by November and fears were entertained that cholera would reach Constantinople, "as it was from the same direction that the last attack came." Advices from the eastern part of Asia Minor of November 15, 1846, indicated that cholera had spread through Mossoul, Orfa, Diarbekir, Aleppo and Damascus, while at Tehran, from November 1 to 7, mortality was so great there was no time for decent burial of the dead. Mortality statistics from the larger cities indicated that at Tehran (population 60,000), between 11,000 and 17,000 perished; Kermanshah, 9,000; Ispahan, 7,000; Reschid, 3,000; Hamadan, 3,700; Mehed, 2,000; Shiras, 750. A letter from Tabriz dated November 14 stated 200 victims fell the first day.[20]

Reports from Persia were no better in 1847; by July, cholera was reported at Tiflis. From that point, it moved southward with horrific casualties, entered Azerbija, the northern province of Persia, before reaching Ooroomiah toward the end of August. It continued to spread westward from Georgia into Turkey, in the direction of Erzeroom. Of a particularly more malignant type than the previous year, the difference was attributed to the earlier season and the "almost unexampled heat of the weather in these regions during the past summer." Complicating matters, "during the present lunar month, which is the Musselman Ramadan, or annual Fast, of a month, the Mohammedans practice the most rigorous abstinence from every species of food and drink during the whole day, and indulge their appetites to repletion, and generally to great excess, during the night; an irregularity which can of course hardly fail to prepare ready subjects for disease." (This method of fasting and feasting was also cited as a predisposing cause of cholera among slaves in the United States. See chapter 20.)

Justin Perkins, the missionary supplying the above information, also noted that "devouring armies of locusts commenced their devastations" a short time before cholera appeared at Tiflis, as though they were harbingers, "ushering in the more awful judgment of cholera." He also observed "an atmospheric phenomenon attendant on the prevalence" of the disease, where an almost unheard-of thick fog covered the lowlands. "The coincidence of the presence of the disease and this dense mist is at least strikingly noticeable in this country." Perkins added that the natives were filled with "almost inconceivable consternation" over the disease they believed to be highly contagious and fired upon those who approached, from fear of contamination. The missionary himself believed that the higher elevations in India, Persia and elsewhere in the East were comparatively safer than the lower lands, likely due to the pestilential atmosphere.

In a postscript to his letter, dated September 4, Perkins wrote, "The ravages of the cholera, in the city of Ooroomiah, have been awful beyond description, during the last twenty five days. On the lowest possible estimate, though absolute accuracy is not attempted, one fifth, at least, of its population, consisting of about 25,000 souls, have been cut down during this period." Another writer from Mossul on the frontier of Persia, October 31, 1847, stated that cholera had appeared "quite unexpectedly" and carried off everyone it attacked. The pasha forbad the sale of fruit to the troops and ordered them outside of town.[21]

Letters from St. Petersburg in May 1848 indicated that cholera "had made its appearance" at Nijui-Novogorod (from April 17 to 24, there were 22 cases and 12 deaths) and Alexandroff, in the government of Wladimir (4 cases and 1 death). At Moscow, from May 23 to 29, 205 persons died out of 464 infected. The number of new cases on May 29 alone reached 89, with 42 deaths. The disease also broke out "with great intensity" at Jaroslau, Robinski, and Kalouga," and appeared to be advancing westward.

The year 1848 continued to prove to be a devastating one. Information from Bucharest in June indicated all political affairs were suspended due to the epidemic; since the seventh, 160 persons were daily attacked, while in Moscow, six hospitals were opened for cholera patients alone. Between June 11 and June 12, of 222 patients, 122 succumbed. At St. Petersburg, a letter dated June 19 indicated 800 cases per day. In a peculiarity of cholera that persisted almost from its first appearance, people (in this case the Moujiks) believed they were being poisoned and several disturbances took place against those they believed were "strewing poison over the provisions exposed for sale in the markets." The situation became so serious the emperor appeared and addressed the crowds, imploring the dissidents to obey the law and report suspicious activity.[22]

Cholera at St. Petersburg, 1848

Date	Total Cases	Fresh Cases	Recovered	Died
July 23	–	153	174	109
July 24	2,986	–	–	–
July 26	2,540	185	258	84[23]

The *Guardian* published a strange report, written by a partner in a Manchester firm from St. Petersburg, stating "a very important discovery has been made here very recently, which clearly proves that the malady is in the air, and that, therefore, quarantines are utterly useless. The air here has had a very singular effect on the magnetic power. Whilst the cholera was at its height, the action of the magnet was nearly neutralized; which, now the disease is gradually subsiding, assumed by degrees its former power. A magnet block, which used to carry 80lb., would, during the worst time of the crisis, not carry above 13lb. Its strength has now increased again to 60lb. The electromagnetic telegraph, at one time, would not work at all."

On an equally peculiar subject, Dr. Andreosky, physician to the Russian forces in Circassia, advocated the use of Elixir of Woronege, an anti-cholera preparation containing naphtha. The dose was 10–20 drops in a glass of wine. The naphtha recommended was not the type ordinarily sold in shops, but the mineral naphtha obtained from Beker, on the shores of the Caspian. "It should be of a white or rose color, and used without previously undergoing the process of distillation." Although the doctor claimed great success in curing cholera, large or repeated doses were likely poisonous.[24]

19

Health and Sanitation

Every person who values health ought to avoid reading Medical books. As Courts tempt men into litigation, so do Medical books persuade them that they are sick and need the doctor. Any body who will sit down and read about "symptoms," will be sure to feel some of the symptoms. Thus fear is aroused, nostrums are resorted to, and imaginary evils become real ones.... When the Asiatic cholera prevailed in our country, hundreds of people were scared to death by it, and hundreds more were killed by camphor, calomel and other powerful medicines taken as preventatives.[1]

In April 1846, English newspapers warned that the "destructive scourge of humanity seems once more on its way to ravage the continent of Europe, originating, as before, in the heart of Asia.... The line of route taken by it appears to be almost due west, northern Persia being the first quarter in which it was noticed." In December 1846, it was observed "the cholera is pursuing its march towards Europe.... The cholera is approaching the Black Sea by the road taken by the caravans, whilst it ascends, in another direction, the banks of the Euphrates and the Tigris, shaping its course toward Syria. Europe, therefore, is menaced on two sides." In November 1847, news was provided that "its march is no longer the same, as it moves from north to east, and very slowly, being the contrary of what occurred in 1831 and 1832."[2]

In a multipart series, "Health and Its Preservation," T.H. Yeoman, M.D., wrote of cholera: "We know little more of its cause or origin than that it is a 'travelling disease,' or one which appears over enormous surfaces of the earth, in a succession of periods, from a certain point; that its advent can be retarded by no human means hitherto discovered; but that it may be modified in severity by certain measures which are under our own direction and control."

Writing that pure air was essential to existence, Yeoman pointed out the danger of living too close to cemeteries where poison exhalations arising from shallow graves were deadly. He urged citizens to remove filth from channels and gutters without depending on the scavenger's cart and advocated sprinkling a solution of chlorine in dark and damp cellars. Deviating from accepted norm, he was also opposed to the use of flannel, inasmuch as it absorbed perspiration but did not allow it to evaporate.[3]

Possibly Yeoman based his theory on exhalations from an incident in Sheffield. The people there suffered greatly from cholera in 1832 and buried the victims in plots set aside for their special interment. Thirteen years later, some children from the workhouse visited the monument erected "to mark the spot for future ages," but immediately afterward a 12-year-old boy named Taylor fell ill and died. Within days, six others were taken ill and diagnosed with cholera. With no other explanation, blame was placed on grounds-keeping work that may have opened fissures through which contagion was emitted.[4]

On the subject of pure air, the Scientific Repository advertised their "Hermetically Sealed

Inodorous Chamber Pails," which would "render the sick room at all times as sweet as a well-appointed sitting room."[5]

Health in the Metropolis: London

Newspapers continued to report outbreaks of cholera in the mid–1840s, but no great panics occurred in London. When attempting to anticipate what the future held for 1848, Lord Morpeth stated that the act of 1832 for the prevention of cholera was in force, and that the act "would enable the Queen, on the least alarm of the cholera, to issue a proclamation for the establishment of boards of health, and it was now under special consideration whether the proclamation issued the last time could be advantageously modified or altered in any respect."[6]

Registrar-General's Returns, 1848
Zymotic, Epidemic, or Endemic Diseases

Date (Week Ending)		Total	Weekly Average (derived from deaths of 1843–1847)
April	2	252	176
	20	238	176
May	6	271	271
	13	263	271
	20	269	176
	27	286	176
June	3	278	176
	10	294	176
	17	289	176
	24	310	176
July	1	347	176
	8	338	257
	15	319	257
	22	390	257
	29	505	257
Total		4,649	3,154

Excess in 15 weeks, 1,495

Cause of death	Week Ending July 22	Week Ending July 29	Weekly Average of 5 summers
Diarrhea	94	173	66
Cholera	21	26	7

Deaths from excess of diarrhea in the last two weeks: 135
Deaths from excess of cholera in the last two weeks: 33[7]

For the week ending August 5, deaths from diarrhea were 141, more than double the average; deaths from cholera, in all its varieties ("cholera infantum, English cholera, cholera endemica, spasmodic cholera and English cholera") were 21. The following week, deaths from diarrhea were 110 (average 66), dysentery 18 (average 7), cholera 19 (average 7). Of the cholera deaths, none were ascribed to "Asiatic cholera," six were diagnosed as "cholera morbus," and the remainder as "English cholera, or cholera infantum."[8]

In the event matters worsened, the *Benbow* and *Devonshire,* two old battleships, were prepared as cholera hospitals, with the *Iphigenia* outfitted should necessity require immediate accommodation.[9]

Laboratories of Pestilence

The worldwide Second Cholera Pandemic drew to a close in 1849. During these twenty years when cholera ran rampant, great strides had been made in public sanitation; but the origin of the disease remained obscure, while vitriolic controversy continued over whether the disease was contagious. Emphasis remained focused on the state of the atmosphere, although scientists had finally begun to factor in overcrowding and the general filth of cities as major contributors.

In 1839, Jordan R. Lynch, M.D., member of the Royal College of Surgeons, London, and medical officer of the West London Union, published a thesis in the *Lancet,* detailing conditions in his district. Over this single square mile, 186,046 inhabitants lived in "the most dirty, narrow, and ill-ventilated lanes and labyrinths of alleys in the city of London, and which are the constant sources of disease and infection—laboratories of pestilence—extending from the Fleet-ditch through Long-lane to Aldersgate-street," including the parishes of Sr. Bartholomew and St. Sepulchre. In perhaps no other paper are conditions better described, nor political and medical science represented:

> There is one alley, Back Bear, running from the Old Bailey to Farringdon street, near which it terminates in a *cul de sac,* and through which there is no perflation, and where two persons cannot walk abreast, and lying below the level of the former upwards of 40 feet, into which place a large mass of life is impacted, every little room containing a family of the poorest and humblest description, and opposite the doors of whom, the offal and ejecture constantly left exposed, and undergoing decomposition, to prevent which no vigilance, no interference, is sufficiently active.

There were laws to correct such nuisances, to be sure, but "they have altogether failed."

> Their reduction to practice is, in the first instance, entrusted to an inquest, composed of tradesmen, who have no idea of the methods calculated to preserve health; men engaged in their business, and in the pursuit of commerce, having little time and less capacity to undertake such an important duty; and, in the next place, the evil, when ascertained, is only remediable at a distant date, by a presentment to the Court of Aldermen, who are too indolent to direct or institute the necessary means of prevention.

To the above, Dr. Lynch exempted the commission of sewers, "who seem deeply alive to the importance of good drainage, and also their excellent and intelligent surveyor, Mr. Kelsey." During the time when cholera and typhus raged, "the localities where the sewers were good were comparatively exempt from attack," but where drainage was deficient, disease was prevalent.

In berating the medical community concerning their ideas of typhus and cholera (the similarity of symptoms and attack "being obvious"), Lynch wrote:

> It is strange that, when the pathognomonic symptoms are so unerring, presenting so uniform a train of phenomena, such distinct and unequivical characteristics, sufficient to cancel hesitation, and to distinguish it from every other in the catalogue of ills "that flesh is heir to," that "the abelest hands and wisest heads" have differed as to the nature, cause, origin, treatment, history, and physiology of this complaint; one refers to it as inflammation of the brain, another to the digestive organs and alimentary canal! One calls with confidence upon pathology, as a confirmation strong of the doctrines which they support; another mocks it as fallacious.
>
> The talent of generalization, or the bump which some men possess [phrenology], when too much developed and abused, has led some enterprising minds to maintain that there is no such thing as essential or idiopathic fever as a general disturbance of the system, independent of local affection, but that all diseases are the consequence of local irritation, disorder, or inflammation. Some deny its

existence altogether; some describe it as a lesion of the nervous system, of the glands of Peyer, of the mucus membranes, of the mesenteric glands; another describes it as the result of animal electricity; another of atmospheric electricity, of the changes in the composition thereof, or of poisons contained therein.

In an excellent summary of the state of the art as it was known in 1839, Lynch discussed the lectures of Francois Magendie (1783–1855), in the College of France, who proved the separation of the serum from the crassamentum of the blood: "The deficiency of water and saline matter was remarked by all who made an examination of the bodies of those who died of cholera." After remarking on the contributions of O'Shaughnessy, Latta and Clanny (see chapter 12), he described Dr. William Stevens' work on yellow fever. Discovering the blood from victims of that malady was always black and "wanting in saline matter," Stevens used tartrate and carbonate of soda ("neutral salts with earthly bases") to treat his patients. Preceding the administration with bleeding, he claimed that out of 343 cases in Trinidad, none were lost.

Believing cholera and typhus to be "effects of the same cause, the latter modified in intensity and in degree by circumstances," Lynch employed common salt with muriatic acid in large quantities of cold spring water "with the most extraordinary success." In three cases he "injected into the venous system the artificial serum of the blood, or its watery part, according to the analysis of Berzelius [Jons Jacob Berzelius, 1779–1848, a Swedish chemist who separated the red material found in blood into a protein called "globin" and a colored compound that he named "hematin," later called "hemoglobin"][10] with the albumen superadded, as suggested by Magendie, to assist the fluid when injected to permeate the capillary system." In two cases out of three the treatment worked; in another patient, "her youth deterred me from making the experiment of the injection."[11]

Debate continued. During the first week of August 1846, twenty-three persons died of cholera, "but it is right to mention that this was English, not Asiatic cholera,"[12] a distinction of little merit. Cholera at Whitehaven in 1845 was attributed to the presence of a large dunghill. Aboard the *Anne Simple*, a ship out of Liverpool lying in port at Honan's Quay, Limerick, several crewmen died. Some alleged cholera as the cause while others asserted poison; more argued their deaths were in consequence of drinking water "which was impregnated with gas tar, which flowed from the cisterns of the gas company into the river at Arthur's quay." In 1846, the registrar-general's report indicated "many thousands were carried off by disease arising from inadequate supplies of water, imperfect sewerage in towns, the open drains and ditches, and the general neglect of cleanliness."[13] While "we have also to thank Cholera for our Public Health Act, which certainly would have remained in the limbo of ministerial good intentions but for its proximity on the continent of Europe,"[14] attention remained on miasma "ascending from the cesspool, called the street-drain, through the sinkhole in that 'sweet back kitchen,' and infecting the air of the whole house."[15]

The Peculiar Case of the Cholera Cabbage

In perhaps one of the most bizarre stories concerning cholera and drinking water, it was reported that at the North Side of the old church of St. Mary, Redcliffe, a portion of land was torn up for the opening of a new street. This property had been used as a burial ground for paupers and cholera victims around 1833. A large quantity of consecrated earth, exceeding 100 tons, was carted away and "pitched down behind a Wesleyan Chapel on the Somersetshire side of the River, in all its holiness and rottonness." Here, amid the "offensiveness of the exhalations," the whole being filled "with animal matter and bones—human remains," the ground was dedicated to raising cabbage plants. "Yes, there they stand, in rows;—flourishing in the remains of the victims of cholera."

The correspondent speculated the enterprise was done for profit, as the vegetables "thrived on the fatness of the soil, and they go readily enough with those who, it is to be presumed, are not aware of the locality in which they are reared. But in the neighbourhood they have arisen to the dignity of a new variety, known as the Cholera Cabbage plant," and many wondered who the profiteers were.

The investigative reporter speculated an undertaker was "engaged insidiously in propagating Cholera through the eating of Cabbages," and suggested the vestry of the parish be required to test the quality of the new variety by eating no less than one plant, to be served at their next dinner. Complicating matters, the parish had a water pipe endowed with property, "which, if let at rack rents, would produce nearly £700 a year; but, upon the system of beneficial leases, does not produce a half that sum." Locals were refused use of this pump, being obliged to draw from a "very uncertain" source, compelling them to go considerable distances and sometimes to even pay for their supply. While the feoffees (trustees invested with a freehold estate to hold in possession for a charitable purpose[16]) made use of water of which "there is no mistake in its quality or its quantity," the poor attempted to fill pitchers from the parish cock (stopcock; handle; pump), which dripped "at a rate of three drops a minute," or they turned away when discovering the spout entirely dry.[17]

Cholera in Great Britain, 1848–1849

The years from 1846 until the end of the decade were spent introducing bills on sanitation and sewers into Parliament, writing amendments, arguing over cost and debating under whose control boards of health should operate. Primary among these was the "Health of Towns Act" (1847) introduced by Lord Morpeth, with the purpose "to remedy what they could, and mitigate what they could not entirely remove."[18] The sanitary commissioners, in their third report (1848), espoused the public sentiment: "past all doubting, that human subjects are easily enough killed off by bad smells. This, however great the ridicule which would have been created by the assertion a few years ago, is now generally believed; and a great thing it is that our faith has been directed into so useful a channel."[19] Indeed, comparing the epidemic of 1832 with Paris (where cholera slew 15,000 people, whereas the city of London did not reach "one-tenth part of that number"), the *Times* proclaimed the "modification was caused by the different habits and food of our population, by the superior draining and ventilation even of our ill-drained and ill-ventilated courts, and, above all, by the greater promptitude, energy, and devotion which was displayed in arresting the incipient progress of the disease."[20] This apparently did not apply to the combined parishes of St. Andrew, Holborn-above-bars and St. George-the-Martyr (combined population 43,600), all of which determined to resist the introduction of public baths and washhouses for the laboring poor.[21]

In October 1848, the General Board of Health warned guardians of the poor and parochial boards that they would be called to enforce the "Nuisances Removal and Diseases prevention act, 1848, 11th and 12th Victoria, c. cxxiii." After reiterating that cholera was not contagious, the Act stipulated that boards abide by the following:

THE MOST CERTAIN PREVENTION of CHOLERA YET DISCOVERED. — FURTHER GREAT REDUCTION IN PRICE.—CREWS'S DISINFECTING FLUID is the best and cheapest.—The IMPROVED CHLORIDE OF ZINC for the purification of dwelling-houses, stables, dog-kennels, ships' holds, cesspools, drains, water closets, &c.; the disinfection of sick rooms, clothing, linen, and for the prevention of contagion. The extraordinary power of this disinfecting and purifying agent is now acknowledged, and its use recommended by the College of Physicians. Unlike the action of many other disinfectants, it destroys all noxious smells, and is itself scentless. The manufacturer having destroyed a monopoly fostered by the false assumption of the title of a patent, has to warn the public against all spurious imitations. Each bottle of Crews's Disinfecting Fluid contains a densely concentrated solution of chloride of zinc, which may be diluted for use with 200 times its bulk of water. Vide instructions accompanying each bottle. It is sold by all chemists and shipping agents in the United Kingdom, in imperial quarts, at 2s.; in pints, at 1s.; half-pints, at 6d.; and in larger vessels at 5s. per gallon.—Agents, Messrs. DREW, HEYWARD, and BARRON, Bush-lane, Cannon-street. Manufactured at H. G. GRAY'S, Commercial-wharf, Mile-end, London.

"The most certain," "improved," "extraordinary power," "recommended by the College of Physicians" and equally important, "further great reduction in price": Who could resist such a pitch? Manufacturers battled one another as certainly as they fought for customers by guaranteeing their product to be the best on the market (*London Daily News*, November 19, 1853).

1. Provide dispensaries operating around the clock with sufficient medical aid to treat cholera patients.
2. Distribute notices stating where dispensaries were located.
3. Provide accommodation for cholera patients who could not be properly treated in their own homes.
4. Provide houses of refuge to families removed from their homes as deemed necessary by medical authority.
5. Provide frequent visitations throughout the parish(s) to investigate their liability to contagious, epidemic or endemic diseases.
6. Apply such medical aid as might appear requisite.
7. Send affected persons to the nearest dispensary.
8. Report daily lists of cholera victims.
9. Provide additional medical officers as necessary.[22]

By October, cholera mortality lists reappeared in the newspapers, prompting the College of Physicians to publish an "important circular":

1. Cholera was very rarely communicated by personal intercourse; quarantine had failed to stay its progress.
2. The disease was most destructive in the dampest and filthiest parts of town.
3. Debility or exhaustion produced increased liability.

4. The public should not abstain from the moderate use of well-cooked green vegetables or unripe, preserved fruits, pork, bacon, or salted, dried or smoked fish.

The circular concluded with the statement that the committee was "unable to recommend an universal plan of treatment" and called upon the rich, "who have comparatively little to fear for themselves," to aid the poor.[23]

As of November 14, 1848, cholera cases stood at 1,015, of which 509 had proved fatal. Of these, 303 occurred in London, 70 in the provinces and 642 in Scotland. The numbers were destined to increase rapidly. For the week ending November 22, the total number of cases had risen to 1,245, and by December 5, it had reached 1,691, with 797 fatalities. By December 28, the registrar-general reported a total of 3,890 cases, with 1,854 deaths.[24]

Deaths in the Metropolis Per Week, 1849

Month		Cholera Deaths
January	6	61
	13	94
	20	62
	27	45
February	3	37
	10	55
	17	49
	24	40
March	3	35
	10	15
June	9	22
	16	42
	23	49
	30	124
July	7	152
	14	339
	21	678
	28	783
August	4	926
	11	823
	18	1,230 (188 from diarrhea)
	25	1,276
September	1	1,663 (234 from diarrhea)
	8	2,026
	15	1,682
	22	839
	29	434
October	6	288
	13	110 (91 from diarrhea)
	20	41
	27	25
November	3	63 (8 from diarrhea)[25]

In 1849, London was divided into 36 districts for registration purposes; districts were divided into 135 sub-districts. Dividing deaths from cholera in the 13 weeks ending September 15, it was estimated that 53 in 10,000 perished from cholera. From all causes, mortality was 116, an annual rate equivalent to 4.64 percent. On the south side of the Thames, 104 of 10,000 died of cholera, three times greater than on the north side.[26]

Scotland was particularly hard hit, recording 10,226 cases, 4,424 deaths and 3,300 recoveries by February 17, 1849. Returns from February 24 indicated a total of 10,759 cases, 4,686 deaths and 3,633 recoveries. By September 1, deaths had been drastically reduced, to 132 per week.[27]

Treatment of the Casual Poor—The Tooting Scandal

An article published in the *Daily News,* under the heading "Seed-Bed of Crime," began:

Thousands of children between seven years and fourteen crowd the streets of London, samples of them turn up in plenty at all our Ragged-schools, who are either orphans, foundlings, or the children of criminal parents, who have deserted them or been removed from the country by force; these know no friends and have no occupation. They live on the *pave* [pavement], and sleep in the gutters. A doorway is a luxury which is denied to them by a vigilant police. As to employment, they sell matches, fusees, tapes, fruit, and so forth in the streets, or hold horses and sweep the steps of omnibuses." In a report of cholera deaths was the following: "M. (eleven years of age), parent unknown, a casual pauper, cholera, nine hours, Sept. 9th. Taken in from Orange-street, *half-starved, stomach full of blackberries.*" How tragic in its brevity! Truly a "powerfully written" volume in a sentence.[28]

On December 8, 1848, an inquest was held in the "board-room" of the Chelsea workhouse upon the body of W. Jones, aged 20. According to the testimony of J. Parrot, nurse, the youth came to the workhouse infirmary in a very low state, suffering from severe vomiting and purging. Jones said before his admission to the casual ward he had not tasted food. He was given four ounces of bread and a drink of water from the common pail, which was standard issue, twice a day (as opposed to half a pound of bread and a quarter pound of cheese at night and half a pound of bread and butter and a pint of coffee in the morning at the police ward). The coroner stated that on the night Jones died, 31 men and two boys slept in the casual ward on a sloping board, 31 feet long and 6 feet, 4 inches wide. They had loose straw to sleep on, which was changed every fortnight and every two persons had one rug to cover them. The verdict was "natural death from cholera," with a request to the board of guardians to apply more effectual means of relief for cholera patients.[29]

One of the most infamous cases of cholera outbreaks at a pauper asylum concerned that at Tooting. After 189 cases were reported, Mr. Grainger, medical inspector, discovered an open, stagnant ditch which passed along the rear of the grounds and to the nuisances arising from the Surrey Lunatic Asylum, a quarter of a mile northeast of the establishment. It was recommended that Mr. Drouet, operator of the Juvenile Pauper Asylum, secure the services of a resident physician and that dead bodies be interred within 24 hours "and not kept for removal by the respective parishes to which the children belonged." At the same time, the inspectors begged "to express their sincere commiseration for the painful and anxious situation in which Mr. Drouet is placed, and hope this fearful visitation will shortly subside."[30]

By January 8, there were 241 cases of supposed cholera reported, with 168 under medical treatment; between 600 and 700 children were removed to workhouses of their respective parishes. A formal inquest, beginning January 12, 1849, was held over the deaths of four children; numerous experts who visited the establishment before and after the tragedies were brought forth to testify. Dr. Grainger remarked that rooms were 16 feet long, 12 wide and less than 8 feet high. In one room there were 5 beds occupied by 11 children, all ill with cholera. In another room, where 18 beds were tightly packed together, 35 boys were ill with cholera, while on the girls' side, one male nurse was responsible for several wards. The breathable air was calculated to be only 136 feet to each child, or the equivalent of that contained in a box 5 feet by 2 inches square, "sufficient to destroy life."

As background, it was stated that paupers in large numbers, both children and adults, were placed by their parishes in such "farming" establishments, where they were "dieted and housed at so much per head." Under the 4th and 5th William IV, chapter 76, the "Poor Law Commissioners" had no positive authority over pauper establishments and the management, not being considered paid officers, could not be subject to liabilities imposed by the act.

Mr. Cochrane deposed that in one "farming establishment" the male casual poor slept three in a bed, in a state of nudity, compelled to wash hands and faces—from 50–60 in number—in two buckets of water that was not changed during the day. At Marlborough House, Peckham, one bucket of water containing soft soap and soda and another of plain water was provided, being changed twice a week; one jack towel, 3–4 yards long, was used for drying.

Most parents were not allowed to visit their sick children at Tooting; those who did were discouraged from walking outside with them for fear the children would run away. To discourage this, boys were sometimes required to wear girls' clothing. Numerous children were brought to testify; comments such as "could not say the whole catechism" or "could not read" were common. All testified they did not have enough to eat, being served a pint of gruel and a slice of bread for breakfast; boys and girls who complained were beaten. Mr. Winch, a member of the Holborn Board of Guardians who had toured the facility on May 9, 1848, testified that the children all stood for meals. He cut up 100 potatoes, all of which were "positively black and diseased." Drouet complained they cost him £7 a ton and he became violent when Winch asked questions of the children, stating that his word on conditions ought to be good enough. A subsequent investigation revealed conditions substantially improved, causing Winch to dryly observe, "There is a peculiarity about our board that if one set of guardians report unfavourably, the next are sure to report the contrary."

The cost to Drouet of maintaining the 1,372 children at his pauper infant establishment, including clothing, was 3s. 1d. per week, per child, occasionally reaching a low of 2s. 6½d., for which he was paid 4s. 6d. per week, per child, by the various parishes, making the enterprise significantly profitable. In addition, children under his care were variously employed in tailoring, shoemaking and garden work.

On January 27, 1849, it was reported that "we, the jury impanelled to inquire touching the death of James Andrews, unanimously agree to the following verdict—that Bartholomew Peter Drouet is guilty of manslaughter." A similar verdict was returned in the cases of the other deceased children, Johnston, Quin and Harper. The jurors added that the guardians of the Holborn Union acted "most negligently in their engagements with Mr. Drouet, and also in their visits to his establishment," but singled Mr. Winch as deserving credit for having brought the case to the notice of the coroner. Ironically, cholera was not cited as having caused their deaths as the medical experts could not agree, many holding to the belief atmospheric conditions were the predisposing cause.[31]

"Mortality occasioned by cholera": France, 1849

The first week of June 1849 saw cases of cholera increasing; by the tenth, 208 new cases were reported, with 119 deaths. In the neighborhood of Paris and Batignolles, the malady was particularly severe. The whole number of cholera patients since the commencement of the epidemic exceeded 700, prompting the municipal administration to solicit private funds for the families of victims. During the last week of August, deaths averaged 43 per day and during the first week of September, the number reached 68. Between September 4 and September 6 alone, 152 out of 154 stricken individuals died, making a total of 10,509 deaths for the year. Coinciding with a drop in temperature, by the 16th, new cases had dropped sharply and by the end of the month, the epidemic was considered at an end.[32]

The Animalcular and the Fungoid Theories of Cholera

Since the first outbreak amongst us of the mysterious epidemic, now, for the second time, spreading apprehension and mourning over Europe, we have had so many speculations, so many theoretical explanations of its nature, cause, and effect, which, from want of substantial proof, have, one after another, fallen to the ground, that the announcement of any actually demonstrative facts in regard to it is calculated to excite unusual attention and interest.[1]

The year 1849 was destined to be the "Year of the Cholera" in Great Britain. The first week of January, the number of deaths was 1,131, or 38 below the average of 5 years. In June, mortality was down to 895, or 68 below average, but numbers rapidly escalated. By the second week in September, the number of deaths registered from all causes was 3,183, or 2,175 over average, with 2,026 attributed to cholera. From the week ending July 7 to the last week of the year, no fewer than 13,321 perished from the disease.

The total number of deaths for 1849 was 68,432, an excess over 1848 of 10,533. Of these, 34,032 were male and 34,400 were female—368 more females than males. In 1848, there were 1,201 deaths in males over females. The number of births was 36,910 males and 35,120 females.

Comparison of Deaths by Age, 1848–1849

Age	1848	1849	Excess of Deaths
0–15 years	28,423	29,978	1,555
15–60	18,663	25,091	6,428
60 upward	10,385	12,979	2,594[2]

Amid the staggering losses caused by cholera, research of a "novel and most important character" emerged through microscopic investigation. The September 23, 1849, edition of *Bell's Life in London and Sporting Chronicle* printed an article concerning the findings of Mr. Brittan, lecturer on anatomy and physiology at the Bristol Medical School. In conjunction with Mr. J.G. Swayne, he observed "the constant occurrence of certain peculiar bodies, hitherto undescribed, as characteristic constituents of cholera evacuations; and, by a furthermore series of experiments, he has succeeded in demonstrating the important discovery of similar bodies in the atmosphere of districts infested with cholera." Eminent "microscopial pathologists" urged Brittan to give them immediate publicity.

Five days later, the *Christian Times* ran the findings of Dr. William Budd, who asserted that "organisms in large numbers infest the drinking water and the air of infected districts. This led him to examine the water from healthy quarters, and "although he found in it a good deal of matter of various kinds, organic and other, in no single instance did he see anything resembling the peculiar bodies in question. He concluded the following:

1. The cause of malignant cholera is a living organism of distinct species.

2. This organism, which seemed to be of the fungus tribe, is taken, by the act of swallowing, into the intestinal canal, and there becomes infinitely multiplied by the self-propagation which is characteristic of living beings.

3. The presence and propagation of these organisms in the intestinal canal and the action they exert, are the cause of the peculiar flux characteristic of malignant cholera, and which, taken with its consequences, immediate and remote, constitutes the disease.

4. The new organisms are developed only in the human intestine.

5. These organisms are disseminated through society, first in the air, in the form of impalpable particles; second, in contact with articles of food; and last, and principally, in the drinking water of infected places.

6. These organisms may probably be preserved for a long time in the air with powers unimpaired; but that in water, which is doubtless the chief vehicle for their diffusion, they soon undergo decay, and moreover—sharing in this the common fate of their tribe—become the prey of beings of a higher order.

Budd's conclusions, taken together, accounted for "all the chief phenomena of the disease" by revealing what happened "as the direct consequence of such conditions." Of more significance, it was hypothesized that if the human intestine was the only breeding place of the poison, and that if it was transmitted from persons affected with the disease, if the poison had been destroyed ("and the destruction of it may doubtless be accomplished by simple means"), malignant cholera would never have been epidemic in England.

The obvious means to "stay the plague" included two actions: to destroy the poison generated by the bodies of infected persons, and prevent, as far as possible, the poison that had already escaped from taking effect. The first initiative was to collect the discharges of the sick "into some chymical fluid known to be fatal to beings of the fungus tribe." Budd's evidence was placed in the hands of the president of the College of Physicians for publication.

In light of the important implications, Mr. Brittan published a paper on his microscopial investigations in the *Medical Times*. He stated that on July 8, 1849, he and J.G. Swayne, a fellow member of a subcommittee appointed by the Bristol Medico-Chirurgical Society, studied two specimens of rice-water feces, and on comparing the drawings they made of them, identified certain bodies depicted in each. Further investigation from July 9–July 30 found these bodies to be present in the rice-water evacuations of cholera patients, "offering the same characteristic appearance that distinguished them from anything" before observed. He became convinced that "a certain relation does exist between the size and number of these bodies, and the time elapsed after the seizure, taken in connexion with the severity of the symptoms. That is to say, they are small and clearly defined in the matter vomited, they become larger and more compound in the dejections; and as the disease progresses favourably ... they vanish as the symptoms disappear, and the motions [bowel movements] regain their natural appearance."

When compared to healthy patients, the researchers were unable to find any of what they called "annular bodies," leading them to consider they were "essentially connected with cholera." (Swayne's studies, made at the cholera hospital Bridewell, were done independently, beginning August 2, and confirmed Brittan's findings.) In determining whether the annular bodies were "cause and agent" or "effect and product," they ruled out the latter "from the fact that they were unlike any of the known healthy or morbid elements of the body, or secretions, and as they were found in the vomited matter apparently in an early stage of development, it seemed probable that they were introduced from without, and would be met with in the atmosphere, &c., of places where cholera was rife."

On July 19, with the assistance of, and an apparatus suggested by, Dr. Ralph Bernard of the cholera hospital, Brittan condensed a drachm of fluid from the atmosphere of a house where five cholera patients had been removed the previous day. He discovered bodies of the same appearance as those represented. The experiment was repeated in a cell in Bridewell that adjoined cells where cholera had been present. The same results were obtained. When attempted in areas without cholera, results were negative for the annular bodies. Brittan and Dr. William Budd repeated the experiments, always obtaining the positive and negative results, employing a "glass of sufficiently high power" (Brittan used a Ross's 1–12th) for the study. The sizes of the annulars were progressive: those in the atmosphere from 10,000th to 3,000th of an inch; in vomit from 8,000th to 5,000th and in dejections, 6,000th to 5000th.

Brittan inferred that the annular bodies of atmosphere, vomit and dejection were but three stages of development of one and the same body, "the light ring round them giving a peculiar cupped appearance which is unmistakable." On September 21, Dr. John Quekett, Royal College of Surgeons, wrote a letter to Brittan, stating that he had reviewed specimens of choleraic vomit and evacuations as well as atmospheric air. He had "no hesitation in stating that in my judgment they are successive stages of development of the same body, which I believe to be of a fungoid nature."[3] Dr. Quekett erred in his judgment: cholera was not a fungoid. But the idea of a microscopic disease put scientists on the right track. Getting away from the persistent idea of atmospheric contamination, however, would prove harder. In a letter to the *London Times,* Dr. Budd detailed more of his research:

> Shortly afterwards, and being at the time aware of this discovery [that of Brittan and Swayne], I detected the same organisms in great numbers in almost every specimen of drinking water which I was able to obtain from cholera districts. First, in the drinking water from Wellington-court, Redcross-street, where cholera first broke out (with any violence) in Bristol; subsequently, in the water of the Float, and in the drinking water from King street in the same city; since then, again, in London from Lovegrove-street, and from the Surrey-canal; and lastly, in drinking-water from the Stapleton work-house; being all places where, at the time the water was obtained, cholera was making dreadful havoc.
>
> This led me to examine a great number of specimens of water from healthy quarters; and although I found in it a good deal of matter of various kinds, organic and other, in no single instance did I see anything resembling the peculiar bodies in question.[4]

"Animalcular and Vegetable Hypothesis Much in Vogue"

Brittan, Swayne and Budd were not alone in their investigation of the causes of cholera. Dr. Holland "threw out a similar suggestion in regard to this and allied diseases; and, moreover, within the last few months, a work has issued from the American Press, *Dr. Mitchell on the Cryptogamous Origin of Malarious and Epidemic Fevers;* and one by Dr. Cowdell, more immediately to the purpose, on the *Fungous Origin of Pestilential Cholera.*"[5] Another London authority, Dr. Alison, found "organic cells" in fluids ejected by cholera patients exhibiting characteristics attributed to plants belonging to the order of fungi.[6]

Perhaps Dr. John Snow made the most significant observations. Snow was the eldest son of a Yorkshire laborer. Apprenticed at age 14 to a surgeon in Newcastle-on-Tyne, he had first-hand experience with cholera when he assisted in the treatment of miners at the Killingworth Colliery in 1831. He attended the Hunterian School of Medicine, Soho, and within two years earned both an apothecary and a surgeon's licenses. In 1843, he earned his bachelor of medicine degree from the University of London. Fascinated with the idea of using ether as an anesthetic, in 1847 he adapted the Julius Jeffrey vaporizer for use in controlling delivery of ether to the patient. As attention turned toward chloroform, he studied its effects and in 1848 published a paper on the theory and practice of anesthesia, *On the Inhalation of the Vapour of Ether in Surgical Operations.*[7]

Snow became fascinated by the conflicting theories of cholera and published his own pamphlet, theorizing that

> having rejected effluvia and the cholera poisoning of the blood, and being led to the conclusion that the disease is communicated by something that acts directly on the alimentary canal—the excretions of the sick contain some material which is accidentally swallowed, either by becoming attached to the hands of persons nursing the patient—or being communicated to the food by the attendants—or perhaps vendors of provisions, and is so conveyed to a distance, or percolates from the sewers into the water of the neighbourhood used for drinking, or for culinary purposes.

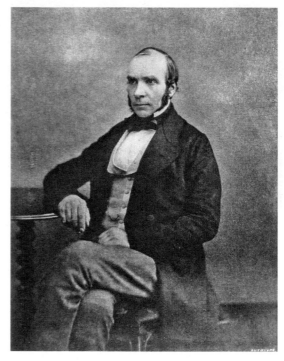

Dr. John Snow, 1813–1858 (U.S. National Library of Medicine).

Snow's idea was "reconcileable with Mr. Brittan's statements," in that fungoid bodies attached themselves to articles of food in cholera districts, water and "by every possible channel," likely from the atmosphere. It would take another epidemic and the assistance of a clergyman for Dr. Snow to divert attention from the miasmic theory to the true source of cholera: water. But they were getting close, as Dr. Budd's words prove:

> As water is the principal channel through which this poison finds its way into the human body (a fact already established by the researches of Dr. Snow, and of the discovery of which he must have the whole merit), so is the procuring pure water for drink the first and most effectual means of preventing its action.[8]

Assailing the Researchers

"The Fungoid Theory of Cholera" of "Messrs. Brittan and Swayne, and the less guarded speculations of their follower, Dr. William Budd," was immediately attacked as failing to account for all aspects of the "mysterious epidemic" of cholera. In an unsigned article that ran in the *Church and State Gazette*, October 12, 1849, a detailed history of "fungoid zoophytes" was elucidated. Described as the "nimble scavengers of nature," their function was described by their name, *funus* and *ago* (to remove the dead), or *fungor* (to execute). Traveling on the wind, they were "invisible house-to-house inspectors" as they multiplied to countless legions under favorable conditions in damp, dark localities. Fungoids were assumed to be responsible for the sweating sickness that ravaged England in the 16th century; immense development of "minute zoophytes, fungoid and infusorial" were believed to taint the air, causing red rain that made it appear the earth was "sweating blood" and being responsible for turning the waters of Egypt "to blood and constituted the first of the seven recorded plagues." During the invasion of cholera in England, Dr. Burnett "found palmella cruenta in abundance, purpling the ground near Oxford, as if red wine or blood had been poured out." The article continued: "It is obvious to remark that the mystery of epidemic causation is only removed one step by the hypothetic recognition of the pestiferous power ascribed to the loemodic bodies. If they cause cholera, how are they themselves caused? What brought them suddenly into existence some half a century since? No problem, indeed, has perplexed philosophers than that presented by the generation of the various entozoa."

Without an answer, the author provided "direct evidence tending against the assumption that they cause cholera." At the Drummond Street cholera hospital, 280 bodies were submitted to post mortem by persons who "had their hands necessarily imbrued in the choleraic secretions," yet none took the disease. The same held true of the Sunpers employed at the cholera hospitals in India to cleanse the closestools and vomiting-pans of the deceased. There was also the experience of Dr. Jannichen of Dresden and M.M. Foy, Pinel and Verat, of Paris, "who actually swallowed experimentally portions of the matter ejected without either of them taking the distemper. "Nor, again, do we find that cholera travels by preference *down* the stream of rivers, as it should do if it were communicated by the loemodic bodies transmitted through the sewers or otherwise into the watercourses. On the contrary, the cholera, in its progress to Europe, *ascended* the streams of the Ganges and the Jumna, of the Tigres and Euphrates, of the Danube and the Volga. It also very commonly traveled against the wind, a course which could hardly be held by floating fungus clouds."

The news was better accepted in the United States, when the *New York Star* reported that Mr. Brittan's experiments (the name was misspelled as "Briton") tended to show that "cholera results from certain animalculae, invisible to the naked eye" and when established, "a specific may be found for the disease."[9]

Among the "assailants" of the Fungoid Theory were writers for the *Athenoeum*, who argued that "persons unaccustomed to microscopic observations" might mistake "normal sporules and cells" for fungi. They argued that the fungi illustrated by Brittan's drawings were discovered in only a few cholera patients, begging the question, "are they not peculiar consequences rather than certain causes?" Furthermore, they had been "sought in vain in the atmosphere of many London localities where cholera has most fatally prevailed. Dr. Cowdell has found one in the perspiration of a cholera patient; and they are said to have been discovered in some of our drains and cesspools."

Unfortunately, the "less guarded speculations" of Dr. Budd, who specifically identified contaminated drinking water (as opposed to miasma) as the culprit in cholera, were particularly singled out for attack. In a letter to the *Dorset County Chronicle*, the Rev. F. Dusautoy remarked:

> Dr. Budd is mistaken in supposing that boiling the water will destroy the vitality of fungi-sporules with which it is impregnated. The Abbe Spallanzani proved, nearly a century ago, that even exposing them in a hot chafing dish would not effect this, nor even alter their size or figure. And does not the mould or mildew (fungi) on jam prove to every housekeeper that long boiling does not destroy the spores contained in the unpreserved fruit. About the same area, but rather before the physiological discoveries of Spallanzani, various experiments were made on spores or sporules of fungi by the celebrated Florentine botanist Micheli; by the Bolognese professor, Dr. Monti; and by M. Bonnet of Geneva; and they also clearly proved that the more minute the sporules, the greater was the tenacious vitality and their adaptation for long preservation.

The reverend also took Budd to task for considering the corpuscles to be *vegetable sporules* and not *animal cytoblasts*. He believed that "cholera corpuscles and other miasmata belonged neither to the animal, nor to the vegetable, nor to the mineral kingdom; but that they must be classed as pertaining to a new and hitherto concealed and undiscovered *fourth kingdom,* even as zoophytes unite the animal and the vegetable creation."

In October 1849, the cholera subcommittee appointed by the Royal College of Physicians, chaired by Drs. William Baly and William W. Gull, published its report on the "Fugoid Theory of Cholera." They stated:

> 1. Bodies presenting the characteristic forms of the so-called cholera fungi are not to be detected in the air, nor in the drinking water of infected places.
> 2. Under the terms "annular bodies" and "cholera cells or fungi," there have been confounded many objects of various and totally distinct natures.
> 3. A large number of these have been traced to substances taken as food or medicine.
> 4. The origin of others was still doubtful but they are clearly not fungi.
> 5. All the remarkable forms were detected in intestinal evacuations of persons labouring under diseases different in their nature from cholera.

Drs. Baly and Gull concluded that the bodies described by Brittan and Swayne were not the causes of cholera, "and have no exclusive connection with that disease." In other words, the "whole theory of the disease which has recently been propounded is erroneous, as far as it is based on the existence of the bodies in question."[10]

Ironically, in a report dated October 14, 1849, cholera broke out at Windsor "with such virulence that her Majesty has resolved not to return to the castle till the disease shall have abated." The area singled out as suffering the worst was called "Garden-court, leading out of Bier-lane, at the bottom of Thames-street, but a few feet above the level of the Thames." In the center of this poor quarter was a small pump, from which water was supplied to all the inmates of the pestiferous court. "The water is strongly impregnated with the stinking water of the ditches and drains by which the pump is surrounded." In a report to the Central Board, it was stated there was "no proper drainage in Windsor" but that the "cesspools scattered through Windsor are more in number than the houses" and that "the annual cost of cleaning these fetid receptacles (mostly uncovered) is one thousand pounds." This compelled them to propose a "solution" whereby cholera patients were to be removed to the gaol, where accommodations were healthier. The move was strongly opposed by the Duke of Wellington, out of regard for his troops stationed there, who had no symptoms of cholera.[11]

In a related subject, a paper written by George Simpson, F.A. Abel and E. Chambers Nicholson on the impurity of well water on the south side of the Thames was published in the *Daily News.* Due to cholera mortality in the district of St. Mary's, Newington, they made an analysis of the public well water, "which, from their supposed purity compared with Thames water, are in common use for domestic purposes." They reported that the wells in all cases were very shallow, from 12 to 15 feet deep, being just below the level of the common sewer. The impurities they discovered were "the same as exist in urinary and excrementitious deposits" and contained a much larger amount of saline substances, especially sulphates and phosphates, with nitrates (never found in pure water), ammoniacal salts and enormous amounts of organic matter.[12]

Investigations in the United States

In a series of investigations and experiments dating from September 1, 1849, Professor R.D. Mussey, of the Ohio Medical College, "discovered in the atmosphere of rooms occupied by cholera patients, *animalcules* in the greatest abundance, and by a series of observations, noted the changes that daily took place, and compared these atmospheric animalcules with those found in the rice-water discharges and muscle of cholera patients.... One of these animals, viewed through a magnifier of 2000 linear diameters, appears about *one-fourth* of an inch long, and moves with a lateral flexure of his body, like a serpent on the ground. These animals exhibit considerable tenacity of life—they are active at nearly eighty degrees Fahrenheit. The atmospheric animalcules survived thirteen days in a loosely corked phial, and the rice-water animals were alive after fourteen days." Hydrant water was tested without finding any animals and the atmosphere of rooms some days after cholera disappeared also proved negative. The atmosphere of rooms occupied by smallpox patients revealed a different species of animalcules.[13]

21

"A dose of magnesia is death"

*If it was known that a foreign enemy had landed at New York, and would, in all human
probability, visit our vicinity, would we not rise as one man, and prepare for his reception?
Surely we would. Then why should we rest quietly until we have the scourge upon us?*[1]

It would hardly be an exaggeration to state that there were as many "cures" for cholera as
deaths. Toward the end of 1848, as the disease continued its ravages across the Midwest, one
Cincinnati physician declared his theory that water, strongly impregnated with calcareous or
magnesian elements, "must have *something* to do with giving activity to the miasm[a] (or whatever it may be called) of this malignant epidemic." As "proof" of his belief, he noted that the
above statement was a common remark in New Orleans. Coming closer to the truth, the
unnamed writer added, "The use of water free from all mineral impurities was, no doubt, the
prophylactic which changed the course of the destroyer...."[2]

In December, newspaper articles began warning of a new epidemic, introduced by immigrants: the packet ship *New York* from Havre brought in 17 cabin and 328 steerage passengers,
of whom 25 had cholera, six having died on the passage. Almost overnight, four new cases
were reported on Staten Island, making 19 cases and 10 deaths since the arrival of the vessel.
This brought out the curious fact that in 1832, passengers aboard the packet *Henry IV* contracted cholera in latitude 43° 30', at exactly the point where it was detected aboard the *New
York*. In Baltimore, the *Silas Richards,* out of Rotterdam, arrived with an infected crew, reporting several deaths on the voyage.[3]

"Real" Asiatic cholera broke out in New Orleans in December, with the first death
recorded on the 12th; by the 16th, five were reported dead. Although the deaths were primarily
found at the Charity Hospital, the unseasonable mildness of the weather elicited much alarm.
Their fears were justified: by December 20, seventy-nine new cases were reported at the hospital. The temperature reached 85° on the 22nd and steamboats leaving port were filled with
passengers running from the disease, leaving the St. Charles Hotel, typically crowded to overflowing, comparatively deserted. The same day, the board of health declared a cholera epidemic.
Deaths averaged between 120 and 150 per day until December 27, when the weather turned
cooler, and by the 30th, daily deaths were down to 84. During the 31 days of the epidemic,
1,285 perished. The board of health proclaimed the epidemic over on January 9, 1849.

As the *Cincinnati Atlas* warned, cholera followed "the line of *passengers, emigrants and
business!*" By December 26, two boats touched at Memphis carrying cholera cases and several
boats arrived at Cincinnati from New Orleans with the disease aboard. Not atypically, the captains positively denied the reports, stating several emigrants died of "dysentery, caused by
change of diet and intemperate eating." By December 30, Mobile registered 50 deaths by cholera
and noted that many steamboats were laid up for want of business to New Orleans and flatboat

operators were selling off cargo at half price rather than risk a trip to that city. On January 4, 1849, Cincinnati reported cholera, some cases originating in the city but most brought in by steamboat. The same held true for Natchez, Vicksburg, Memphis and Louisville.

The greater number of passengers headed up the Ohio to the mountainous regions of Pennsylvania. Between New Orleans and the mouth of the Ohio, the *Peytona* had 11 deaths, with a large number of people "lying prostrate" on the deck. Those boats remaining on the Mississippi arrived at St. Louis carrying cholera with them. The *Grand Turk* reported 11 cases during the trip with four deaths, while the *Andrew Fulton*, arriving on the same day, had seven cases with two deaths.[4]

Cooler temperatures in New Orleans lowered the death rate but isolated cases continued until the return of hot, sultry weather. By late March, reports such as that from the *Star and Banner* (March 30, 1849) began appearing: "The New Orleans steamers of the past two or three days have again brought the Cholera up the river. On the *George Washington*, previous to her arrival at Memphis, there were fifteen deaths, and on the *Creole* three deaths." The rising waters of the Mississippi that submerged half the city exacerbated the spread of disease; among the victims was General Gaines, at 80 years of age the oldest officer in the army. The *Joan of Arc* arrived in Cincinnati from New Orleans on June 10, carrying 300 passengers, mostly Germans. Twenty-five cases of cholera and 17 deaths were reported. Two days later, the city reported 62 new cases and 12 deaths.[5]

The "Western Cholera"

Like cholera itself, arguments over diagnosis, treatment and nomenclature were epidemic, recurring whenever circumstances were favorable. In 1849, the disease prevalent in the West and Southwest was considered different from that which struck the United States in 1832. Then, victims often died within 24 hours, but seventeen years later, symptoms were considered milder, with greater chance of the victim's recovery.[6] The idea of "Western cholera" became a favorite with editors, being used by such illustrious newspapers as the *National Intelligencer* and the *Buffalo Commercial*, the latter claiming the strain extended beyond the Mississippi and Ohio rivers to all the larger towns of the country, as they were "more or less exposed" to atmospheric influences.[7] The *Star and Banner* (PA) warned the Western cholera could, under the right circumstances, assume the more virulent form of the "original disease," while a correspondent for the *New York Sun* believed cholera was contracted by steamboat passengers drinking river water of the Mississippi, "which produces a most deadly disease of the bowels even in healthy seasons." His opinion was "confirmed by the fact that many of the patients recover after they arrive in regions where the water is pure and healthy. The Mississippi water contains a vast amount of decayed vegetable matter, and living animalculi, and it is the opinion of many distinguished physicians that cholera is propagated by animalculi, existing both in air and water, when in an impure state." While not using the new name, the *Toledo Commercial Republican* and the *Cleveland Herald* remarked that the prevailing disease had assumed the character of a "billious diarrhea."[8]

Likely those in St. Louis would have disagreed. Cholera came early to the city from passengers fleeing New Orleans; by January 13, 1849, the board of health advised citizens to abstain from eating fish and vegetables, prompting the Roman Catholic archbishop to suspend the obligation of abstinence from fresh meat on Fridays until further notice. For the week ending May 16, deaths totaling 193 were reported. Especially hard hit were emigrants on the steamboats:

33 cases with 21 deaths were reported on the *Mary* "after she left the city for Council Bluffs where she was conveying a load of Mormons from New Orleans."

Those passing through the "Gateway to the West" on their way to the gold fields in California were advised that the land route was preferable to traveling by steamboat because of the probability of cholera on shipboard. A letter written from Independence, Missouri, February 8, 1849, gave added impetus by adding, "I do not believe that cholera can exist on the plains—the atmosphere is too pure."[9] Unfortunately, those who hurried away by land were not exempt; so many cases of cholera followed in their wake the disease became styled "California fever."[10] A letter dated Independence, May 13, indicated 54 deaths in camp, with reports reaching as far as 80 miles from the city. A second letter of the same date remarked, "All the Californians have pretty much left in affright: the Cholera rages so extensively among some of the immigrating parties, that they do not even stop to bury their dead. Corpses are found, wrapped in their winding sheets, lying along the road, in heaps of five and six together. The scene on every side is painful and horrible in the extreme." Among the more prominent victims was Moses Harris, a mountain guide, who died at Independence.[11]

Another of the many tragedies was the Reverend Davis Gobeen, formerly of Columbia, Pennsylvania. Migrating west, he and his brothers purchased a tract of land in Lebanon, Illinois, and were instrumental in starting a college or seminary and were engaged in the medical profession, drug business, editing and newspaper publishing. Struck with "gold fever," they sold their property and made it as far as Independence before the reverend fell victim to cholera.[12]

The travels of Dr. Israel Lord from St. Louis to Sacramento in 1849–1850 provide a firsthand account of the hardships such pioneers suffered. The opening line of his May 6 journal entry summed up what so many others experienced: "We left a dead man by the name of Middleton on the levee at St. Louis, and thought we had left all the cholera with him. We were grievously disappointed, however." Taking a ship to St. Joseph, Lord noted, "we had on board ten or twelve different medicines, put up and labelled 'Cholera Specific.'" Once he was on the overland route, his entry for June 2 mentioned the discovery of a man prostrate from cholera lying on the dry bed of a ravine, abandoned by his company from Hannibal. Already abandoning all thought of California, the victim hoped to attach himself to a team going east.

Eight days later, Lord described "a great many graves, and seen any quantity of clothing, bedding, wagon tire, old iron, etc. thrown by the side of the road. The cholera is only a few days ahead of us, and the clothes of all who die seem to be thrown away."[13]

Many 49ers traveling by water to San Francisco opted to take the overland route through Panama before catching a mail packet or other ship up the Pacific Coast. Most came to rue the decision, as they were plagued as much by disease as prohibitive costs. Two early adventurers from Buffalo wrote home from Cruces on January 8, 1849, opening their letter with this dire observation: "Here we are, in the midst of Asiatic Cholera. Six cases have occurred in this small place since yesterday, nearly all proving fatal; three cases were among the passengers by the *Falcon*, from New Orleans, and three among the natives." After taking six days to reach Cruces from Chagres, the writer complained that mules were very scarce and dear. "The fact is, the rush of passengers have taken the muleteers by surprise, and they have become so frightened by the Cholera that they pay any price for saddle mules to get over to Panama, only 8 miles—half that way the mud is full knee-deep."

A young woman who arrived on the *Falcon* wrote home on January 14: "I add a few lines ... to conjure you not to let any one of our friends come this route to California, unless he has a good constitution, a large share of patience and perseverance, and great deal of courage—moral and physical—and a *very full purse*. These are absolutely necessary to get along. They have, too, on the Chagres river, a species of cholera, brought on by exposure, drinking the water, and eating the fruit. We lost ten of our company by this disease, which generally terminates fatally in a few hours."[14]

For those remaining in St. Louis, unlooked-for disaster struck with unmitigated fury. On May 17, 1849, the steamboat *White Cloud* caught fire, quickly spreading to the *Edward Bates*. Before the flames could be quenched, numerous wooden buildings along the waterfront were engulfed. Before it was all over, St. Louis sustained $3,000,000 in property damage.[15] Adding to the panic, cholera took its deadly toll, with 231 cases and 131 deaths reported on May 22. Complicating matters, the *Atlantic* arrived carrying 300 emigrants, of whom 65 had cholera and 10 had already expired. For the week ending the twenty-ninth, 118 fatalities were recorded. Matters would get worse. By June 25, cholera deaths reached 691 over a seven-day span. For the week ending July 19, six hundred thirty died from cholera, but by July 26, only 229 deaths were registered.

By mid–August, the *St. Louis Union* estimated that cholera interments in the city during the epidemic reached 5,000–6,000; including outlying districts, the newspaper placed the actual total at 8,000, noting "the city is filled with orphans." As the disease tapered off across the Midwest, mortality counts for the epidemic were staggering: in Cincinnati, alone, for the eight weeks ending August 9, a total of 4,628 cholera deaths occurred. Even President Taylor, on a tour through the Northeast, was reported to have suffered a slight case of cholera at Carlisle, Pennsylvania, while former President James K. Polk reportedly died of cholera on June 15 at Nashville. Among other prominent victims were Horace Greeley's 5-year-old son and Colonel Jack Hays, the Texas hero. Henry Clay also suffered a bout of cholera on July 3, but it was hoped "competent physicians" would arrest it without difficulty.[16] The *St. Louis Organ* wrote this of the situation:

> When disease comes with the death warrant in his hand, demanding almost immediate execution it is sad enough.... But sadder, sadder far is it to behold the poor, answering the same preemptory summons, without the ministrations of friends, or even, in many cases, those remedies which may alleviate suffering, if they cannot cure disease. But saddest of all it is to behold, with the destitute, the scene after death. There lies the unshrouded and uncoffined body, evidencing in all its ghastliness, the struggle it has just passed through, deserted of every one, save, perhaps, a heart broken wife, or weeping children, without means to purchase that covering which protects, for a little while, the body from contact with the cold sod; or to command that sable vehicle—the last that shall ever convey our bodies—to take it to the house appointed for the dead, there may be seen that widowed woman, wringing her emaciated hands in agony of despair.[17]

When death was not so graphic, victims treated with large doses of narcotics often displayed death-like symptoms. To avoid the too-common tragedy of premature burial, one physician recommended applying a heated iron to the surface of the body. If a blister appeared, the person was not dead; "if there be no blister hope may be banished."[18]

A letter published in the *Cincinnati Chronicle,* under the heading "Dreadful Mortality on the Missouri" indicated:

> The accounts of the cholera ravages on the Upper Missouri are heart rending; on the *Monroe* 87 died—all the officers died except the 1st clerk, they were refused all aid except at very exorbitant rates; the burial of one man cost him $200—at least they found that sum on him and kept it. They died in the sheds and out houses, some on the banks of the river; their contortions and torturing shrieks unheeded by the almost barbarians. This occurred at Jefferson, Mo. Deaths almost as numerous have occurred on other boats, and reports from the caravans states that its ravages are increasing. The physicians still disagree as to the remedies to be used.

In more succinct language, it was reported "cholera has broken out among the Kickapoo Indians and proved very fatal, most of them have abandoned their homes and have left for the plains."[19] A notice from St. Louis, September 3, indicated cholera was raging among the northwestern Indians "to an alarming extent," while disappearing among the southern tribes and those on the South Arkansas River: "The Indians along the Missouri river continue greatly incensed against the whites for introducing the epidemic among them, and were committing daily murders on the inoffensive inhabitants out of revenge." The situation, no less sympathetically reported by the *Buffalo Express*, stated that near Mackinaw, the bodies of 21 Indians were found on the beach. With typical 19th century callousness, the article added, "The Indians were on their return home from payment [government remuneration], and had no doubt indulged in excesses of all kinds, which brought on the cholera."[20]

Accounts of African American deaths were equally terse, differing little in tone from reports 17 years earlier. In early June 1849, a one-line report stated, "The accounts from the Mississippi plantations of the death of slaves by cholera are distressing—on some plantations as many as 90 have died." A letter from a Louisiana planter the same month stated, "I think it probable that the cholera has destroyed a full tenth of the slaves of Louisiana. My children have lost fifteen, whilst I have lost but one man." In explaining his slight losses, the writer, also an "eminent physician," said he treated his chattel with calomel and morphine at night and asserted that "no person will take the cholera whose liver is in healthful condition."

In a letter to Zachary Taylor, dated May 3, 1849, Dr. A.G. Goodall, late Surgeon, 7th Regiment, U.S. Infantry, provided the president with his theory on cholera, stating there was little doubt the disease was "wafted in currents," affecting persons "predisposed to it by their containing in their system matter or air of a similar nature with that floating in the atmosphere. We find *the negro* more subject to it than the white man; *the white man* more than *the white woman*. The negro has more nitrogen and less oxygen about his person than the white man. It is this superabundance of nitrogen which I take to be nearly allied to the remote cause of cholera."

A writer for the *Cincinnati Gazette* noted that from 10 to 25 percent of slaves along "The Coast" of Louisiana were carried off by cholera, while another exchange reported an estimated 10,000 slaves had died of cholera in southern cities. From a British perspective, the *Patriot* reported, "The state of feeling existing between the slaves and slaveholders in the Southern states is represented to be very bad, and has been much increased by the desire of the latter to exclude the free blacks from the slave districts. The ravages of cholera had lessened the slave population by some twenty thousand, increasing the market value in Maryland and Louisiana." Under the heading "Demand for Slaves," the *Baltimore Sun* added, "It is estimated that ten thousand slaves have died of cholera in the Southern cities and on plantations. These the planters will, of course, deem it necessary to replace. The supply will be, as usual, principally from Maryland and Virginia, creating an increased temporary demand. Slaves are already said to be held at a high value."[21]

Slavery, of course, was not limited to the United States. Cuba, with its vast sugar and coffee plantations, was particularly dependent on such bonded labor. In 1848, official records indicated that during a ten-week period, there were 16,000 interments at Havana, with attrition heavily seen in the slave quarters. In April 1850, Havana suffered 300 cases with 150 deaths; for the week ending May 8, the city averaged 94 deaths per day. The following month, as 50 persons died per day, the slaves were removed to the interior, leaving business "quite prostrate." In 1852, heavy rains were to be responsible for an increase of the disease. Matters would only get worse. In a letter dated October 11, 1853, it was noted that in the sparsely peopled district between Matanzas and a point below Sagualo Grande (20 leagues in extent) 18,000 slaves had died from cholera. Some attacks lasted only one hour before death followed.[22]

By 1853, slave labor had diminished to such a degree that "persons of great experience and capital" were prompted to fill this void by fresh importations. After Spanish and Cuban authorities refused to act, Lord John Russell ordered the British Admiralty to dispatch several swift steamers to Cuba in an attempt to check the increased revival of the infamous traffic.

Disgracefully, the first evidence of this movement was seen in the shipyards of Baltimore and other American ports. Constructed with fittings used to hold human beings, clipper ships swift enough to outrun cruisers avoided the more heavily trafficked Havana and put in at smaller, less-frequented ports. From Cuba, these ships sailed to Africa, filled their holds with slaves and quickly returned.

The same year, the *Lady Suffolk* landed 1,287 African slaves in Cuba: upwards of 300 died on the passage from a form of cholera generated "from the crowded state of the hold." Those who survived the passage soon died on the plantations, their half-buried bodies "poisoning the atmosphere."[23] Cholera persisted throughout 1853, with two reports from October emphasizing slave deaths. The first noted many estates were depopulated, with mortality as high as 200 on some plantations, while the second stated that as many as 16,000 slaves died during the year.[24]

Dr. Bird's New Cholera Remedy

In writing of a cure by Dr. J.H. Bird, the *Chicago Journal* declared "the excitement caused by the discovery has been heightened by the success it has met with, in cases where almost every citizen has witnessed or experienced its effects, in the premonitory symptoms of the cholera."

This "cure," postulated by Bird and W.B. Herrick (editor of the *North Western Medical and Surgical Journal*), came about when they read articles by a German chemist who declared that influenza depended upon the presence of ozone in the atmosphere. Based on the historic precedent that influenza preceded cholera, they sought an agent that would prove deleterious to ozone. Research indicated that "cholera never prevailed in the vicinity of sulphur springs, or in situations where this substance abounds; hence the conclusion, that sulphur might be, and probably was the antidote for cholera."

Working with Dr. Blany, the three physicians tested sulphur on themselves and their patients, concluding that it entirely dissipated choleric symptoms. A correspondent of the *Chicago Tribune*, June 1, 1849, eagerly wrote that Bird's name would "soon be on every tongue," because "if this remedy is what it is supposed to be it will instantly attract the attention of the whole civilized world." The specific Bird proposed was a combination of powdered charcoal to 4 parts sulphur, formed into a pill. One dose of 4 grains was said to check premonitory symptoms, and, repeated every 3–4 hours, "entirely dissipates cholera symptoms."

Word did indeed travel quickly. The *Buffalo Courier* carried a story of the positive effects, reporting that after the pills revived a patient in Chicago who had "no pulse," a telegraphic dispatch was sent to New Orleans, advising of the remedy and requesting it be tried there. The following day, a reply was received pronouncing that the treatment had "the desired effect." By June 16, in consequence of the demand for sulphur cholera prescriptions, crude brimstone had risen from $28 to $34 per ton in New York. (Brandy also witnessed an extraordinary increase in price as people substituted it for malt liquors in the belief that it was a preventative of cholera.) Although Dr. D. Francis Bacon, editor of the *New York Day Book,* denied sulphur could possess any property neutralizing ozone and if administered was "a very severe and drastic cathartic" superinducing an attack of cholera, the newspaper exchanges that traded information among one another "fairly swarmed" with the cure.

For those who did not know what ozone was, the *Alexandria Gazette* published an article stating that it was discovered by Professor Schonbein, the inventor of gun cotton. It was "generated by the passage of electricity through the air, and is the cause of the peculiar odor perceived during the working of an electric machine, or after a stroke of lightning." Ozone was "generated by exposing common phosphorus to moist air" and, according to Berzehus, was of "no particular element, nor any combination of known elements, but is oxygen gas peculiarly modified."

By June 27, advertisements stated "Doctor Bird's Sulphur and Charcoal Specific, for Cholera, Cholera Morbus, Diarrhea, & c." were offered for sale in Ohio, 1 shilling per bottle, while in Poughkeepsie, residents were using "Dr. Bird's Sulphur remedy" with the happiest effect. Interestingly, Dr. Adrian R. Terry, of Detroit, made a chemical analysis of Bird's pills, discovering they actually contained "a notable portion of morphine or one of its salts." He concluded that Bird's cure using sulphur and charcoal was "absurd; the fact that the pills contain morphine, deprives him of the right to draw support for his theory from the results of his practice."[25]

At the same time, a doctor in St. Louis declared cholera to be caused by carbonic acid, for which he administered a medicine of his own making. One astute editor added the following in brackets: "If Dr. White really possesses so valuable a secret as a specific for cholera, a reward far more great to the heart of a great man would be secured by *giving it* to the world, than by any pecuniary advantage he might derive from selling his secret to a few physicians in St. Louis."[26]

"Is it safe to go to New York?"

The 1849 epidemic of cholera in New York was believed to have begun on May 17, at No. 20 Orange Street. In order to get a better idea of conditions there and in surrounding pestholes, the assistant editor of the *Day Book*, in company with the health warden and the police, made a tour. At the rear of No. 20, they "descended into a low, damp and filthy basement, where a scene of human misery and degradation, beyond all power of description, presented itself." In the main room, a female had just died and her drunken companions were washing the body for the grave. Their operations "were enlivened by ribald jokes, and the idiotic gibberings and laughter peculiar to far gone drunkards of the lowest caste." Other rooms held women, "the traces of humanity scarcely visible upon faces which once might have been handsome, but now bloated by intemperance, disfigured and blackened by violence, and so besotted and stupified as to be apparently unconscious of our presence, or the more unwelcome visitation of Death." In one corner, a woman clung piteously to her dying husband, while their sick child cried for buttermilk to quench his burning thirst.

Proceeding to Anthony street, the group then entered the garret of No. 146, discovering a small child, ill with cholera; its parents had died of the same disease and had been buried the day before. Nearby, a drunken man uttered "insane ravings" in French and English; before leaving, the visitors were obliged to have him removed to the Tombs to protect his wife and dying child from his brutal assaults. The editor ended his description by sadly observing that "amid the noise and fighting, and cursing of drunkards, was the spirit of the child passing away. Far better so, than to live a living death."[27]

Once started, death tolls rose quickly. Numbers, however, varied wildly. In an interesting study by the *New York Herald* (August 26, 1849), statistics from the board of health were compared to those provided by the city inspector.

Board of Health		City Inspector	
Week Ending	*Deaths*	*Week Ending*	*Deaths*
June 2	21	June 2	29
June 9	91	June 9	121
June 16	100	June 16	145
June 23	110	June 23	152
June 30	186	June 30	286
July 7	137	July 7	317
July 14	274	July 14	484
July 21	281	July 21	714
July 28	314	July 28	692
August 4	455	August 4	678
August 11	283	August 11	423
August 18	219	August 18	389
August 25	167	August 25	233
Total	**2,682**	**Total**	**4,818**

The total difference in reported deaths was 2,136.

Comparison of General Mortality between 1848 and 1849

1848		1849	
Week Ending	*Deaths*	*Week Ending*	*Deaths*
July 22	299	July 21	1,409
July 29	402	July 28	1,352
August 5	368	August 4	1,273
August 12	338	August 11	1,011
August 19	351	August 18	968
August 26	321	August 25	749

This presented a difference of 133 percent mortality in 1848 and 1849.

On his visit to New York, a correspondent from the *Philadelphia Inquirer* confessed to a lack of words to describe a scene he witnessed among the hills on Second Avenue, "where one would suppose disease could hardly reach." There, a number of rude shanties had been constructed by the indigent and laboring poor, but when cholera was discovered, that section of houses was fired and destroyed. Among those left homeless was a father who was left to die in the open with no friend to administer aid. "His body exposed, with no protection but the covering furnished by a maniac wife, remained until late last evening, for the hogs to feed upon."[28]

Stories such as that prompted the question, "Is it safe to go to New York?" The *Express* responded that the city was "as healthy as any in the Union," adding, "it is just as safe as it is to go to Boston." This prompted the *Boston Courier* to counter that with its "stagnent pools," beef boiling establishments and cattle yards, the "foetid odors" created "an atmosphere not safe for human beings to breathe," leading to cholera "vapors charged with miasma." Its conclusion: "New York would be very healthy if there were not such abundant cause of disease in it."[29]

In November, the New York Sanitary Commission issued a final report on the Cholera Epidemic of 1849, dating it from May 10 to October 1, or a total of 143 days. They concluded the following:

1. The cause of the disease appears to exist in the atmosphere.
2. The disease generally gives notice of its approach by some preliminary symptoms.
3. Symptoms are ordinarily under the control of medicine, and, being arrested, further development is checked.
4. There are agencies generally required for its appearance: filth and imperfect ventilation, irregularities and imprudences in the mode of living and mental disturbance.

The committee "commenced and perfected a thorough purification of the city," while "they *endeavored to wake up an extra amount of* MORAL COURAGE *as the* BEST PREVENTATIVE AGAINST DISEASE." In addition, they opened five hospitals, but these proving insufficient, they opened the public schools as edifices for hospitals.

Breakdown of Cholera Deaths, NYC, 1849

Type of Cholera	Deaths Attributed
Cholera asphyxia	5,017
Cholera infantum	901
Cholera morbus	226
Diarrhea	615
Dysentery	949
Inflammation of the stomach and bowels	344
Other diseases of the stomach and bowels	34
Mortality from bowel complaints	8,064
Total	**15,219**

The report added that on July 11, Professor Ellot commenced experiments on the atmosphere as public attention was drawn to a "peculiar principle called 'ozone,'" which was asserted to be the probable cause of the pestilence. He concluded "that no such peculiar principle or condition existed in the atmosphere at the time."[30] Mortality in New York City had reached 1,235 in 1832 and 336 in 1834.[31]

Cholera: The "Caleb Quotum" of Diseases

A small article that ran in several newspaper exchanges offered the following "Effects of the Cholera":

> Judging from the New York *Mirror*, this is the Caleb Quotum of diseases, for "it cleans the streets, makes men temperate, reduces the price of strawberries, raises the price of beef, allows sallad to go to seed, raises the price of lime and sulphur, thins the theatres, crowds the churches, shuts off the soda fountains, injures the hotels, benefits the doctors, gives oysters and lobsters a holiday; and furnishes editors with a topic to write about."[32]

The "Caleb Quotum" referenced (also spelled "Quotem") referred to a jack-of-all-trades, taken from a character in a play by Colman called *The Review, or Wags of Windsor*, 1808. Colman borrowed the character from a farce by Henry Lee (1798) entitled *Throw Physic to the Dogs*.[33]

As bad as cholera was, Americans could not refrain from adding a little humor to the grim statistics. One play on the myriad cures appearing in the newspapers came from "an excellent physician":

Dr. Common Sense

Tincture of Conscience, Continence and Contentment	3 scruples
Essence of Soap and Rubhard	3 pounds
Spirits of Courage	3 drams
Oil of Happymint	40 drops
Tincture of Hope and Home	12 ounces
Aqua *pure*	Quantity Sufficient

To be taken daily with thankfulness, exercise and laughing good nature.[34]

The *Boston Post* had its own prescription: "Take half a pint of hen's milk, two ounces of beeswax, and mix them in a hog's horn, stirring well with a cat's feather; then roll the mass in pills about as big as a piece of chalk, and as long as a stick, and swallow them crosswise." In one instance an exchange editor found this less than amusing, writing, "The editor of the Boston Post has a reputation for wit and pleasantry; but there is no wit in jesting with the cholera, and treating it as a hoax, or some imaginary complaint.—The foregoing item is simply flat and disgusting. The man who could pen it, while thousands were falling by cholera, around him, and all over the country, is destitute of all sympathy for his kind, or respect for the feelings of the bereaved."[35]

Apparently on a more serious note (one certain to have the approval of Frances Trollope, the English visitor famous for her critique of life in the United States, most especially the inhabitants' habit of spitting, and author of *Domestic Manners of the Americans* [1832]) came the article "A Cholera Producer":

> It is ascertained, by numerous experiments, that the habit of frequent spitting is among the leading promotives of cholera. A close observer, in this and other countries, lays down as a rule, that where there is most spitting there is most cholera. Some very curious evidence of this fact are gathered, and will soon be laid before the public.[36]

If that did not ruin a reader's day, then the note that Welch, Delevan & Nathan's circus company, which had planned to perform at Eaton and Dayton, was unable to offer a full performance on account of the cholera death of one artist and two horses, surely would. At Buffalo, Spaulding's circus was denied a permit, leading to this conclusion: "It's a bad season for circus companies."[37] Slightly more uplifting was the case of cholera at Philadelphia. A woman was suddenly taken ill and a doctor sent for. He diagnosed a severe case of Asiatic cholera and treated her, but in the course of the afternoon another physician attended her and delivered a beautiful baby daughter.[38]

Matters were not going well for practitioners of the healing arts in 1849. Dr. Pierce, a well-known clairvoyant lecturer, issued handbills offering to tell by clairvoyance, "to a moral certainty, whether an individual had any predisposition to cholera or any other disease," and professed his ability to cure, "without fail," all who applied to him. Unfortunately, two days later he died of cholera. It was observed that during his sickness, "he made use of none of his own remedies." In a parenthetical note, the editor added, "He had too much sense to do that."[39]

On the subject of water, a project was put forth to bring "Saratoga Waters" to New York City in glass pipes. The plan proposed to mold bricks with semicylindrical grooves in their sides, and in those grooves to place a glass tube, the space between the glass and bricks being filled with cement. The estimated cost of the work was $1,000 per mile, or $180,000 in the aggregate. "The project seems somewhat fantastic, but it may not prove so in the end. The object of it is to secure the benefit of the mineral waters of Saratoga."[40]

In the category of "Curious, Interesting and Alarming," the "thirteen years' locusts" made their appearance in 1846, having last been seen in 1833, when cholera was prevalent on the

Mississippi. Local superstition had it that the insects had a "C" on their wings, "the initial of the great scourge of nations." Unfortunately, no savant at the time thought to preserve the wings for future generations. But in 1846, the letter "W" (the initial of dread war) was noted on the extremity of their outer wings, each locust having two pair. The same year, cholera among horses was treated with olive oil, a "specific" for Asiatic cholera among humans. In 1850, the abundance of flies in New York and Baltimore was considered a good sign, as they were considered scarce whenever cholera prevailed.[41]

Along with the amusing and the fantastic came a "Remarkable Cholera Story" from Bangor. On September 29, Mrs. Hangley, wife of an Irish laborer, died of cholera. Her death was followed by the death of their 7-year-old daughter. While waiting for a child's coffin to be prepared, the grieving father had returned home, "when the supposed dead child stretched forth her arm, with the exclamation, 'Oh, father, I have been to heaven, and it is a beautiful place!'"

The child revealed that she saw her mother in heaven taking care of many children, among whom were three children of her Uncle Casey. Her sister objected that only two of Uncle Casey's children had died of cholera, but the child persisted, saying, "Yes. I saw three of them in heaven and mother was taking care of them. All were dressed in white, and all were very happy, and the children playing. Oh! it was beautiful there; and I shall go there again next Sunday afternoon at four o'clock." She also said that her Aunt Lynch "would be there tomorrow."

News soon reached the family that another child of Mr. Casey had died. Although Mr. Hangley tried to cheer up his daughter, she stated she had no wish to live, "but preferred returning to her mother." Her aunt died exactly as the child had said she would and although the family physician stated the girl would get well she followed her mother, niece and aunt that Sunday. The *Bangor Whig* concluded, "Such are the simple facts which we leave for the present without comment or attempted explanation."[42]

22

"Cleanliness is the very vaccination of cholera"[1]

THE LONDON MILLENNIUM—Fifty years hence London will scarcely recognise itself. Nay, for all we know, the traveller who has been making the tour of the world, and returns after some score of years, will be astonished by the change which will have come over this dingy metropolis of ours. What with ... a new board of health, new sewers, and all the other improvements we are promised, there is no limit to the spendour which may presently make London the most beautiful.... As for our sanitary condition, we shall have no sewers breathing forth pestilence, for the very refuse and filth, which is now so horrible and offensive, is to be turned into gold. Cholera will be a terrible spectre of the past, a plague of which fathers will tell their children, as the wanderers in the desert told their descendants of the plagues in Egypt. In short, physicians will have lost their occupation, and the air of the Strand will be as pure as the air of Highgate.[2]

The years 1850 and 1851 were interspaced between the second and third cholera pandemics. The general good health of the metropolis was responsible for a decrease in the importation and consumption of brandy, which "was to be expected from the unusual supplies in consequence of the cholera of 1849." The total importation in 1850 was 3,237,464 gallons, compared to 4,479,549 in 1849.[3]

Of significant import to medical researchers of the time was Dr. Stephenson Bushman's book, *Cholera and Its Cure: An Historical Sketch* (1850). After a review of the two major cholera outbreaks in England and the treatments employed, he concluded that the mortality of cholera had not been diminished a single iota: "Nay, more, I fear experience in hundreds of thousands of cases has not advanced us one step beyond the ignorance of uncivilised nations. The mortality in every part of Europe, and under every variety of medical treatment commonly employed, has been the same.... Nearly half of those attacked have been cut off in every part of the world. This is a sad conclusion, and holds forth a fearful prospect to the mind."

After noting "confidence was claimed for a drug because it was extensively used in India, where cholera slays its hundreds of thousands, uninfluenced by the intangible charm," Bushman pointed out the same disease was imported to England, "where some forty or fifty per cent of those attacked with cholera have died." Bushman advocated the discovery of Dr. William Stevens relative to the action of neutral saline substances on the blood. This, he proclaimed, "proved cholera *can* be mastered, and its mortality reduced to an insignificant per centage." (Stevens, of course, was not the only advocate of saline. In 1849, Mr. Lamplough, a London chemist, published "Pyretic Salts," promoting the use of effervescing salts for the treatment of cholera. By 1868, Lamplough's "Pyretic Saline" was advertised in Jamaica, using statistics from Stevens' research and noting it had been used most effectively in Africa and London.) Stevens apparently suffered considerable persecution from the medical community in consequence of his discovery, with many of his statements falsified to the public. If that were true, wrote a reviewer for *Lloyd's Weekly Newspaper* (September 1, 1850), "many thousand lives have been blindly sacrificed."

Although absent from England for many years, Dr. Stevens had endeavored to procure from the government, from the central board of health and from the College of Physicians, an inquiry into his work at the prison. In a 70-page introduction to his book, *Observations on the Nature and the Treatment of the Asiatic Cholera* (1853), he stated that in certain reports "the grossest falsehoods, the object of which was, to laud one system of treatment at the expense of the other; that of Dr. Stevens was represented as having caused a mortality of 88 per cent in all the cases in which it had been used, whereas that adopted by the favoured party had reduced the mortality to 30 per cent!" He added that "on the faith of an investigation of a few minutes duration, conducted, not only with indecent haste, but with a degree of levity that shocked the witnesses (some of them magistrates) who described it, *and began and ended in the absence of Dr. Stevens*, the new practice was condemned by the Board of Health, and a series of machinations emanated from within, and was carried out by that body, calculated greatly to injure its reputation. It is chiefly to be ascribed to those machinations, that a treatment which well deserves to be ranked as a specific for cholera, is, even to the present day, practically known to comparatively a small portion of the Medical profession."

With the publication of the new book in 1853 and the surrounding charges against the venerable British institutions, considerable excitement was occasioned by Stevens' work, not the least from the fact he had substantial testimonials to back his claims. The late King, Christian VIII of Denmark, had extended his royal munificence to Stevens in a gift equivalent to a liberal independence for life for having, among other medical and surgical benefits, introduced the saline practice into the Danish West India Islands. The "visiting justices" of the Coldbathfields (also written as Cold Bath Fields) Prison had also presented him with a piece of plate of the value of 100 guineas. Nor could Stevens' medical credentials be doubted: in 1834, in the honored company of Dr. Hume and Sir Astley Cooper, he had received the degree of doctor of civil law at Oxford. Stevens' "vital electric salts" were presented at the Great Exhibition, "resembling the saline ingredients in the blood" and were prepared by Mr. Lamplough.[4]

"Cholera Months" Around the World

In 1849, the final year of the Second Cholera Pandemic, there appeared to be little relief for Bombay. August was set down as the "Cholera month," with a death count of 127, broken down as follows:

Mortality by Different Classes, Bombay, August 1849

Christians (including natives)	26
Jews	None
Mahometans	33
Parsees	None
Hindoos not eating flesh	1
Hindoos eating flesh	67
Chinese	None

While the Jews and Chinese made up only a small percentage of the population, it was a cause of wonder that the Zoroastrian body in Bombay, who possessed numerical strength, suffered no casualties.[5]

While vitriolic arguments continued in Great Britain over the treatment for cholera, Dr. Musgrove, practicing in Bombay, observed, "It has long been a matter of surprise to me, not merely that any should oppose the administration of cold water, but that it has not long ere this taken its place as the first and most powerful remedial agent.... That, in this disease ... the urgent cry for *water, water,* has been disregarded." His plea was heard, as the Cholera Hospital Committee addressed a letter to the government, recommending Dr. Musgrove's plan be given a 2-year trial.[6]

Later the same year, devastation caused by cholera was reported in the province of Guzerat "which appears to have been almost unprecedented." The article noted that while the English press held that the disease moved slowly in a regular progression toward the West, in India, there was "a total variance with this theory, as the cholera breaks out in places hundreds of miles apart, and apparently without any rule of the kind."[7] One "rule," however, remained a constant theme. In 1851, the outbreak of cholera at Bombay was attributed to the steam frigate *Ajdahe,* lying in the harbor. When she left, "the epidemic also disappeared."[8]

The following April, cholera was so prevalent at Akyab (present day Sittwe, Burma) among the native population that those employed on the public works were unable to continue working, forcing the British superintendent to suspend the projects until reinforcements were sent from the presidency.[9]

In 1852, when inquiring into the renewal of the East India Company's charter, which expired in 1854, several objections were raised in the House of Lords. Although representatives of the company presented a laudatory picture, Mr. Herries noted that the natives themselves considered "their condition was one of hopeless misery ever since they came under English rule." One of the primary injustices complained of was the article of salt, "essential to the people not merely as a necessity," but used in the "prevention and cure of diseases in India, where the cholera has become the normal condition, owing, probably, to the restriction in the use of salt, and according to the evidence of medical men, it seldom took off the rich, but made fearful ravages in the ranks of the poor." The East India Company had placed an unjust tax on the commodity and prohibited the people from making salt under heavy penalty, "the object being to keep up a most unjust monopoly." The matter was taken under consideration.[10]

In 1849, reports from Cochin, China, indicated that cholera made its appearance in September in rural provinces and quickly spread in a northern direction. The greatest malignity occurred in October, after which it diminished but remained an ever-present threat. "In the royal province the most moderate and trustworthy estimates state the number of victims at 20,000," although some stated the death toll as high as 100,000, and it was thought that in other provinces losses ranged from 10,000 to 15,000. The greatest consternation prevailed over the usual care and respect for the dead, with corpses thrown out into the fields, in some places obstructing streams, and persons struck with the malady were cast away before life had departed.[11]

Although Ningpo, China, suffered severely from cholera in 1820–1821, it did not prevail epidemically until the autumn of 1852, when it was recognized as *kioh-kin-tiau,* or "the disease which 'contracts the tendons of the leg,' the name given to cholera." Chinese physicians believed cholera arose from derangement of the three *ying* (stomach, lungs and kidneys) relying on stimulants and cooling remedies. Among the remedies was a mixture of the juice of fresh ginger, various aromatics and bitters. Ginseng was also recommended, but as it was expensive, it was generally dispensed with. Acupuncture, piercing the tips of the tongue, fingers, toes and particularly the popliteal space, was performed by thrusting a silver needle to the depth of an eighth of an inch and leaving it "during the space of time occupied in six inspirations, and the dark blood would flow from the incision," tending to "restore the equilibrium of the dual powers." These methods brought relief but failed to treat the consecutive fever, "and hence the mortality was very great."[12]

In the first half of 1850, cholera raged with such virulence in Siam (killing 70,000–80,000 persons) priests warned the king that the plague had been caused by the sacrilegious conduct of foreigners in killing fowls, ducks, pigs and domesticated animals. Consequently, the king ordered every foreigner to make offerings in the temple in expiation of their offense. The French ministers refused and were deported to Singapore, while the bishop was excused as some of his converts offered sacrifices in his name.[13]

"Some remarks relative to the Cholera"

Tracing the spread of cholera, reports indicated that from June 1 to August 1, 1848, it traveled from St. Petersburg to Berlin and was predicted to reach London by January 1849.[14] During this period, the "mysterious disease" stretched its "gigantic arms from the Red to the White Sea." In a note from Constantinople, August 27, 1848, the writer indicated that the disease had existed there for nearly a year, with quarantines, sanitary cordons and disinfectants instituted in vain. Although of a mild type, this strain turned malignant in August and during the last week of the month, 1,100 deaths were registered.[15]

By the end of December 1848, fresh cases were breaking out at St. Petersburg, while the official journal of Poland offered a list of mortality that totaled 51,214 cases, 26,985 recovered and 23,560 deaths.[16] At Venice, summer statistics indicated that upward of 400 new cases were reported daily, resulting in a per diem death toll of 233.

The year 1849 harbored no better statistics. Of Carthagena, Colombia, South America, it was written "the miserable state of this unfortunate place was beyond description, as starvation, filth, and disease, were rapidly thinning the inhabitants." In 29 days, 900 persons out of a population of 10,000 perished of cholera, with fatal cases reaching 90–100 daily. Authorities ordered the frequent discharge of cannon in the hope of destroying the impregnated state of the atmosphere.[17] Local history believed that a man had died after fishing at sea, unleashing the epidemic.[18] In 1850, reports from the Andes at Bogota (elevation 7,800 feet) noted that cholera was prevalent there, higher by 6,000 feet than the point yellow fever had ever passed.[19]

The city of Monterey, Mexico, suffered a cholera epidemic in March 1850, the governor dying from the disease on the 10th. Mortality quickly escalated to 200 per day and the disease rapidly spread to the mining town of Jaemel. By May, it had reached Mexico City, destroying so many lives that great secrecy was maintained concerning mortality, which prompted one resident to place the death toll throughout the country at 20,000. While members of the congress absented themselves, the governor issued a proclamation forbidding the introduction or sale of fruit, most vegetables, butter and pork, depriving the poor of their ordinary meals. This only increased the misery as proprietors of "fondas" merely raised their prices, forcing the poor to eat only what they could grow.

On June 7, an uncoffined young woman was buried alive, but fortunately she was placed in a shallow grave. Twelve hours later, when she came to her senses, she was able to dig herself out; this incident (which received wide notice in the newspapers) prompted the governor to give orders that no interments could take place until 24 hours had elapsed after decease.

Toward the end of 1851 and in early 1852, authorities at Mazatlan refused passes to Americans who wished to pass through Mexico because of cholera raging through the country. Nearly 2,500 deaths were reported at Guylecan in three weeks, while the two-year drought caused a failure of the grain crops, creating famine, exacerbated by the law prohibiting the import of food from foreign ports. During the prior three years, it was estimated that at least one-third of the population had died by disease.[20]

During 1849, letters from Algeria stated that Oran lost 700 soldiers and 3,700 civilians from cholera, exclusive of Jews and Moors, amounting to a sixth of the population. Business was suspended and the usual deterrent of firing cannon was attempted to allay the disease. Thirty condemned offenders were employed in digging graves of the bodies collected every evening in carts. Among the dead were 200 tirailleurs, 80 soldiers from the 2nd African chasseurs, four Sisters of Charity and four surgeons.[21]

The Third Cholera Pandemic began in 1852. Reports as early as April indicated the disease had broken out with severity in Persia. By May, the disease had progressed as far west as Upper Silesia and by summer, within an 8-day period, in the town of Landsberg (population 800) 60 deaths were registered.

In 1851, Warsaw had a population of 164,115, but the new epidemic of cholera in 1852 reduced it to 160,000 by August; reports indicated that 400 fell ill every day and half died. By August 11, new cases reached 479 and the following day 485 were reported, with casualties of 175 and 170 respectively and 1,319 still under treatment. A committee was formed to relieve the "miserably destitute," and the Jewish congregation distributed 9,000 portions of tea "without any regard to distinction of creed, and 600 meals at noon to the destitute of their own faith." The epidemic was believed to have started at Lasak after excavations began in the cemetery where victims of the 1832 cholera epidemic were interred. Almost immediately, the workmen became ill, every one of them dying, and from that time the disease spread "with more than ordinary mortality."

By August 24, new cases at Warsaw were reduced to 226 daily; by August 29, the total number of fatalities was placed at 5,000, while in Posen, 89 were attacked, of whom 36 died. By September 30, reports indicated there had been 2,571 cholera cases with 1,356 deaths. Similar statistics were reported for other cities, with medical aid "almost impossible to procure." At Danzig, of every five attacked four died.

**Cholera Mortality in West Prussia (Population 405,000)
for 1852 with Comparisons to Previous Epidemics**

Year	Deaths
1831	3,624
1837	3,624
1848	1,941
1852	5,215

The city of Marienburg, which lost only 271 in 1831, lost 1,529 in 1852.[22]

In a final summary dated September, the medical board of Poland indicated cholera reached the small town of Zioszew, east of Kalisch. On the 29th, it reached Warta, east of Kalisch, and on the 31st it appeared at Sieradz. After ravaging those places for a fortnight, it appeared almost simultaneously at Zgierz, southwest of Lowic and at Kalisch, close to the Prussian frontier. In a short time, it spread with intensity in all directions, falling with severity upon Warsaw. This was considered peculiar, as the disease sprang up in the westernmost districts of Poland without apparent conducting or connecting cause from places in Asia. Secondly, it revisited two or three times places where it had apparently ceased to occur. The number of towns affected was 154, with a total number of cases to September 5 of 46,500, with 21,000 deaths. By October 16, the epidemic was considered over.

CONCLUSIONS DRAWN BY MR. GRAINGER, MEDICAL SUPERINTENDING INSPECTOR, ENGLAND

1. The epidemic of 1852 in Poland and Germany was the most severe and fatal ever occurring in Europe.
2. Cholera was advancing toward Berlin and Hamburgh along the front of Posen, West Prussia and Silesia.
3. The disease, in all essentials, was the same as former epidemics.
4. The disease was preceded by an unusual amount of diarrhea, gastric fever and intermittent fever.
5. As a rule, there was premonitory diarrhea.
6. The premonitory diarrhea was controlled by proper treatment.
7. In collapse, medical treatment was unavailing.
8. The poor neglected premonitory diarrhea and consequently did not seek medical treatment until in a state of collapse.
9. There was reason to believe cholera would become epidemic in Berlin and Hamburgh.
10. There was reason to believe cholera would reach England as part of a great epidemic.

As though prophetically, reports dated August 30 indicated that cholera had broken out at Berlin in a very virulent form, 37 of the first 52 cases proving fatal. Concurrently, Hamburgh suffered 160–180 cases, two-thirds of which proved deadly, most "confined to a wretched quarter of the town, in which 800 poor English sailors lodge and spend their time when on shore."[23]

Cholera in the West Indies

Sometimes it takes a village to raise a child and at others it requires the efforts of a journal to get results. In the case of aid for cholera victims in Jamaica, the perseverance of the *London Daily News* (acknowledged by the *Patriot*) prompted the Colonial Office, "at the eleventh hour," to send medical assistance to the beleaguered island.

Already, by January 1850, several estates were without laborers; in Port Maria, one-third of the population were "swept away," while at Kingston, out of a population of 40,000, it was estimated 5,000 had perished. In the West Indies, "25, 50, and even 90 per cent. of the inhabitants of some towns are represented to have fallen victims."[24] Little had improved by the end of October and as late as December, 100 deaths a day were reported at Kingston, causing the board of health to cease making mortality lists. Spanish Town, Port Royal, St. Andrews and St. Thomas were in similar condition, the number of dead exceeding the availability of coffins.

Because of the epidemic, the House of Assembly suspended business before passing the Cholera Relief Bill for the various parishes, with 10,000*l* placed at the disposal of the central board in Spanish Town. The governor called them back in session and with a reduced quorum it passed.

By February 1851, fresh cholera cases had almost entirely vanished, but the question of additional labor for plantation owners persisted. In June 1852, the subject was brought up in the House of Commons but was unresolved. Two months later, the Jamaica Association of

Liverpool pressed the issue, stating that the production of sugar, once amounting to 150,000 hogsheads annually, would be reduced to 35,000 in 1852. One plantation owner opined that the British government had a moral and political obligation to supply laborers, "by means of immigration, under proper regulations, from the continents of Africa and Asia." The delegates also demanded a decrease of the duties on British colonial produce.[25] Problems with "labor" persisted into 1854 as cholera passed into the Windward Islands from Rio Janeiro via St. Thomas, where 300 blacks died within 10 days.[26]

Cholera appeared in St. Thomas on December 23, 1853, prompting one letter writer to remark, "Our lovely island seems doomed to become the place where that awful pestilence, the cholera, shall work its most dreadful and fatal work." In 17 days among a population of 12,000, there were 690 victims. "With very few exceptions, the disease has been confined to the colored population, and of this class, the majority who have died were dissolute, or crowded together in filthy and ill-ventilated rooms." It was believed cholera was brought to St. Thomas by the emigrant ship *Atlas*; from there, it introduced the disease to Vandyke's Island, Nevis, Tortola and St. John's. A month later, the same author reported 1,263 deaths in town and 273 in the country.[27]

The cholera epidemic of 1851 started in the Canary Islands on May 31 at San Jose. By June 4, the diagnosis was definitive and by the seventh, numbers had increased rapidly from 5 per day to 20. On June 8, the scourge broke out in full force, driving the inhabitants out of town, so that by the 10th only 4,000 out of 16,000 remained. Between June 10 and June 12, deaths reached 100 daily, overwhelming hospital staff with the dead and dying. The situation became so dire soldiers chased the few remaining men, compelling them to lift bodies and dig trenches. The course of disease proved short-lived, but by June 18, nearly 1,000, or one-fourth of the population, had perished.[28]

"The Triumph of cholera is complete"

The summer of 1853 brought dreadful news from Copenhagen. Since June 12, there had been 427 persons attacked by cholera and 234 died. In consequence, Danish steamers plying between Copenhagen and Settin were ordered to perform four days' quarantine at Swinemunde. On July 24 alone, 230 new cases were declared with 131 deaths; since the commencement of cholera, 3,831 cases were reported with 2,041 deaths and 848 cures. Among the victims were nine physicians, including Dr. Witthusen of the king's household, the celebrated painter M. d'Eckenberg, and Baron de Holstein, intendant of the Theatre Royal.

A letter noted the list for August 3 had 146 new cases and 97 deaths, "or, from the commencement, 5,999 sick, of whom 3,219 have died. The *Koln Zeit* openly proclaims that the epidemic is the direst punishment of heaven against the Danes for their resistance to the German movement in the last four years!" The writer continued: "In Sweden the authorities are quite sublime in their absurdity. In spite of the strict quarantine the cholera has broken out with virulence in Ystad, whereupon the men of Gotham in office have drawn up a double *cordon sanitaire*—one round each house "infected," and another round the whole town. The consequence is that the poorer classes are suffering dreadfully, provisions rising daily in price. In fact there will soon be a famine in this place. Of course a panic has seized the whole province, and makes matters ten times worse. But the people are quarantine-mad."

The correspondent of the *London Morning Chronicle* reported August 22: "The triumph of cholera is complete. The pitched battle between this disease and the quarantine system has been fought out." Norway was compelled, "contrary to its own wishes," to follow suit and despite everything, the disease reached Christiania and other parts of Norway, while Sweden was "completely at its mercy," being enveloped in a net as the disease spread from Stockholm in the north to Ystad in the south, and from Gothenburg in the east to Carlskrona in the west. At the same time the disease wore down in Denmark, the total as of August 18 being 7,121 cases, with 3,854 deaths. The island of Amazer, close to Copenhagen, however, continued to suffer, cholera having "carried off nearly 5 per cent. of the population in one or two parishes." The march of the disease was said to have been "from Persia direct" to Copenhagen, ultimately forcing 30,000 to flee the city, with the only carpenters in the streets carrying coffins and omnibuses conveying loads of corpses to the burying grounds. "On Sunday *one hundred and seventy coffins were lying in the churchyard exposed to the broiling sun, and had lain there since the Thursday previous.*"[29]

23

"Our hopes that England may escape are less sanguine"

In London, our water has to be doled out by companies, who, for a scant supply, charge a high price, and pocket large profits—the dead are still interred in the midst of the living— the refuse of above two millions of people is left to run into the Thames, poisoning its waters, and wasting the rich aliment which ought to fatten the soil.[1]

It did not take a soothsayer to predict that cholera, once again raging in India, would soon reach England. Newspapers were filled with such predictions and they were right: but no one could have imagined the total devastation—or the medical discovery—that would change the landscape of the world.

The Third Cholera Pandemic is generally considered to have run between 1852 and 1859. "Summer cholera" in England appeared during the end of July 1852, but diarrhea was the "reigning disease," proving fatal to 110 children and 15 adults, eight of whom were elderly.[2] These deceivingly low numbers brought good news to stockholders in life insurance companies, which had suffered great losses during 1849. During the visitation of cholera that year, mortality from the epidemic in Lanark, Dumfries and other shires "told powerfully on the funds of insurance offices," creating, according to the common expression, a "run upon them" during July and August. Rather brutally, one report stated, "The number of deaths from cholera among persons whose lives are assured is computed by a high authority at but one in every thousand; testifying that carefully selected lives, like those of persons assured, are not so liable to the malady as less valuable lives." However, "pressure of the times, and the large sums absorbed in railway and other forms of speculation" led to an extensive surrender of policies.

Proving that the exercise of "great caution in accepting proposals" for life insurance policies was wise, in its first year of operation, the Aegis Life Assurance Company issued a dividend of 5 percent in 1850.[3] That would soon change.

The Graveyard Nuisance: Pestilence Invited

Throughout the 1840s and 1850s, the subject of noxious emanations (miasma) seeping through cemetery soil became a "grave" concern. During one meeting of the Metropolitan Society for the Abolition of Burials in Towns, one report stated "churchyards were so overgorged that half-rotten bodies were upturned to make room for fresh ones, which compromised not only general subjects, but those who died of malignant cholera." Another noted "it was quite a systematic and rule-of-three affair—dig a hole, put them in, and take them out again." Unfortunately, burials were big business: the Bunhill-fields cemetery, opened during the plague of 1665, had since realized £1,000,000 revenue.[4]

Nor was London unique. A typical graveyard in Glasgow, less than half an acre in size, had, in 1847, a total of 2,269 bodies buried, and in 1848 upwards of 3,000. The magistrate reported "there have been, within the period of five years, the aggregate number of 10,000 bodies buried in this small spot" and concluded "in the vicinity of the ground there have been more deaths from cholera than in any other parts of Glasgow." One witness added, "The mound in which fever patients had been interred last year, was now being opened on one side for cholera bodies; and there was a vapour arising from the pit, on frosty days, which was offensive beyond all description."[5]

In 1850, there were 200 private burial sites in London and from these "came pouring forth by day and night the noxious gases from decomposing human remains, amounting in one year to upwards of two millions and a half of cubic feet—that the air breathed by the two millions and a quarter of human beings in the metropolis was considerably affected thereby," and that a case was made for the total prohibition of interment in the city. This resulted in the Metropolitan Interments Bill of 1850 (Extramural Interments Act), offering compensation to the clergy for loss of fees, while permanently incorporating the General Board of Health with unlimited power to close existing, and to purchase new. burial grounds.

Little was accomplished. Lord John Manners introduced the Burials Act, giving the government and parochial authorities the power to close graveyards that proved a nuisance. The demand for extramural interments (burials outside London) prompted the formation of the London Necropolis and National Mausoleum Company," which obtained an act with the power to purchase ground for an extensive cemetery on the elevated portion of Working-common, closely adjoining the South-Western Railway. Situated 27 miles from London, 2,000 acres were provided for interments. This grandiose scheme offered enough room for the 50,000 who died in London to lie undisturbed for centuries, with churches, reception rooms, lodges, the "hotel" (containing catacombs and monuments for the dead), walks and seats for the living. The main objection to the plan lay in the railroad fee of 2s. 6d that was prohibitive to the poor.

Without that as a viable alternative, burials within London continued as usual, providing one interested person to suggest that graveyards all be paved to secure the city from "influences of animal putrefaction."[6]

Sanitary Evils: The Water Supply

The idea that water and cholera were connected was not new in 1849. During a meeting to discuss the metropolitan water supply, Mr. Horne cited statistics from medical officers stating that "where there was a plentiful supply of water the cholera had touched lightly."[7] The registrar-general's report for the week ending December 8 accompanied the returns with a diagram that exhibited cholera mortality in the London districts with the average elevation of each[8]:

Cholera in the Districts of Nine Water Companies

Grand Junction Company: Waters of the Thames at Kew supplied the sub-districts of Paddington, Hanover-square and May Fair and the greater part of St. James, Westminster. Mortality from cholera was 10:10,000 inhabitants.

West Middlesex Company: Waters of the Thames at Hammersmith supplied Marylebone and Hampstead. Mortality from cholera was 17:10,000 inhabitants. In Hampstead, mortality was 8:10,000.

Chelsea Water Company: Waters of the Thames at Battersea, much below Battersea-bridge and below the Chelsea Hospital supplied the Belgrave sub-district of St. George (31:10,000), Hanover-square and the districts of Chelsea (55:10,000) and Westminster (71:10,000). Mortality from cholera was 56:10,000.

Southwark Company: Water of the Thames at Battersea, still lower down the river supplied the districts of Wandsworth (111:10,000), St. Olave (183:10,000) and Bermondsey (194:10,000). Mortality from cholera was 156:10,000.

Lambeth Water Company: Waters of the Thames between Waterloo Bridge and Hunderford Suspension Bridge supplied parts of the districts of Lambeth (115:10,000), St. Saviour (166:10,000), St. George (Southwark) (168:10,000), Newington (145:10,000) and Camberwell (102:10,000). Other parts of these districts were supplied from Battersea by the Southwark Company. Mortality from cholera was 131:10,000.

Southwark and East Kent Water Companies: Rotherhithe was supplied by the waters of the Thames from Battersea and the Ravensbourne and partly from ditches and wells, into which drains and cesspools soak. Mortality from cholera was 268:10,000.

East London Water Company: The Lea supplied the districts of Poplar, Stepney (49:10,000), Bethnal-green (95:10,000), St. George in the East and Whitechapel. Mortality was 69:10,000.

New River Water Company: The Amwell and Lea supplied water to Islington, Shoreditch, St. Luke, Clerkenwell, London City, West London, East London, Holborn, St. Giles, the Strand and St. Martin-in-the-fields. Mortality was 48:10,000, least in Clerkenwell (19:10,000), near the head of the reservoir (96:10,000) in West London on the edge of the Thames.

The newspaper continued:

Arranging the 12 groups of districts in the order of mortality, it appears that the mortality from cholera was lowest—or 10, 17 and 23 to 10,000 inhabitants in districts which have their water chiefly from the Thames so high as Hammersmith and Kew. Upon the other hand, the mortality was highest—or 131, 156, and 268 to 10,000 inhabitants—in the districts which have their water from the Thames so low as Battersea and the Hungerford-bridge. The districts of the New River occupy an intermediate station.

For those unacquainted with the Thames it is necessary to state that the contents of the greater part of the drains, sinks, sewers, and water-closets of 2,200,000 people, after stagnating in the sewers, are poured daily into its waters—which spread over more than 2,000 acres in the midst of the inhabited parts, and are increasingly agitated by the tides—which ascend to Teddington, and carry the matters into the thickest waters below London-bridge, and a mile and a half above Battersea-bridge, twice a day. The large Chelsea sewers open into the Thames above the point at which the water is taken up from the Thames by the Southwark and Chelsea Water Companies; but the suction pipe of the Chelsea Company extends into the centre of the stream. The water, it is said, is filtered by all the Thames water companies.[9]

The nine water companies furnished 270,581 private dwellings with 44,388,332 gallons per diem. From this gross supply was deducted for daily flushing 492,350 gallons and 753,707 gallons for watering roads. The number of dwelling houses supplied by the various companies amounted to 270,581. The total number in the metropolis (ascertained by income tax assessments) was 288,037, leaving 17,456 houses (6 percent) without a water supply.[10] While the need was great, there was always an eye for profit. The proposed Wandle Water and Sewerage Company, hoping to gain an act permitting them to supply the inhabitants south of the Thames, had capital of £300,000, with 30,000 shares selling at £10 each.[11]

The proposed water company faced an uphill battle. Since 1849, when the importance of obtaining pure water gained public attention, two select committees of the House of Commons were called—one in 1851 under Sir James Graham and another in 1852 under Mr. Beckett. The vested interest of the existing water companies, which owned a monopoly, presented evidence "favourable to the existing state of things," while others advocated an entire change. An act (15 and 16 Vict., cap. 84) was finally obtained in 1852 "to make better provision respecting the supply of water to the metropolis." Unfortunately, its terms were long-range. The act stated that after August 31, 1855, it would not be lawful for any company to supply London with water from any part of the Thames below Teddington-look, or from any part of its tributary streams below the highest tidal point. Not surprisingly, the monopolies remained in place, leaving undisturbed "large masses of invested capital."[12]

This tied in with the cry for better sewers. In the text *Exposition of a Plan for a Metropolitan Water Supply*, two civil engineers called for water to be taken from a pure portion of the Thames, softened by the process of Dr. Clarke, and brought to London in cast-iron pipes and noted that nowhere should large quantities be stored.[13] In addition, waters of the Thames between London Bridge and Chelsea were so low that steamers drawing less than three feet of water were grounded amid the earth, mud, gravel and dirt brought by the sewers.[14]

One locale singled out for notoriety was Jacob's Island, where houses were constructed over a stagnant ditch. Many privies were constructed over this and outbreaks of cholera were excessive. In a report on Bermondsey, Mr. Bowie gave medical testimony that "the supply was wretchedly defective, and the water very impure." He continued that women dipped "water with pails attached by ropes to the backs of houses, from a foul foetid ditch, its banks coated with a compound of mud and filth, and strewed with offal and carrion; the water to be used for every purpose, culinary ones not excepted." In the summer, crowds of boys also bathed in the putrid ditches, "where they must come in contact with abominations highly injurious."[15] (Charles Dickens made Jacob's Island infamous by his descriptions of living conditions there; subsequently, his writing was considered "over-coloured," with Sir Peter Laurie asserting no such place existed. In light of the above, one editorialist observed, "Mr. Dickens's description is almost as applicable now as when he wrote it."[16]) At the same board of health meeting, Dr. Gavin remarked as follows:

> The connexion between foul drinking water and cholera was established by irrefragable evidence. The cases where the connexion was most clear, were where the parties had been recently drinking water taken from pumps near to, and contaminated by, the matter of cesspools: but whenever the water was contaminated so as to be nauseous, diarrhea was invariably present, and affected every person in the habit of drinking such water. I am not aware of any valid exceptions to this law.... I have traced, in many instances, the unsuspected cause of the development of cholera in the state of drinking-water. When it is recollected that the water of the poor is nearly always exposed to the noxious gases and agencies which arise from privies, and the slow decomposition of the refuse in their yards, and also from those in their close, offensive, and impure dwellings, it will at once be understood that such water produced much and severe diarrhea during the period of cholera.[17]

In his annual report, John Simon, F.R.S., F.P.C.S., medical officer to the city commissioners of sewers, offered "little new," citing cholera as a disease "proportionate to removable causes," adding "if the deliberate promises of science be not an empty delusion, it is practicable to reduce human mortality within your jurisdiction to the half of its present average prevalence."[18] Science was, indeed, at the doorstep: Mr. Gavin and others had made the "connexion," but it required more definitive proof to finally separate the idea of "noxious gases" from contamination by drinking water.

Cholera in Newcastle-on-Tyne

As close as scientists were to the final cause, an editorial in the *Patriot* (September 15, 1853) aptly sums up conditions in England, and by example the state of the world:

From a Return just printed by order of the House of Commons, we learn that, since the creation of the General Board of Health in 1848, its annual expenditure (after deducting the amount repayable from local Boards) has been 4,813*l.*; the number of Board meetings held, 1,000; the number of letters received, exclusive of letters and returns relating to epidemics, 27,172; the number of letters, & c, despatched, 93,580; the representations made to the Board for assistance, and complaints as to public nuisances, 2,167; local reports, 720; legal opinions given in answer to questions from Local Boards, 1,430; and 20 volumes of General Reports. After so much expense, so much letter-writing and printing, and such a vast amount of legal wisdom, it is extremely mortifying that the Cholera, in revisiting its old quarters, at Newcastle, Liverpool, and even the Metropolis itself, should find them not swept and garnished, but in as foul and feculent a condition as it could possibly desire.

On August 31, 1853, cholera broke out at Newcastle, which was destined to become "the headquarters of cholera." One of the resolutions adopted by the board of guardians was that the police *"request (!)"* residents not to throw night soil out the windows, eliciting a howling of indignation from newspapers.[19] The *Church and State Gazette* (September 30, 1853), noting "so has it ever been in times of epidemics, human nature always being the same," published 30 "Incidents of the Epidemic," among which were:

7. Appearance of a placard seriously proclaiming the Asiatic cholera to be a myth—moonshine! A mere creature of the imagination! Sanitary stories all fudge! The excessive mortality solely the offspring of "fear!"

...

11. Burial-operations retarded by a monopoly of the Incorporated Company of Sextons, Diggers, and Bearers. Rival bearers coffining the dead to secure a job.

...

21. Lawyers busy making wills—never busier. Law, Medicine, and Divinity—all set in motion by Disease and Death.

...

23. A funeral procession pausing at a public house to indulge in that most popular of "preventatives"—a dram.

Mortality from Cholera and Diarrhea at Newcastle and Gateshead, 1853

Date		Newcastle Deaths	Gateshead Deaths
September	14	59	–
	15	121	110
	21	935	227
	28	21	20

Mortality tapered off and by October 11, the total mortality at Newcastle stood at 1,477 and at Gateshead, 498. After 52 days since commencement at Newcastle, 4,668 cases were reported with 1,528 deaths. Significantly, the "Registrar-General's Quarterly Report" noted that in 1848–9, Newcastle was supplied with water that was relatively pure, but by 1853, the city was supplied "with water containing a strong solution of the contents of the sewers." In the same report, Dr. John Snow stated, "Water into which sewers flow, or which is navigated by persons living in boats, or which is in any other way contaminated by the contents of drains or cesspools, should be entirely disused."[20]

Getting closer to a true preventative, Dr. Lyon Playfair recommended boiling water as the most effective means of avoiding injurious results. He added that it should be used immediately after cooling and kept in a closed vessel. He also suggested the water be filtered through "animal charcoal" as well as through porous stone or gravel.[21]

24

Following the Pestilence
The United States Through the 1850s

*Shall the streets be cleaned? It would be easier to tell who built the pyramids than who cleans the streets;—
less of a job to say whether or not the moon is inhabited, than whether said streets are or are not swept;—
easier to say what is the price of building lots on the shady side of one of her volcanoes, than to indicate
what it would really cost to clean them. Yet the City [New York] pays bills for the latter purpose, and
plethoric bills too.*[1]

In many respects, New Orleans was both the starting and ending place for cholera in the
early 1850s. Putting it succinctly, a newspaper notation contained the following: "There were
537 deaths in New Orleans during the month of December [1849], of which 111 were from
cholera. This disease, notwithstanding the season, maintains its hold upon several cities in the
south, and south west, and upon the steamers on some of the rivers. It will be very apt to make
another tour North next summer."[2] In its summary for 1849, the board of health reported
9,862 deaths, of which 3,176 were from cholera, the worst month being March, with 813 fatal
cases.

By April 3, 1850, one sentence summed up the state of affairs: "The number of interments
at New Orleans to the 23 ult. [March 23] was 284, of which 189 were from cholera." The
malady persisted throughout the summer but, as the *New Orleans Delta* observed, new outbreaks usually occurred toward the end of the year: by December 7, 1850, although the disease
was not considered "in epidemic form," 106 persons died from it, 53 of them in the Charity
Hospital. During 1851, total cholera deaths at the Charity Hospital reached 140 but in 1852,
the number was reduced to 70.[3]

December 1853 would prove more deadly. In a letter dated November 22, the writer indicated that Asiatic cholera had broken out "in the most malignant form." At the Charity Hospital, 87 persons were admitted, with 11 deaths, all of which terminated within 12 hours. Total
mortality, including private practices, was placed at 26. By December 10, another report indicated that as soon as the yellow fever disappeared, cholera took it its place, "destroying nearly
as many lives as its predecessor." Three days later, the toll lay at 111, "a decrease of 160 from
the preceding week." January 1854 would prove more healthful, with a mere 20 deaths attributed to cholera.[4]

"The Cholera has once more made its appearance...

among the emigrants...." The sentence might just as easily have ended with the words
"along the waterways" or "across the Plains." The fact was, there was no place to hide.

If there was cholera in New Orleans, it was sure to find its way along the inland rivers. The *Millanger* reached Madison, Wisconsin, on December 8, 1849, with "several deaths" occurring onboard during her passage up; the *Constitution* arrived at St. Louis at the end of December carrying 200 German and 80 Irish and English passengers, 18 of whom died en route. As the disease maintained its hold, it appeared at Thiadeaux in early February 1850 among slaves belonging to Virginia and South Carolina traders.

By April, as hundreds of victims were felled in New Orleans, the disease reached as far up as the mouth of the Ohio; reports quickly came from Cincinnati that steamboats plying the trade between those two cities carried death aboard. As many as 10 died on the *Cincinnatus* in the latter city, while New Orleans laborers on the levee and those of the "lowest walks of life" continued to suffer greatly. The *Dutchess*, *La Fayette* and *Belle Key* all had cholera deaths on the passage to Louisville, and by May 10, cholera was introduced to St. Louis by "the mass of emigrants brought up from New Orleans." The *St. Louis* brought 700 passengers, of whom all but 114 were on the lower deck, and lost 13 on the trip; the *Missouri* carried 500 emigrants and suffered 12 fatalities. She was followed by the *Iroquois* with 300 more. Authorities rapidly established quarantine on Arsenal Island below the city.[5]

Not surprisingly, magistrates were hesitant to say an epidemic existed ("seventy-four interments in a week, out of a population of eighty thousand, is by no means large or unusual"); they were less sanguine about cholera in the wagon trains headed for California. On May 7, 1850, the *Republican* carried a letter from one traveler advising that "cholera has broken out in Dr. Clark's train, in its most malignant form," adding he was fearful it would extend to Marshall's train of about 60 persons.

By June 23, Cincinnati had recorded 649 cases, with a daily average of 29, and at Louisville on the 25th, there were 45 cholera burials, the greater part of the victims having been among those just arrived from foreign countries. On July 9, Cincinnati had 65 cholera deaths, the *Gazette* remarking that a feature of the disease was that it attacked all classes as opposed to previous years, when only those who lived "imprudently or uncleanlily" fell victim. Among those of the "better class" was President Zachary Taylor, who, on July 8, 1850, was reported to be "very low" from Bilious Cholera Morbus. He died July 10, at Washington, D.C., attended by his physician, Dr. Witherspoon.

While numbers continued to escalate in St. Louis and Cincinnati, cholera ("or as some would have it, the milk sickness") on the upper Missouri prevailed to such a great extent among emigrants that many teams turned back on account of it. News was worse for those moving through the Plains for California, where 250 deaths were reported for the first two weeks of June; some wagon trains were passed "in which almost every individual was prostrated by disease, or already dead."[6]

The Geological Theory of Cholera

One theory on the origins of cholera held that the disease prevailed more generally in limestone regions as it was supposed that carbonate of lime with which ground water was impregnated was an "exciting cause." Acting on this belief, the board of health of St. Louis ordered handles to be taken from the pumps to prevent their use. David Christy, in a letter to the *Cincinnati Gazette* from Oxford, Ohio, Oct. 20, 1849, posed a different idea based on geological theory.

As Christy explained, in nearly all limestone districts the rock was interstratified with marlite—a mixture of lime and clay. The limestone rock was impervious to water, but joints and fissures in the strata allowed rain and melting snow to penetrate the earth, often to great depths. But when rock was interstratified with marlite, it was unable to reach any greater depth because of the compactness. Therefore, water ran off into springs or wells, carrying with it the putrid matter of decomposing animal and vegetable substances. In diluvial districts, where soil rested on sand and gravel, water penetrated the soil and diluvial, or flood, districts before reaching the marlite or limestone, becoming filtered of all putrid matter. In sandstone regions, rock was generally interstratified with shale—sand and clay intermingled—which was more porous than marlite. As the water of sandstone penetrated to an even greater depth, it was even more filtered and thus more pure.

In limestone regions where wells were filled with murky surface water from runoffs, the unfiltered liquid not only carried decaying matter but also the filthy portions of alleys and streets. In these areas, cholera was far more prevalent than in others where water was saturated with lime but the wells were filled from deeper, more filtered sources.[7]

Mortality in St. Louis
Comparative Figures from 1849 and 1850

	1849		
Total Deaths	Cholera Deaths Week/Number	Most Deadly Week/Number	Least Deadly
8,431	4,144	July 16/639	December 24/31
	1850		
4,595	872	July 31/216	February 19/35[8]

The end of 1851 saw similar reports of deaths along the waterways. Typically, cholera broke out in New Orleans in December, reaching to Gainsville on the Pearl River, the first time it had ever been seen in the pine woods, while "every boat arriving at Cincinnati from New Orleans has more or less cholera aboard." Although "mostly confined to emigrants," numerous reports of slave deaths came from Louisiana and Alabama.

By November, emigrants to California on the south side of the Platte were attacked by cholera, with 2,500–3,000 falling victim between the frontiers and Fort Laramie. The disease soon reached San Francisco. By Christmas, 135 deaths were reported there, while in Sacramento, the numbers reached 1,000. In consequence, gold miners determined to remain in the mountains during the winter instead of retreating to more comfortable city life. The California *Cherokee* noted, "There is probably not a population in the world which is so liable to an epidemic, as the motley tribe gathered in the golden region. Their prodigal habits of living, and the reckless exposure incidental to a new country, are like tinder for the cholera match." For the gold-crazed nation, however, this was considered good news, as the Yuba mines were said to yield $8–$10 per diem per man.

The year 1851 saw more of the same. The *Thibodeaux (LA) Minerva* remarked on the spread of cholera through the plantations, with mortality confined to the "black population," which was considered great. By mid–May, the malady was frequently reported on steamboats navigating the lower Mississippi, but it reached as far up as Alton and Galena. The *St. Louis Republican* cautioned people against "setting down as cholera what seems to be a new phase of ship fever," a disease "confined to emigrants." Quarantine Island overflowed in June, forcing buildings to be fastened with cables to prevent their being swept away, and those detained were transferred to a steamer chartered and anchored nearby.[9]

The *St. Louis Intelligencer* observed on June 25 that, although cholera was rare among the settled areas of the city and had nearly ceased at Jefferson Barracks, the disease was seen in immigrants from Europe "who drink the muddy water of the Mississippi." For the week ending July 14, cholera interments reached 149; neighboring Alton continued to suffer from high water and cholera, although a local physician persisted in calling the malady "ship fever," a term not associated with "epidemic" and thus calculated to inspire less fear. This was particularly important, as the groundbreaking ceremony for the Pacific Railroad was held in St. Louis on July 5. Citizens were warned to shy away from "Cholera Bombshells" (watermelons) being sold for a penny a slice.

During January 1854, fourteen large steamboats were compelled to put in at Cairo (a low, swampy, sickly place at the junction of the Ohio and Mississippi rivers) in consequence of the suspension of navigation. Two thousand passengers, chiefly emigrants, were set ashore, many of whom died from cholera and yellow fever. In March, cholera broke out among steamboats transporting emigrants from Georgia to Texas, leaving 12 whites and 20 blacks dead. It was stated that the disease first attacked the Negroes, attributed to the fact boats were too crowded and the "filthy condition of the negroes' department on board."[10]

From the Indian Country

Not atypically, in 1849, Indian agent Mr. Childs at Wolf River, in Northern Wisconsin, reported that cholera was raging among the Menominces [*sic*] to an alarming extent, which he attributed to a change of diet, they "having principally subsisted during the summer upon fish, until they received their rations of salt pork, &c. [from the government], which they have indulged to excess, accompanied with the liberal use of whiskey."

In June 1851, Indian agent Burt was engaged in collecting various tribes at Fort Mackay for a convention. Among those were the Cheyennes, Kiowas, Comanches and Arapahoes. He was unable to meet with Col. Summer's command, however, as the troops were proceeding slowly on account of cholera. Between eight and ten soldiers died daily and in consequence, the traders and teamsters deserted.

Conditions were worse for the Rocky Mountain tribes. At Fort Berthold (225 miles below the mouth of the Yellowstone), a letter dated August 30, 1851, from an agent of the American Fur Company stated that the Gros Ventres had recently suffered from violent colds that led into cholera, causing 16 deaths within 48 hours. Had he not provided them with medicines, he believed he would have been killed or driven away and the fort destroyed. He finally prevailed on them to remove to the plains, which they did. At Fort Clark (300 miles below the mouth of the Yellowstone), in a letter dated September 1, the company agent reported that after a severe attack of influenza, cholera broke out among the Arickarees, killing 62 within days. Two attempts were made to kill the agent, as the Indians charged the whites "with the introduction of the disease among them" and regarded him as one of the evildoers. He was frequently called upon for goods to cover the dead and in some instances was "compelled to accede to the demand."[11]

Mortality Aboard Emigrant Ships

While inland cities continued to report large numbers of cholera deaths among immigrants, the disease was so horrific among those leaving Liverpool and other European ports that public attention was finally drawn to the tragedy. In November 1853, the packet ship *Washington* arrived at New York from Liverpool, reporting 100 deaths and 60 fresh cases. Preceding her were the *Charles Sprague* (passage from Bremen, 45 deaths) and the *Winchester* (from Liverpool, 79 deaths). Between September 9 and November 26, a total of 17,400 passengers arrived from Europe among whom had occurred 1,300 fatalities, primarily from cholera. Health officials at the Quarantine Grounds, New York, stated symptoms as "a day or two of diarrhea, followed by vomiting and purging, spasms, collapse and death within six or twelve hours."

In 1849, John Lea of Cincinnati attributed shipboard mortality to "the calcareomagnesian properties of the water [which] unite with the miasm of cholera—a diarrhea ensues, more water is taken, and death soon closes the scene." Right, but for the wrong reason, he rationalized that fewer deaths occurred in ships from Bremen because of the "purer quality of water furnished at that port." Arguing that rain or boiled water was a prophylactic for cholera, he felt that if passengers drank only tea, coffee or table beer they would escape the disease. (In 1852, a French medical commission at Paris asserted that rainwater was a prophylactic for cholera, observing that the disease had never proved epidemic in any city where rainwater was exclusively used. The *Galveston Citizen* asserted its city afforded the "strongest possible evidence of the truth of this statement.")

Lea followed up his "Geological Theory of Cholera" in an 1850 article published in the August 1850 number of the *Eclectic Medical Journal*. Maintaining the idea that certain mineral properties in the water (lime and magnesia) caused cholera, he traced epidemics in the United States from 1832 to 1849, arguing the disease could be avoided by the exclusive use of rain or boiled water.[12]

After giving a thorough and at times graphic account of conditions aboard emigrant vessels and making a good case for the appearance of disease from foul food, water and air, A.C. Castle, M.D., surgeon dentist, lost his credibility by declaring the occult force behind mysterious epidemics to be "electric aberrations in terresto-electricity." He was not alone: many physicians of the 1850s were of the opinion that disease was "occasioned by a pestilential vapour or atmosphere hovering over or passing across the Atlantic."

Sea captains did not offer explanations, but many advocated a cure consisting of one tablespoon of common salt and a teaspoonful of red pepper in a half pint of hot water. On a related topic, the *Charleston Standard* traced the prevalence of cholera in that city to an indulgence in oysters gathered from brackish, not salt, water.[13]

Poor Houses, Cholera Hospitals and Visitations

Expectations for cholera outbreaks in 1854 were almost sanguine, with the *Logansport Journal* (June 17, 1854) noting, "There is little doubt but that the disease will make the regular tour that usually follows its appearance in the country. Experience has lessened its terrors, for science has done much toward stripping it of its fatality." In Chicago, 142 deaths from cholera were recorded in June, with similar numbers in St. Louis, Toledo, Cincinnati, and along the Western waterways. In Brooklyn, for the week ending July 15, there were 84 cholera cases, 35 of cholera infantum and 15 identified as cholera morbus. In Philadelphia, for the week ending July 15, sixty-nine deaths were from cholera and 85 from cholera infantum.

At Niagara Falls, gruesome reports of cholera among workers on the canal and Suspension Bridge in July 1854 made all the national exchanges. With 50 men declared dead in a short period of time, management offered $3–$4 per day for any who would stay on the job but found no takers. Later, when the bodies of two laborers were discovered in a nearby shanty in a state of decomposition, a reward of $30 was made to any who would bury them, but again there were no takers. Finally, a number of shanties were burned down, but visitors to the Falls were "not over numerous." The same month, near Scales' Mound, 12 miles from Galena, cholera broke out among 300 men working on the Illinois Central Railroad; ultimately, more than half died. As the ground they worked was 450 feet above the Mississippi and the air was pure, the explanation of how cholera appeared remained a mystery.[14]

While New York City newspapers were constant in their vituperations of the Epidemic Cholera Hospital on Franklin Street, complaining that those suffering from contagious diseases were admitted among the cholera sufferers and that the peace of the neighborhood was destroyed by the clanking of hammers nailing up coffins, affairs were even more horrendous at the Erie County Poor House in Buffalo. In the Insanity Building, 19 cholera deaths (out of 53 inmates) were recorded in 36 hours, exceeding the total mortality of the city and its 80,000 inhabitants.

Upon investigation, the board of health found insufficient ventilation and a starvation diet beyond which "Dickens ever ascribed to a parish workhouse or to Dotheboys Hall." For breakfast, a piece of bread about 3[qm] square by ¾" thick, a little salt pork and coffee made from barley and sweetened with the cheapest molasses was served. Dinner was the same as breakfast without the coffee, and supper consisted of bread and tea. After remonstrance from the house physician, a ration of beef broth was provided. This broth was made from refuse from the slaughterhouse where certain shanks of beef were purchased as 12½ cents apiece. The shank was boiled in enough water to give 30 patients a pint of broth each. During winter and spring no vegetables were provided and since the appearance of cholera, no vegetables of any kind were issued, resulting in another death, from scurvy. The article from the *Buffalo Commercial Advertiser* concluded, "We have no word of censure for the Superintendent in charge. We leave the facts with the people."[15]

"The Workings of Cholera"

While most authorities considered cholera "a periodic epidemic, naturalized to this country," the idea that the disease was caused by decayed vegetation, putrid miasma or some "undiscovered phenomena of electrical action" persisted. In 1854, one author considered cholera "to be no longer a proper source of greater apprehension than is felt at ordinary malignant dysenterys and other summer diseases."[16]

Few inroads were made, and those that were went ignored. The same year as the above appeared, Dr. J. Philip Hobbs, of Memphis, addressed the mayor of Nashville, stating that the exclusive use of cistern water would "entirely and exclusively" cause cholera to disappear. The editor of the *Nashville Gazette* corroborated this by observing that in 1849, when the disease was at its worst, those who used rainwater exclusively were free from it. A "Correspondent" to the *Pittsburgh Gazette* also believed cholera was spread through water: he suggested that after a long drought reduced the Allegheny "to a feeble stream," heavy rains spread sediment from filthy gutters into the reservoirs, causing an epidemic.[17]

In 1855, the Sanitary Commission of Bavaria published the report of Prof. Dr. Max von Pettenkofer, which was not only distributed "in hundreds of thousands of circulars" in that place but also received praise in the United States. Among his findings were the following:

1. There was no cholera-catching matter (contagion), but the disease could be conveyed from one place to another.

2. Cholera always took its course along passages of trade (rivers and roads).

3. Elevation above or below sea level was immaterial to reception of the disease.

4. The air contained no cholera-catching matter and therefore the disease did not follow the direction of the wind.

5. Cholera was not carried forth by or spread through water.

6. The earth received and developed cholera-catching matter from the excrements of cholera patients.

7. Excrements of patients in privy vaults or closestools generated the catching matter and were the real cause of the disease.

8. Gasses were developed by the decomposition of organic matter, particularly excrements, penetrated the earth, rose to the surface and caused fevers and cholera.

9. Cholera was always transported and spread by a sick person and in no other way.

10. The cholera could be kept in a person for 28 days, which accounted for the spread of cholera to distant places.

11. To prevent infection, closestools were to be rendered harmless by sulphate of iron or green copperas; chloride of lime was insufficient because it only purified the air and did not destroy cholera poison.

12. Clothes soiled by excrement should be burned, never soaked.

13. There was no other means of preventing cholera than by rendering harmless the decomposition of human waste.[18]

In the final meeting of the special committee of the board of councilmen, New York, May 1857, Dr. Wynne presented a thorough study of street cleaning around the world with a view toward improving health. Unfortunately ignoring studies such as that cited above, he concluded that increased miasma from rotting vegetation directly affected mortality from fevers, dysentery and cholera.

Bills of Mortality, New York City

Year	Percent of Deaths Annually
1810	1:46
1815	1:41
1820	1:37
1825	1:34
1830	1:39
1835	1:41
1840	1:39
1845	1:37
1850	1:33

Wynne suggested that to defray the cost of street cleaning, the refuse matter collected be sold as manure, as was done in England.[19]

25

"The Grand Experiment"

The well is simply a pit sunk in a porous soil, and that the surface water of the street, saturated with the manure of the road, permeates the sides of the well; this, in truth, is the source of the water supply.—Dr. Thomson's report to the Medical Officers of Health, 1858.[1]

In 1854, Leeds would have the distinction of being the first district to report a cholera outbreak, but it was Golden Square in Soho that would ultimately become famous for its unintended contribution to the cause and prevention of this deadly disease.

Two special meetings of the Leeds poor-law guardians met on March 4 and 6th to discuss 13 cases, six of which had already proven fatal. The disease was first reported among workers in the flax-spinning mill of John Wilkinson and Co., known for its "salubrity, cleanliness, ventilation and care of the operatives." The original cause was assigned to the flax that emitted a strong, peculiar odor. Dr. Gavin, who was sent to investigate, attributed the cause to the River Aire that flowed past the mill, and to a large manure depot on the opposite side. By March 17, the disease abated after attacking 40, sixteen of whom died.[2] On behalf of the College of Physicians, Drs. Baly and Gull were deputed to prepare a report, Baly writing on cause and prevention and Gull on cholera's morbid anatomy, pathology and treatment. In reviewing the conclusions in their paper, "Report on the Cause and Mode of Diffusion of Epidemic Cholera," the *Morning Chronicle* (March 27, 1854) wrote:

A council of war, it is said, always counsels a retreat. Official or deputed responsibility seems generally to lessen the freedom and decision of most men. Perhaps originality of view depends upon actual observation, and a man who is set down to arrange and decide upon the observations of others is not in the best position to strike out new theories or indulge independent thoughts. Caution is the motto, running into over-caution. Except in some propositions of strained or questionable character, the influence, power, and delegated skill of the College of Physicians has arrived at no more satisfactory opinion upon cholera than that, "All that we know is, nothing can be known."

Dr. Baly presented six theories, of which only three were broadly discriminated, the others being combinations or variations of the same:

1. A morbific condition of the atmosphere, requiring predisposition of the patient to be affected by it.
2. A morbid matter not produced in the air but in the body of the sick, affecting others by transmission.
3. A morbific matter produced in the air but reproduced by the sick and contagious.

Dr. Gull's treatment on the subject provided nothing more than that which was already well established, prompting the *Chronicle* to make an astute observation: "It is much more satisfactory in a literary and logical than in a practical sense, seeing that patients who get nothing but cold water do pretty nearly as well as those for whom the whole pharmacopoeia is laid under contribution; while those who are favoured by the most active resources of art, die in greater numbers than those who are left alone."

Simultaneously, Dr. William B. Carpenter published a ten-part thesis, ultimately concluding that cholera was caused by air tainted by subterranean emanations. He recommended free ventilation, avoidance of overcrowding, abstinence from stimulants, wholesome diet and attention to the bowels.[3]

These two publications were clearly a step back from the forgotten proof that saline injections were a positive cure and that water, not air, was the conduit. Ironically, it was the editorialist from the *Morning Chronicle* who ultimately proved correct: an independent man who dared pursue his ideas would discover the route of cholera.

Two Steps Back, One Step Ahead

If the reports cited above represented two steps back, the time was fast approaching when medical science would take one bold step forward. In the interim, deaths from cholera increased from 5 for the week ending July 15 to 847 for the week ending August 26, 1854. Of these, the majority were confined to the south side of the Thames.

In what might be considered a lateral move, on July 31, 1854, the House of Commons debated the renewal of the Public Health Amendment Bill, which included a continuance of the board of health. Lord Palmerston argued that the threat of cholera required "instant directing actions" furnished by the board of health. Lord Seymour countered that the board "had not acted with the caution, prudence, and forbearance" required. He also assailed its constitution, which he considered could never be satisfactory while one of its three members was an unpaid amateur "whose principle was centralisation." The vote divided, 65 for and 74 against, and the bill was lost.[4]

With cholera deaths increasing to 1,287 for the week ending September 2, the situation became inflammatory. The *Morning Chronicle* (August 17, 1854) editorialized that, while science had proven that removing nuisances could make the disease disappear, the subject had not been widely acted upon: "Indeed, to judge from the reports of the REGISTRAR-GENERAL, it might well be doubted whether a stupid fatalism, or a sceptical distrust of all human knowledge, was the predominant motive of conduct among men upon whom all the terrible experience of the past has made no impression."

Lord Seymour, Sir Benjamin Hall (MP for Marylebone and a proprietor of ironworks in Wales) and others immediately brought forth and passed a new act reforming the General Board of Health. Hall assumed the presidency and began his duties August 13, although not without contention. The *Press* (August 19, 1854) complained: "The time is singularly ill-chosen for the appointment of Sir Benjamin Hall as head of the Board of Health, a feeble Ministry having been inducted to place an ignorant and arrogant man at the head of a department of which he can possibly know nothing, to get rid of a troublesome opponent." Drs. Sutherland and Granger were immediately employed as medical inspectors for the metropolis; Dr. Gavin became medical superintendent of the General Post Office, and Mr. J. Borlase Childs served as the surgeon-in-chief of city police.[5]

Dr. John Snow and the Broad Street Pump

Three words exemplify the phenomenal discovery of how cholera was actually transmitted: "Soho," "pump" and "Snow." The first indicated location, the second transmission, and the third, investigator.

In the 1690s, Soho emerged as one of London's most fashionable districts, but by the middle of the 18th century, as the wealthy and titled moved westward, artists emerged, eventually sharing space with slaughterhouses, manufacturing plants, brewers, tripe boilers, and the working poor. All would prove equal in the eyes of disease, however, as a five-month-old daughter born to Sarah and Thomas Lewis fell ill on Monday, August 28, 1854, vomiting and expelling watery, green stools. Five days later, she was pronounced dead by Dr. William Rogers. Under cause of death he wrote, "diarrhoea and exhaustion," unknowingly setting the stage for one of the most fascinating investigative discoveries in the history of medicine.[6]

Within 48 hours of the Lewis baby's illness (the incubation period of *V. cholerae*), black flags were raised, indicating the presence of cholera. Once started, numbers increased rapidly. On September 2, the same day the baby died, John Rogers, medical officer of health, St. Anne's, was proceeding from Walker's Court up Berwick Street to visit cholera patients when he encountered "one of the most sickening and nauseous odours it has ever been my misfortune to inhale." Looking down into a gullyhole he saw the house of a well-respected surgeon named Harrison. Later in the day he was informed that the doctor had just died, prompting him to remark, "That gullyhole has destroyed him." Rogers subsequently learned there had been seven seizures and six deaths in the vicinity. A neighbor living at No. 6, Berwick Street told Rogers that he had previously applied to the sewage commission to trap the gully and was told he must pay for it himself.[7]

The same day, newspapers reported that cholera had broken out with extreme virulence at Broad, Berwick and Poland streets. People collected outside, relating horrors, while customers mobbed chemists' shops, pleading the urgency of their "cases" so as to be allowed to take precedence at the counter. At one druggist's, 300 pennies' worth of camphor was sold in a few hours, some eating it while others used it as a disinfectant. Stretching into 2:00 a.m., workers at an undertaker's shop were busy; outside, a crowd watched with morbid excitement "the hasty knocking together of the coffins" and calling out the names of the dead: "The crowd was terror-stricken. When they spoke, it was in a half whisper, and above all you could hear the sharp rattle of the hammers."

Incredibly, on that infamous September 2, the *Daily News* published a letter merely signed "A." The author wrote, "As people were poisoned in London by the water they drank in 1849, so they are poisoned now in 1854; and they are poisoned in a direct ratio with the degree of impurity of the water. The Thames is polluted by the sewers which run into it.... Mortality and impurity of water are so closely and constantly related that they must be considered in the light of cause and effect." The writer continued by stating the theory was advanced by Dr. Snow, who concluded "that the disease is propagated by something which passes from the inside of one person into that of another, which it can only do by being swallowed."

In a letter published in the *Medical Times and Gazette*, Snow himself detailed his work of making inquiry in every house in the Southwark and Lambeth districts where cholera had occurred to the 19th of August, finding that only 11 houses were supplied by the Lambeth Water Company, while 81 houses received water from the Southwark and Vauxhall Company. Since both utilities supplied water to "the rich and the poor indiscriminately," yet the numbers of cholera cases were wildly divergent, Snow concluded "it is evident, therefore, that in the sub-districts to which the inquiry has extended the people having the improved water supply enjoy as much immunity from cholera as if they were living at a higher level on the north side of the Thames."

Although adding that water provided by Southwark and Vauxhall (S&V) was "not worse, either physically or chemically," than that generally supplied, it went through "a coarse kind of filtration before it is distributed, and it passes with careless observers for being quite clear, though it is not so in reality." By comparison, the Chelsea Water Company obtained its supply from almost the same part of the Thames but filtered their water much better, which resulted in much less cholera in their district.

By Sunday morning, a scene "heartrending in the extreme" presented itself: children crying and calling for their parents; men and women huddled together, afraid to enter their dwellings; fights outside chemists' shops, made worse by the fact a chemist and his assistant had died during the night. Readers surrounded every placard on the walls containing directions for persons attacked by cholera. Crowds surrounded medical men, petitioners praying they visit their homes.

Toward nightfall, mortality had become so great it became necessary to remove the dead. Covered vans called from house to house and picked up corpses wrapped in sheets and blankets: "There were no followers of the bodies, no signs of grief, but a terrible silence reigned. Policemen, holding camphor to their mouths, warned passers-by not to travel certain streets."

By Monday, September 4, inhabitants commenced flying from the neighborhood. Nearly all shops were closed and hearses carried coffins on their roofs, the insides of the vehicles being closely packed. By afternoon, many vehicles were drawn by brown instead of black horses, for the usual animals had been "knocked up by repeated journeys to the graveyard." Cabs, too, were employed, coffins placed inside. Undertakers' men refused to work unless brandy was supplied, "and even then their pale faces showed the fear with which they performed their labour."

Crowds gathered outside physicians' residences, pleading for visits. In one typical scenario, it was related that a lad came for the doctor, as a young woman had taken worse. A visit was promised but he returned 20 minutes later to say the poor girl had died. At one time, a medical man was reported dead (two did die) and the fear of the crowd multiplied. While the medical attendants seemed "perfectly bewildered," more "strange and ominous" were the black mourning clothes worn by everyone.[8]

The districts of St. James's parish, Westminster and St. Ann's (also spelled "Anne"), Soho, bordering on Golden Square, Berwick and Broad streets, were watered with a solution of chloride of lime and zinc, while the dispensary fell into debt £400, with a balance of only £5, prompting the board of guardians to form a committee to receive contributions for the purpose of relieving destitute families. Messrs. Huggins and Co., brewers of Broad Street, offered an ample supply of hot water for the purpose of cleaning houses.[9]

On September 7, as the number of cholera cases increased in the parish of St. James, the board of guardians ordered a house-to-house visitation to inspect for nuisances; the president himself visited Dufour's Place, Broad Street, Silver Street and other infected areas "to allay alarm by his presence."[10] At the same time, the General Board of Health issued ten "simple suggestions" for prevention of the disease, using virtually the same verbiage as in 1849. Dr. Henry Mayhew's theory of "Ozone," also from 1849, received new press and Dr. George Johnson's "new treatment of cholera, by castor oil," was lauded. (A subsequent investigation of Johnson's treatment by the General Board of Health reported that in 89 cases, 68 proved fatal, 15 recovered and 6 remained uncertain.)[11]

THE CHOLERA PREVENTED by the Destruction of all Noxious Effluvia.—CREWS'S DISINFECTING FLUID.—Recommended by the College of Physicians and the London Board of Health.—The Cheapest and Strongest Chloride of Zinc. Quarts, 2s.; Pints, 1s.; Half-pints, 6d. Sold by all Chemists, Druggists, and Shipping Agents, and at Commercial Wharf, Mile End, London.

"The free use of disinfectants is highly desirable, as a preventive of cholera. We can confidently recommend the article known as 'Crews's Fluid.' It is a strong solution of the chloride of zinc; it is, moreover, cheap as well as highly efficacious. For general use, it may be diluted with about two hundred times its volume of water."
—From the Medical Circular, August 9, 1854.

Crew's Disinfecting Fluid was composed of chloride of zinc, but other products containing bromide and iodine were also marketed for disinfecting purposes. At mid-century, disinfectants were classified by their physical properties. Solids included lime, dry earth and ashes; mixtures containing mineral acids and solutions of the salts of almost all metals were fluids. Gaseous disinfectants, including ozone, became widely popular as did nitrous and sulphurous acids. Imponderables, such as heat and light, were also included as disinfectants (*The Morning Chronicle,* London, September 5, 1854).

Adding to the difficulty Snow would face in proving his theory, another letter to the editor began this way: "The cholera cases in St. James's parish appear to have baffled the most eminent of the medical men, and the most virulent of the cases have occurred in the neighborhood of Broad-street and Carnaby-market." Espousing the popular idea of noxious gasses escaping through a local sewer constructed through a cemetery, the writer quoted from Harrison's *History of London* (1776, p. 532): "Carnaby Market stands on part of a piece of ground formerly distinguished by the name of Pest-field, where was a lazaretto for the reception of persons seized with the plague in 1665, and at a small distance from it was a common cemetery, where some thousands of persons were buried in that calamitous year." A subsequent response from "An Inhabitant of St. James" contradicted this, writing that the sewer did not traverse any part of the pest-field. Rather, he believed cholera was caused by a change in the sewer line that had previously run down Marshall Street straight to the Thames. The commissioner of sewers had diverted it 50 yards higher up through Broad Street with a flow insufficient to carry away heavy matter originating from the slaughter- and cow-house at the sound end of Marshall.

A third letter from J. York, an inhabitant of Golden Square and the local surveyor, agreed with "Inhabitant." He argued that as the district had previously been exempt from cholera the present epidemic was caused by the fact the sewer at the lower end of the street had turned into a cesspool, "by reason of the current of water having been diverted from it by the recent new sewer operations." Into the old sewer were discharged an immense mass of animal matter and refuse, putrefying into gasses that contaminated the air.[12]

William Farr was responsible for compiling the weekly mortality tables widely distributed in the newspapers. A firm believer that statistics were a useful tool in correlating data with disease, he was instrumental in obtaining accurate records later used by John Snow. A believer in the theory that cholera was caused by miasmic influences, he included elevations above the Trinity high-water mark in an effort to prove those living in the putrid fog along the riverbank were more susceptible. As Steven Johnson indicated in *Ghost Map* (pp. 101–102), this was a case of "correlation being mistaken for causation": those living at higher elevations were safer because their distance from the Thames made them less likely to drink contaminated water.

The average value for houses in the area encompassing Golden Square was £128, markedly higher than most other sub-districts. Water was supplied by both the Grand Junction and the New River companies.

Cholera Deaths, St. James, Westminster

District and Subdivisions	Elevation in 1851	Population Sept. 2	Week Ending Sept 9	Week Ending Sept 16	Week Ending
Berwick St	65	10,798	31	133	25
St. James Sq	40	11,469	8	5	2
Golden Sq W	68	14,139	63	149	40[13]

On September 18, 1854, engineer J. W. Bazalgette presented a report to the commissioners of sewers: "From personal inspection and special inquiry, since the late fearful outbreak of cholera in the district of St. James's, I find those houses which were properly drained into the sewers have been remarkably exempt from the epidemic, and that it burst with unmitigated violence on the overcrowded houses, with overcharged cesspools and obstructed drainage."[14]

The Waterborne Theory of Cholera

As important as sewers were to the general health of a district, Dr. John Snow believed the key lay in the water people drank. As one of England's leading anesthesiologists (see Appendix I, "Cures") Snow had dismissed the idea of miasma as the cause of cholera, concentrating on the waterborne theory. Having already determined vast differences between that carried by the various water companies, he needed to determine which specific company delivered to the cholera-plagued area of Golden Square. The problem would prove nearly impossible, as the water pipes from both the S&V and Lambeth were inextricably tangled and local residents were indifferent to which company the bill was paid.

There were four water pumps in the immediate vicinity, but the 25-foot-deep Broad Street pump was closest to the deadly outbreak. On the surface, this pump seemed the least likely to be the cause as it maintained a reputation as having the sweetest-tasting and (by inference) the purest water. In order to isolate this pump as the source of contagion, Snow made a mental map of the area, determining those residents most likely to use it. Referencing Farr's data and by knocking on doors and through the course of his medical practice, he eliminated the three other pumps by proving the deaths of those living nearest them (who might be supposed to obtain water there) were actually in the habit of drawing water from the Broad Street pump.

Second, he needed to address the question of why there had been so few fatalities among the 535 inmates of St. James's Workhouse, 50 Poland Street, and among the workers at the Lion Brewery, 50 Broad Street: if so many individuals remained unaffected after drinking water from the pump, his theory could not stand. Investigation quickly proved that the workhouse received a private supply from the Grand Junction Water Works and that the brewery had a private pipeline and a well on the premises. In addition, the owners informed him that rather than drink water their employees subsisted on rations of malt liquor.

Fully aware that he must attribute all cholera deaths to the pump or face intense scrutiny and ridicule from his medical brethren tied to the miasma theory, Snow faced one seemingly unexplained cholera death: that of Susannah Eley. A resident of Hampstead, it was extremely unlikely she would have had access to water from the Broad Street pump. Snow interviewed her sons, who operated a factory in the vicinity of the pump, and what they told him must surely have caused goose bumps: on account of the sweet taste, they were in the habit of sending their mother water from the Broad Street pump. The Connection was made.

Ultimately, Snow established that of the 83 deaths from Golden Square, 73 lived closest to the Broad Street pump. He confirmed 61 drew their water from that source, leaving only six unaccounted for. Of the ten cases who had lived outside Snow's boundary, eight had a reasonable connection to the pump.

On September 7, authorities of St. James's Parish held an emergency meeting. John Snow addressed them and presented his data. The following day, in an unheralded act that went unnoticed by the press, the Broad Street pump handle was removed, effectively preventing water from being drawn. More deaths would occur over the next week, but the worst was over. In all, nearly 700 people living within 250 yards of the pump died in a two-week span, causing the *London Observer* to observe, "Such a mortality in so short a time is almost unparalled in this country."

Cholera Deaths, St. James, Westminster

District and Subdivisions	Week Ending Sept. 23	Week Ending Sept. 30
Berwick St	196	3
St. James Sq	17	–
Golden Sq W	262	4[15]

John Snow's connection between water and cholera should have immediately changed the world, but it did not. As with the theory expounding the use of saline to cure cholera, it came at the tail end of the epidemic. With the number of cases subsiding, public interest waned and no one wanted to talk about deadly diseases, even if they had occurred in the very recent past. Authorities ultimately remained unconvinced of Snow's data and his conclusions, finding it safer and easier to maintain hold of their preconceived notions of poison air and sanitation reform. A report read to the court of sewers on September 26 centered on the reconstruction of the sewer that led to the "elongated cesspool" in Broad Street, where drainage from the slaughterhouse caused "lethal effects of its miasma." In defense, the chairman, Mr. Jebb, denied sewers had anything to do with the spread of cholera in the St. James's District, stating the real cause "was the filthy and undrained state of the houses."[16] Even curate Henry Whitehead, who had conducted his own investigations and published a pamphlet, "The Cholera in Berwick Street," shortly after the epidemic, did not subscribe to Snow's proofs.

Determined to prove the doctor wrong, Whitehead conducted research over a four-month period, reaching into April 1855. Instead of disproving Snow's waterborne theory, however, he grudgingly began to accept it. But it was not until he accidentally linked a crucial piece of evidence that the pieces fell into place, providing the answer even Snow did not have: how the epidemic began in the first place.

The Lewises' daughter fell ill on August 28; their home was directly outside the Broad Street pump. Interviewing Mrs. Lewis (her husband had died of cholera two weeks after the outbreak began), Whitehead learned that she had soaked the baby's diapers in pails of water before emptying them in the cesspit in front of the house—less than 3 feet from the pump well. The implications quickly being realized, the local surveyor, Johosephat York, was ordered to dig into the cesspit. He concluded its fluid matter had been draining into the well for a considerable time. If this were correct, removing the pump handle on September 8 came too late to help victims of the epidemic but certainly prevented a second outbreak, as on that date Mrs. Lewis had dumped water contaminated by her dying husband's clothing into the cesspit.

In January 1855, John Snow published the second edition of his 1849 pamphlet, "On the Mode of Communication of Cholera," enlarged and expanded to include the history of the disease and his investigations of the 1854 Broad Street epidemic. In what is now known as the "Grand Experiment," he correlated cholera deaths during the 1848–1849 and 1854 epidemics to the water supplied by the S&V Company, concluding, "If the effect of contaminated water be admitted, it must lead to the conclusion that it acts by containing the true and specific cause of the malady." Far from being successful, the work cost him £200 to print, from which he recovered a scant 200 shillings.

A reviewer for the *Morning Chronicle* concluded, "Whether his theory be sound or not, Dr. Snow deserves credit for the number of facts he has brought to light upon a subject of the deepest interest to all, and we cannot help thinking that his labours will be productive of some useful results." A review in the *Builder* concluded, "The peculiarity of Dr. Snow's theory is, that it is not produced by simple contamination, but that the actual matter of the cholera through the dejections of the patient is thus transmitted."[17]

To date, there is no explanation of how the Lewis baby contracted *V. cholerae*; there were cases in London, but most at the time were located south of the Thames. Nor is there an explanation why the epidemic ended so quickly. Steven Johnson (*Ghost Map*) speculates that cholera having killed so many people, there were not enough fresh sources seeping into the water supply to replenish the organism, or that the water, free from organic matter, eventually starved the bacteria remaining in the dark depths of the well.[18]

"Death in the Pump"

In January 1855, the board of health undertook "the investigation of the meteorological, chemical, and microscopial condition of the air and waters of London," including inquiry into the "defects of our sanitary organisation, and the results of different systems of medical treatment."[19] A medical council consisting of three bodies was appointed: Committee for Scientific Inquiries (Dr. Arnott, Dr. Baly, Dr. Farr, Mr. Owen, Mr. Simon); Treatment Committee (Dr. Alderson, Dr. Babington, Dr. John Ayrton Paris, Dr. Tweedie, Mr. Ward) and Committee for Foreign Correspondence (Dr. Babington, Mr. Bacot, Sir James Clark, Mr. Lawrence). In September, a report of inquiries was presented to President Benjamin Hall. Much of the text concerned "the impure conditions of the London atmosphere." One particularly disturbing paragraph stands out:

> The extraordinary irruption of cholera in the Soho district, which was carefully examined by Mr. Fraser, Mr. Hughes, and Mr. Ludlow, does not appear to afford any exception to generalisations respecting local states of uncleanliness, overcrowding, and imperfect ventilation. The suddenness of the outbreak, its immediate climax, and short duration, all point to some atmospheric or other widely diffused agent still to be discovered, *and forbid the assumption, in this instance, of any communication of the disease from person to person, either by infection or by contamination of water with the excretions of the sick.*[20]

Nearly a year later, a small blue book was published, containing the report by the medical officer of the board of health. In "Report of the Committee for Scientific Inquiries," Mr. Simon, medical officer of the General Board of Health, stated that a comparison between water supplied by the Lambeth and Southwark and Vauxhall companies indicated that supplied by the latter "was not only brackish with the influence of each tide, but contaminated with the outscourings of the metropolis, swarming with infusorial life, and containing unmistakeable molecules of excrement." It continued:

> An experiment, at which mankind would have shuddered if its full meaning could have been prefigured to them, has been conducted during two epidemics of cholera on 50,000 human beings. One half of this multitude was doomed in both epidemics to drink the same fecalized water, and on both occasions to illustrate its fatal results; while another section—freed in the second epidemic from that influence which had so aggravated the first, was happily able to evince, by a double contrast, the comparative immunity which a cleanlier beverage could give. By this experiment, it is rendered in the highest degree probable, that, of the 3,776 tenants of the Southwark and Vauxhall Company who died of cholera in 1853–54, two-thirds would have escaped if their water supply had been like their neighbors'; and that of the much larger number-tenants of both companies-who died in 1848–49, also two-thirds would have escaped, if the Metropolis Water Act of 1852 had but been enacted a few years earlier.[21]

It was not until August 1858 that an investigation into the quality of water supplied from London pumps concluded, revealing "fearful and startling" disclosures. Written by John Simon, it was inspired by an agitation arising from proceedings adopted in the parish of Marylebone by Dr. Robert Thomson. After completing an analysis of pump water, he found that it was "strongly mixed with the surface drainage of the streets, and the percolations from the sewers, as likewise being strongly impregnated even with gas, which had escaped from the gas-pipes beneath the street."

"As in all such movements," the editorialist for the *Morning Chronicle* (August 24, 1858) noted, "strong objections were got up on the old-fashioned plan, 'infringement on the liberty of the subject,' and then a little bit of the canting dodge, 'What prevents the poor man from having a drop of water?'" Although locals described the water as "pellucid and beautiful" and insisted on drinking it over Thomson's defense that it was more impure than when he examined it in 1856, the majority in the vestry overcame the public's "nonsensical objections" and closed the pump.

Dr. Druett, medical officer for St. George's, Hanover Square, also analyzed water from the Park Street pump, finding it to contain "yellow flocculent organic matter, which I believe to have been faeces." He added that a storm might flood such wells with sewage, "and thus we might have diarrhoea or cholera." Dr. Lankester, medical officer for St. James, "in which parish stands the notorious 'cholera pump,'" added this:

> The organic matter found in the surface wells of London are of precisely the same nature as those found in rivers, which are the receptacles of house-sewage. The most observable difference arises from the fact that the water passing into the wells undergoes a process of filtration, so that the animal matters are more perfectly dissolved and decomposed than they are generally in the river waters. Hence the surface well waters are cleaner, whilst the carbonic acid of the decomposed matter makes them sparkling, and the nitrates they contain gives them a pleasant coldness to the taste. Nothing could be better adapted to lure their victims to destruction than the external qualities of these waters, hence the worst of them are the most popular for drinking purposes. The most impure water in this parish is that of the Broad-street pump, and it is altogether the most popular. The large amount of mortality from cholera in this parish in 1854 arose from the popularity of that water, persons sending from a distance to obtain it, and dying of cholera wherever it was drunk.

After Dr. Griffith of Clerkenwell district observed "that the idea of drinking the excretions of other human beings is sufficiently repulsive to counterbalance the attractive physical qualities of pump water," Simon's report concluded that remedying the evil could be accomplished by removing all pumps and filling up wells, while at the same time connecting stand pipes with the water companies' mains to provide pure water.[22]

John Snow, who had achieved the breakthrough of definitively connecting cholera to contaminated water in the Broad Street pump, was not mentioned in Simon's study. Perhaps the greatest acclaim in his lifetime came at a meeting of the British Medical Association in 1856, when Benjamin Ward Richardson introduced a motion of thanks to him for the discovery. Richardson was supported by Edwin Lankester and William Budd, who stated the entire priority of his own investigations belonged to Snow.

On June 9, 1858, Drs. Richardson and Snow attended a meeting; the following day, Snow was seized with paralysis. Attended by Drs. Murchison and Budd, Snow's condition continued to deteriorate, and he died on Wednesday, June 16, at the age of 46, unmarried and childless. The obituary of the Great Experimenter in the *Medical Times* stated, "His name was known to the profession chiefly in connection with chloroform" and added, "He is well known as having devoted great attention to the investigation of cholera, and his views regarding the propagation of the disease by drinking impure water are familiar to the profession,"[23] less than a sterling tribute. It was left to history to accord Dr. Snow the immortality he deserved.

26

The Crimean War and Beyond

It is much to be feared that but few, very few of us, take more than a hurried account of the immense sacrifice of human victims offered up daily to the sanguinary and insatiable god of war.... If we lament anything, it is the comparative inaction of the allied troops. If anything excites our disapprobation, it is that greater injury, that more remediless ruin, has not been inflicted upon our antagonist's forces.... But who thinks of Cholera abroad? Who lays it to heart that it has visited our fleets, both in the Black Sea and in the Baltic, the crews of which it has almost decimated in a few hours?... And then, how little thought we take of surviving relatives and friends—the anguish and the utter desolation of soul with which fond parents or loving children, tender wives, or sisters, or lovers, will be doomed to receive the curt information concerning him upon whom, perhaps, their chief hopes have centered, "Died of Cholera."[1]

The Crimean War (October 1853–February 1856), known in Britain as the "Russian War" and in Russia as the "Eastern War" or, more generally, as the "Eastern Question," stemmed from conflict between the Russian Empire and an alliance between France, the British Empire, the Ottoman Empire and the Kingdom of Sardinia over the future of the weakening Ottoman Empire.

After the coup d'etat in France in 1851, Napoleon III demanded the Ottomans recognize France as the sovereign authority in the Holy Land. Russia quickly disputed this claim, prompting France to send the *Charlemagne* to the Black Sea, eventually achieving a treaty with Sultan Abdulmecid I that confirmed France and the Roman Catholic Church as supreme Christian authority in the Holy Land. This prompted Russian tsar Nicholas I to place troops along the Danube.

Negotiations between British Prime Minister Lord Aberdeen's government and the other three powers—France, Austria and Prussia—met in Vienna and drafted a peace plan that was acceptable to Nicholas I but rejected by Abdulmecid I, who considered it too vague. Abandoning diplomacy, the sultan declared war on October 23, 1853, and moved on the Russian army near the Danube later that month. In the Battle of Sinop, November 30, Russian warships destroyed a fleet of Ottoman frigates, prompting France (March 27, 1854) and Britain (March 28, 1854) to declare war on Russia.[2]

This did not mean the nations were ready for war. The *Medical Circular* of March 30, 1854, began thusly: "No military or medical arrangements have been made in the horrible country known as Dobrudscha." Cholera was already decimating Russian troops. As cholera was little understood, military men believed it could be produced "artificially by compressing together ... large masses of soldiers, and that, under certain conditions, cholera, after being a while in a district, becomes contagious.... Though the infinitesimal treatment [homeopathy] of cholera, and other quackeries, have made much noise in Russia, the best observers believe that in confirmed cholera and collapse all treatment is alike ineffectual." The article ended by pleading for more medical men.[3]

In June, Allied troops landed at Varna. In consequence of cholera raging at the supply base in Gallipoli, all ships arriving from there or the Dardanelles were subject to quarantine. In July, after landing troops at Gallipoli, the steamer *Indus* went on to Varna. When Marshal St. Arnaud released her early from the mandatory ten days' "incubation," he received a formal protest from the Turkish government.

Complicating matters for both sides was the presence of disease at home. Between July 6 and July 12, 101 cholera deaths were reported in Paris; from July 13 to 16th, there were 31 deaths. From July 17 to August 2, six hundred thirty-three fresh cases were reported with 301 deaths; from August 14 to 16th, eighty-one more died, making, from the commencement in November 1853, a total of 4,884 cases: 1,862 recoveries, 2,508 deaths and 514 under treatment. Deaths continued to mount, reaching 150 per day in Paris, with 4,000 dead reported at Marseilles, Burgundy and Dijon suffering most.

Reports dated July 28 indicated that cholera had broken out at Genoa, with 124 cases and 51 deaths, and quickly spread to Leghorn, Florence and Naples. By early August, the city was in panic, exacerbated by rumors that medical men were attempting to poison the Genoese through drugs obtained at apothecaries' shops.

At St. Petersburg, amid a cholera outbreak, Count Woronzoff Dashkau, grand master of ceremonies at the Imperial Court and a privy councilor, and Senator Tolstoi, also a privy councilor, became victims. On July 9, there were 670 cases and 30 deaths and on July 10, there were 55 cases with 30 deaths. By the 14th, 113 new cases resulted in 46 deaths.[4]

Cholera at Varna affected British troops during July, particularly among the officers, including the Duke of Cambridge and Lord Dupplin, but French troops suffered greater casualties. The transport of troops was also affected, as a French troop transport steamer from Marseilles was forbidden entry at Piraeus and was sent on to Gallipoli, but not before four cholera patients were secretly landed. A week later (July 16), the disease appeared in the town near the French camp; by the 20th, twenty-four out of 30 attacked had died.[5]

On July 18, 1854, at a council of war in Varna, the Allies resolved to prepare for an invasion of the Crimea, but as siege artillery and other munitions were lacking, the expedition in the Black Sea was delayed until August 15. Because of the violence of cholera, the date was postponed. Amid the "daily loss of life by cholera," it was hoped the army might "open up more cheering prospects." The article continued: "It might easily have been foreseen that the prevalence of cholera in Europe would seriously aggravate the miseries of war. It has appeared not only at Varna, but at the Piraeus, at Gallipoli, at Adrianople, and in the steam-ships lying in the Bosphorus with troops from England."

A correspondent from the *Morning Chronicle* wrote on August 10 that two battalions of Zouaves and Bashi Bazooks chased the Cossacks to within a few leagues of Kostendje, at the mouth of the Danube, but on July 29, before an attack, the dreadful visitation of cholera "fell on the soldiers like a thunderbolt." The Bashi Bazooks lost one-fourth of their number in four days, some falling from their horses "never to rise again." As soon as he heard the news, "which no one had for a moment anticipated," Marshal de St. Arnaud sent vessels to return the Zouaves (out of 1,200, only 480 survived and out of 10,000 troops of the line, 4,000 were left in the marshes of the death swamp) back to Varna, later remarking in defense, "The flight of the Russians, the cholera, and fire—here certainly are three disasters which I could not have been expected to calculate on."

The French also brought off their forces from Kostendje, having lost, by one estimate,

7,000. A correspondent noted that "without exaggeration, the French bury their dead in fifties." Another eyewitness wrote that as the Russians suffered greatly from the same cause and left behind pits where bodies were piled 8–10 deep. The horrendous losses to disease were attributed to the poisonous condition of the water, "all the wells being filled with dead bodies of Turks and Russians." A private soldier in the Grenadier Guards wrote home to his mother in graphic terms that would be echoed ten years later during the American Civil War:

> The cholera is very bad. We are burying ten or so every day. They are buried very differently from the way in England. They are sown up in a blanket, and put in a hole; and since we left Aladyn, the natives have dug them out on purpose to get the blanket, and have left the bodies exposed to the weather, the wild dogs, and many other animals, such as jackals, &c. The healthiest men seem to go first.[6]

Reports from troops on the Black Sea were hardly less encouraging. After 3 three-deckers, 4 two-deckers and some steam frigates put to sea for a change of air, isolated cases of cholera were seen on the *Trafalgar*, but after two days, the disease broke out "in all its fury in several ships simultaneously." In 24 hours, 50 men died on the *Britannia*, and 30 more in the next 20 hours. Cholera at sea, the British medical report continued, was more frightful than ever. Imagine "1,000 men narrowly caged up" between decks at night, with a heavy sea obliging them to close all the ports, and breathe the most stifling and fetid atmosphere at such a time. Fifty or sixty robust men in the prime of life, are suddenly, almost in an instant, struck with the death-agony, raving, perhaps, or convulsed, in the midst of this dense mass of sleepers." The report noted two remarkable points: not a single officer suffered and cholera "picked and chose among the ships." The *Britannia* lost 100; the *Trafalgar*, another three-decker, 35; the *Albion*, a two-decker, 50; the *Furious*, steam corvette, 17.[7]

On July 19, 1855, Dr. Sutherland, chief sanitary officer in the Crimea, wrote that British troops had been concentrated at Balaklava, observing, "Nothing could be worse than its condition.... All our efforts have been unavailing to save the place from cholera." In defending himself from accusations of unburied carcasses and filth, he added it was not worse than "entire villages I could name in our own country, and it was about on a par with the district where knackers' yards, private slaughterhouses, and unwholesome trades exist in the Borough, and where cholera was so fatal last year." He concluded with a timeless plea:

> War at best is, in one word, "misery." We cannot gild it; it is an abrogation of civilisation for a time, and those engaged in it have to return to primitive habits, and to learn the lesson of ages—I mean physically. Hence, to have an army furnishing the smallest percentage of deaths we must begin military training early. If England will go to war she must consent to study and prepare for it, or to be ready for it. Had we recognized this necessity more we should not have had to pour out so many unavailing regrets and unjust recriminations.[8]

In November 1855, as troops were moved into Scutari, one writer noted that cholera appeared to be "a sort of tribute levied upon every body of men newly imported into the country." Germans suffered worst, being "completely tainted, and have the germ of the malady strong among them," while among the British, 39 officers and 1,203 men were hospitalized with disease. Worse news came from St. Petersburg, where troops were decimated by epidemic cholera, one writer stating that for the previous several years the disease had not ceased a single day: "The number of cases may vary, but the malady never disappears." He added that cholera also raged in Finland, the Baltic provinces, Poland, the Crimea and in the Caucasus.[9]

As the world dragged slowly toward peace, an English physician named Dr. Pincopp from the Scutari hospital suggested that surgeons of the English, French, Sardinian and Turkish armies meet at Constantinople to exchange information on what they learned. From this, they planned a permanent medical association of all nations, by which it was hoped more human lives could be saved.[10]

And Around the World

The year 1854 brought frightful ravages. At Mauritius, a small island off the African coast near Madagascar, 170 out of 273 cases proved fatal; at Barbados, by July 27, cholera was said to have killed 16,817 persons, or nearly one-ninth of the entire population. Horror stories of bodies being interred wrapped in tarred sheets and without Christian burial were rife; in Grenada, after 1,500 succumbed, the dead were consumed by fire. At St. Lucia, 100 deaths at one place was not uncommon, and by August, the disease had spread to Trinidad.[11]

The total number of cholera cases in France from July 17 and August 2, 1854, was 633; 301 died and 217 were discharged. Between August 14 and 16th, there were 156 cases with 81 deaths. From November 1853, there was a total of 4,884 cholera cases, with 2,508 deaths and 1,862 discharged. From July 10 to 29th at Marseilles, deaths exceeded 100 daily, making the general mortality in France 50 percent.[12]

By September 3, 1855, there were 46,480 cases in Lombardy; of these, 13,153 recovered and 22,987 died. Statistics were worse in the province of Brescia, where 8,338 died out of 17,428 cases. At Genoa, out of 1,040 infected, 590 were fatal. From June 10, there were 1,900 cholera victims recorded in Dantzic, of whom 1,200 died; in Stettin, out of 631 cases, 347 terminated fatally (137 recovered).

On the cholera trail, the disease made an appearance at Para, traveled via a Portuguese vessel to Bahia and finally arrived at Rio de Janeiro.[13] Accounts from Florence indicated that 11,000 died during the month of August 1855, reducing the population from 100,000 to 60,000 by death and flight. Numerous reports of people being buried alive filled the newspapers; one survivor who disinterred himself told the tale of being buried with 10 others, several of whom lay twitching beside him.[14] So prevalent was the fear of premature burial that in 1869, news of a French physician's invention to determine death became important news. His technique involved dropping Belladonna in the eye: during life, the pupil dilated; in death, it did not. He recorded the operation using a camera with ordinary photographic paper that unrolled from a spindle for 10–15 minutes. After that time, if no variation in the pupil was detected, the subject was known to be dead.[15]

During August 1856, official returns from Lisbon indicated more than 500 deaths from cholera in a single week; cholera also appeared at Madeira, supposedly brought in by an infected ship. By mid–August, 5,000 cases were reported, most untreated from a lack of medical men, forcing the Portuguese government to dispatch a warship there with several practitioners and apothecaries, all of whom "received a handsome remuneration." The following year, the path continued into Sweden, killing 5,000. Norwegians fell next, before the disease ascended northward by the coast of the Gulf of Bothnia. In 1858, cholera in Honduras claimed 5,000 lives, originating, it was said, by the opening of cholera graves from 20 years earlier.[16]

The Medical Literature

While hope existed for a learned "Medical Association," medical literature of the times fell short of recognizing the advances made by saline treatment or the transmission of cholera solely by contaminated water. Richard Hassall, M.D. (1854), promoted castor oil and fresh air; Dr. Thomas Allan (1854) argued that there was no "presumptive evidence" to support any theory, but entertained the idea that heat, moisture and conditions of soil and atmosphere assisted in its development. Dr. Henry Stephens, in *Cholera: An Analysis of Its Epidemic, Endemic, and Contagious Character* (1854), oddly supported an "antiseptic theory" whereby drugs "which have the power of preserving dead animal or vegetable substances from decomposition" (such as mercurial preparations, kreosate, arsenic, nitrate of silver, vinegar, cinchona and alcohol) would cure cholera. James Arnott (1854) proposed the use of extreme cold for the treatment of epidemic cholera; Dr. Granville (1854) used statistics to prove that cholera was "an inexplicable visitation" from Heaven that did not, "in reality increase the average rate of mortality." In 1855, James John Garth Wilkinson, M.D., pleaded for the homeopathic treatment of cholera, stating that out of 1,875 cases treated according to that system, only 169 died; a "Pedestrian" wrote *Plague Cradles of the Metropolis* in 1855, arguing cholera was caused by poisonous vapor; and Henry Wentworth Acland, M. D. (1856), argued for improvements in spiritual and temporal living conditions for the poor. The only mention of saline treatment came in an advertisement for a pyretic saline preparation advocated by a Dr. Turley and sold by Dr. William Stevens.[17]

While taxes on windows, coal, candles and soap were removed in an effort to improve health, as late as 1858, an inquest into the death of Richard Billingsley, waterman, was attributed to "Asiatic cholera, brought on by inhaling the noxious vapours of the Thames."[18] Innumerable meetings were held on the "State of the Thames," and everyone had a theory on how to purify it; little overall success was achieved. One tongue-in-cheek editorial noted the following:

> The obituary of the London daily newspapers may shortly be expected to contain an announcement something like the following: "We regret to announce that in consequence of the frightfully foetid state of the river Thames, the banks and water, the greater number of the members of the House of Lords and Commons are ill from Asiatic cholera, and as the public are aware, the mortality has been so serious, a sufficient number cannot now be mustered to form a House, Parliament has therefore been shut up for the present."[19]

The Third Cholera Pandemic ended in 1859, but it would not be long before another outbreak occurred, as too little sanitation had been accomplished and authorities continued to argue over the cause.

In accordance with the Public Health Act of 1858, the British Privy Council was empowered to make inquiry into the outbreak of disease. Mr. Simon superintended the 1860 report, part of which detailed "the Thames nuisance" and the "diarrhoeal districts of England," noted to be increasing and of "appalling severity." Those towns habitually suffering an excess of mortality from diarrhea and cholera were Coventry, Manchester, Salford, Nottingham, Birmingham, Dudley, Leeds, Wolverhampton and Merthyr Tydfil. In all, two circumstances stood out: impure water drinking and an atmosphere tainted by decomposition, especially human refuse.[20]

In 1861, Dr. Letheby issued a report to the commissioners of sewers, headlined by newspapers as "The Poisonous Wells of the City." Remarking on the same idea Snow found in his research at Golden Square, that clear and remarkably cool water was presumed to be pure, he disputed the notion by stating that London pump water used by the laboring classes was incredibly contaminated.

> The quantity of organic matter in them ranges from 1.5 grains per gallon to 8.8; the common salt, from 2.7 to 25; the sulphate of lime, from 2 to 29; the alkaline nitrates, from 2.1 to 24.6; and the combined ammonia, from 6.5 to 2 grains per gallon. The results show that the City wells are not only charged with decaying organic matter, but also with the saline products of its oxydation: the

ammonia, for instance, is a sign of *present putrefaction,* and the alkaline nitrates, of a *past;* besides which, the existence of so large a quantity of common salt is suggestive of the *filthiest impurities,* as, for example, the fluid matter discharged from the human body and the percolations from cesspools and sewers.[21]

Not surprisingly, another pandemic was on the horizon. While it was estimated that a single visit of cholera in London cost one million sterling, the toll on human life would prove incalculable.[22]

27

The Fourth Cholera Pandemic, 1863–1879

A physician, in company with others of the profession, thus boasted: "I was the first to discover the Asiatic cholera, and communicate it to the public."[1] A jovial doctor, on being asked, "How do you treat the cholera?" replied, "I treat it with contempt."[2]

In 1863, the subject of deodorizing and disinfecting sewage was brought to the attention of the municipal commissioners of Bombay by staff assistant-surgeon P.G. Hewlett. To eliminate the "gasses emitted from putrefying animal and vegetable matter," he suggested the use of carbonic acid during the cholera season. The idea was favorably received, placing the city in a superior state to Calcutta, but attention to the drainage of the city remained a matter of concern.[3] In 1868, Hewlett, the health officer of Bombay, reported great improvement in public health, citing the reduction of cholera deaths between 1864 and 1867 as 5.9 per 1,000; 3.5; 0.4 and 0.1, resulting in a scant 111 deaths for 1867.[4]

Among the poorer classes of Calcutta, one favored treatment for cholera was that of "quassia inoculation," developed by Dr. Honigberger and performed by two of his native assistants. Medical authorities took a different view: Dr. Stovell, principal inspector-general, Bombay, wrote that in his view, quassia was "a species of empiricism which may serve for a time to influence the minds of the ignorant native population" but when used alone prevented the use of more conventional measures.[5]

From Shanghai, 1863, Florence Nightingale wrote she was sorry to say that cholera had made its appearance again, noting, "I am afraid we shall have such another summer as the last. We are losing men fast; not a day passing without one or two dying from it. I was in charge of funeral parties three nights running last week, and fearfully sudden are the attacks.... You really can have no idea of what Chinese dirt is, and they are commencing to leave their coffins about again in hundreds. The other night when going round the garrison guards, the stench was overpowering, and very nearly made me ill, and we cannot go a hundred yards without coming upon a lot of them.... The soldier dies in the East—not at the cannon's mouth, but at the mouth of a sewer."[6]

In 1865, many pathologists attributed the outbreak of cholera in Arabia ("Hedschaz, the Holy Land of Islamism, and notably in the cities of Mecca and Medina, and upon Mount Ararat") to the "Kourban-Bairam" (Feast of Sacrifice), which yearly drew 700,000–800,000 pilgrims. Crowded conditions, the "murderous character of the climate," the fact the dead were "hastily shuffled under the desert sand," and the "prejudice" not to change clothes (upon returning home, these garments were cut into pieces and distributed as memorials; clothes of the dead were preserved for the same reason) was added to the offal, blood, bones and entrails of 2,000,000 sacrificed sheep, creating a "glowing atmosphere" of deadly miasma.

The Kourban-Bairam was celebrated in the first week of May, and when cholera broke out, 100,000 died within a fortnight. Worse, the sick carried disease with them, changing traditional routes of contagion over Arabia to Alexandria, Istanbul, Southern France and Italy. This prompted Porte authorities to establish a sanitary commission compelling Turkish physicians to introduce more precautions in religious practices of the pilgrims while still adhering to principles of the Koran. Later in the year, the president of the General Sanitary Department for Egypt, Colucci Bey, called upon European powers to assist in preventing further cholera epidemics as it was "far beyond the competence of the Egyptian Government or even of the Porte."[7] Mortality at Alexandria on July 3 reached 228 and fell on the 4th to 176 and to 118 on the 5th. At Cairo, during the same period, deaths were reported between 300 and 500 per day.[8] To prove the theory that cholera was caused by a "peculiar state" of the air, two balloons were sent up, one from a village untainted by cholera and the other from Alexandria. Hanging from them were quarters of meat. The one floating over Alexandria returned completely putrefied while the other remained perfectly fresh.[9] Reports from Constantinople dated August 9 indicated mortality exceeded 1,500 for the week, attributed to raw fruit and shallow graves disturbed by starving dogs.[10]

In March 1865, conflicting reports from St. Petersburg of a strange disease (alternately referred to as "the worst kind of cholera" or a plague of a "typhodial [sic] character") struck with force. The first symptom was a cramp in the nape of the neck extending into the cerebellum, followed by rapid death. The Berlin correspondent of the *London Times* called it a "malignant species of *febris meningitis spinalis*," or recurrent fever, that began in September 1864, reaching a mortality of 30–60 percent. Dr. Charles Murchison referred to it as a "relapsing fever," while the Rev. J.F. Francklin of Whaplode, Lincolnshire, reported a similar disease in his parish referred to simply as "the illness." Another authority likened it to "congestive or spotted fever" that had struck Federal troops during the Civil War.[11]

Significantly, although camp hygiene had not progressed much further than that practiced during the Mexican War (1846–1848), where the ratio of death from injury and disease was 1:7, cholera did not play a major role in the American Civil War. Diarrhea and dysentery were the primary bowel diseases, from which 44,558 Union soldiers perished, compared with 110,070 combat-related deaths.[12]

One point of historical trivia from the Civil War bears mentioning. Augustus Stanwood of Maine was a paper manufacturer. Because rags were in short supply, he resorted to a practice common in the 1850s: using contraband Egyptian mummy bandages that could be obtained more cheaply than ordinary cloth rags. Stanwood could find no way to bleach the resin-coated cerements white and so gro-

The American Civil War was widely reported in England and garnered great interest. Hoping to capitalize on this, John Jackson promoted Worsdell's Compound as "The Great American Remedy." Letting testimonials prove the efficacy of his product, Jackson's carminative (meaning "to allay pain and dispel flatulence") contained the home remedy blackberry brandy as his prime ingredient. Medicines with high alcoholic content were often a substitute for liquor obtained in bars and carried none of the stigma of alcohol consumption (*East London Advertiser*, July 11, 1863).

cers used his product to wrap food. When a cholera epidemic broke out, the source was traced to the paper mill, where the workers had been handling the mummy wrappings.[13]

The Imperial Medical Society of Marseilles, registering 30 deaths per day during September, declared cholera had been brought from Egypt. Between September 18 and 19, 1865, eighty-seven deaths were recorded, throwing townspeople into a state of panic; in neighboring Segue, after 20 died in a single day, 8,000 of a population of 12,000 literally took flight. A similar situation was seen in Madrid as "fugitives rushed into the trains" to escape.[14]

The year 1866 saw more of the same. Daily mortality figures in Paris during July, although considered "moderate for so populous a city," were: 19th, 116; 20th, 142; 21st, 106; 22nd, 89, 23rd, 92; 24th, 94; 25th, 90; and 26th, 86. Perhaps more telling was the story of a French mayor, who, upon being notified to take precautions, had graves dug in sufficient number to accommodate the whole population. A less gruesome situation but more violent, riots broke out at Amsterdam when authorities cut short the annual fair on account of cholera.[15]

A Lover of Coincidences

In 1865, there was likely some consternation in England with the success of Meyerbeer's opera *L'Africaine*, as one sage drew the conclusion that cholera outbreaks in France always followed the production of the composer's works. As "proof," it was pointed out that *Robert le Diable* appeared in 1831, *Les Huguenots* in 1836 and *La Prophete* in 1848, all cholera years. The same fatal attendant waited on *L'Etoile du Nord* and *Le Pardon de Ploemel* (*Dinorah*), but his minor works did not provoke as great a devastation.[16]

Less coincidentally, Dr. Letheby, medical health officer for the City of London, traced the path of cholera in his "1865 Sanitary Report." In previous epidemics, the disease came prominently from India and moved in a northwesterly direction through Persia and along the waters of the Caspian Sea to Astracan, before traversing Russia by the Volga and reaching Moscow. After halting for the winter, the disease again moved in a northwesterly direction, arriving at St. Petersburg by June or July. It then branched off in two directions: northwesterly through Finland and by the Gulf of Bothnia into the north of Sweden, where it died out, and southwesterly and via the Baltic into Sweden, Prussia and Denmark and then across the German Ocean into the eastern coast of England.

On this occasion, however, the course of the epidemic was confined almost entirely to the eastern shores of the Mediterranean, acquiring its virulence among the pilgrims at Mecca and Mount Ararat. After the pilgrims dispersed, epidemic cholera appeared at Alexandria; by June, it moved inward, via the river, to Cairo and returned via the eastern arm of the Nile, to Damietta, where it proved remarkably fatal. The path then crossed the eastern extremity of the Mediterranean to Smyrna and shortly afterwards turned back upon Cyprus. By early July, cholera had reached Constantinople, Ancona, Italy, Malta and Sicily. Letheby concluded there seemed little tendency to move north and westward toward Europe, but warned that in the spring of 1866, if cholera again appeared at Constantinople, it could creep along the eastern coast of the Black Sea and take its usual route by the Danube into Europe and reach the western states of Germany. It might also reappear upon the northern shores of the Mediterranean and travel into Italy, France or Spain.[17]

Letheby's worst-case scenario came to pass, and by May 1866, cholera appeared at Liverpool; towns immediately applied to enforce the Disease Prevention Act by establishing quarantines. That the quarantines did not work was proven, as the disease spread into the east of

London, affecting Whitechapel, Bow and Stepney. The poor law board put local boards of guardians on notice to enforce extensive regulations, but England's preparations for staving off another epidemic proved grossly inadequate. Death tolls of 904, 1053, and 781 were registered between the weeks ending July 28 and August 11.[18]

As the disease waned in October, nothing had been accomplished, either in medicine or law, to prevent another epidemic. As the *Nonconformist* cried on October 31, "The legislature must no longer be content to pass stringent Acts, but must provide an agency capable of carrying them into effect." The last scene was painted by "A Cholera Hospital Widow":

> A man in the prime of life occupies [a hospital bed]; he has matted locks, damp brow, hollow eyes, and quick-coming but feeble breath. Those eyes so sunken are wide open, the pulse has fallen, and the natural heat of the body is decayed and spent.... His bare arms are blue at the elbows, and on the backs of his hands are stripes and streaks of a deep blue; his chin, clean shaven, but rigid and ghastly, is thrown up in the air.... For worn and wasted as he is, the brain is clear; and the eye, fixed though it be, is full of intelligence.... We must all face death alone; the end of the battle of life is with each of us a single combat. Pray Heaven that you and I bear it as bravely as did this poor stranger.[19]

Overleaping Seas and Countries: The Fourth Pandemic in the United States

On February 26, 1866, "An Act to Create a Metropolitan Sanitary District and Board of Health Therein" passed the New York state legislature, empowered to both create and administer ordinances relating to the preservation of public health.[20] There would be much work to do, for by August, Dr. Elisha Harris, its corresponding secretary, reported that cholera had "rapidly overleaped seas and countries in its approach to our country." Without intermittent steps or long delays, epidemics had already appeared in New York, Cincinnati, Louisville, Tybee Island, Savannah, and upon military transports on the Mississippi and in Galveston harbor.

In Cincinnati, 60–90 lives were lost daily, while the overcrowded and filthy quarters occupied by the poor in St. Louis, "the great centre of Western commerce," flanked by undrained and stagnant pools, made confinement of the disease impossible. By mid–August, 806 cases had already been registered. Chicago and several towns upon the western railroad lines "gave probability to the opinion that Cincinnati, Louisville and New Orleans" were major centers of dissemination. The report added that the French and Negro quarters of New Orleans were ravished but predicted Boston, Providence, Newark, Baltimore and the inland cities of New York and Pennsylvania were in a "good state of readiness" to combat the epidemic.[21]

In post–Civil War America, when the *New York Times* reported cholera among the Negroes at the Freedmen's Hospital and in Carolina, the writer also felt free to add: "Here is the opportunity now for the Abolitionists to show how much they really care for and sympathize with the negro. They were ready enough to come down in the Winter months to a mild pleasant climate ... for which they were well paid, and lived comfortably. But let us see how many Abolition 'Howards' and 'Florence Nightingales' will come South at this time of the year to nurse and care for the poor darkey?"[22] Reports from New Orleans, August 27, indicated cholera was abating in the city, but showed no diminution on the plantations, where the "Negroes" were convinced they were being poisoned by the whites and refused to take their remedies.[23]

As in Europe, the newspapers were full of speculations on the origin, prevention and cure of cholera. The favorite theory, noted the *New York Times*, was that choleraic germs were distributed in the water. It was suggested to boil the water or drink hot coffee and tea. Unconvinced, the newspaper added there were also the "blue mist" and "dirt" theories. As if to confirm the former, in September, Nashville physicians affirmed that during the cholera ravages, a "misty blue vapor, hardly visible, without any perceivable smell, hung over the town, being densest in the filthy places.... This statement agrees with that of other cities, including Memphis, and is believed to be present in all places scourged by this malady." At Cincinnati, flies died on the streets and the gutters were covered with a green scum, while the atmosphere was dry, heavy and sickening. In a more dangerous situation, at Philadelphia, the city council refused an appropriation of $20,000, prompting the board of health to give notice it would no longer remove nuisances from the streets.[24]

Cholera cases decreased during the summer, but despite the lateness of the season, mortality suddenly escalated: At Nashville during the last two weeks of September, 554 deaths were registered out of a population of 20,000. What was more staggering, between August 1 and mid–November, 7,000 cholera deaths were recorded in the cities of Cincinnati, St. Louis, Nashville and Memphis. October proved the most deadly month in Chicago, when 1,175 out of a total cholera mortality of 1,581 were registered.[25]

Cholera in New York City, 1866

The first case occurred on May 1, killing Mrs. Jenkins, a 35-year-old woman living in a tenement-house on Third Avenue and Ninety-third Street. By June 6, the disease had manifested a tendency to occur in groups as a "house epidemic," with causes attributed to saturated clothing and the infected excrements of the cholera sick. By July, there existed in New York and Brooklyn certain "well-marked cholera fields" where the "virtue of the epidemic" was attributed to the soil or local atmosphere. By August 1, the number of cases had advanced from 25 to 30 per day. Reaching a high point on August 4, rates slowly declined until October 10, when the epidemic was considered over. In his report to the board of health, Dr. Harris drew a number of conclusions:

1. Neither the "house epidemics" nor cholera fields were solely the result of local origin or domestic causes.
2. When property was not properly disinfected, cholera gained a foothold; when disinfection was prompt, the disease was arrested.
3. In 362 houses brought under sanitary control, cholera did not spread beyond those previously infected.
4. Overcrowding, bad ventilation, dampness, filth, neglected water closets, common privies, street filth and defective drainage aided in the spread of disease.
5. One-half of victims who reached the "cold stage" died, and no method of treatment had any positive effect upon cholera in collapse.
6. Choleric diarrhea preceded full-blown outbreaks.
7. When cholera was left to contaminate an area, outbreaks followed.

Between May 1 and November 30, 1,215 persons died of Asiatic cholera in New York City. Harris concluded the disease was introduced by passengers aboard the *Atlantic, Virginia, Peruvian, Union* and *Bavaria* ships and that more than 50,000 emigrants from Europe arrived at Castle Garden from areas where cholera was present at the time of departure. Under the heading "Sanitary Deductions," he concluded "that the diarrhoeal excrets of the sick when impregnating the soil, the drinking water, or any kind of decomposing matter, especially that of privies, cesspools, sewers, drains, and the ground about dwelling houses," constituted "the only means for propagating and spreading Asiatic cholera."[26]

Putting Out the Sparks: The International Sanitary and Weimar Conferences

In 1851, at the invitation of the French government, the first International Sanitary Conference (ISC) was held in Paris. The six-month debate between experts from most European powers and the Ottoman Empire (which had formal or informal control over Muslim lands in the Middle East) centered on how to keep cholera out of Europe. Debate during the Second ISC, held in Paris in 1859 and attended by delegates from the United States, concerned quarantine but little was accomplished.[27]

The Third ISC, held at Constantinople in 1866, determined that the disease was primarily spread by pilgrims attending annual Hindoo festivals and recommended strict quarantine at all seaports of the Red Sea. This did not meet with much acceptance, as authorities considered the expense too great and the probability of success too slim. In 1867, a world conference held at Weimar sought to replace the suggestion of quarantine with more practicable measures. Reports set down by these scientific physicians were based on "special investigations, experimental, microscopial, and chemical" studies. Sir John Simon of England, an adherent of Pettenkofer's theory, that cholera was dependent on the different qualities and states of local soil, demonstrated the prevalence of the disease with maps, showing how cholera coincided with the want of cleanliness, pure water and disinfectants; attendees agreed that if all countries were careful to "put out the sparks," or remove local causes by enforcing these plain prescriptions, cholera would be starved out, eliminating the need for quarantines. Dr. Harris also forwarded a paper sketching the recent success of the New York Board of Health.

Without specifically delving into the cause or communication of cholera, members generally held that cholera was propagated and spread by an infective poison of the excremental discharges of the sick that could be destroyed by certain chemical agents. Among the best and least expensive were copperas and carbolic acid; St. Louis was cited as an example of how the system worked when officials acted soon after the arrival of a cholera patient in the spring of 1867. After making house-to-house visitations, the board of health put down disinfectants, eradicating the disease and making the city one of the healthiest and safest in America. (As an indication of how fast matters changed, by late September, 100 deaths per day were reported from St. Louis. One special dispatch noted that deaths arose "from the indiscreet conduct of the Board of Health, in rescinding the order relating to the sale of vegetables, &c." In defense, Mayor Thomas stated that, "from its geographical position [St. Louis was] the empire city of the West, and of the Mississippi valley, being easy of access by steamboats and railroads" and the only place "within 300 miles where hospital treatment existed," and thus became "the resort of large numbers of the sick and afflicted, not only of the people of Missouri and Illinois, but of Kansas, Iowa, Indiana, Kentucky, Tennessee and many of the southern states.")

CONCLUSIONS AND RECOMMENDATIONS

1. Efforts to arrest and prevent cholera by disinfectants should be continued in the most energetic manner.

CHOLERA. — JOHNS'S PATENT PERMANENT STUCCO WASH.

— The attention of SANITARY BOARDS, Boards of Guardians, Barrack Masters, and the public generally, is directed to this WASH, which has been adopted in some of the largest Hospitals and Asylums, as being a cheap, readily applied, and efficacious non absorbent for all rough surfaces likely to retain miasma. It dries quickly, does not wash off, and may be exported to any climate.

In Casks of one to five cwt. each, ready for use.—Manufacturers, PHILIP HARE and Co., 22, STEEL-YARD, UPPER THAMES-STREET.

John's Patent Permanent Stucco Wash was another example of the plethora of products rushed to market as the concept of disinfecting buildings to prevent the spread of cholera became generally accepted. As with many ads of the time, the manufacturer appealed to those who clung to the idea of poisoned air by promising his wash would stick to rough surfaces likely to retain miasma (*London Daily News*, November 15, 1853).

2. Disinfection should be done by sanitary authorities in a compulsory manner after excremental matter was gathered and kept from being cast about.

3. When entire localities could not be disinfected, concentration was to be throughout places where cholera had previously visited.

4. Disinfection should be performed at the proper time and infected areas were to be continuously disinfected.

5. A combination of sulphate of iron (copperas) and carbolic acid were the best disinfectants.

6. Infected clothing should be boiled in water or chemically treated with "zinc vitriol" (sulphate of chloride of zinc).

7. Disinfection of sewers and drains should follow the trial of Mr. Sauvern's method (similar to that published by McDougal, who used a combination of carbolic or coal-tar preparations, in a cheap form).

8. Infected houses should be vacated and the inhabitants removed.

9. Groundwater should be kept clean and disinfected; all drinking water should be pure or disinfected by boiling.

An editor for the *Edinburgh Evening Courant* concluded with the following: "Henceforth municipal remissness will be unable to shelter itself behind the alleged variance of medical opinion as to its counteracting agents, and all cases of neglect must be visited with the severity appropriate to every breach of a simple and universally recognized duty."[28]

On August 11, 1866, under the sanction of the Privy Council, Dr. Burdon-Sanderson began experiments "to conclusively establish the communicability of cholera," following the course adopted in 1854 by Professor Thiersch, who concluded cholera "possessed a peculiar contagiousness." In both studies, strips of paper were steeped in cholera matter at certain intervals after its removal from the body during life or after death to represent every stage of decomposition. White mice were used, as their digestive systems were considered close to that of humans.

After the cholera matter killed one series of mice, their bodies were devoured by a second series; it was found these bodies communicated the original form of disease in undiminished virulence, with mortality as high as 57 percent. Sanderson concluded, "We have, therefore, evidence that the disease produced in mice by the administration of cholera material in small doses can be readily communicated from the affected animals to others of the same species, and that when so communicated it is quite as fatal as when received primarily."

Sanderson's Study on White Mice, per 100 Animals Employed

Period of Decomposition	Number Affected	Number Died
1st day	11	8
2nd day	86	32
3rd day	100	21
4th day	71	57
5th day	40	24
6th day	0	0

The researcher added that the liability to attack was of greater importance than mortality, making the 3rd and 4th days of highest significance. He also reported that during the month of November he achieved negative results, leading to the supposition that temperature was critical to the transmission of the disease. Experiments with guinea pigs, hedgehogs, pigeons and dogs did not yield any important results. In reviewing the studies, John Simon noted the positive results "would retain their full value in regard to the animals experimented on, even if all other animals should prove insusceptible of the influence; and the value in explanation of the facts of human infection, is, in my opinion conclusive."

Already an ardent supporter of Pettenkofer's soil theory, Simon took Sanderson and Thudichum's subsequent experiments a step further by suggesting the results were "dependent under varying conditions of *time* and *place*," drawing his own conclusion that the two great governing influences for the spread of cholera were the height of wells and the determination of water levels in the soil."[29]

Moving even closer to enlightenment, at a meeting of the American Institute, Professor Vornderweyde remarked that many diseases ascribed to other causes, including cholera, were actually produced by animaliculae and soon the discovery of parasitic life would be proven by microscopic analysis.[30] The 1867 Medical Congress at Paris proved less helpful. Authorities concluded cholera was not contagious but originated where large numbers of people collected under bad hygienic or atmospheric conditions. Declaring crowding was the principal cause, they suggested individuals in an infected district should be scattered and their clothes disinfected.[31]

"The gross ignorance of the population"

Epidemic cholera raged in the southern Italian provinces during the summer of 1867, reaching 13,983 cases by late August, with 8,337 deaths. Equally distressing were local riots, occasioned by the belief that the disease was caused by poisoners. Numerous reports of "savage atrocities" from Milan, Salerno, Calabria and Potentino cited instances where druggists or those thought to "blow poison through keyholes" were dragged from their homes, beaten and dismembered.

Of Rome, it was written that filth "at the corner of every street is kept up as a national institution. All over the south of Europe, in some of the French departments, and throughout Spain and Italy, the same contempt for sanitary measures; the same disregard for the common decencies of life, are observable; but still the very centre of all uncleanliness is Rome, and habits unworthy of human beings linger."[32] As if in acknowledgment, thunderstorms washing up filth from the streets caused "poisonous vapors," leading to 50 deaths per day. Official reports indicated that from May 4 through mid–August, 2,800 cases resulted in 1,458 deaths.[33] In Rotterdam, on August 12 after the *kermesse* was held, 388 cholera cases were reported by September 8, and 245 proved fatal, while in the China's northwestern provinces, the monthly mortality rate rose from 8 : 1,000 in October 1866 to 13 : 1,000 in October 1867. Mortality from cholera in October was given as 5,339, compared to 726 from the same period in 1866.[34] News was little better at "Buenos Ayres," where a recurrence of cholera that claimed 3,000 lives in 1867 made a comeback in the spring of 1868. It was said to have swept down the Parana from the pestilential quarters of the seat of war, while as far away as Belgium, from September 1867 until February 1868, cholera was said to have claimed 27,340 lives.[35]

"Facts Regarding Cholera"

In 1869, the *Delhi Gazette* offered a short resume of facts known regarding cholera:

1. Cholera was an ancient disease, being mentioned in the Sanskrit *Nidan* of Siesruta, then called "Vishuka."
2. Fatal epidemics of cholera may occur anywhere in the world.
3. Sporadic cases can only be explained by admitting the malady may arise or be reexcited into action by favorable circumstances.
4. Once it has originated, the malady may subside or spread.
5. When it is spread, sufficient time has passed for human intercourse to take place between the sites.
6. Cholera follows great lines of traffic.
7. It prevails more in low, damp localities, where sanitation is poor; inspiration of an impure atmosphere localizes cholera.
8. Impure water has a powerful influence over the intensity of cholera as proven by Drs. Acland, Sutherland, Budd and Snow. Unwholesome food or the injudicious use of purgatives act as a determining or predisposing cause of cholera.[36]

During 1867, the strength of the British Army in India was 34,603 until the close of the year, when 6,000 were sent to Abyssinia. Of that total number, 1,071 died, 479 as a result of cholera, especially at Rohilcund and in the Punjaub. By contrast, soldiers' wives and children suffered a mortality of 96.91 per thousand. In the disgraceful gaols of Bengal, mortality was 56.65 percent. By November 1869, four hundred natives a day were dying from cholera in the northwestern provinces, with 70 percent of those attacked perishing.[37]

The 1870 report on the sanitary condition of Shanghai was worse. Prepared by Dr. Jamieson, it described scorching heat, uncontrolled prostitution and low grogshops as contributing evils, but his primary emphasis centered on the lack of sanitation. Beginning with the European community, he described their stately homes built on alluvial plains, making drainage impossible, and the absence of wells from which to draw pure water.

In the native city, open privies were backed up, creating cesspools that reeked of poisonous vapors; slime-covered ditches were receptacles for filth; and open spaces were converted into ash pits where decaying ordure, dead animals and rotten vegetables festered. Additionally, canals that intersected the city were not cleaned, resulting in a great spread of waste during high tides. Jamieson called for new sanitary measures by showing how the excreta of cholera patients found its way into the water used for drinking and cooking.[38]

Cholera in Sub-Saharan Africa

The first of two 19th century cholera visitations in the Senegal and Gambia river valleys occurred during the Fourth Pandemic, 1868–1869. During November and December 1869, the French colonial capital of Saint-Louis registered nearly 100 deaths per day; by the time the disease subsided, 1,112 Africans and 92 Europeans had died. Another epidemic began in June 1869 and lasted until the beginning of 1870.[39] A letter to the *Lancet* described conditions at the cholera cemetery at Bathurst from May 29, 1868, noting that trenches holding cholera victims were so shallow, arms and legs protruded: "The stench from the exposed bodies was horrible."[40] Further information stated that cholera had killed 1,823 out of 4,600 natives of Santa Marie de Bathurst. Of the 25 white settlers, only one was attacked.[41]

The island of Zanzibar suffered from cholera visitations in 1821, 1836, 1860 and 1869. During the last six weeks of 1869, there were a reported 15,000 deaths, including a number of American seamen. The island had recently been made familiar to Europeans as the place of residence of Dr. Kirk, one of the men communicating with Livingstone, and 20 other Europeans lived there for the purpose of trade. The population of Mohammedan Arabs amounted to about 100,000, most of whom lived in town. During the outbreak of cholera that included the mainland, 13 English people and Americans died, while 30,000 natives perished. It was said that caravans from the interior laden with ivory and spices were abandoned on the plain as merchants fled for their lives.[42]

Cholera in Russia

Reports dating from December 1869 at Kieff indicated that Asiatic cholera carried off patients within hours. The same swift action was seen in St. Petersburg, as people died "while walking in the streets." The *Official Messenger* reported 26 cases at Orel on January 13, 1870, and 27 more the following week, of whom 14 died. Small outbreaks were seen in the government of Minsk (Russian Poland) at the end of December and early January, and the disease was also seen at Kursk and Smolensk, in western Russia. By March, "instantaneous deaths" were being reported at Moscow.[43]

28

The Water We Drink

The Thames along the bridges and far below the Pool became putrid; those who accidentally fell into its filthy waters were poisoned rather than drowned, London lived over an open sewer, and but for the fortunate circumstance that the House of Commons was placed on its banks, and that no lime-washed blinds could keep the horrid effluvia from the palace of Parliament, the Thames might still be a stinking drain. Awful lessons helped the warnings of sanitary reformers.[1]

Science and sanitary reform were advancing. In September 1869, at a meeting of the British Medical Association at Leeds, Sir William Jenner positively stated that two of the most fearful diseases, cholera and typhoid fever, were "mainly if not entirely propagated by the drinking of contaminated water." Almost simultaneously, Dr. William Budd of Bristol read a paper before the Sanitary Section of the Social Sciences Congress. In what had the potential to revolutionize medical practice, he stated (1) The vast brood of infectious, or "self-propagating" diseases, furnish the great field for preventative medicine; (2) The same diseases furnish preventative medicine its greatest opportunity.

Grouping together smallpox, measles, scarlet fever, whooping cough, typhus, enteric fevers, cholera and other infectious diseases in the category of self-propagating, Budd calculated that in 1863 (an average year), 10,049 out of 69,983 deaths were attributed to infectious diseases. In 1866, when cholera prevailed, the ratio was 19,626 out of 81,808. Adding consumption to the list raised the proportion to two-sevenths of the whole. When the list was finalized, he determined that infectious diseases would actually account for nearly a third of all deaths and half of concurrent sicknesses.

"Each infectious disease," he stated, "is caused by a specific entity of its own; the living body is the soil in which this entity grows and multiplies, and from which issues the seed for future crops." To prevent infectious diseases, the seed of infection must be destroyed as it issued from the body of the already infected man: "The whole case is ripe for action; the law of spreading is made out, the conditions of prevention are clear; the measures required are for the most part easy of execution, and, when not so, may be defined in the simplest terms.... All that is needed is the fitting organisation to give effect to knowledge, and this organisation can only be supplied by the State controlling or compelling individual action for the general good."

Budd called for an enlarged and greatly empowered government body to enforce sanitary legislation, "and to do away with that form of liberty to which some communities cling, the sacred liberty to poison unto death, not only themselves, but their neighbors. What we have is a small Board of able men.... What we want is a standing army, well-trained and ably commanded."

Even as he spoke, Budd must have known what he proposed was the same battle waged by vaccinationists—and lost. Despite overwhelming evidence that vaccination prevented small-

225

pox, anti-vaccination leagues in Europe and the United States argued successfully that mandated health laws usurped personal freedom. Even the editor of the above article concluded

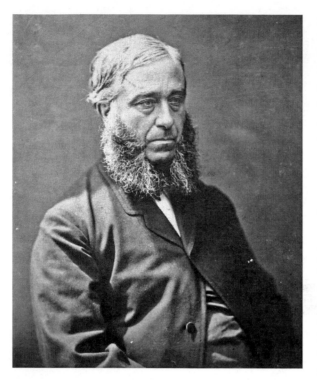

Dr. William Budd, 1811–1880 (U.S. National Library of Medicine).

"There are some things even worse than infectious diseases which a nation may fear—and among them is this, the handing over of every man's health, whether he likes it or not, to a 'standing army' of State-authorized medical practitioners with compulsory powers."[2] Science and sanitary reform were progressing: society would have to go a long way to catch up.

Cholera Is Coming: International Preparations

The *Police Gazette* of St. Petersburg, July 18, 1871, provided a summary of the current cholera epidemic, giving 67 new cases: 33 cured, 27 dead. Since the appearance of cholera on August 29, 1870, the aggregate totaled 6,072 cases, 3,040 cures, 2,485 deaths. At Moscow from March 13 to mid–August, 3,568 cases were diagnosed, with 1,643 deaths.

Fear of a major epidemic was so great life insurance companies in Berlin and Prussia began selling policies as protection. Alarm throughout Europe was immediate, with sanitationists anticipating its advance through Germany into the British Isles and the United States. Newspapers on both continents published statistics, dire predictions and preventatives: when the first cases were reported at Konigsberg, authorities in New York City began spreading lime over the streets. Simultaneously, the "pestilential fly," which many believed to be a harbinger of cholera, appeared, increasing anxiety.

By September 10, 1871, the number of persons attacked by cholera in the Baltic provinces numbered 2,517 civilians and 84 soldiers. Of these, 1,273 died, 620 recovered and 708 remained under treatment.[3] Although isolated cases were reported at Hull, England, brought by emigrants from North Germany en route to the U.S., New York reported that of 110,000 emigrants arriving within the past three months, none were infected. At Italy, in conformity with the International Sanitary Conference (ISC), quarantine of ships arriving from the Sea of Azov and the Baltic was implemented.

By July 26, 1871, cholera had reached Elburg and Danzig and deaths from diarrhea in London rose to 487, with 28 more attributed to Asiatic cholera. A week later, however, hopes that an epidemic might be avoided that season made the rounds of the press.[4] Russia did not escape as easily. Reports for August 3, 1872, indicated that at Kieff, 1,300, or nearly half the number of sick, died, while at the capital, from June 23 to August 3, there were 896 cases, 367 deaths and 133 cures.[5] The following October, the malady resurfaced at Vienna, striking 75–

115 per day with a 50 percent mortality, while at St. Petersburg, from August 18 through September, 326 new cases were reported, with 135 deaths.[6]

Cremation

The problem of how to properly dispose of human remains became a major issue during the cholera era. Many feared that decomposing bodies interred below ground contained germs which polluted the soil and water or emitted noxious gasses. Conversely, leaving bodies unburied was an even greater threat. During the epidemic raging at Bangkok, Siam, in September 1873, reports that 2,000 corpses awaiting "incremation" at one temple alone and numerous bodies floating in the Menam River were a cause of spreading contamination. A typical response published by a London medical journal noted "the immense number of corpses burned by the Hindoos, who are compelled by the worship of Brahma to burn their dead, is the real cause of Asiatic cholera. The poisonous gases generated in this way hover in the air during the day, but at night sink into the lower atmosphere, mixing with the water and the various kinds of food, and permeating the lungs in the process of respiration."

These concerns added interest to the study of scientific cremation promoted by Sir Henry Thompson, professor of clinical surgery in the University College, London. His method involved placing a body in a light wood shell and then in a suitable outside receptacle. It was then slid into a reverberating furnace, a cylindrical vessel 7 feet long by 6 feet in diameter and heated to a temperature of 2,000°F. "During the first few moments gasses were abundantly given off, but by passing through a heated chamber of fire-bricks, laid lattice fashion, they were rapidly oxidized, and neither smoke nor gas escaped from the chimney." The process required one hour, leaving five pounds of ashes for a 227 pound body. Using the 1849 study of Dr. Lyon Playfair, Thompson estimated this method would prevent 2,500,000 cubic feet of gas from 52,000 interments (reaching 80,000 by 1874) from polluting the atmosphere.[7]

An adherent of the theory that decomposing bodies contaminated groundwater, in 1876, Dr. Francis Julius LeMoyne built a crematorium on his own land outside Washington, Pennsylvania, then called Gallows Hill. The project cost $1,500 and consisted of a simple 30 × 20-foot brick building with an oven he designed so flames would never touch the body.[8] By 1881, the *New York Tribune* observed, "The world moves slowly in the direction of Dr. Le Moyne's hobby, but it does move." The article said "Buda-Pesh and several other Hungarian towns have decided in favor of cremation," while "increased familiarity" in Italy and England had made the idea more popular. While scientific and religious men argued the merits, one newspaper concluded that "in the end the question is likely to be decided by the necessities and convenience of the living rather than by any sentiment or prejudice concerning the dead."[9]

In order to investigate the Asiatic cholera epidemic of 1873, the New York Board of Health sent Dr. John C. Peters on a tour of southwestern cities. His insightful study revealed that a Russian ship from Odessa brought it to New Orleans, with the first case reported in February. It traveled up the Mississippi on steamboats; few reports were made by crews in the belief the disease was merely the less-fatal cholera morbus. Peters believed that personal contact of the virus in the stomach was necessary to communicate the disease: "there was no cholera without contact with cholera poison, and that not through the air, but by being taken in food or drink." The disease was also transferred from soiled clothing or towels to hands, and by hands to the lips, where it entered the system. He recommended hand washing with water and carbolic acid, as well as disinfecting clothing, as a means of prevention. By these means, "cholera may be stamped out, unless in some way it gets into the water; then the epidemic is fearful."[10]

In subsequent and, fortunately, widely reprinted interviews, Dr. Peters shot down Dr. Bell's theory that cholera was confined to the lower portion of dwellings (see Appendix I, "Cures") by remarking it was "undoubtedly an error; in fact, his whole theory of cholera being superinduced or springing from miasma is nonsensical." On the subject of food, he stated, "improper diet renders the attack more fatal, but does not cause cholera," On the idea that fear caused cholera he added, "Fear of cholera may produce profuse diarrhea and exhaustion, and may kill a person who has the virus in his system more quickly, but cannot produce cholera. The idea of fear causing cholera, as a general thing, is purely fallacious."

In stressing that "the use of thoroughly boiled water is the safest water beverage," Peters warned that water sources should be zealously guarded and that severe punishment be inflicted on these who fouled tributaries. He added that cholera pollution of wells, springs, fountains, pumps and small streams was "too common in all parts of the world" and was the most productive source of severe local outbreaks. Toward that point he added that "every stricken town is the guardian not only of the lives of its own citizens, but is responsible for the damage done elsewhere, as each cholera patient is a source of danger to others."[11]

By a joint resolution passed in March 1874, the secretary of war was directed to detail a medical officer to collect statistics on cholera. Surgeon Ely McClellan was selected and completed a 900-page report published in August 1875. His findings were similar to those of Peters, although he stressed cholera originated "alone in India, and is thence carried to all parts of the world." He also noted cholera was *frequently communicated through the atmosphere of infected localities, and by the use of water contaminated with the poison*," concluding that one attack was no protection from future attacks. In his annual report (1875), Dr. J.M. Woodworth, supervising surgeon of the Marine Hospital Service, reported that acids were the best antidote to cholera poison, diluted sulphuric acid taken internally being a valuable prophylactic. Unlike international authorities, he recommended rigid quarantine to prevent the disease from entering the United States.[12]

Although New Yorkers complained the "agitation" of newspapers suggesting cholera was on the horizon "keeps strangers from town and greatly injures business here," and they complained sanitary reform meant little more than "old street-dirt moistened into a disgusting mass of mud by the sprinkling-carts,[13] the American Health Association, meeting in the city in November 1873, had greater concerns. Figures released for the cholera season of 1873 revealed total fatalities of 5,475, with Tennessee having the highest number. Reasons were not difficult to determine. At Memphis (which had no organized board of health until July), the disease was so severe trade was suspended, costing the city several million dollars. Even worse, the potter's field was situated on the banks of Wolf River, just above the Holly Waterworks. This area was considered "the foulest place of foulest stenches on the continent," where shallow graves were often washed away, revealing piles of corpses heaped together in various states of decomposition. Just above the pumps sat a major butcher-house from which a chute ran into the river with the blood of slaughtered hogs and cattle, while hoofs, horns and entrails decomposed at the water's edge. On reaching Memphis, the Wolf River water merged with that of Gayoso Bayou (receptacle of all the sewers), before passing through the heart of the city. At Nashville, a spring used as a major source of water was found to contain, among other things, hair-pins, old boots and pieces of leather, broken lamps, knives and three bottles labeled "poison," complete with death's heads and crossbones.[14]

What made the cholera visitation of 1873 unique was that after striking Memphis, the

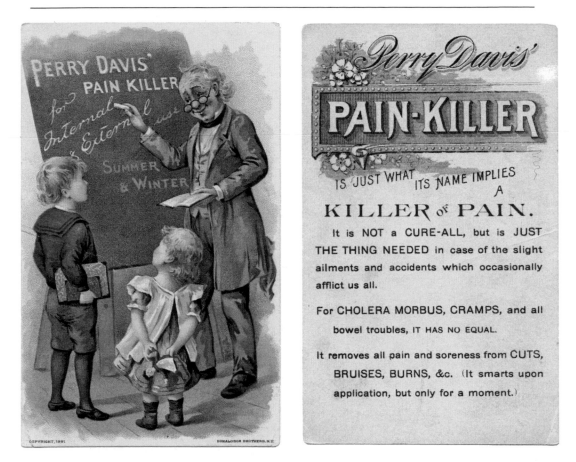

Left: **This is an 1890 chromolitho trade card for Perry Davis' Pain Killer. The product was not just a painkiller but a cure-all for nearly everything! Advertising claims changed very little throughout the 1800s. The danger, of course, was that these concoctions did not cure cholera morbus and a belief in their powers often prevented people from seeking professional help.** *Right:* **Back of the Perry Davis card (Authors' collection).**

disease took an erratic course, jumping over cities while spreading through small towns; when it crossed the Ohio, cholera attacked Mount Vernon, Indiana; while in Missouri, the small town of Louisiana fell victim. In both instances, Cincinnati and St. Louis were spared. Unfortunately, while cities were generally better prepared for defense with adequate sewer systems, villages had no ready means of disposing of the poison.[15]

One novel method of reaching the sick and destitute was practiced in New York using the "Floating Hospital of St. John's Guild." A large vessel, supplied with physicians, took on patients at various landing sites, offering free meals, examinations and treatments. One such voyage up and down the Hudson on August 19, 1874, aggregated 1,478, including 380 nurselings, 431 mothers and 667 children between the ages of two and six, aged people and cripples. Doctors diagnosed 293 cases of cholera infantum, 73 cases of Marasmus and 640 cases of debility from impure air and improper nourishment. One problem with the idea was reported from England, where the Floating Cholera Hospital at Lowestoft was sunk by the high tide.[16]

For those with an eye toward prophesy, the monk Tranquil Wolfgang, who died in 1873 at Munich, predicted there would be a terrible cholera outbreak in France in 1878, and that a cure for the disease would be discovered in Bavaria. On a similar subject, *Appleton's New Encyclopedia* (1875) discoursed on the cyclic reappearance of cholera, based on attendance at "Hindoo" festivals. According to the study, numbers at Hurdwar increased every three years, with the 12th attracting more than 3,000,000 pilgrims. Beginning in 1756, major epidemics were seen in 1759, 1768, 1781 and 1817, when the first worldwide cholera epidemic was recorded. These statistics indicated a "juggernaut" outbreak in 1877, supplemented by a Hurdwar cholera epidemic in 1879.[17] If Wolfgang the monk were correct, however, a cure for the disease would have been discovered in the interval between the two disasters.

Cholera in India during 1876–1877 was particularly severe, with many reports indicating horrific loss of life along the Bombay and Baroda Railway. At Golwood, a village of 200 people, disease killed half in three days. By the spring of 1877, nearly 4,000 deaths at Madras were attributed to cholera. Reported numbers were worse at Akyab, Chitagong and the islands along the coast, where it was claimed the disease took 50,000 lives. According to official tables, total cholera cases in Bombay for 1881 reached 30,966 cases, with 14,282 fatalities.[18]

According to a report by Dr. D.B. Simmons ("China Imperial Maritime Customs Medical Reports for the Half-year Ended 30th September, 1879"), Japan enjoyed immunity from cholera between 1862 and 1877. On September 5, at Yokohama, a man appeared with cholera. It quickly spread to neighboring women, attributed to the fact that after leaving a nearby temple, they rinsed their mouths with what Simmons believed to be contaminated water. The disease appeared again in 1878–1879, introduced by passengers aboard two steamers.[19]

As the Fifth Pandemic ground slowly to a close, cholera struck Morocco with unimagined violence toward the end of 1878, causing the country to be cut off from its neighbors. Hundreds were reported starving in the streets of Tangier as business came to a standstill.[20]

International Cholera Conferences

The first question debated by 300 members attending the 1873 Medical Congress of the International Exhibition, Vienna, centered on whether the cholera infection was spread by contact. With four dissentions, the group adopted the resolution that "the cholera is a contagious disease." Further discussion centered on the best means to prevent its extension, concluding quarantine should be "effective, and yet not oppressive." Prolonged dialogue failed to settle how this might be accomplished.

The same year, Dr. Tholozan, physician to the shah of Persia, addressed the recrudescence of the malady, believing

> that Asiatic cholera in Europe, as in India, can manifest itself in its three forms, endemic, epidemic, and sporadic. Its introduction into Europe has always given rise to violent and general epidemics when the period of immunity has been sufficiently prolonged. And after these epidemics have subsided, and apparently have become extinct, the disease may resume its activity and give rise to new regional or general epidemics, which have all the original violent characteristics of the pestilence. In a word, Asiatic cholera when introduced into Europe manifests, so long as it persists, the same phenomena which distinguish the disease in India.

Dr. Pelikan, director of the Imperial Medical Department of Russia, concurred, based on his belief the outbreak at Kiev in 1869–72 was of European origin developed out of the epidemic of 1865–70. Dr. Fauvel, French Academy of Medicine, shared this view. However, John Netten Radcliffe, British Medical Department commissioner, disagreed. He argued that at the period of the Crimean War, the principal route between Persia and Europe, via Russia, was from the

Caspian ports of Persia and through Transcaucasia and its ports into the Caspian, and by the highway across the Caucasus to Astracan. A second route ran from Tabriz through Turkish territory to Trebizond, and thence by the Black Sea.

Since 1864, however, traffic had largely been diverted to routes traversing Transcaucasia to the coast of the Black Sea at Poti and from there to ports of South Russia. This led to Baku becoming a port of import for the produce of the Caspian provinces of Persia, instead of, as formerly, a port chiefly for the transmission of Persian produce to Astracan. To further develop the traffic from Persia along the Poti route, the Russian government proposed a railway from Poti to Baku. This, Radcliffe concluded, had created a path for cholera directly into Europe during the prior three years and when completed would make the "contagious current" of cholera "current in Europe."[21]

At the invitation of Count Andrassy, the world's leading scientists agreed to meet in Vienna on June 15, 1874, at the Fourth ISC (also called the "International Conference" or "International Cholera Congress") to discuss terms of an international treaty respecting measures of quarantine during a cholera outbreak and the nomination of a permanent commission to study causes of the disease. As with the first three meetings, agreement was difficult, as any quarantine was nearly impossible to achieve.[22]

Epidemiology

"It is, indeed, to be regretted," noted a writer for the *New York Herald* (September 27, 1871) "that the literature of cholera has not been equalled in its advance by the scientific and exact pathology of the disease. But there is no room nor reason for discouragement." The author's optimism was based on the fact that microscopists, including Macnamara, Budd and Tyndall of England, Lister of Edinburgh and Pasteur of France, were all entertaining similar theories concerning cholera. Among those stated by Macnamara were the following:

1. The cause of Asiatic cholera is invariably a portion of the *fomes* of a person suffering from the disease.
2. The organic cause of cholera may be preserved dry for years.
3. Water is the most common medium of its diffusion.
4. Cholera-infecting matter is solely capable of producing the disease.

Experiments by Professor Chauveau of Lyons and Dr. Sanderson, medical officer of the Privy Council, concluded that contagious fluids of infectious diseases, when diffused through an animal membrane, lose their contagious property, while the portion that does not pass through retains it. They concluded that the essential and active principles of contagion reside in "the solid gelatinous particles to which the term microzyme is applied." Water was found to be a peculiarly good medium and repository for microzymes, which often resided there even if they could not be detected by microscopic analysis. Sanderson warned that "filtration exercises no perceptible influence on the zymotic power of water," and he revealed by experiment that blood and body fluids, when passed directly into his test solution, gave no trace of zymotic properties, demonstrating that "all septic and putrescent diseases come, not from within, but from without the body."[23]

In 1872, the *World* ran a multipart series on cholera. In the installment entitled "Epidemiology" (August 4, 1872), it summarized:

The only point of agreement has been the somewhat vague proposition that the cause and carrier of cholera is a material ferment or poison capable of rapidly multiplying itself; but concerning the nature and modus operandi of this poison there is infinite difference of opinion. One learned gentleman holds that minute microscopic particle of animal matter—depraved "protoplasm," so to speak—are at the bottom of the mischief, emanating from the body of a sick person, and by their evil communication corrupting the good manners of the tissues of any sound man whom they may encounter.

In a discussion of the "Germ Theory," the *World* noted that the idea originated in 1849, when Drs. Budd, Brittan and Swayne each published descriptions of peculiar cyst-like bodies observed in excretions of cholera patients, Budd adding that he found "cholera fungi" in the water of infected districts. After these papers were discredited by the Royal College of Physicians, the germ theory was set aside until 1866, when Professor Hallier reported finding the cysts noted by his predecessors. He supposed them to be the mature plant, containing minute "spores" which escape from the parent cyst and break up into fine granules known as "micrococcus." These granules grew into nucleated cells which arranged into chains and soon afterward gave off branching filaments whereon were borne new cysts. Hallier believed the choleracyst might originate as a parasitic growth in the rice plant, being thence transferred to humans, and that the excreta from cholera patients contaminated soil, conveying the fungoid spores to graminaccous plants.

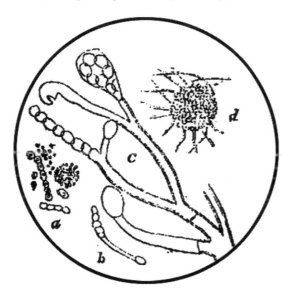

This illustration demonstrates the various stages of a fungoid cyst, which were considered in 1858 to be the "seed vessels" of the mature, microscopic plant found in English water. As they mature, the cysts developed a number of "spores," which, escaping from the parent cyst, break up into fine granules known as "micrococcus." These granules grow into nucleated cells that arranged themselves in chains, soon afterward giving off branching filaments on which were born new cysts. In the diagram, "a" represents the growth of nucleated cells from micrococcus; "b" the formation of a filament; "c" a highly developed cyst bearing filament; "d" a form of germination sometimes observed in the cyst (*New York World*, August 4, 1872).

By 1874, the Frenchman M. Tellier purported the idea that cholera was propagated by "invisible germs conveyed in the air or in water," and after being taken into the alimentary canal found conditions favorable for rapid multiplication. Dr. Simon of London clung to a similar theory, noting that "foul water and foul smells" were necessary to give cholera its full malignity.[24]

Can We Live Forever?

The 1880s proved a watershed in the history of cholera. Until this point, the scientific community was dominated by men such as Max von Pettenkofer, who postulated that although humans carried cholera germs, the germs were harmless unless fermented in the soil. Defending his ideas in an article written for *Popular Science Monthly* (1881), Pettenkofer noted that episodes of cholera on ships at sea (where influences of soil were far removed) were explained by the fact only persons who came from certain places were attacked, while passengers from uncontaminated areas had no symptoms although they were exposed to the same food, water and air. He added that sea voyages were regarded as pro-phylactic as they separated passengers and crew from infected ports.

Louis Pasteur's early work centered around the idea that Pettenkofer's "fermentation" was caused by a living organism carried in the air. Widening his scope, in 1868, Pasteur dis-covered bacilli in diseased silkworms and developed a system for their eradication that was credited with saving the Italian silk industry in 1883. By 1880, he had turned his attention to "chicken cholera," not only isolating the causative germ but also developing a technique for immunity. (Pasteur's research was detailed in the September 1883 issues of *Faneter's Journal* and *Science Monthly*. He stated his belief that the "vaccine virus" inoculated into the birds pro-tected them from cholera and throat ulcerations known as canker, croup and diphtheria.) Repeating the technique with rabies, Pasteur provided the world a cure for hydrophobia.[25]

Pasteur's lecture at the international medical college, London, in 1881, was widely circu-lated. In it, he avowed that vaccination could be used against a wide variety of contagious diseases, including fevers, cholera and hydrophobia and possibly measles, scarlet fever, diph-theria and typhus. Pasteur described the process, which was similar to Jenner's smallpox vac-cination:

> A drop of blood from a person sick with cholera is placed in a close glass vessel containing clear strained, recently boiled broth, made from chicken or other flesh. Great precaution is taken to exclude the organic germs floating in the air; in fact the glass neck of the vessel is closed with a plug of cotton, or is drawn out in a lamp flame and hermetically sealed. The glass vessel, or flask, is kept at a tem-perature of about 55 degrees Fahrenheit. Its contents at first become turbid from the growth of the *microbes* nourished by the broth, but at the end of a couple of days the thickness of the broth disap-pears because the *microbes* have ceased to develop and have fallen to the bottom of the flask, and things will remain in this condition for months without either liquid or sediment undergoing any visible change, provided the atmospheric germs are kept excluded. After an interval of a month the flask is shaken to mingle its contents, and a drop from it is placed in a second flask, containing fresh broth. A crop of *microbes* is produced as before, followed by the same clearing of the liquid and falling of sediment. The interval of a month's waiting is repeated, and a drop from this second flask is employed to produce *microbes* in a third, and so on until there has been, say, a dozen crops of *microbes* raised. At the end of the process it will be found that the "cultured *microbes*" are innocent, and, when introduced into the veins, fail to produce cholera, as their uncultured ancestors did, yet, at the same time, they prevent the one vaccinated from catching the cholera. In a word, the cultured *microbe* can be used to vaccinate, and thus protect the person for all time to come.

Putting his technique to the test, the French government gave Pasteur 50 sheep on which to experiment in the hope he could prevent splenic fever, a disease destroying these animals at a cost of $50,000 annually. After vaccinating 25 with cultured microbes, he inoculated all 50 with the uncultured splenic microbe: the 25 vaccinated sheep resisted the infection while the 25 unprotected animals died within 50 hours. By 1881, twenty thousand sheep and numerous cattle and horses were vaccinated, with good results.[26]

During a tour of the United States in 1882, Dr. Declot, an associate of Pasteur, lectured that their latest investigations proved that "there were parasitic beings which were born with us and placed in us the germs of diseases which were falsely termed hereditary, but were really the results of this parasitic action." They believed "all ills were caused by living organisms, whether in the animal or the vegetable": in surgical operations, "these little germs produced either the local erysipelas, or the deadly and general erysipelas." Declot's point was proven at Bellevue Hospital, New York, when his antiseptic treatment cured a patient of pyaemia. He observed that if his method had been used, it would have saved President Garfield's life (who suffered from blood poisoning after being shot by an assassin on July 2, 1881), adding that

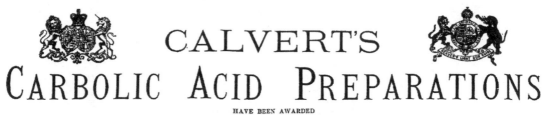

Carbolic acid was used as an antiseptic and disinfectant. By 1880, when cholera had been classified as a "disease of filth," hygienists believed proper sanitation was the best preventative. Calvert's preparations (a tumblerful of acid to a garden can of water) were used to disinfect rooms, bedding and clothes. Calvert's was also "most deadly and disagreeable to serpents," and at a time when many believed the origins of cholera came from poisoned air, Calvert's was promised to destroy "the miasma and morbid germs in a vitiated atmosphere" (*The Colonies and India* (London), July 3, 1880).

when parasites were all destroyed by a purified carbolic acid, there was no reason "why we should not live always, and the days of Methuselah come again to the children of men."[27]

Jakob Henle, a pathologist at Gottingen University, Germany, developed a series of rules for proving that a microorganism was the cause of a disease. His most famous pupil, Robert Koch (1843–1910) further defined them into what became known as "Koch's postulates":

1. The microorganism had to be isolated from a diseased subject.
2. It had to be used experimentally to induce the same disease in an animal.
3. The microorganism had to be isolated from that diseased animal.
4. The experiment had to be repeatable.
5. The microorganism had to be present in all diseased subjects.

By 1876, Koch successfully isolated the anthrax bacillus and between 1871 and 1881, he published a number of works on the principles of bacteriological investigation, including the staining of bacteria with aniline dyes and the use of microphotography. On March 24, 1882, he delivered an address, "The Etiology of Tubercular Disease," before the Physiological Society, Berlin. After announcing that one-seventh of all human deaths were due to tubercular diseases, he announced the discovery of the tubercle bacillus, the cause of tuberculosis. He also pointed to the grave danger of inhaling air in which particles of dried sputa of consumptive patients were contained. A second article noted the research proved the "remarkable testimony to the profound sagacity which enabled Dr. Budd to see the essential similarity between tubercle and the [eruptive] fevers in question, notwithstanding the enormous superficial unlikeness which distinguishes them."

Interestingly, in a letter to the *London Times* conveying the above information on Koch, Professor John Tyndall defended his animal experimentation by writing that the noisy "fanaticism of the moment" must not block investigations for the good of mankind. The first public Anti-Vivisection meeting in France was held in Paris in September 1863. After it was noted that nothing had ever come of animal torture, someone questioned, "And Pasteur?" One member replied, "Hypotheses, hypotheses! Nothing certain!"[28]

29

The Fifth Cholera Pandemic, 1881–1896

A single bacterium in suitable conditions may cause an outbreak of cholera in Egypt; an outbreak of cholera necessarily delays the settlement of the country, and the departure of the British troops. This delay subjects international relations to a prolonged strain, and affords a constant chance of complications, which may affect Turkey, France, India and Russia. Thus it is conceivable that a single minute creature, invisible except through a powerful microscope, might change the course of political events, and even involve two continents in war.[1]

Cholera appeared at Mecca in 1881, and by early November had taken the lives of 214 individuals. Much press was given to the fact that water from the Holy Well of Hagar that pilgrims drank for purification had been analyzed by Dr. E. Frankland of the Royal College of Chemistry, South Kensington, and found to contain "sewage more than seven times as concentrated as London sewage," with no less than 579 grains of solid matter per gallon. As it was known "excrementitious matters" propagated cholera, Frankland wrote, "it would scarcely be possible to provide a more effective means for the distribution of cholera poison throughout Mohammedan countries."[2]

By 1882, in consequence of the outbreak at Sumatra and the appearance of cholera on the island of Padang in the Straits of Malacca near Singapore, the International Sanitary commissions at Constantinople and Egypt ordered quarantine of all vessels coming from the Dutch Indies and Singapore and warned they were prepared to order a prolonged quarantine of pilgrim vessels coming from the Indian Ocean at the entrance to the Red Sea.

Conditions did not improve: cholera appeared at Damietta, Alexandria and Port Said, prompting the governor of Algiers to issue an order on June 30, 1883, prohibiting pilgrimages to Mecca, while rumors circulated that the Suez Canal would be closed. Spain and France placed blame for the deteriorating situation on England, claiming a lack of governmental foresight and control in the area and ignoring the resolutions adopted by the Sanitary Conference in favor of their shipping and commerce. (Closing the Canal would deprive British shareholders of their monetary returns.) International tensions increased as the French became more vocal over the Suez Company agreement to allow the British fleet free access to the canal as a basis of operations against Arabia.[3] By July, the Sanitary Commission, comprising General Wood, Baker Pasha and General Stephenson, undertook the operation of establishing three more hospitals and an ambulance corps as well as purifying Cairo, but the commission opted not to quarantine either that city or Alexandria.[4]

Death tolls from cholera at Java (East Indies) in 1882 were said to have reached 80 percent, marking the third time in eight years the country had suffered an epidemic. By September,

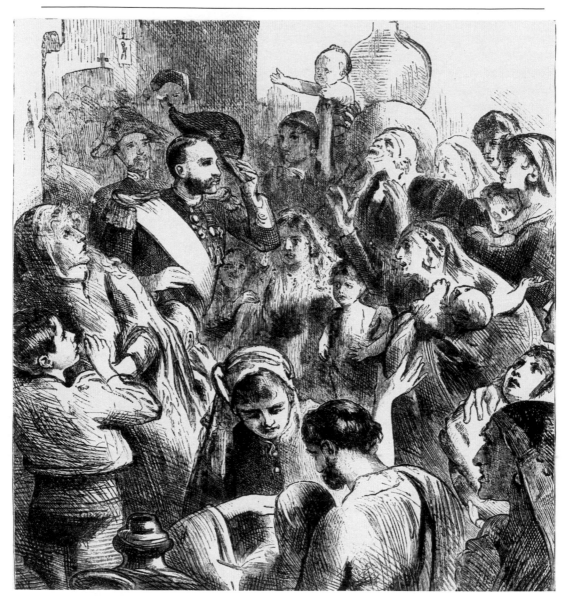

"King Alfonso Visiting the Sufferers from the Cholera," 1886. Alfonso XII of Spain had a reputation for being benevolent and sympathetic and it was not uncommon to hear stories of him visiting cities ravaged by cholera. The role of monarchs in reaching out to their people (typically by gifts of money for the oppressed) or by making personal appearances during epidemics was generally credited with uplifting depressed spirits and infusing new courage during troubled times (Authors' collection).

cholera had struck 449 in the Philippines. A colonial possession of Spain, the islands, with a population of 7,500,000, were particularly valuable, exporting 3½ million pounds sterling worth of tropical produce to England and the United States. By September, 300 cholera deaths occurred daily at Manila, eventually taking 12,000 lives, while at Yloilo, it was reported that 4,550 deaths had been recorded during a two-week period. On the other side of the world, cholera struck Chiapas, Mexico, leaving so many dead the bodies had to be burned, while at Tonala, 60 deaths per day were registered.[5]

International Scientific Investigators

The dire situation in Egypt offered a prime research field for scientists and the opportunity for governments to enhance their own reputations in the field of discovery. Louis Pasteur obtained a grant of 2,000*l*. from the French Chambers to conduct a mission investigating whether cholera was due to a microscopic animal in the human body. The mission consisted of Drs. Roux, Thuillier, Strauss and Nocard, whom Pasteur hoped would be protected by the hygienic precautions he set down for them. The British sent Drs. Henry Crookshank, M'Nalty, A.F. Wilkins, Armand Leslie, F.E. Taylor, A. Honman, F.G. Thrapp, C.F. Parker and J. Cantlie.[6] Germany sent Dr. Koch and assistants, including Georg Gaffky and 50 mice. They arrived on August 24, 1883. Unfortunately, the teams came too late, as the epidemic had died down and the Frenchmen returned home.[7]

By October 1883, newspapers were filled with news that Dr. Koch had discovered the cholera germ. The bacillus was described as bearing a close resemblance to the thread-like bacteria found with glanders in horses. The bacteria was located in the walls of the intestines of those who died from the disease but was absent in those slain by other diseases. Koch sent home a comprehensive statement of his findings to Prince Bismark, requesting permission to continue his quest in India.

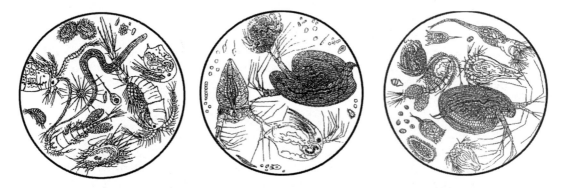

Left: **What did English drinking water of 1858 look like under a microscope? The answer was not one calculated to prompt anyone to take a sip of that refreshing beverage. This illustrates a sample taken from Thames water at Brentford (*London Illustrated Times*, May 8, 1858).** *Center:* **Sample of cistern water, New River, East London.** *Right:* **Sample of cistern water, Hampstead, West Middlesex.**

In a bit of gamesmanship connected with politics and national pride, the reticent physician allowed his preliminary findings to be "prematurely announced because M. Pasteur and other investigators are at work in the same field and Dr. Koch could not take the risk of being anticipated in his scientific quest."[8]

Koch and his team went on to Calcutta and by January 7, 1884, succeeded in identifying and producing a pure culture of the microorganism that was labeled the "comma bacillus." (This became known as the pathogen *Vibrio cholerae 01*, linked to the fifth and sixth pandemics. A second strain, *Vibrio cholerae 01* El Tor, named after the medical inspection and quarantine station port at Sinai on the Red Sea, was identified by Armand Ruffer in 1897. The strains that caused the first four pandemics, as well as earlier cholera-like diseases before 1817, have never been determined.)[9] On February 2, Koch announced this as the cause of cholera. On his return to Germany, he was greeted by the emperor and acclaimed as a scientist whose work was "a brilliant testimony to the persistence and thoroughness of German science."[10] But there were others addressing the same issue.

Who Discovered Vibrio cholerae*?*

Although Robert Koch was given credit for being the first to discover *Vibrio cholerae*, the Judicial Commission of the International Committee of Bacteriological Nomenclature awarded that honor to the Italian scientist Filippo Pacini for his work in 1854. In fact, Koch's discovery failed to conform to his own postulates as he failed to reproduce the disease in animals, his announcement resting on the assumption that normal procedures did not apply. (Cholera is virtually impossible to reproduce in animals.) Richard J. Evans argues persuasively in *Death in Hamburg* that German nationalism and politics promoted the scientist to international fame. Evans added that Koch's work changed the face of medical research by eliminating the need for meteorologists, statisticians and others vital to the miasmatic theory while changing the emphasis from social hygienists to bacteriologists, concluding, "Koch's achievement was to reinterpret contagionism in terms compatible with medical professionalization."[11]

Contemporary authorities also credited Dr. Bohm for discovering germs in the dejecta and intestines of cholera victims in 1838, and again by Drs. Brittain, Swayne and Hughes Bennett in 1849. Pouchet, Davaine and Pacini found them in 1854 and 1856, as did Drs. Dundas, Thompson and Hassell. Hassell was also credited with providing fixed points of practical value in treating the disease, announcing that rice-water discharges were always alkaline and prone to putrefaction. In 1861, Dr. Macnamara added confirmation to the theory that persons with strong digestion and plenty of gastric juice in their stomachs were unlikely to contract cholera.

In 1871, Dr. Nedwetsky revised conventional wisdom by announcing quinine would not kill cholera, thus proving the disease did not come from malaria. Further testing also indicated camphor, laudanum (tincture of opium), carbolic acid, tar, and calomel did not kill the germs. However, studies with dilute mineral acids—nitric, muriatic and sulphuric—quickly killed the majority of germs. As these dilute acids made a "pleasant and graceful drink," their use was recommended. Nedwetsky also found tannin or tannic acid, gallic acid and alum were effective. Sulphate of iron required too concentrated a solution to be used in humans; chloroform killed some but not all germs, while chlorine water killed them at once. "Medicus," a frequent contributor to the *New York Times*, added that oil of peppermint was a good germicide, while common table salt or muriate of soda not only killed germs but acted as a preservative for beef and pork. Koch himself demonstrated that cholera bacilli were readily killed by drying, a fact significantly important to the rag importation trade.

In 1884, newspapers indicated there was "no little excitement" in learned circles that Professors Finkler and Prior of the University of Bonn claimed an equal share with Koch on his discoveries. Koch was "forced to recognize the justice of their claim at the Imperial Board of Health." Simultaneously, Dr. Dudgeon, a London homeopathic physician, gave credit to Hahnemann, founder of the practice, who, in 1831 "suggested that the contagious matter of cholera consisted of excessively minute invisible living creatures," advocating camphor, which he held to be a "potent cholera baccilicide."[12]

In 1884, it was noted "there is a drawn battle between the followers of Dr. Koch and the Pasteurites." Koch declared the "comma" bacillus was the primordial cause of cholera, while those following Pasteur admitted the existence of the microbes, but believed cholera produced the microbes. One editorialist put it succinctly:

If Dr. Koch's experiments in inoculating with microbes had produced cholera his theory would be perfect. However, it must be borne in mind that certain animals present a refractory action and resist disease. In order honestly to test Dr. Koch's theory it would be necessary to inoculate a man, and, of course, an experiment of this kind is out of the question. With this objection Dr. Koch's theories are generally approved of.[13]

Aware of the political implications of Koch's discoveries, Pasteur published nine anti-cholera rules: he stressed that all table water should be boiled and half filled in bottles; before drinking, it was to be aerated by shaking. Water pitchers were to be heated to 150° C before use; wine should be heated to 55° and drunk from cups freshly plunged in scalding water; all food should be thoroughly cooked, while underdone flesh and raw vegetables promoted cholera. Bread was to be toasted hard before eating; all sheets and clothes were to be scalded and rapidly dried; water for toilet purposes was safe only when it had been first boiled and then diluted with thymic acid; hands and faces should also be washed with this mixture. Tableware was to be taken straight from the boiler or oven to the dinner table. The "least practicable rule" was the requirement, meant for health care workers, to wear a mask made of two thin sheets of brass with a layer of phenolized wadding between, designed to destroy cholera germs passing through it.[14]

The news was not universally well received. No less an entity than the *New York Times* (August 24, 1883) ran an article denouncing Pasteur's rules by sarcastically noting that if cooled water became contaminated by cholera, it should be consumed at the boiling point, hot wine would become "lifeless," meat should be cooked until "nearly dried up," bread had to be burned to a crisp and masks must be worn to ensure immunity from disease. Calling Pasteur a "medical humorist who is ridiculing the popular alarm concerning cholera," it decided that rather than follow Pasteur's dictates "most people will decide that it would be preferable to die of cholera." Another editor noted, "Next we shall hear that cholera morbus can be prevented by vaccinating a person with a little virus from the end of a cucumber." As an explanation to the French "discovery" that married men were less liable to contract cholera than were bachelors, a third declared that as cholera germs were destroyed by boiling, the news came as no surprise, "married men generally being kept in hot water, there is no chance for the cholera germs to work destruction."[15]

Perhaps worse was another article from the *New York Times* entitled "Farewell to the Bacteria Scare," which described the findings of a Buffalo physician named Gregg, who asserted that bacteria were always present in blood, and, of more significance, were not living microorganisms but simply particles of fibrine. If true, the author remarked, all theories based on living bacteria would have to be thrown away.[16]

While the *New York Times* was ready to throw out Pasteur's research, the makers of "Warner's Safe Cure" happily avowed "the truth remains that the germ theory is the correct one," promising their remedy put the body in condition "to kill these germs before they obtain a hold on the body."[17]

As early as 1831, the question of cholera being transmitted in rags was an open debate. In 1879, Professor August Hirsch of the German Cholera Commission lectured on his belief that the infection of the Turkish army by troops from Baghdad and a consequent communication of these germs to the Russian army was impossible. Instead, he stated the plague was transmitted by infected blankets and clothing taken as booty. In 1883, when Pasteur and Koch focused world attention on germs, the idea that Egyptian rags were responsible for introducing cholera into England and the United States took on new life. In describing how cholera traveled, "Medicus," a frequent contributor to the *New York Times*, considered diseased wanderers and

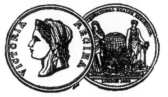
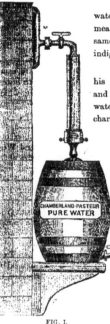
In 1883, Louis Pasteur advocated all table water be boiled before consumption to destroy cholera germs. The idea was immediately ridiculed, one writer remarking that the preventative was worse than the disease. By 1886, the scientist had altered his view. When promoting the Chamberland-Pasteur water filter, the advertisement specifically stated boiling destroyed the taste of water, rendering it "indigestible"— the point taken by his detractors (*The Colonies and India*, London, June 18, 1886).

soiled clothing the two most common causes of distant outbreaks, while the *London Echo* warned that if 56 bales of Egyptian rags aboard the *Favian* were allowed to land, the government would be guilty of "mad indifference." Ironically, the House of Commons actually prepared orders in regard to the rags but never issued them, as the ship, with cargo intact, sailed for America. Interviewed by a Boston reporter, the importing firm of Train, Smith & Co. used Pettenkofer's theory that soil was a great disinfectant to deny the danger. Egyptian rags, he explained, went through a "natural disinfecting process" by lying on the sand for "months sometimes" before being baled for shipment.[18]

Unfortunately for him, Pettenkofer's stance was rapidly falling into disrepute. In Germany, Robert Koch superseded him on the Cholera Commission, stressing quarantine and disinfection, particularly of soiled clothing, which he believed should be destroyed or boiled to kill cholera germs. He further noted that cholera developed only in alkalis, a small quantity of acid being sufficient to prevent their growth.[19]

Other tenets were reinforced in 1885, when Pasteur's cholera treatise was translated:

1. Cholera found its home in India, where it was never absent.
2. It was of germ origin, with the power of self-multiplication in blood and secretions.
3. The germs that produced cholera were the products of animal decay, excretions and sewer matter. Finding their way into the drinking water, they were the cause of many outbreaks.
4. Cholera germs required from 1 to 4 days to incubate and only tenants the same house for 12–14 days.
5. It was not contagious in the proper sense of the word, but secretions were full of infection and soiled clothes retained the infection for weeks or perhaps months.
6. It spread rapidly in filthy districts and had not been known to cross the desert or Indian Ocean; American epidemics were traceable to immigrants.
7. Cholera was not dependent on the wind, although telluric and aquatic conditions appeared to influence its movements.
8. It had been known to stop short of regions where drought existed.
9. Sporadic cases had occurred in the U.S. without any contact with imported disease.
10. Cholera violence had diminished in the last 60 years.
11. Habits of decency and cleanliness were the best preventatives.[20]

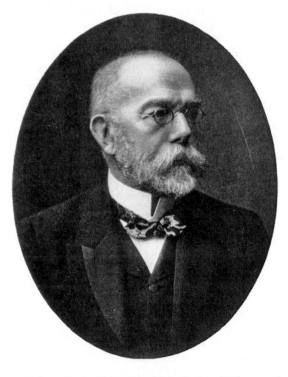

Robert Koch, 1843–1910 (U.S. National Library of Medicine).

Fallout and Debate Over the "Comma" Bacillus

Koch's inability to infect animals with cholera and thus conclusively prove his theory caused "his stock to fall," preventing universal acceptance and spawning numerous others to promote their own discoveries. Dr. Vincent Richards, a British surgeon residing in India, made headlines when he announced that by experimenting on pigs he had succeeded in transmitting the disease. This was quickly tempered when it was discovered he had not inoculated the animals with cholera bacilli: his claim lay in the belief that the diarrheal discharges of cholera patients contained "a virulent poison," in the nature of a chemical compound rather than a living organism.

More significant, British cholera commissioners Drs. Klein and Gibbes issued a report contradicting nearly all of Koch's theories. Klein, already infamous for showing his contempt of Koch by swallowing cholera bacilli and living to tell the tale, announced their research showed the "comma" bacilli in diseases other than cholera and that autopsy findings often revealed low concentrations of the bacilli, whereas Koch stated they were always present in immense numbers. The report caused a "decidedly antagonistic" response against Koch in France, where the disease was raging. Dr. Ricord announced his own theory that infection came from the air, while Dr. Bosche Fontaine also grandstanded by swallowing pills made of cholera dejecta. (Koch responded by stating the "experiment" was useless as bacilli could not survive the ordeal of passing through the acid secretions of a healthy stomach in that the germs were digested as well as the food.) One American humorously put the situation into perspective by writing, "The mistake Dr. Koch made was in not giving his comma-shaped microbes a barbed wire, unpronounceable name of ten zigzaggy syllables." Perhaps unwittingly restoring his good name, in 1886 Koch declared that his comma bacillus died in beer as a result of the ingredients being thoroughly "cooked" and the destructive powers of its alcohol. The declaration was "hailed with delight."

Dr. Chapman, another British authority, came out with a book, *The Scientific Treatment*

The manufacturer of Eno's Fruit Salt clearly had the multinational city of London in mind when they wrote this advertisement. With directions that came in sixteen different languages, they appealed to the agrarian population by using simple farming expressions: comparing cholera and fevers to "ugly weeds" and promising disease poison could not "take root" and that their product "prepared the soil" to resist the "seed" of poisoned blood and sick headache. With the illustration of a healthy, innocent child pointing the way, the "mystery" of sickness was solved (*Bell's Life in London and Sporting Chronicle*, November 17, 1883).

of Cholera, repudiating the bacilli theory and stating his belief that cholera was essentially a disease of the nervous system. Pettenkofer also published a book reaffirming his old theory, avowing that clay soils in relatively dry conditions were most likely to assist in outbreaks, while rain-soaked earth had not enough "bad air for the animal germs to breathe." In an article for the March edition of *Popular Science*, he went further, disavowing Snow's work based on the Broad Street pump water, claiming the test could not be reproduced during an 1854 epidemic at Munich.

Drs. S. Maurin and Lange of Marseilles claimed a "mucor" to be the "missing link" in the propagation of cholera, which, while "sporifying," gave birth to the bacilli of Koch, while a Marseilles commission announced it could trace a cholera patient's condition by an hourly examination of the blood. Alternately, French physicians Reitsch and Ricati announced they succeeded in transmitting cholera to animals using Koch's microbes, thus proving his theory. Contrarily, the pair also identified the bacillus in persons who had never had cholera, leading the *New York World* to observe, "The bacillus is vindicated, and the terrible Asiatic scourge is as much a puzzle as ever."[21]

The Fifth International Congress on Hygiene opened at the Hague on August 21, 1884, with the hope it would serve as a "Council of War to combat the cholera." Quarantine was denounced as "injurious and useless," while a proposal was unanimously passed expressing the desirability of a new international sanitary conference and the creation of a permanent international scientific committee to act against epidemics. It also passed a resolution in favor of an International Sanitary Code. Holland was asked to pass the views of the Congress to other governments.[22]

The same year, Florence Nightingale, "the Crimean heroine," wrote to the *New York Herald* that "cholera is not communicable from person to person" and that the sick "do not manufacture a 'special poison' which causes the disease." Arguing isolation and quarantine "fatally aggravate the disease," she affirmed "the only preventative is to put the earth, air and water and buildings into a healthy state by scavenging, limewashing and every kind of sanitary work, and if cholera does come, to move the people from the places where the disease has broken out, and then to cleanse." She concluded: "The real danger to be feared is in blaming somebody else and not our own selves for such an epidemic visitation."[23]

Cholera Makes the Rounds

Cholera made its dread appearance at Shanghai in May 1883. By September, when Dr. Jamieson made his report, he noted that the number of fatal cases of diarrhea and dysentery were larger than any half year since 1874, while cholera among the Chinese was extremely virulent, causing death in 2–3 hours. Interestingly, in 1884, water supplied by the Shanghai Waterworks Company, reputed to be pure and clean, was shunned by the locals on the grounds the water was an innovation unheard of before, it interfered with the livelihood of water-coolies, and it was poisonous. The situation became so dire, the operators appealed to the American consul-general for redress. He, in turn, applied to the magistrate of the Mixed Court, who issued a proclamation, mildly defending the water.

The year 1884 was destined to bring grim news to the world. By April, death rates from cholera in Calcutta were as high as 49.9 per 1,000, while on June 24, evidence of cholera outbreaks at Yangstun and Pekin and isolated cases at Tokyo made headlines. The day previous, French officials had officially confirmed an outbreak at Toulon, although the first death occurred

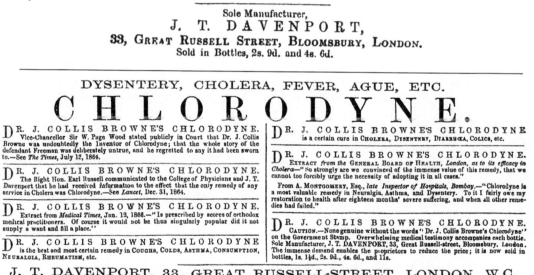

Top: Dr. J. Collis Browne's "Chlorodyne" gained respectability by having been invented by an ex-army medical staff member and was promoted, in a round-about way, by the director-general of the Army Medical Department. (To avoid any negative connotations that might arise from the product, or because they were not compensated, authorities asked to comment on a specific medicine frequently used the expression "I have seen it used," rather than "I have used it.") To increase sales, Browne offered three stages of disease where the chlorodyne had proven effective (*Cape and Natal News, South African Colonies,* London, January 15, 1863). *Bottom:* Still advertising in the *Cape and Natal News* (London, December 1, 1866) three years later, Dr. J. Collis Browne relied on more specific testimonials to promote his medicine. Not surprisingly, the first of seven statements declared Dr. Browne to be the sole inventor of chlorodyne. Competitors frequently stole successful products and most ads of the day bore warning for consumers to beware of imitations and look for specific markings on the packaging, such as stamps or engravings, to avoid "counterfeit and worthless preparations."

on June 4. Authorities in Paris, Rome, Vienna, Madrid and as far away as San Francisco immediately announced plans for protection and quarantine.

Early explanations for the spreading epidemic were attributed to the cheap sale of apricots, while Americans pointed the finger at Marseilles, a city known to be the pathway of cholera and having introduced it into the United States via immigrant ships in 1866. From Washington, Secretary Frelinghuysen announced mail from France and Italy was to be enclosed in tarred sacks to prevent contamination.[24]

As a growing panic developed in France, reports of June 30 confirmed cholera at Saluzzo, Piedmont, Italy. The appearance of the disease in India and China prompted Odessa authorities to institute a quarantine, while the Spanish and Algerians entered into bitter quarrels over the former's quarantine of ships from that city. In the United States, the request of Rep. King of Louisiana for $200,000 to prevent the introduction of cholera became a hot news item. Matters worsened after Dr. Koch announced he had isolated the same microbes in Toulon as he had in Egypt and India, thus pronouncing the disease to be Asiatic cholera.[25]

Health officials at Marseilles indicated that by July 29, eleven thousand deaths were attributed to cholera. They classified the nativity of the victims as 798 Frenchmen, 322 Italians, 13 Spaniards and 9 Greeks. Despite intense sanitary measures, recurrence of the disease there and at Toulon was attributed to the fact that the harbors were artificial: old ports were no more than estuaries, dredged out into large docks with narrow outlets to the sea, while new ports were spacious but enclosed by miles of breakwater. Into these ports, the entire volume of city sewage was poured. As there was no tide to maintain the circulation of seawater, it grew foul and pestilential. Scientists believed the dredging of a disused dock at Toulon during April and May developed the seeds of the epidemic, originally imported from Saigon, China, by the French transport *Sarthe*.

Complicating matters was the widespread dislike of physicians (a phenomenon frequently seen in other countries, as well) among the "lower class," who believed the doctors were "instigated to help the cholera along in order to get rid of the surplus population." Calling them *empoisonneurs* (poisoners), a mob accosted several doctors outside the Pharo Hospital at Marseilles. Unsuccessful medical treatments did not aid the cause: those tried at the Pharo included inhalation of oxygen and ozone, intravenous injections of artificial serum (patients died of anemia) and electricity. In reviewing the situation, Dr. Koch strenuously objected to water flowing through the streets (used to wash away filth) as he believed moisture festered the development of the disease. He objected also to the use of disinfectants generally. By August 6, however, the disease was thought to be waning, having claimed 1,800 victims.[26]

That hope proved deceptive as new cases continued to mount; worse, microscopic examination of water drawn from infected areas revealed vast colonies of cholera microbes. In a lecture at Berlin on August 8, Koch affirmed his belief that the delta of the Ganges was the real home of the disease and stated his belief that an improved water supply was the best means of checking the disease. Frank H. Mason, United States consul at Marseilles, added the depressing thought that "science and medical skill have made but little substantial progress" and noted the "rigor and deadliness" of the present attack when compared to the 1865 epidemic.

By late August, mortality returns at Paris were 1,092, down from 1,196 the previous week, while cholerine remained prevalent. Citizens departing the city in one week were 27,654, leaving it nearly empty: one travel agent in England estimated tourism was off 80 percent, which was bad, he noted, for France, but good for English watering places.[27]

As the summer wore on, cholera continued cutting its deadly swath. At Naples, from the first outbreak up to October 1, there were 10,121 cases with 5,370 deaths, primarily at Naples.

Rather than trust doctors, peasants sought relief in superstitions, including allowing sheep into sickrooms on the belief the wool absorbed the disease. People also resorted to burning

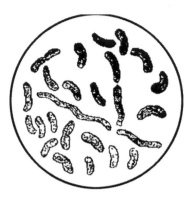

sulphur in the streets to ward away disease. Statistics from the *London Times* indicated that since the outbreak at Toulon began, European mortality from cholera had reached 14,132, with 7,974 from Italy, 5,798 from France and 360 from Spain. The cost to the Italian government was placed at one million and a quarter pounds, predicted to rise to three million if the epidemic lasted another two months. Economic factors also played a role when Spanish authorities at Alicante furiously denied any cholera existed there for fear it would drive away visitors from their annual fair. Not everyone was so uncharitable, as the Paris Telephone Company granted the use of their offices for calling assistance for cholera patients.

This illustrates the "comma bacillus," magnified 2,500 times. It was found in "myriad swarms along the intestines of persons who have died of the scourge. It is also found in waters and in the earth during cholera epidemics" (*Wellsboro* [*PA*] *Agitator*, April 14, 1885).

As cholera slowly decreased across Europe, one, perhaps spurious, article reminded everyone that the disease remained foremost in people's minds. It was said that newsboys in Paris sold a special paper called *L'Anti-Trac* (The Anti-Scare) as "the only journal which doesn't mention the cholera." For a penny, purchasers received four blank sheets of paper.[28]

The first case of cholera reported at Nagasaki, Japan, came on August 19, 1885; by September 4, there were 830 cases with 406 fatalities. By May 1886, the disease had spread to Kioto and Osaka. At Hiroshima, it was discovered that plum vinegar was fatal to cholera microbes and it was used with success. According to the *Japan Gazette*, cholera cases from January to August 1886 were 59,000, with 37,000 being fatal. Official returns for July alone set the number of deaths at 36,000 out of a population of 250,000. At Shinshua, in the province of Keishodo, 5,000 died and at Torai, 6,000 more perished in one month. September brought no relief, as 34,908 new cases occurred, with 23,774 deaths. At Seoul, Korea (spelled "Corea" during the latter half of the 1800s), the July death toll was placed at 38,600.[29]

During July 1889, cholera struck again in Persia, reaching Bagdad by August 24. At that place, from August 20 through August 31, death rates ranged from 200 to 400 per day. By September, the disease had traveled to the Euphrates and the Tigris and into the Persian Gulf. International authorities warned that if the Russian government did not take proper measures, all Europe would be exposed.

European sanitary measures ultimately proved successful in keeping cholera away but devastation in Russia and Japan was horrific. In September 1893, the United States consul at Odessa reported that for the week ending August 12, there had been 2,183 cases and 768 deaths in the various governments of European Russia and that recent news indicated the disease had appeared in Egypt. By September, the world read with horror that cholera was striking at Moscow, Warsaw, Kasan, Kursk, and St. Petersburg. Putting a name to the numbers, the great composer Pyotr Ilyich Tchaikovsky was believed to have died of cholera on November 6, 1893. There was little relief, and the toll at Volhynia in September 1895 numbered 4,269 cases and 1,701 deaths.

Casualties were excruciatingly higher in Japan. Introduced from China by returning soldiers, in the six months ending October 10, 1895, reported cases were 52,218, resulting in 36,075 casualties, an exceptionally high mortality of 69 percent. Cholera quickly passed the barrier of the Red Sea and appeared at Damietta and other places along the Nile delta, while epidemics at Tangier and Tetuan, on the coast near Gibraltar, were caused by pilgrims returning from Mecca. The pilgrim quarantine station of El Tor, at the northern end of the Red Sea, and that on Kamaran Island were in poor condition, with isolation "purely nominal," and rules adopted by the International Sanitary Conference concerning pilgrim fleets were not enforced.[30]

Reports also surfaced in 1895 that cholera had reached Honolulu, carried by some of the 588 Chinese immigrants from the *Belgic* out of Yokohama. The immigrants were placed on Quarantine Island, a lowland of 30 acres, half a mile west of the harbor and separated by shoal water.

A private letter from Buenos Aires dated December 10, 1886, observed that the cholera dead were "removed to the outskirts of the city, piled up like cross-ties and burned." During that month, reports indicated 700 cases with 352 deaths, with similar daily numbers from Mendoza. By March, another eyewitness reported 40,000 deaths in the Argentine Republic, 19,000 in Buenos Aires alone. Fearing contagion at its borders, Chile imposed quarantine and passes on the Argentine frontier were closed, but the disease "surmounted all barriers" and reached the Pacific slope. Fearing the "horrible scenes of 1850 and '51," Jamaican authorities prepared for an onslaught, sadly aware that quarantine was of little use.

As the disease traveled northward in South America until reaching the Isthmus of Panama, quarantines were established in El Paso by authorities who feared the Mexican Central trains would bring it into California and Texas. Once cholera was established, authorities supposed it would quickly reach New Orleans and advance up the Mississippi and along the seacoast of the South.[31]

How Far We've Come

While the average American of the mid–1880s watched death tolls mount in Europe, the depression in Wall Street was coupled with Asiatic cholera "by some grumblers who do not hesitate to attribute any unfavorable condition in the stock market to the latest sensation." Conversely, monopolists of the telephone and telegraph companies used the scare to advantage, claiming that New York State law dictating they expend great sums of money to bury wires underground would cause undue health concerns, as digging trenches would agitate cholera germs, endangering public health.

Other financiers were investing profits in science. In May 1885, the Carnegie Laboratory at 26th Street and First Avenue, New York, opened. The building, erected with $50,000 given by Andrew Carnegie for pathological investigations, housed a laboratory with the identical apparatus used by Dr. Koch; scientists were to study cholera, typhoid and pneumonia. In July 1885, a pathological laboratory in connection with the New York Polyclinic School of Medicine opened under the supervision of Dr. Frank S. Billings. Containing "seeds" of cholera, typhoid and smallpox, courses were recommended for all health officers.

Complementing these were numerous scientific journals. The August number of the *North American Review* offered five articles on the subject "Can Cholera Be Averted." One of the authors, Dr. John C. Peters, wrote that cholera germs "thrive enormously in alkaline fluids, containing decomposed organic matter, when aided by warmth; and of course the stomachs and bowels of those afflicted with foul stomachs and bad digestion." Mineral acids, he noted, "counteract this alkaline condition, act as antiseptics and disinfectants against the decomposing

Goods will be shipped and receipts taken in good order, and no breakage or loss that may occur in transit will be allowed.   Pay no money to salesmen without our written authority.   This bill becomes due immediately when the purchaser suspends payment, removes, is closing out, or refuses to receive the goods.

CHICAGO ___ NOV 4 1898 189__

L. C. Ford,

Lima, Mont.

Bought of E. C. DE WITT & CO.,

PROPRIETARY MEDICINES,

203 & 205 LA SALLE AVE.

This bill is NET at maturity.   It is subject to a Discount of 4 per cent IF PAID WITHIN 10 DAYS FROM DATE OF INVOICE.

This bill is due and payable ___ *1/2 6 mos; 1/2 9 mos.*

Quantity				PER GRO		
1/	Gro.	De Witt's Little Early Risers (the famous little pills)...		19.20	9	60
1/2	Gro.	" Witch Hazel Salve (cures piles)...		24.00	12	00
1/3	Gro.	" One Minute Cough Cure, medium...		48.00	16	00
1/	Gro.	" One Minute Cough Cure, small...		24.00	12	00
	Gro.	" Colic and Cholera Cure, large...		48.00		
	Gro.	" Colic and Cholera Cure, small...		24.00		
	Gro.	" Stomach Bitters, large...		96.00		
	Gro.	" Stomach Bitters, small...		48.00		
1/6	Gro.	" Toilet Cream, large...		24.00	4	00
	Gro.	" Toilet Cream, small...		14.40		
	Gro.	" La Grippe Specific, Large...		96.00		
	Gro.	" La Grippe Specific Small...		48.00		
	Gro.	" Veterinary Witch Hazel Salve...		48.00		
1/4	"	" *Cough Cure Tog*			4	00
1/	"	" *Kodol Dyspepsia Cure*			4	00
					61	60

3 BOXES, WEIGHT *194* LBS.

Via. *C & N. W.* R R

Compare this with the expense bill rendered
to you by Transportation Co.

The above goods are shipped and billed to you in accordance with the terms of your signed order, for which accept our thanks.

Two of the preprinted items on this November 4, 1898, invoice were for colic and cholera cures, large and small sizes, indicating the frequency in which they were sold. As items on the form were sold by the gross, E.C. DeWitt was likely a supplier to smaller pharmacies in Illinois and the Midwest. It was not uncommon to see tonics marketed for both colic and cholera as both diseases shared somewhat similar symptoms and one appeal of patent medicines was that they "cured" a wide variety of diseases (Authors' collection).

material, and kill all the germs or microbes." He suggested "one pound of corrosive sublimate in 500 pounds of water," which, when drunk, killed all the germs in the system, or when used externally, disinfected clothing and discharges. Phosphoric acid was also recommended as a safe and tolerably certain preventative and curative.

One of the most interesting manifestations of a cholera scare came in April 1886, when reports from Cleveland began circulating that a mysterious "thick blue fog" was issuing from the earth. Residents reported seeing the same manifestation during earlier cholera outbreaks. The story made the exchanges and appeared all over the Midwest, prompting one editor to note, "Cleveland has of late been afflicted with the craze of 'saloons open on Sunday.' Isn't it barely possible that therein lies the cause of things looking so 'blue' about the otherwise umbrageous city?"[32]

With all the sad financial and scientific news, there still existed room for some typical American humor. When a father was asked if he were afraid his son would fall victim to cholera during a planned trip abroad, he answered, "No, indeed; he is a member of a base-ball club, and his friends inform me that he was never known to catch anything."[33]

There was still much serious work to be accomplished during the final decade of the Fifth Pandemic. One of the most difficult problems scientists faced was the inability to make a rapid determination on whether cholera was present in water. Robert Koch had already noted that cholera vibrios always presented their long axes in the same direction, so that a group of them resembled a shoal of fish swimming in a slowly flowing stream. He considered identification of this phenomenon an absolute diagnosis for true cholera. However, it was often difficult to identify this under the low-powered microscopes of the time. Koch provided the answer by discovering that in Dunham's peptone solution (1 percent peptone and ½ percent sodium chloride), the vibrios multiplied so quickly their presence could be readily identified in as little as 6 hours. This new test was also useful in rapidly detecting the presence of cholera in "carriers," or those without symptoms who carried the bacillus within their bodies.[34]

Ilya Ilyich Metchnikoff, a Russian biologist (May 15, 1845–July 15, 1916), created a breakthrough in immunology when he discovered amoeba-like cells that engulfed foreign bodies such as bacteria. He called these cells phagocytes (from the Greek word meaning "devouring cells") and named the process phagocytosis. Recognizing these phagocytes were the first line of defense against acute infection, being one type of leukocyte, or white blood cell, he formed the theory of immunity (1892).[35]

The Sixth Cholera Pandemic,
1899–1947

A new generation has sprung up since the scourge last visited our shores, and we are apt to look upon it, as we do upon earthquakes and plagues in general, as something remote from our daily life—an improbable, almost impossible contingency, with which it is scarcely worth while to reckon. To realize even partially the terror which "King Cholera" is capable of inspiring, it is necessary to visit the East.[1]

Louis Pasteur read a paper by Dr. Gamaleid of Odessa before the Academy of Paris in 1888. A student of the Pasteur method, Gamaleid had studied in Paris before returning to Russia and developing what was believed to be a cure for cholera by the inoculation of the cholera virus. At this point, it had been tried only on animals, but hope existed it would have the same effect in humans. By 1900, the hope remained unfulfilled. British sanitary commissioners reports from 1896, 1897 and 1898, on the subject of what was termed "anti-cholera inoculation" among coolies and soldiers in India, were "decidedly in favor of the operation," yet the reports qualified all positive results by stating it was not possible to determine how far protection went, as complete statistics were lacking.

The English were more vocal about the success of their sanitary efforts in Egypt. After enumerating the struggles and overall rejection of their practices, the "unswerving heroism" of their inspectors, although crippled for want of money, succeeded in preventing drainage from mosques running into the nearest water supply. Under the Mosque Decree of 1892 (the first legislation on the subject), 470 mosques in provincial towns were dealt with, while without legislation, in 1898, in 2,000 mosques taps and reservoirs were substituted for the medahs or ablution basins formerly used. Under the leadership of Sir John Rogers, cemeteries were also removed from the center of villages and 20 hospitals and 46 dispensaries were opened.[2]

Opposite, top: "Davey's Differential Expansive Pumping Engines." This side elevation view of a hydraulic pump was particularly effective in hilly districts where water accumulated at a height on one side of a valley could be made to pump water to a higher elevation either on the same side or the opposite one, there to be stored for use or employed for giving motion to machinery. *Middle:* "Compound Differential Pumping Engine—Plan." This sketch illustrates the compound pumping engines, force pumps and separate condenser used in Davey's system. The engine had cylinders 35 and 60 inches in diameter and a 6-foot stroke. The pump rams were of gun-metal, 12½ inches in diameter. *Bottom:* "Differential Hydraulic Pumping Engine." At the bottom of the pits, 300 feet below the main engines (see preceding illustrations) are placed a pair of hydraulic pumping engines. The engines were capable of lifting 1,000 gallons a minute to the main engines. The main engines forced the water to the surface and supplied power through the column to the hydraulic engines. By this system, the main engines were kept out of danger of flooding. As coal became more expensive, hydraulic engines took on more importance and improvements in engines utilizing the motive power of flowing water garnered much interest in the 1880s (All photographs, *London Iron*, October 23, 1875).

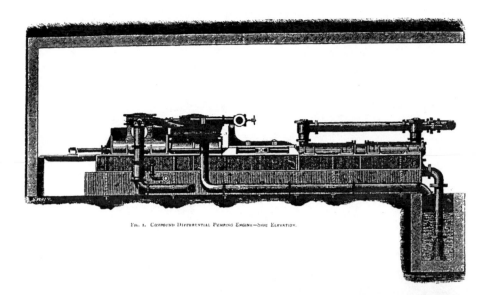

FIG. 1. COMPOUND DIFFERENTIAL PUMPING ENGINE—SIDE ELEVATION.

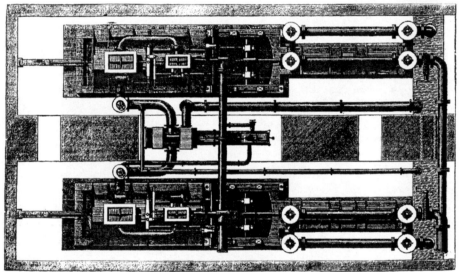

FIG. 2. COMPOUND DIFFERENTIAL PUMPING ENGINE—PLAN.

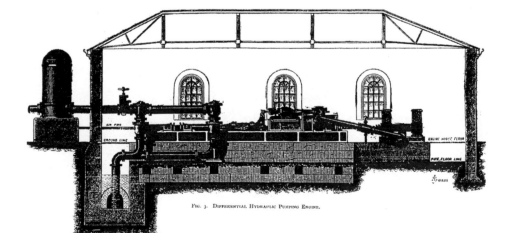

FIG. 3. DIFFERENTIAL HYDRAULIC PUMPING ENGINE.

Results in Hamburg were no less impressive. The cholera epidemic of 1892 killed as many people as all the other cholera epidemics of the 19th century combined, destroying 13.4 percent of the population.[3] The epidemic was caused by contamination of the water supply, and Professor Georg Gaffke and Robert Koch were involved in stemming the disaster. Aiding them was a young American, Dr. Dunbar, of St. Paul. He eventually became responsible for the 700,000 inhabitants, under the title "director of the Hamburg Institute." Facing a historic crisis from the fact Hamburg was situated in a low, flat section at the head of the Elbe tidal water without access to other water, Dunbar became involved with construction of a filtration plant, put into operation in May 1893. The plant occupied two islands in the Elbe, where 28 large basins, each one capable of supplying the city for a day, were situated. A pump lifted the water into the first series of basins, where it sat for 24 hours before being drawn off into a second series, where it percolated through filtering beds built with clay, concrete, brick and cement. Containing 40 inches of sand and gravel, the system produced clean water reportedly better than that of any other city in the world.[4]

Ozone Water Treatment

Sand filtration remained the preferred method of water filtration but a new method lay on the horizon. Ozone, once considered a cause of cholera, took on a new and different significance in 1886, when a scientist named de Meritens recognized its power to disinfect polluted water. Several years later, the German firm Siemans and Halske constructed a pilot plant at Martinikenfelde, Germany, to put the idea into practice. The discovery in 1889 that ozone was effectual against bacteria (including cholera and typhus germs) gave similar projects new impetus.

In 1889, the French chemist Marius Paul Otto expanded his studies of water sterilization by ozone by creating the Compagnie Provençale de l'Ozone (renamed Compagnie Generale de l'Ozone in 1919, and Compagnie des Eaux et de l'Ozone in 1929). The first full-scale application of ozone in drinking water treatment came in 1893 in the Netherlands. Two municipal plants were constructed in 1899, one at Blankenberg on the Belgian coast and the second at Joinville le Pont, near Paris. Both failed, owing to the inability to maintain the electrical equipment and the "breaking down of dielectrics." The Dutch scientist A. Vosmaer invented the method of producing the silent brush discharge without dielectrics, which so impressed Dr. Clifford Richardson that in 1899, he recommended the Vosmaer system for water purification supplied to workers on the Panama Canal.

Sanitary engineer J.J. de Kinder, in charge of the Vosmaer ozoning plant at Nieuwersluis, Holland, remarked that the operation purified 120,000 gallons of water daily, reducing bacteria from 85,500 cubic centimeters to 1–3 centimeters. Simultaneously, organic matter in solution was largely reduced, and the foul odor and disagreeable color entirely disappeared. German scientists Drs. Ohimuller and Prall confirmed these findings in independent research. They concluded as follows:

1. Water treatment by ozone achieved a remarkable destruction of bacteria and was superior to separation of bacteria by sand filtration.
2. Cholera and typhus bacilli were destroyed.
3. From a chemical standpoint, water was affected only insofar as the oxidability was reduced and free oxygen increased.

4. Ozone was of no importance from a technical or health affecting consideration.
5. Taste was not affected.

Professor Soper of Columbia University, New York, added that, as ozonization was not a straining process, simple filtration was indispensable.

Advantages of Ozone Treatment Over Sand Filtration

1. Ozonization gave absolute bacterial purity: filtration did not.
2. Ozonization installation cost ⅙ less and operation ¼ less.
3. An ozonization plant could be built in a few months; filtration plants took years.
4. Ozonization machinery covered a few hundred feet; filtration plants required acres.
5. With ozonization, the nearest body of water could be purified; with filtration this was not possible in the neighborhood of large cities.
6. With ozonization, the degree of purity was constant; filtration was imperfect, intermittent and dependent on the care of attendants.
7. An ozonization plant output could have its capacity doubled at slight cost in little time with a reduction of the ratio of operating expenses; in filtration, costs were doubled and years of preparation were required.
8. Ozonization provided absolute sterilization; filtration was imperfect.
9. Ozonization destroyed the bacillus causing cholera and other summer diseases; filtration did not appear to affect it.
10. Ozonization destroyed the spores of crenothrix which filled water mains with organic growth and diminishes capacity.
11. Ozonization freed water from objectionable color, odor and taste.
12. Ozone aerated and regenerated water.

Plants were constructed in Wiesbaden (1901) and Paderborn, Germany (1902), Niagara Falls, New York (1903), St. Petersburg (1905) and Nice, France (1906). Their numbers grew rapidly and by 1915, there were 49 European plants.

Research conducted during World War I on poisonous gases led to the development and use of inexpensive chlorine for water treatment, curtailing ozone plants, but by 1936, there were nearly 100 plants in France and 30–40 in other parts of the world. Communities preferring the improvement in taste and odor by ozone continued to use the process and in the 1960s, the widespread introduction of new applications, including the addition of ozone during early stages of treatment (preozonation), where before it had been the end stage, increased its popularity. In the 1980s, concern over chlorination by-products generated new interest and it became the method of water treatment for cities such as Los Angeles.[5]

Too Many Wars

The "next generation" had little to fear at home, but encountering cholera on foreign shores proved to be another matter. American intervention in the ongoing Cuban war for Independence ultimately led to the Spanish-American War in 1898. The major medical concern at the time was typhoid fever encountered by troops engaged in the United States' attack on Spanish possessions in the Pacific. Ultimately, this led President McKinley to issue a "Procla-

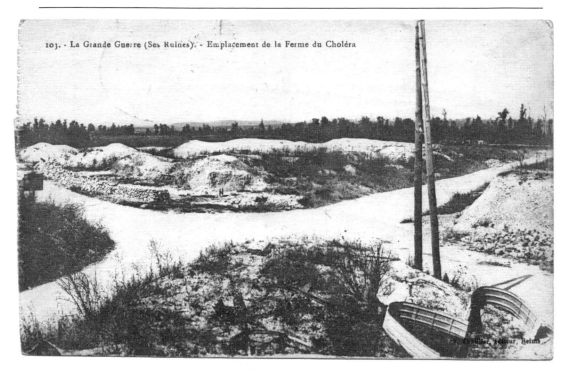

103. - La Grande Guerre (Ses Ruines). - Emplacement de la Ferme du Choléra

This postcard image reveals a cholera burial ground at Berry-au-Bac, France, during World War I (Authors' collection).

mation of Benevolent Assimilation of the Philippines" on December 21, 1898. Complex political negotiations broke down between the U.S. and revolutionaries and fighting erupted on February 4, 1899. A severe epidemic of cholera during the Philippine-American War (1899–1902) in 1902 was responsible for the deaths of many of the estimated 34,000 Filipino soldiers and 200,000 civilians.[6]

According to Surgeon General R.M. O'Reilly's report on the U.S. Army for 1902, there was a death rate of 15.49 for 1,000 of the entire force, as compared with 13.94 for 1901. The total number of cholera cases in all the Philippines was 485, resulting in 386 deaths, or 7.57 percent per 1,000 troops serving there. O'Reilly noted that cholera had not appeared among American troops since 1866, when it destroyed 1,629 soldiers. The report indicated that "utmost precautions" were taken to prevent the spread of disease and that nearly every case among Americans "resulted from a willful or careless violation of standing orders." Were it not for cholera, the death rate for 1902 would have shown improvement over 1901.[7]

The headline in the *Boston Globe* EXTRA! 5 O'clock (March 5, 1903) read, "New Antitoxin. Dr. Flexner Made a Very Valuable Find. Says It Will Kill the Germ of Cholera Infantum." The announcement stated that Dr. Simon Flexner of the Rockefeller Institute had discovered an antitoxin that would destroy cholera infantum. The next step, involving Flexner and Dr. J.H.M. Knox of Johns Hopkins, would be to perfect a serum that the former indicated would be ready before the end of the year. Response to the news was mixed: one expert hailed the discovery (if true) as having the advantage of saving poor as well as wealthy infants while a second observed that genuine instances of cholera infantum were rare, most actually suffering from infant diarrhea.

Work on a viable serum would continue for decades. Flexner (1863–1946), who pioneered in field investigations of infectious diseases, discovered a bacillus causing a common form of dysentery that was named after him; he also developed the Flexner serum for treating meningitis.[8]

The Pan American Sanitary Bureau was established in Washington in 1902. The following year at a meeting of the International Sanitary Conference, delegates agreed in principle that a permanent health bureau should be established. In 1907, in Rome, it was decided to establish the Office International d'Hygiene Publique (OIHP) in Paris. The committee met in 1908, and thereafter twice a year, except during World War I.[9]

Marching Toward World War I

The year 1904 brought probably exaggerated reports of 300 dying per day in Teheran while cholera was spreading throughout northern Persia. By January 1905, the disease had traveled over Syria, Mesopotamia and Persia, across the Caspian Sea into European Russia and onward to the Volga, prompting the German government to send a circular for resisting the spread of the disease to its confederated states. Quarantine and sanitary measures failing, by September, isolated cases were reported in Hamburg, Berlin and Warsaw.

Between August and October 1905, there were 14,713 cholera cases reported in the Philippines, with 553 deaths. The disease reappeared in Manila in June 1906, attributed to the endemic nature of the disease and the fear harbored against health officials, causing them to underreport sickness. Worse were warnings from health authorities that the Hedjaz Railway, constructed for the benefit of pilgrims going to Mecca and Medina, would aid the transmission of disease by allowing them to go overland to Damascus and by railway to Mecca without health inspections. Similarly, the railway would facilitate the spread of cholera in India by providing a more direct route, carrying back the disease to Constantinople and Turkey.[10]

Matters were grave in St. Petersburg during 1908. Toward the end of August, several cases occurred, but it was not until September that authorities acknowledged the presence of cholera. Exacerbated by a lack of sanitary reform, sewage thrown into the canals contaminated the drinking water, infecting the workmen, cab drivers and porters. This enabled cholera to gain a foothold in all quarters, catapulting St. Petersburg to first place among infected Russian cities. Matters quickly deteriorated as hospitals prematurely discharged patients, creating "walking centers of infection." Soon, isolated cases reached the Winter Palace, palaces of the nobility and the Imperial Opera House.

As corpses piled up outside graveyards, students at St. Petersburg University voluntarily underwent vaccination, after which they drank a solution containing cholera germs in an effort to test the efficacy of the procedure. A movement was even started to insist physicians be clean-shaven after it was alleged their patriarchal beards were liable to spread cholera germs. As the economy crumbled, one news service adroitly stated the only industries to flourish were chemical manufacturers and pickpockets.

Cholera quickly reached Odessa, the most important port on the Black Sea, and Surgeon General Wyman ordered quarantine for Russian immigrants shipping for the United States. Epidemics raging in Shanghai, Amoy and Hankow, China, indicated 60 victims at the latter place were dying daily. By October, 30,000 natives had perished at Hankow. In the Philippines, extraordinary measures were taken by Governor General Smith to combat the growing infestation there but nothing stopped the plague. By August 1909, British sanitary authorities declared Rotterdam an infected port.[11]

Amid ongoing news of cholera in Russia, little notice was taken of the passing of Robert Koch at Baden on May 27, 1910, of heart disease. One of the most laudatory came from a four-paragraph obituary written by the Associated Press. It noted he "became distinguished as an investigator of micro-organisms, but probably gained most renown as the discoverer of the bacilli of tuberculosis and cholera.... His first writings, covering investigations of anthrax and the etiology of traumatic infective diseases, marked an epoch in medicine and placed bacteriology on a scientific basis."[12]

As Europe trembled in fear over a projected spread of the disease, cholera in Russia claimed nearly one-half of those afflicted, reaching 90,000 cases by October 5. Experiencing similar accusations to those leveled against Russia, the Italian government was accused of "permitting the scattering of infection everywhere, rather than admit the presence and extent of the epidemic, for fear that it would frighten away tourists. The Italian government censorship permits nothing to go over the telegraph lines regarding the cholera." Likewise, in both countries, the populace believed authorities were out "to kill the patients," a belief that led to riots and incendiary destruction.[13]

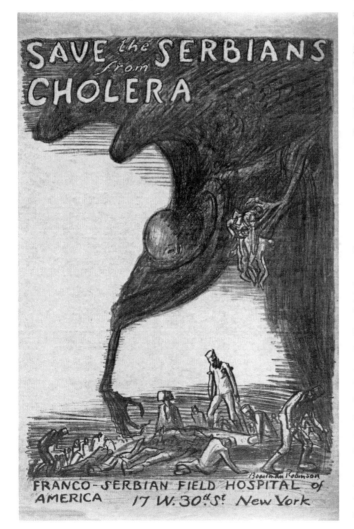

"Save the Serbians from Cholera." This widely distributed poster depicted the Franco-Serbian field hospital of America as the deadly arm of monstrous cholera reached down to steal victims from life to death (Authors' collection).

The Balkan Wars

The First Balkan War (1912–1913), preceding World War I, was fought between the Balkan League (Bulgaria, Greece, Montenegro and Serbia) and the Ottoman Empire. By November 1912, cholera cases among Turkish troops holding the line of fortifications at Tchatalja in front of Constantinople had reached a reported 500 per day, with a total of 6,000 already stricken. Simultaneously, the disease presented a formidable opponent to the Bulgarian advance, limiting their ability to occupy the city.

While editorials were written stating "under the rules of modern warfare, no humane commander would take his troops into an infected zone ... [nor] would a commander possessed with the least spark of humanity attack an enemy with men who were infected with a deadly disease," cholera numbers rose exponentially to 1,000 per day with a 50 percent mortality. Turkish officers regarded further resistance at Tchatalja impossible but felt it equally improbable for the Bulgarians to occupy the Turkish positions without endangering the whole army.

Horror stories arising from the cholera camp at San Stefano, where sick soldiers from Tchatalja were sent, shocked the world and hopes were raised late in the year when a cessation of fighting was called to allow diplomacy to achieve peace. Although fighting was resumed in February 1913, the Treaty of London temporarily ended hostilities by creating an independent Albanian State from the Ottoman Empire.[14]

The Second Balkan War began June 16, 1913. Dissatisfied by results of the Treaty of London, Bulgaria attacked Serbia and Greece. Although Greek forces had escaped cholera in the first war, the disease broke out among soldiers concentrated at Saloniki. Greek authorities obtained a supply of cholera vaccine from Germany and established hospitals near the line to prevent the spread of the disease by soldiers being transported to a base hospital. After cholera infected the civilian population at Saloniki, the military took charge of the situation and controlled it.

Realizing the danger of spreading cholera among civilians by carriers returning home after the conflict, physicians took advantage of prolonged peace parlays to hold Greek troops in camp from September to November, believing the infectious period lasted 60 days. Efforts by the Romanian Army to prevent the spread of cholera concentrated on the use of a three-part vaccination. The first injection consisted of 7 drops of vaccine, followed in five days by 15 drops and ten days later by a third injection. At least one month was required to establish immunity. Studies indicated that a treatment of only one or two injections failed to protect, requiring the full course to be effective.[15]

World War I and the Aftermath of War

After the assassination of Archduke Franz Ferdinand of Austria on June 28, 1914, a month of diplomatic maneuvering between Austria-Hungary, Germany, Russia, France and Britain (the "July Crisis") ensued. This did not prevent Austria-Hungary from declaring war on Serbia on July 28, 1914. Russia and Germany immediately mobilized. On August 2, Germany invaded Belgium and attacked French troops, declaring war on Russia the same day. The United Kingdom declared war on Germany August 4.

In late September, reports of cholera among Austrian soldiers who had returned wounded from Galicia caused one Canadian newspaper to opine, "Before the prospect of a scourge of cholera spreading over Europe the horrors of war, even on German lines, pale into insignificance." In response, by mid–October, Dr. Bruno Buffon of the Austrian Army, who had studied cholera during the Balkan War, began inoculating the troops against the disease, utilizing 120,000 packages of serum received from Vienna. The period of immunity was given as three months. Horror of a different type occurred at Metz, where it was reported that a French doctor poisoned the wells with cholera microbes. Captured by the Germans, he was tried and shot.[16]

The *American Medical Journal* warned that increased moisture and seepage of surface water carrying cholera germs came in close contact with human beings, and an epidemic among soldiers appeared likely. Headlines screamed, "War Brings on the World That Worst Scourge of Mankind, Asiatic Cholera." Combating the disease ran the gamut from protection by the

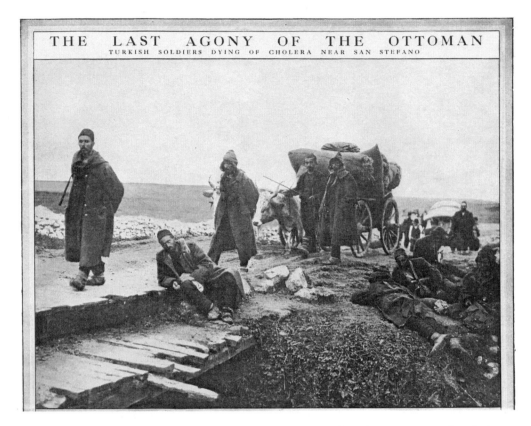

THE LAST AGONY OF THE OTTOMAN
TURKISH SOLDIERS DYING OF CHOLERA NEAR SAN STEFANO

"The Last Agony of the Ottoman: Turkish Soldiers Dying of Cholera Near San Stefano." Photography changed the face of war, putting human visages to mind-numbing death figures. Images such as this, printed in the *Graphic*, November 30, 1912, conveyed the tragedy of cholera victims from the Balkan War (1912–1913), causing international sensation. The misery of men at the prisoner of war camp at Tchatalia led to renewed calls for peace negotiations.

Haffkine vaccine to whitewashed coal. As described by William G. Shepherd, a news correspondent traveling the road from Vienna to Galicia, along wayside railroad stations piles of whitewashed coal, depot platforms and pathways were all covered with a white disinfectant used to fight germs which Russian prisoners carried into Austria-Hungary. In another report, Shepherd wrote:

> We come to a cholera hospital along the road. It is an old farm house. The scene in the yard is indescribable.... All about the yard, lying on straw under the trees through which sunshine filters are inanimate men, sick of cholera.... I've seen men hanged; I've seen men executed at the wall, but this sight that I have happened upon by accident in Galicia is one of the most piteous that the sun could ever shine upon or that a human being could ever behold..... One figure and a blanket, an unshaven soldier whom the priest has been unable to rouse, writhed and tossed about. The priest hurried over to that corner of the yard and stood with outstretched hands and uplifted face, with a Red Cross doctor standing hopelessly by his side, until the writhing ceased with a sudden jerk and the soldier of Austria came to his end.

During the first year of war, Austrian prisoners introduced cholera into the Italian lines. Infection spread rapidly and within a few weeks, more than 10,000 cases among prisoners and troops was documented. Prompt efforts by sanitation officers who ordered drinking water sterilized, infected camps burned and flooded areas with corrosive sublimate kept mortality under 2,000. The following spring, several small epidemics started, but totals were kept below 2,000, with greatly reduced mortality. At Warsaw, removing bodies hastily buried near wells and in "heaps just under the surface near houses" helped contain cholera.

In the spring of 1915, the *Buffalo Inquirer* asked, "Would an epidemic of cholera end the war? If so, would an epidemic of cholera be welcome?" Noting cholera killed as fast as war, the newspaper speculated that a raging disease that destroyed soldiers and civilians alike would at least "spare the handiwork of centuries," forcing nations to cease fighting each other and unite in battling pestilence. That hope, if indeed it were one, was quashed by a report by Dr. Pottevin, chairman of the Parliamentary Committee on Hygiene, France. He stated that the decomposition of thousands of cadavers in the trenches of war offered "no grave menace." Professor Legroux of the Pasteur Institute confirmed the findings, stating, "Any dangerous microbes or putrefying bodies are themselves destroyed by others which develop during decomposition. The odor and the flies annoy the soldiers but the cadavers constitute no source of danger."[17]

Surgeon General Blue issued a report for the fiscal year ending June 30, 1915, reviewing the world distribution of cholera. Among those areas listed were Austria-Hungary, Ceylon, China, Egypt, Dutch East Indies, India, the Philippine Islands, Russia, the Straits Settlements, the Balkan Territory, Germany and Indo-China. Cholera was also found in 23 German prison camps, Silesia, Brandenburg, Posen and Zirka, and was traceable to the seat of war in the East. The new infection in the Balkan territory may have originated from the endemic infection of Austria-Hungary or from Turkey, where the disease was prevalent in 1914 and 1915.[18]

By September 8, it was reported that within the previous 20 days there had been 7,427 cholera cases in Austria, 3,295 of which were fatal; the disease was also said to be widespread at Galicia and that measures to combat it "have proved insufficient, isolation is impossible and contamination is spreading." Information at the Vatican warned that cholera and typhus "threaten to reap more victims than the war." During the same period, the American Red Cross announced doctors and nurses would be removed from the battlefield due to lack of funds. During their work in Serbia alone, the organization had supplied 358,783 pounds of sulphur, 700,000 bi-chloride tablets and 12,200 doses of cholera vaccine.[19]

By August 5, 1916, Tokyo declared quarantine against the port of Yokohama, where 52 cases surfaced; by the 15th, that number had reached 109. The disease was believed to have been imported from cargos loaded at Manila or Hong Kong aboard the steamer *Hawaii Maru*.

After the armistice in 1918, the disorganization of Russia, coupled with the revolution and civil war (1917–1921), removed whatever health defenses had been established. Cholera quickly devastated Petrograd and spread through the eastern shore of the Baltic. By April 1920, the Red Cross reported, "Ten thousand cases of cholera now exist among the refugees in the crowded territory of the Crimea, with the number of new cases doubling daily." During the previous three weeks, the disease had "defied all measures of repression" and threatened to penetrate every corner of the Crimea. By December 24, the Jewish Telegraphic Agency reported that the disease among Russian refugees in Constantinople was "daily assuming more serious proportions." Echoing a familiar theme in August 1921, Dr. N. Semashko (also spelled Zemashko), commissioner of public health for the Soviet government, stated sewers and water supplies were in terrible disrepair, while the "mass migration, as if it had been maliciously planned," distributed the infection from place to place.... The starving population of Volga is moving to the south as an avalanche, sowing on its way infection and death." Semashko advocated stationing "vaccination squads" at every railway station to vaccinate travelers or require certificates that they had undergone the procedure.

Fragmented reports from Moscow officials indicated 75,000 cholera cases had occurred between January and August 1921, forty-seven thousand of which were seen between January 1 and July 15, with 15,000 cases in June alone. Overall death rates were substantially higher due to widespread famine.

Letters dated September 1921 stated that throughout the area where fighting between Turks and Armenians during the past winter had been severe, cholera and starvation were killing an average of 25 young and old per day. By October, districts along the Volga had further deteriorated, with the death rate of cholera victims estimated at 50–75 percent.

The League of Nations was formed after World War I. One of its goals was to "endeavor to take steps in matters of international concern for the prevention and control of disease." It was presumed all existing international bureaus would be incorporated into one organization, but the United States objected. Not being a member of the League, the U.S. preferred to keep the Office International d'Hygiene Publique (OIHP), of which it was a member, separate. Therefore, between the World Wars, these two independent health organizations, along with the Pan American Sanitary Organization, coexisted.

In early 1922, the league sent a commission to Russia, reporting one positive fact, that "scientific studies in behalf of public health were pursued with the utmost zeal," and suggesting the government conclude a sanitary convention and an anti-epidemic strategy with adjoining countries. The council also noted that all Mediterranean countries trading at Black Sea ports were in grave danger from cholera. By July 18, Dr. J.L. McElroy, district physician for the Americas Relief Administration, warned that Europe's greatest cholera epidemic was raging in Odessa (2,000 cases) and the Ukraine 500,000 cases) with a death rate of 60 percent.

Dr. A. Schlesinger of the German Red Cross warned that refugees pouring into Germany from Polish, Latvian and Estonian borders sought passports to the United States, where they would be risks in spreading cholera to American shores. While this prompted the usual outpourings of fear in the United States, it did not stop aid efforts. In 1923, Herbert Hoover, chairman of the American Relief Administration, announced that cooperation among agencies had provided $70,000,000 for Russian Relief, more than 10 percent going to medical purposes. In the areas where starvation was rampant, 7,000,000 persons were inoculated and vaccinated, producing "an astonishing decrease in the high incidence of cholera, typhoid, para-typhoid and smallpox." During the summer of 1921, in the Kazan District, 170 cases were reported daily; after providing 350,000 inoculations, by 1922, the number had been reduced to a total of 276 cases. At the time, this inoculation campaign was the most extensive single preventative medical effort ever undertaken.[20] News was no better in other cholera hotspots. Of the 30,000 pilgrims passing into Calcutta from Daugor Island in 1919, many contracted cholera, 20 of which died. Complicating the situation, the cause was blamed on underfeeding due to the high cost of food.

The same year, reports continued to surface of cholera epidemics from all parts of China and Manchuria. For a three-week period ending August 31, there were 3,567 cholera deaths reported at Harbin, exclusive of Russian and Japanese victims. The numbers would have been worse but for the sudden stop and termination due to the technique of infusing isotonic solutions of saline (as suggested by Sir Leonard Rogers of Calcutta: sodium chloride, 120 grains; calcium chloride, 4 grains; Potassium chloride, 6 grains; distilled water, 1 pint) into patients' veins.

Called "the dead but living plague" by the Chinese, flies were still believed by many people, including foreign missionaries, to be the principal carriers. Nor had science mitigated the belief in West China that the scourge was a visitation of the Supreme Being as punishment for sins.

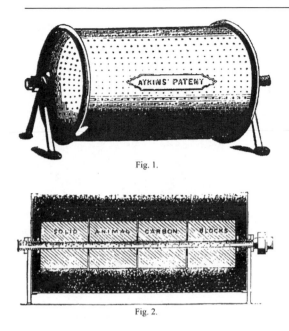

Fig. 1.

Fig. 2.

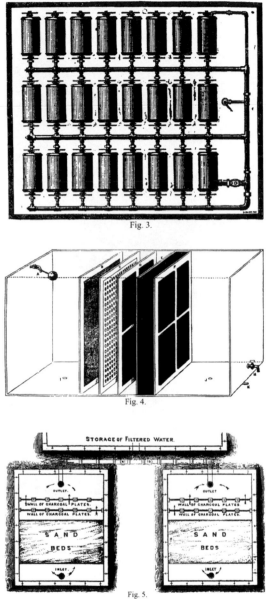

Fig. 3.

Fig. 4.

Fig. 5.

Recognized authorities stated that animal charcoal served to purify 136 times its weight of impure water, while vegetable charcoal purified only 116 times its weight. Atkins' Patent System of filtering water (Figure 1) utilized molded carbon blocks created by pulverizing animal charcoal mixed with Norway tar. The combined material was then amalgamated with liquid pitch and the whole kneaded into a homogeneous plastic mass and then molded into slabs or blocks (Figure 2). These were employed chiefly in cylindrical forms and so arranged that the percolation was from the external periphery inwards. The center of the blocks being hollow, they formed a tube where the purified water flowed for use. The bulk of impurities formed on the outside of the block, which could be removed and washed for reuse. A system of interconnected blocks allowed for a greater capacity of water (Figure 3). Figure 4: For hospitals, barracks and buildings where a larger capacity of filtered water was required, the Atkins system employed molded carbon plates presenting a large superficial area. Water passed through a series of frames: the first was covered with fine wire gauze, followed by separate frames of carbon plate, with or without the intervention of a bed of pure loose animal charcoal. There might also be a double frame containing a sheet of felt compressed between two perforated plates of sheet copper and zinc. Figure 5: Overhead view of the Atkins system with filtering sand beds for large-scale use. In 1873, this system was used by British forces stationed on the west coast of Africa and was adapted for use by the British Navy and Army (all figures from *Iron* [London], December 13, 1873).

Warring factions around Chengtu, Szechuen, the richest province in China, added to the misery, as frightened civilians abandoned sanitary precautions imposed by foreigners, raising death tolls above 1,000 daily. In the famine-stricken districts of Pekin, where underfeeding was believed to lead to cholera and little girls were sold "for the price of a small Chinese mule" to raise money for food, death tolls climbed.[21]

In the years following World War I, the world was never free of cholera outbreaks, principally in India and China, where the disease remained endemic. Although early reports indicated 1926 would have fewer cholera mortalities than 1925, temperatures reaching 102°F on August 6 exacerbated conditions at Shanghai and the Pootung (Potung) district, where reports indicated a daily mortality of 1,000. By September, the port of Tsingtao was declared infected, keeping American squadrons ship-bound. While sanitary measures were credited with reducing fatalities, massive parades honoring temple idols and the "Dragon King" were seen at Shaohing as desperate people expressed themselves in the ways of their ancestors. Blame for the outbreak was directed toward the "disgraceful state" of the Chapei Waterworks, where filter beds had been allowed to grow filthy and settling tanks contained deep sediment of "slime and living creatures."[22]

Conditions were mirrored in the Behar district of Bengal, India, where epidemics occurred in 1924 and 1927, the latter of which was considered the worst cholera outbreak in decades. By December, 30,000 cases had been reported in Bengal alone, with mortality estimates running as high as 15,000. In 1929, major flooding through the Syhlet and Cachar districts of Assam, British India, contributed to cholera among the inhabitants of a 5,500-square-mile area.[23]

Cholera outbreaks in the Philippines in 1925 were followed by worsening conditions in the spring of 1930, when the islands of Cebu and Bantayan were hardest struck. The disease spread to Manila, where "public antagonism" was said to be a factor complicating the enforcement of sanitary regulations. Eventually, the Red Cross reported 3,500 deaths from 5,000 cholera cases across the islands. Between two and three million people were given the "cholera prophylactic" to bring the epidemic under control.[24]

Quarantine Revisited

The International Sanitary Conference held in Paris in 1926 set new rules for quarantine, stipulating that printed material need not be subject to sanitary measures, but section III, article 13, provided measures to be used at ports and on the departure of vessels. Those measures concerning cholera provided that authorities were obliged to take measures: (1) to prevent the embarkation of persons showing symptoms of cholera and those in such relations with the sick as to render them liable to transmit the infection; and (2) to see that drinking water and foodstuffs taken on board were wholesome and that water used for ballast be disinfected if necessary.[25]

The advent of air travel also posed serious problems. In 1929, the England-to-India air route cut travel from 21 days to 6, while the *Graf Zeppelin* reached Los Angeles from China in 2½ days. As Pettenkofer warned in the last century, such short voyages allowed a carrier of disease to reach his destination without showing signs of illness, increasing the likelihood of an international spread of cholera. While article 13 pertained to ship travel, voyages by air were far more dangerous. One suggestion from 1929 posed the possibility of quarantine officers flying out to board a plane or dirigible in midair and climbing a rope ladder to enter the craft. If disease was found, an officer could divert the craft to a detention field. At the time, the United States quarantined for cholera, yellow and typhus fevers, plague, smallpox and leprosy. Airship quarantine stations were located in Buffalo, Albany, Los Angeles, Brownsville, Texas, West Palm Beach, Miami, San Diego, San Juan, Nogales, El Paso, Newport, Vermont, Key West, St. Paul, Newark, Detroit and Seattle (two).[26]

The Epidemiological Intelligence Service of the League of Nations instituted a different preventative by creating a radio network capable of distributing news of medical outbreaks around the world. By 1926, with its field headquarters at Singapore (the strategic center of the Far East), data was received from British North Borneo, Ceylon, China, Dutch East Indies, the Philippines and the Straits Settlements, Camaran, El Tor, Jeddah and Mecca. Singapore cabled the facts to Saigon; the message was received by the French wireless station of Ste. Assise and relayed to the Eiffel Tower. Paris telephoned the information to Geneva, where a health bulletin was broadcast to the world. It was hoped this news would allow countries to coordinate sanitary efforts to prevent the spread of disease.[27]

In the United States, Surgeon General Hugh S. Cumming operated a chain of quarantine stations along the nation's borders and coasts, with agents stationed abroad to conduct inspections of would-be immigrants. For this work, Congress annually allotted 11.5 million dollars, paying 10,000 officers and employees, 4,600 of whom were state or local officials.[28]

Bacteriophages

In 1917, the French-Canadian scientist Felix d'Herelle discovered "bacteriophage," a bacterial virus, at the Pasteur Institute in Paris. This anti-microbial agent was far more potent against bacteria than any agent at the time and was able to selectively destroy many pathogenic bacteria, including *Vibrio cholerae*, without damage to the host cell. D'Herelle developed the concept into specific treatments that, for a time, revolutionized medical science.

Phage suspensions were administered by both topical application and systemic administration through oral routes or injection or both. When introduced into the water supplies in high epidemic areas, they also proved highly effective in disease prevention. In 1927, an epidemic of Asiatic cholera was halted within 48 hours after prophylactic delivery of phage; using traditional interventions, the time factor would have been 26 days. According to d'Herelle, the region where the phage had been used became progressively cholera-free for several years. Capturing the imagination of the world, by 1928, d'Herelle was hailed as the conqueror of cholera for having succeeded in reducing mortality in parts of India from 62 percent to 8 percent. Large drug manufacturers, including Parke-Davis, Lilly, Abbott and Squibb in North America and Robert and Carriere in Europe, marketed phage as a therapeutic preparation and it became a commercial success. Sinclair Lewis' 1925 novel, *Arrowsmith*, was based on d'Herelle and the scientific events that led to phage treatments; d'Herelle held the post of director of Bacteriological Services for the League of Nations and also served as a professor at Yale.

Although it was little understood, by 1930, specialized bacteriophage (meaning "bacteria eater") was credited with curing dysentery in Brazil, bubonic plague in Egypt and Asiatic cholera in India. During World War II, the German army used phage therapy and it was alleged that German troops occupied Georgia, Soviet Union, to seize one of d'Herelle's scientific centers.

In 1941, Drs. Albert P. Krueger and E. Jane Scribner of the University of California published findings on bacteriophage in the *Journal of the American Medical Association*, stating its importance in the treatment of cholera and dysentery. Although they concluded "the germ killing virus" had little effect on other diseases, functioning in a very restricted field, they confirmed the "bacteria slayer's" usefulness in Oriental countries, particularly India.

Unfortunately, d'Herelle was a derisive figure who refused to compromise or blend his findings with more standard scientific beliefs, including those of Metchnikoff, Jules Bordet and Ehrlich, the founders of immunology. Accusations that his field trials had not been carried out in a rigorously controlled manner, d'Herelle's idea that findings of "bacteriologists of the laboratory," including Koch's postulates, had to be revised and his insistence in the fundamental role of phage in the process of natural recovery led to the eventual abandonment of phage by American and European researchers, although it continued to be used in Russia for decades and has never been completely abandoned.[29]

Cholera in the 1930s

Europe and the United States remained free from cholera epidemics, but China continued to be plagued by serious outbreaks, complicated by flood and famine. After the Yangtze overran its banks in 1931, thousands of Chinese believed they had angered the Dragon God and waited stoically for the river to sweep over Hankow, Wuchang and Manyang. It was estimated 35,000 square miles in Hupeh Province and 22,000 square miles in Hunan Province were under water, with the destitute there numbered at 5,000,000 and 2,000,000, respectively. Sanitary authorities made arrangements to inoculate at least 100,000 against cholera, but low supplies made that task nearly impossible. Dire conditions were also reported throughout Southern Persia in 1931, particularly at Basra, Irak (Iraq), as 1,960 cases were registered, with 1,202 fatalities.

A year later, cholera had become epidemic as the Hwang Ho (Yellow River), running from Northeast Tibet to the Gulf of Pechihli, inundated Shensi, a province of 8.5 million people. Charges were made against contractors dumping garbage into the Whangpoo River, from which three municipalities along the lower course drew their water. At Sian, Shensi Province, the trade crossroads of Asia, streets were covered in powdered lime but serum for inoculations remained inadequate. By October 13, 1932, Dr. J. Heng Liu, director of the bureau of public health, declared the cholera epidemic the worst ever witnessed in China, with a mortality of 27.5 percent and placed death numbers for the summer at 30,000.

Temperatures above 100°F in North China worsened conditions in 1933, and in 1934, the League of Nations was called upon to help alleviate further spread of cholera at Foochow. The *Kansas City Star* reported that representatives of the league assembled a parade carrying large figures of the "wicked cholera devil" and the "good angel of boiled water" through the city. When the epidemic came, villagers outside the city suffered from the disease but those who had followed the message escaped.[30]

31

Cholera in the World War II Era

Cholera is such a horrible disease and epidemics spread so fast that the mere mention that a person has cholera is nearly enough to start panic in the Middle East. In this case, the dread was sufficient to make the natives beg for the vaccination needle, which they normally shun as if it were a lesser plague.[1]

During World War II, there were only 13 cases and two deaths from cholera among American troops. This was attributed to a strong emphasis on sanitation and well-developed and well-executed disease control methods.

Even before the United States entered the war, the surgeon general's office had identified two fields of interest: preventative measures and research and investigation. On October 22, 1941, a conference of experts prepared resolutions for protecting American troops, including the use of immunization procedures. These resolutions became the basis for practices adopted by the War Department. Arrangements were made to obtain new strains of *V. cholerae* from East Indian and Egyptian sources for study and possible use in preparing vaccines. Similarly, before the cities of Manila and Hong Kong fell, the Canadian Public Health Association took the precaution of obtaining sufficient cultures to create vaccines for their troops.

In February 1942, all U.S. military personnel stationed in or traveling through areas of epidemic typhus or cholera were required to be immunized. Personnel were warned, however, that vaccination provided incomplete protection of relatively short duration and was to be considered an adjunct to other control measures. That said, a study under the direction of R. Adiseshan, director of public health, Madras, determined that those immunized were "at least 10 times less susceptible to [cholera] than an unimmunized population."

The greatest cholera threat to American troops was to those serving in the China-Burma-India theatre, especially near Calcutta. Despite ever-present outbreaks, the army reported no cases of the disease, although such was not the case with Indian and British troops. Except for immunization directives, very few administrative actions were specifically directed against cholera. However, other gastrointestinal infections (diarrhea and dysenteries) approached critical levels in 1944.

In the spring of 1945, a severe epidemic of cholera struck the native population at Calcutta, prompting an intensive educational campaign among soldiers. Other measures included an emphasis on immunization, rigorous inspection of foodstuffs and food-handlers and enforcement of strict sanitary discipline. Conclusions from this theatre indicated that opportunities for exposure to the disease were present at all times and much of the protection afforded soldiers was attributed to the effectiveness of the cholera vaccine. American troops assigned to the China section of the China-Burma-India theatre faced essentially the same threat from cholera as those in India. Routine immunization and sanitary measures were enforced with equal success.

In the summer of 1945, outbreaks of cholera seriously threatened military units in various parts of Free China, the first of which occurred in Chungking. A report generated by the medical director indicated many American installations were "very unsatisfactory," with serious defects in sanitation and protection of water supplies. Corrective measures were apparently successful, as no cases of cholera were reported.

The only two outbreaks of cholera among American troops appeared shortly thereafter, the first in late July 1945, among personnel stationed at Liangshan Air Base, attributed to cakes and cookies from a local bakery. Six cases were reported; case histories revealed that several of the victims had not received timely six-month stimulating vaccinations.

The other outbreak occurred at Chihchiang during the first week of August 1945, involving staff from the 547th Quartermaster Depot Supply Company. Attributed to contaminated water, seven cases were reported with one death. American troops in the Southwest Pacific Area were exposed to cholera by the movement of Japanese soldiers throughout Southeast Asia, including Indo-China, Siam, Singapore and the Philippines. Preventative measures were taken and no incidents occurred.

In summary, fortunate circumstances, preventative measures and the fact most United States personnel in the India-Burma-China theatres were not engaged in ground combat to any significant degree led to the extremely low incidence of cholera in World War II.[2]

"It is cholera rather than cannon that is causing concern...."

War of a different type than guns and bullets attacked civilians during the decade of the 1940s. Reflective of the times, these years were described in terms of battle and casualty lists. In the "campaign" against the disease near Lucknow, India, in 1941, anti-cholera inoculations were given to 50,704 people in one week. Like battle, cholera "broke out" in northern Thailand in 1943; 379 lives were "claimed" in Calcutta during September 1943, with 456 others "killed" during the first ten days of October. The "enemy" famine was "decisively defeated" in Bengal in 1944, but Major General Douglas Stuart, commander of the British-Indian troops, reported they were "now confronted by a formidable disease enemy" and promised 9,000,000 Bengalese would be immunized against cholera and smallpox by the end of March.

From the beginning of July until mid–September, 16,800 people died of cholera in the United Provinces; altogether, 34,000 were taken ill during that period, with the death toll reaching 1,900 in a single week. Cholera and malaria in the province of Bihar claimed 42,000 victims up to July 31, adding 6,000 more in the first three weeks of August. The pre-monsoon cholera epidemic in Calcutta in 1945 was attributed to "lax and dilatory" dealings of the Bengal authorities, with an average number of cholera deaths in the province placed at 53,266 annually.

Matters did not improve after the cessation of hostilities. Refugee camps in Delhi in 1947 were reported jammed with thousands of Muslims seeking military protection from Hindu-Sikh violence, while a 10 percent mortality of 400 cholera cases was registered in the Kasur camp in the Muslim sector of the Punjab. By February 1948, cholera claimed 1,374 lives in Madras, Calcutta and Bihar. Nearly 300 more died at Allahabad, where three million had gathered for a religious ceremony and the committal of Mohandas K. Gandhi's ashes to the river.[3]

The lead paragraph of a 1950 newspaper article stated the following: "New Delhi, Dec. 18 (AP)—The bodies of hundreds of dead and dying Indians today were reported strewn in roads around a village in Orissa state as cholera raged among seekers of a 'divine all cure' medicine distributed by a 12-year-old cowherd [shepherd]." According to the report, "hundreds of thousands of enthusiasts" in the previous six weeks had crowded into the village to get the herbal medicine of powdered tree bark that the healer, Nepal Baba, was said to have received by divine dispensation. An official committee concluded the medicine was "not effective" and forbade further pilgrimages to see him. To counter the subsequent panic, the government sponsored mass inoculations and tragically, mass cremations among the 40,000 who had hoped for a miracle cure.

The following year, cholera raged in Mandalay, 500 miles north of Rangoon, where daily death tolls averaged forty-two. Complicating matters, there was only vaccine sufficient for 50,000 out of a population of 200,000. Unsanitary conditions in Calcutta, exacerbated by Hindu refugees from the Pakistan state of East Bengal, added 142 more lives to the mortality list.[4]

The situation in China was equally devastating. In 1940, the epidemic at Shanghai was so bad, Japan declared quarantine against ships from that area. By September, 5,000 Chinese living in the coastal regions of Fukien province died from the disease that claimed 75 percent mortality. By 1941, at Siu Lam, Japanese soldiers spent weeks vaccinating civilians in an effort to control cholera in refugee camps. The contagion was also present at Hong Kong, where mortality climbed to near 100 percent.

A year later, epidemics raged among refugees from the invasion of Burma and China that began when these displaced people poured into Kunming, leaving hundreds stranded and dying along roadways. Two months later, reports indicated infected refugees in the overcrowded city reached 5,250; feverish efforts by the Chinese Red Cross and mission hospitals resulted in inoculation of 150,000, but not before another 4,000 had perished in the Japanese-occupied Tengyueh, in western Yunnan Province. By August, Japanese soldiers also numbered among the victims.

A September 1943 headline read, "Cholera and Plague Wage Guerilla War Against Japanese" in the Southwest Pacific. Cholera not only appeared in Japanese-occupied Peking and Tientsin, but the disease, uncontrolled in Thailand since June, appeared in the Philippines. Five months later, reports from Chungking indicated "a million Chinese have died of famine and cholera in Kwangtung Province," depopulating 80 percent of some villages. News grew worse in 1944, when cholera appeared among refugees escaping the Kweilin area for Liuchow. Making matters more serious, the airstrip used by American combat planes was threatened by Japanese bombers to the point where the combined threat caused speculation that the loss of the base might affect 20,000 tons of U.S. military supplies flown into China each month.

By a moderate estimate, 4,000 cases of cholera broke out in Chungking during the first three weeks of June 1945, prompting Dr. James Watt of the U.S. Public Health Service to hurry there to fight the disease. Although no U.S. military personnel were affected, all possible humanitarian efforts were made to alleviate the suffering.[5]

The World Health Organization

In April 1945, world representatives met in San Francisco to establish the framework for the United Nations. At this time, Brazil and China proposed the creation of an international health organization. In February 1946, the secretary-general ordered a conference for this purpose and delegates met in Paris from March 18 to April 5. They presented their constitution to the International Health Conference in New York City, which ran from June 19 to July 22,

1946. On the basis of these proposals, the constitution of the World Health Organization (WHO) was signed on July 22. The conference also created an "Interim Commission" to carry on the work previously undertaken by the Health Organization of the League of Nations and the Office International d'Hygiène publique (OIHP), established in 1907.

For several years, the Health Division of the United National Relief and Rehabilitation Administration (UNRRA) and the Interim Commission of WHO assumed responsibility for international sanitary conventions and for international epidemiological reporting. (The Interim Commission ended at midnight on August 31, 1948, immediately succeeded by WHO, whose constitution had come into force on April 7, 1948.)[6]

In March 1946, the UNRRA announced cholera was raging throughout south China, where more than 1,000,000 persons were threatened. Enough vaccine was flown to Canton to immunize 200,000, with the eventual goal being 100 percent. The U.S. Navy also delivered enough vaccine to cover 250,000 persons in Hankow, as repatriation vessels from China to Japan carried more than 400 cholera cases. By May, the U.S. chief surgeon prohibited Americans from eating Japanese seafood due to the danger of contracting cholera. Repatriates from China also introduced cholera into Korea, where 1,212 cases were reported in June 1946, with 651 deaths.[7]

Cholera broke out in Sharkia, Egypt's northernmost province (which extended to the Suez Canal zone, where thousands of British troops were stationed), on September 23, 1947.

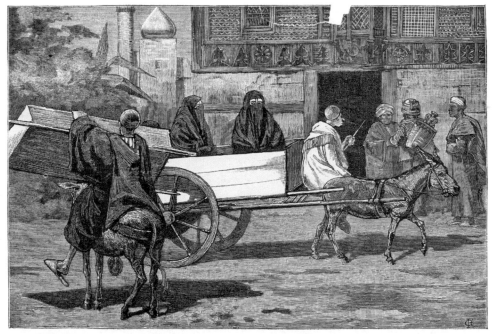

HOW CHOLERA IS SPREAD IN EGYPT—MOURNERS RETURNING FROM A FUNERAL IN THE COFFIN

"How Cholera Is Spread in Egypt—Mourners Returning from a Funeral in the Coffin." Every culture had traditions when it came to honoring and burying the dead. Friends of pilgrims who died in Mecca frequently cut the dead man's clothes into small pieces and distributed them to family members on their return home; the Irish held feasts around the corpse; washing and kissing the body and even relatives sleeping in the same chamber were all means of spreading contagion. Ancient rituals were nearly impossible to break despite warnings from health authorities and admonitions from religious leaders (*London Graphic*, August 4, 1883).

By September 26, the UP reported from Cairo, "panic-stricken crowds nearly mobbed vaccination centers today, begging physicians to save them from cholera—that is spreading swiftly in an epidemic in the Nile River valley." With only enough vaccine for 60,000, the government sent urgent appeals to the United States, Britain and South Africa for all they could spare, while notifying all foreign countries it was a "cholera infested area."

Although the United Nations Security Council was unable to reach agreement on Prime Minister Nokrashi Pasha's demand for the withdrawal of British troops from the Nile Valley, the report of 2,606 cholera cases in the first 21 days of the epidemic, with the resultant 568 deaths, caught international attention. As medical experts warned the disease would spread quickly through the Middle East if help were not immediate, the international community heeded the call from the World Health Organization. Aid arrived not only from the above countries, but also from Soviet Russia, France, Italy, Holland, Switzerland, Lebanon, Syria, Iraq, Brazil, Sweden, Poland and China.

With hospitals under military control, Egyptian troops sprayed DDT as a disinfectant over contaminated areas. In an attempt to prevent unauthorized sales of "remedies," black-market traffickers in anti-cholera supplies were made liable to a three-month imprisonment and a £500 fine (about $2,000). These efforts did not prevent the governments of Palestine, Syria, Lebanon, Iraq and Turkey from establishing quarantine against Egypt. They also instituted their own inoculation campaigns, requiring vaccination certificates of travelers.

Well aware that the last cholera epidemic in 1902 (reportedly caused by Moslem pilgrims returning from Mecca) extracted a toll of 35,000 lives in six months, the Egyptian government also took the extraordinary step of canceling the pilgrimage for the present year. In 1948, the high commissariat of the Spanish zone of Morocco also banned all residents of the Spanish Moroccan protectorate from participating in Mecca pilgrimages.[8]

WHO developed a two-pronged attack against cholera in Egypt: the most immediate need was to control the epidemic and prevent its spread; the second was to eradicate the disease entirely. On the first front, travel restrictions to Palestine and Saudi Arabia were put in place and vaccinations were given to residents of Jidda, the seaport where Moslem pilgrims converged during their trips to Mecca and other holy cities. Pilgrims were also subjected to vaccinations and other safeguards before they were allowed to leave. Passengers to the United States were also required to have vaccination certificates, while luggage was inspected and occasionally sterilized. On arrival in the U.S., the Public Health Service, under the direction of Dr. G.L. Dunnahoo, quarantined passengers and crew for five days if cholera was aboard.

As one explanation for the cholera outbreak in Egypt, Dr. William F. Petersen borrowed a page from history by suggesting sunspots as the culprit. He stated, "During periods of sunspots with resulting disturbances of the weather people are more unsettled and move around more. They have less resistance because of the strain put on them by variable weather and they have contacts with other people, making possible the spread of disease." On the positive side, Petersen avowed that more geniuses would be born during these periods of solar turbulence.[9]

Cholera at the Midpoint of the 20th Century

Five diseases were subject to international quarantine in the 1950s: cholera, plague, typhus, smallpox and yellow fever. India was considered the prime focus of cholera, and ships wishing to enter American ports with that disease aboard were subject to fumigation. This was accomplished by placing canned cyanide-impregnated discs throughout the vessel. Combined with teargas meant to drive people away, the discs, once exposed to air, released gas very slowly. The danger of this technique was demonstrated in New York, when 13 stowaways failed to heed or did not hear any warnings and were later found dead.

Those traveling abroad in 1956 were warned that cholera vaccination was frequently required by countries where the disease was endemic, while the U.S. Public Health Service recommended immunization for all those going to or through an infected area.

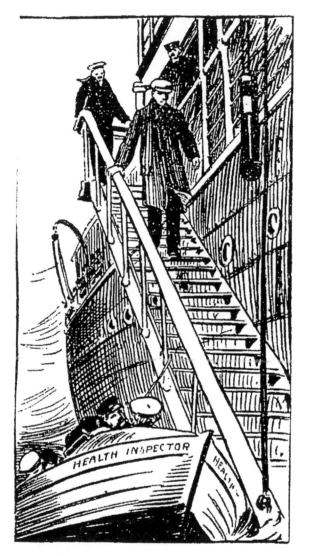

"Health Officer Leaving Suspected Vessel After Inspection." In order to guard New York ports of entry where ships from known cholera areas around the world disembarked passengers, health officers were required to inspect crews, immigrants and even the food and water they consumed. If any signs of disease or germs were discovered, the entire manifest could be quarantined; after the travelers' recovery, it was within the power of the health inspector to return them to their native country (*Cannelton [IN] Enquirer*, October 31, 1908).

Reports in September 1953 indicated 870 deaths from cholera in north Kwantung Province, China. The following year, an influx of refugees fleeing flood-stricken areas of Communist China introduced the disease into the former Nationalist capital. Cases quickly escalated to 1,000 cases, creating a severe epidemic.

India, however, remained the focal point of cholera outbreaks. In June 1953, officials indicated 200 deaths per day in Calcutta. Prognosis remained grim as analysis of waters from the Hoogly River revealed large quantities of germs, believed to result from peasants throwing bodies into the river. Inoculation programs reached 4,000 per week out of a population of three million, although many refused treatment.

Flooding in 1954 created new epidemics, reaching into East Pakistan, where melting snow combined with monsoon rains brought starvation and death. At the request of the Pakistani government, the 37th and 163rd Medical companies flew in from Korea, setting up headquarters at Dacca. Formed into 76 "shot teams" composed of two American medics and two Pakistanis, they inoculated people against cholera and typhus and sprayed fields with DDT.

The cholera season began in April 1955, and by mid–June, authorities indicated 150 people were dying daily at Calcutta. Traced to a leakage in the water main in the Kidderpore area, the problem was repaired but the epidemic continued. The dread disease lasted into May 1956, setting a world record in the number of victims per capita. By July, an estimated 2,000 more deaths were reported in the East Indian state of Bihar, while Korean officials listed 600 deaths, including 20 soldiers, occurring just north of the truce line.

The devastation of cholera continued into 1957, claiming 9,000 more Indian lives between September and November; conditions in Ceylon also reached the breaking point, prompting the government to appeal to President Eisenhower, who promptly sent the Navy to deliver vaccines and supplies. Bad news persisted into 1958, when unfiltered water used to supplement Calcutta's regular supply spread cholera into the middle-class living areas, claiming 500 more lives. Numbers were worse in East Pakistan. By early April, as the death toll climbed to 15,000–20,000, American, Russian and Canadian teams were rushed into the country. Vaccine was also sent by India and Australia, but as conditions worsened, WHO predicted it would take an additional two years to bring the epidemic under control.[10]

In August 1958, WHO termed the cholera situation throughout Asia "the most serious in years." From January 1958, the communiqué listed 48,729 cases and 20,687 deaths in areas including India, East Pakistan, Thailand, Cambodia and Burma. Cholera was also found in Nepal for the first time since the beginning of the century. Ultimately, WHO reported cholera was worse in 1958 than at any time since 1953, when 242,000 cases were reported. About 93,000 cases were reported in 1958, compared to 64,000 in 1957.

Aiding the fight against cholera in Thailand, Americans introduced revolutionary "hydrospray guns" for inoculation in 1957. Drs. Edward Anderson of the navy and Adrian Mandell of the army instructed locals in the new tool that allowed physicians to immunize patients twenty times faster than by using traditional needles. The "gun" also eliminated errors by administering correct dosages, while its speed made the operation practically painless. Unfortunately, more needed to be done. In 1958, during the June–December cholera period, Thailand experienced 11,582 cases with 1,747 deaths; between January and March 1959, there were 4,200 cases with 358 deaths, prompting a medical team from Walter Reed Army Hospital and 12 members of a navy medical research unit to visit the stricken area.

By September 1960, West Pakistan officials stated 5,000 people suffered from cholera during the year, resulting in 700 deaths. The origin of the epidemic was traced to Jammu, Kasmir, where the epidemic began around early July. Iranian authorities attempted to seal off the border with Pakistan to avert the importation of disease from that country and Afghanistan, but, finding it impossible, they evacuated 5,000 inhabitants.[11]

Cholera and Cholera Research

Between 1951 and 1959, Sambhu Nath De made the crucial discovery on the pathogenesis of cholera, finally proving the third of Robert Koch's postulates after 75 years: the comma bacillus obtained from cholera victims could cause disease in an animal model. In 1959, at Bombay, N.K. Dutta, Pause and Kulkarni also developed a rabbit model demonstrating disease symptoms were caused by a toxin.

De and Chatterje's groundbreaking article in 1953 demonstrated that living *V. cholerae* cultures introduced into the intraperitoneal cavity of a rabbit and later into the lumen of a rabbit's ligated intestine, altered the permeability of the intestinal mucosa and thereby caused fluid secretion. Prior to this, scientists searching for systemic or lethal effects had obtained conflicting results administering stools of cholera patients or toxic preparations derived from *V. cholerae* to different animals using a multiplicity of techniques:

The prodigious work of De & Chatterje was followed by a demonstration that the pathogenicity of some strains of *Escherichia coli* was very similar to that of *V. cholerae*, and such strains were what we know today as enterotoxigenic *E. coli*. The discovery of the cholera enterotoxin and its effect on intestinal permeability, the demonstration that bacteria-free culture filtrates of *V. cholerae* are entertoxic and the development of a reproducible animal model for cholera are milestones in the history of the fight against the disease.[12]

Army medical experts were also involved in clinical cholera research. In 1943, Lt. Maurice Landy and three coworkers (Lt.-Col. Newton W. Larkum, Elizabeth J. Oswald and Sgt. Frank Streightoff) reported a solution to the problem concerning the effectiveness of sulfonamides, first discovered in Germany in 1936. Sulfa-guanidine drugs had proven highly effective in treating cholera but researchers discovered that much higher doses were required than anticipated. Landy identified p-aminobenzoic acid (PAB), a new member of the vitamin B family produced by various disease germs as food; if sufficient numbers were present, they served as a protectorate, sometimes sustaining the ability to withstand 20,000 times as much sulfonamide as the original germs.

"In other words," Landy explained, "though scientists have expected that the germs must produce some kind of sulfa-resistant material, exactly what it was and how it worked had never been proven." His first step was to perfect a test whereby one half of a billionth of a gram of PAB was detected. "Our next job will be to prove what the other micro-organisms, such as the germs of cholera, dysentery and pneumonia produce to repel the deadliness of the sulfanomides. The rules of biology are usually consistent, so I feel these germs produce a substance similar to PAB. When it is known exactly what each germ makes, a method for tearing down the organism's ability to turn out such a substance will be the ensuing step."[13]

The following year, a bulletin from the American Medical Society carried an article by Dr. Joo-se Huang, of China, who reported success treating 21 out of 22 cholera patients with sulfa-guanidine. By contrast, treatment with kaolin and the injection of salts resulted in a 26 percent death rate. (Kaolin, a mud product of the erosion of igneous rock—aluminum silicate—had been used to treat cholera in China for centuries, administered orally or as an enema. Its action was two-fold: engulfing and then carrying away bacteria and absorbing poisons to prevent them from entering the bloodstream. Adding aluminum hydroxide to kaolin made a mixture useful in treating ulcerative colitis and stomach ulcers.)[14]

A new sulphonamide (sulfonamide) compound called "six-two-five-seven" (or 6257), derived from sulphathiazole and formaldehyde, underwent trials in Madras, India, in 1948. The *British Medical Journal* reported that Dr. S.S. Bhatnager, of St. Xavier's College, Bombay, achieved "remarkable" success in 82 out of 85 patients but cautioned "it would be rash to assert a panacea for cholera has been obtained. Nevertheless, results are so striking they merit further investigation." The same year, Drs. Harry Seneca, a research associate at Columbia University's College of Physicians and Surgeons, and Edward Henderson, director of the clinical research division of the Schering Corporation, New Jersey, announced a new drug named phthalyl-sulfacetimide. Tests on more than 500 cholera patients in Egypt during the epidemic of 1947 proved effective.[15]

In the early 1940s, Japan controlled 90 percent of the world's agar, one of the most vital necessities for the maintenance of public health. A gelatinous substance derived from certain seaweeds, agar was used for testing the purity of water and milk and diagnosing typhoid, diphtheria, strep and staph infections and for the growth of cultures used in creating vaccines for bubonic plague, cholera and whooping cough. Not only did the Japanese harvest agar off their own shores, it was believed they also exploited secret beds off the Southern California coast.

To counter the threat, Robert H. Tschudy and Marston C. Sargent of the Scripps Institute began experimenting with other seaweeds. In 1943, they announced four new types that would provide agar sufficient for American needs.[16]

Another development in the field of medicine came from the Franklin Institute; it was announced in 1945 that a potent, single-dose cholera vaccine had been developed under the direction of Drs. Ellice McDonald, Robert A. Jennings and Richard W. Linton. The liquid culture required a minimum of equipment and no special skills; a technician in a field station could produce 65,000 doses of serum within 4–5 days. Under the old system, cholera vaccine was grown on solid material and three injections were required, a serious drawback when individuals refused to return for the second and third shots. By simulating conditions occurring in cholera-infested intestines, the researchers were able to produce a profuse growth in a liquid medium; its components included salts, casein, trypsin, glucose and distilled water. "American Relief for India, Inc.," sponsored by Lord Halifax and Sir Girja Bajpai, was to introduce the vaccine to the Bengal population.[17]

Contributions to cholera research by the United States Navy began in Cairo during the 1947 epidemic. CDR Robert Allen Phillips, first commander of the Naval Medical Research Unit 3 (NAMRU-3), discovered a lack of protein in a victim's stool that indicated no disruption of the gut mucosa. He concluded "that all of the pathological features of the disease could be explained by the diarrhea alone. This conclusion anticipated the discovery of the cholera toxin by a decade." Giving infusions of sodium bicarbonate to normalize blood pH, Phillips reduced case fatality from 20 percent to 7.5 percent.

In 1958, Phillips became commanding officer of the newly reactivated NAMRU-2 in Taipei. Offering the team's services to the Thai Ministry of Health, they confirmed the previous Cairo IV therapy results and invented an army cot with a hole under the buttocks to allow discharges to drain down for accurate measurement and hygiene. In 1960, the NAMRU-2 team continued their research at Taipei, first garnering the respect of the natives by participating with Buddhist priests in prayers before beginning their day's research.

Covering the Far East in mobile teams comprising mules, jeeps and light planes, NAMRU-2 injected thousands with smallpox, cholera and tetanus vaccines. By utilizing little more than salvaged equipment and carefully calculated IV solutions, team members were able to greatly reduce mortality that typically ran 5–60 percent. By 1966, the case fatality rate for cholera treated with the navy method of IV therapy was 0.6 percent and was reduced to zero with expeditious treatment.

After the 1958 outbreak at Bangkok, Phillips proposed a United States field team assist him. He was joined in 1959, with investigators from the National Institutes of Health and Jefferson Medical College. Dr. Robert Gordon of the NIH used IV radioactive povidone to confirm normal gut permeability, proving that cholera was not an invasive disease.[18]

In 1956, Dr. Sanders T. Lyle of Texas Christian University received a $10,000 grant from the National Institutes of Health to conduct research on cholera. The bacilli used came from the Campbell Hospital in Calcutta, isolated there from the 1953 epidemic. Frozen in a vacuum and sealed, the cultures were brought back to life by thawing and adding broth. Working with Dr. Lyle were Christine Pierce, Jeannine Scott and Johnny Barnett. The project involved infecting rabbits in an effort to find a vaccine. In 1959, Dr. Theodore E. Woodward of the University of Maryland became a team member of a research group sent by the National Institutes of Health under the auspices of the Southeastern Asiatic Treaty Organization to study the cause, prevention and treatment of the ancient scourge.

The same year, Dr. Yoshikazu Watanabe was sent on a McLaughlin Foundation postdoctoral fellowship to the University of Texas to develop a more effective vaccine against cholera. An advisor on serological problems for the U.S. Army in Japan, Watanabe hoped use of a new technology at the university that isolated toxic substances electronically rather than chemically would aid him in the development of a vaccine that covered 10 percent of the population then resistant to current vaccines.

On the natural front, a doctor at Calcutta's Chittaranjan Hospital reported success against cholera by administering the juice of an indigenous herb, *Coleus Aromaticus*, claiming the new medicine reduced mortality to less than 5 percent against the city's death rate of 26.5 percent.[19]

32

The Seventh Cholera Pandemic
"No country is safe from cholera"

For the seventh time in the annals of medical history, King Cholera is marching out of Asia into the Middle East and reaching its fingers into Southern Russia and Western Europe. Next to the Black Plague, no communicable disease is more terrifying to people than cholera.... The scourge of antiquity, cholera has once again emerged as a major health problem internationally.[1]

The official start of the Seventh Cholera Pandemic began in 1961, which proved to be a busy year. In August, the first cases at Hong Kong since 1947 prompted half a million cubic centimeters of vaccine to be shipped from the United States, Britain, India, Australia and Sarawak. The disease was believed to have been introduced across the "Bamboo Curtain" from Celebes, Indonesia, due to the shifting Chinese population and the movement of troops. Social workers estimated case numbers rose into the hundreds in less than a week. Peiping Radio grudgingly admitted some deaths occurred in Kwantung Province but claimed victims died of "vibrio paracholera," not true cholera, a technicality medical authorities considered "splitting hairs."

By September, despite a massive vaccination campaign, disease erupted in the Philippines, quickly claiming 750 lives. Again, doctors argued over whether it was cholera, gastroenteritis or a new disease called "choleriform enteritis." By mid–January 1962, the epidemic, now called cholera "El Tor," had become endemic.[2]

Endemic Cholera in the Philippines, 1961–1968

Year	Mortality
1961	1,405
1962	1,682
1963	433
1964	1,518
1965	493
1966	572
1967	193
1968	260[3]

After massive flooding in 1972, seventy thousand residents were inoculated against cholera, but contaminated drinking water aided the spread of both cholera and gastroenteritis.[4]

Nor was India immune. While a majority of the 400,000 citizens of Banaras submitted to inoculations, orthodox Hindu priests and their followers relied on religion, organizing guards to watch the streets against entry of the Goddess of Cholera. Following tradition, the faithful made an idol of the goddess with wheat flour and secretly smuggled it out of town under the belief the spirit would take the disease with her: guards watched to ensure no one from a neighboring village brought it back. Similar to other times and other religions, one priest stated cholera was attributed to "god's anxiety to test the spiritual discipline of the people."

In 1963, WHO declared that cholera remained the number-one killer in diseases subject to international quarantine, having been reported in Taiwan, West Pakistan, Afghanistan, Iran, Southern Russia, Iraq, North and South Korea, Burma, Cambodia, South Vietnam, Malaysia, Singapore, Nepal, Thailand, Uzbekistan and Hong Kong. While cholera deaths in 1960 totaled 11,216 (a drop from 1950, when 130,481 deaths were recorded), by 1965, WHO indicated that the El Tor strain had spread to almost all Asian countries and was on the verge of reaching the Middle East and Eastern Europe. (El Tor had become generally recognized 30 years earlier in Indonesia. At the time, it did not appear to have the same severity as classical cholera, but spread more rapidly and produced long-term carriers. By 1965, however, as experts argued over whether it was a completely different disease or merely a variation, it was feared its virulence had increased, as victims seemed to have less natural or acquired immunity.)

WHO's 1965 prediction proved to be accurate, as Iran, which had been free of cholera since 1939, reported 2,704 cases by mid–October. The following year, at an international conference on cholera control, Francisco J. Dy, regional director of WHO, stated that within a span of five years, cholera had claimed 76,000 lives out of 260,000 cases in 23 countries. By 1967, WHO warned "no country is safe from cholera."

The year 1968 marked WHO's 20th anniversary. With 129 members (as opposed to 53 at its founding), the organization was credited with checking the spread of cholera. Much more work needed to be done, however, as fears continued to be entertained that Europe was at risk. Complicating matters, the voluntary reporting system in which nations were obliged to participate was less than perfect, as proved in 1970, when WHO was forced to admit the disease was spreading more rapidly than indicated by official notification.

The new cause for concern lay in the fact simultaneous outbreaks appeared in Israel, Libya and Lebanon as well as in Astrakhan, an important Soviet city on the Caspian Sea, straddling the uncertain border between Asia and Europe.[5]

The World Wages War on Cholera

In 1970, with new outbreaks of cholera appearing in Egypt, Syria, South Korea and the Soviet Union, an international effort began to end the trail of death. The campaign included the research laboratory in Dacca, the Southeast Asia Treaty Organization (SEATO), the United Kingdom, Australia and various American agencies, including the Agency for International Development, the National Institutions for Health (NIH), the National Communicable Disease Center in Atlanta, Georgia, and the Maryland Department of Corrections, where human volunteers took part in an NIH-sponsored series of tests to develop an effective cholera vaccine.[6]

Countries Considered Infected with Cholera, 1971

Africa	*Asia*
Algeria	Burma
Cameroon	India

Africa	*Asia*
Chad	Indonesia
Dahomey	Malaysia
Ghana	Nepal
Ivory Coast	Pakistan
Kenya	Philippines
Liberia	Oman Sultanate
Mali	South Vietnam
Mauritania	Yemen[7]
Morocco	
Nigeria	
Niger	
Sierra Leone	
Togo	
Upper Volta	

In 1976, a *Washington Post* article by Stephen S. Rosenfeld ("Famine, Epidemics Covered Up to Save National Pride" in the January 29 *Register,* CA), reported as "unquestionable truth" allegations leveled against WHO in the booklet "The Politics of Starvation," written for the Carnegie Endowment for International Peace. Rosenfeld charged that WHO, "eager to continue its 'long-term projects' in Ethiopia, went so far as to suppress information of a cholera epidemic spreading across international boundaries into neighboring states," adding that "Guinea hid a cholera epidemic in 1969."

WHO countered by stating no cases of cholera were reported to it from Ethiopia in 1973, nor were any cases identified from neighboring countries; in 1970 and 1971, there was a cholera flare-up in Ethiopia that was quickly reported to WHO and requisite supplies were sent; in 1969, cholera was discovered in Guinea and announced by WHO radio. On the issue of "speedy provision of assistance," WHO acknowledged room for improvement and offered to take part in meaningful dialogue.[8]

Although the number of cholera cases reported to WHO in 1977 represented the lowest number in seven years, as of May 10, 1977, seven African nations and eight Asian nations remained infected. Putting the numbers into perspective, the Centers for Disease Control (CDC) suggested cholera was actually more prevalent but had become so endemic countries stopped reporting it. Not surprisingly, data suggested that sickness around the world would fall by 30 percent if people in underdeveloped countries could be given pure water. Targets set for the United Nations (1971–1980) were for 60 percent of city-dwellers to have house-water connections and 25 percent of rural people to have safe water. Unfortunately, experts estimated it would require $21 billion to reach pure-water targets and $14.5 billion to provide adequate excreta-disposal facilities. The cost was many times WHO's annual budget of $140 million.[9]

Predictably, more cases of cholera were reported worldwide in 1978 than in any year since the pandemic started in 1961. The disease was also more diffuse than at any time in the prior 18 years, being identified in 40 countries, including the United States.

Worldwide Cholera Statistics from the CDC

Year	*Cholera Cases*
1976	66,020
1977	58,087
1978	74,632[10]

Cholera in the United States, 1965 and Beyond

The first American cholera case in more than 50 years struck an unimmunized worker at Walter Reed laboratory, Washington, D.C. On June 1, 1965, he assisted in the injection of 45 guinea pigs with vibrio cholerae organisms. During the procedure, he noted liquid leaking from a tube in the injection apparatus about 18 inches from his face. He came down with symptoms on June 3. On July 20, the D.C. Health Department revealed a second technician had been diagnosed with cholera. Both victims recovered.

A similar accident was reported in February 1977, when Dr. Edward Nelson came down with cholera after being contaminated when a rubber line leading from a large fermenter burst, spewing culture into the lab at the University of Texas Southwestern Medical School. Dr. Richard Finkelstein explained there was no chance of the disease spreading but these accidents underscored the danger of working with dangerous diseases, even under controlled conditions.[11]

In August 1973, the first naturally occurring case in 62 years appeared in Calhoun County, Texas, where a 51-year-old man came down with cholera after eating at the Port Lavaca motel. At the hospital, the patient went into shock and required resuscitation. Dr. James Thompson recognized the symptoms and administered tetracycline and fluid replacement, saving the man's life by his astute and rapid diagnosis. The CDC confirmed the findings and sent an investigative team to seek the source of the infection. Suspicion centered on an Indian ship in harbor and the proximity of the Mexican border, where the disease was known to exist, but it was never satisfactorily explained.[12]

Isolation of cholera bacteria in the fall of 1976 and the spring of 1977 in Chesapeake Bay, Jones Falls, Baltimore and the Baltimore harbor marked the first time cholera had been detected in United States waters where there was not an outbreak of the disease. Concentrations were low and microbiologist Rita R. Colwell suggested they might be important in the ecology of the Bay, as the bacteria digested chitin that made up the hard shells of many aquatic animals. "Without them, undigested matter would clog the Bay and estuaries," she said.

Cholera was also found in raw sewage in the Cajun country of south Louisiana during August 1978, infecting several people. Officials quickly identified crabs caught in a 75-mile coastal stretch from Mud Lake to Pelican Island as the source of contamination. In all, eleven people were sickened in a three-month period. By the spring of 1979, more locations of cholera-infested water were identified, threatening the Louisiana fishing industry. That April, cholera bacteria were also discovered in the coastal waters of St. Bernard Parish and in the sewers of Jefferson Parish, a suburb of New Orleans. Scientists concluded cholera bacteria had "survived in Louisiana for years but nobody knew about it."[13]

Studies conducted at the Cholera Research Laboratory in Dacca, Bangladesh, contradicted the belief that to be diagnosed with cholera a patient had to exhibit rice-water-like diarrhea. New studies indicated that only 2 percent of victims evinced such symptoms and as many as three out of four cases produced no diarrhea, highlighting the danger that they might unknowingly spread the disease through their stools.

With that in mind, the CDC focused on the outbreaks in Louisiana. The rare phage, or biological fingerprint, of cholera that was discovered during the Port Lavaca outbreak in 1973 proved identical to that found in 1978. Although not predicting an epidemic, authorities warned that cholera was likely in the United States to stay. Their prediction proved correct as isolated cases appeared in League City, Texas, and North Florida in 1980; Beaumont, Mid-County, Jefferson and Orange County, Texas, and on an oil rig on a bayou south of Port Arthur in 1981. Twenty-two cases were ultimately diagnosed, 17 from the oil rig, making it the largest common-source outbreak in the United States during the 20th century and "winning" for the Gulf Coast the dubious title of "Cholera Capital."

In 1984, several cholera cases in Houston were attributed to eating oysters, prompting the precautionary measure of burying 40,000 pounds of oysters in a landfill. The same cause was blamed on a case of cholera in Georgia in 1987. The same year, a congressional report warned the nation's waterways pose "a serious threat to seafood consumers." That threat appeared in Colorado in 1988, again in a man eating raw oysters harvested from a "contamination-free" area of the Gulf of Mexico. Between August and December, five other states reported cholera linked to that mollusk. A single case appeared in Philadelphia in 1989, and the same year, an Oregon dairy farmer's accusation that his land had been polluted by disease-carrying water containing salmonella and cholera sued under the Resource and Recovery Act, the case reaching the U.S. Supreme Court.

The numbers and sources of contamination continued to mount. In 1990, a Syracuse, New York, woman recently returned from the tropics brought back a case of cholera, while illegally imported crabmeat from Ecuador sickened eight New Jersey residents in 1991. Complicating the problem, the same cholera bacteria that killed thousands in South America was found in oyster beds in Alabama, closing the reefs indefinitely and dealing a financially crippling $4 million blow to the oyster industry. The bacteria were traced to ballast tanks of three ships in Mobile Bay. No fatalities were reported, but microbiologist Jim Bell, working on the North Saskatchewan River, Canada, identified new drug-resistant organisms, meaning high doses of antibiotics would not kill them. More seriously, these organisms possessed the ability to transfer their resistance to other organisms in the water.[14]

Wash Basins, Breast Milk and Fluoride

In 1972, a widely publicized case of international contamination brought attention to the very real danger of contracting cholera from food. After an outbreak occurred in Australia, suspicion centered on meals served to economy-class passengers aboard a Qantas jumbo jet that had taken in supplies at Bahrain. The jet arrived at Sydney November 4; less than a week later, 56 people were being treated for symptoms of the disease. Although Qantas officials had been notified on October 28 that cholera was present at Bahrain, they were satisfied the company's "stringent food preparation precautions would prevent any contamination." WHO authorities later confirmed the Australian outbreak and small outbreaks of cholera in New Zealand and Britain were the result of the Bahrain-prepared food.

Another problem surfaced in 1978, when Dr. Charles Rondle at the London School of Hygiene and Tropical Medicine approached the question of why cholera appeared in peculiar places such as the Dordogne area in southwest France and the Essone district in the north. His team discovered that these and other spots where cholera had inexplicably appeared were all beneath the paths of regular flights from India to the West. Although airlines typically held toilet refuse in tanks for disposal at airports, wastewater from sinks was routinely discharged into the air. Bacteria was capable of withstanding subzero air and Rondle found enough bacteria was released when a cholera victim washed his hands to contaminate the ground. He suggested airlines lace washbasin waste with disinfectant and provide medical soap for passengers. The CDC considered Rondle's findings hypothetical or coincidental but by 1990, reports still surfaced linking this practice with cholera outbreaks, reports supported by a WHO report

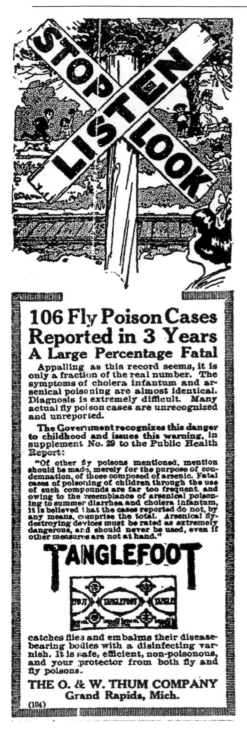

indicating a low risk to swimmers from sewage dumped at sea.[15]

As the world approached the 21st century, both new and old questions were raised about what was and was not healthy. A study in 1978 centered on an unusual cholera epidemic in the Middle East. This study became the first to link bottle-feeding with the disease. The Bahrain case study, conducted by Drs. Ann Kimble and Robert A. Gunn, working as consultants to WHO, discovered that between August and October, nearly 750 people were stricken by cholera, of whom 81 were under the age of one year. Attention was drawn to the high incidence of disease among infants fed commercial formula mixed with water as opposed to breast-fed babies. Researchers concluded that bottle-fed infants were deprived of some immunity to cholera from their mother's milk, particularly in the first days of nursing and that they were more exposed to cholera bacteria from the water.

Two other topics still debated today are the potential risks from chlorinated and fluorinated water. The use of chlorine in city water systems became widespread early in the 1900s and by 1980, it was used in 80 percent of America's drinking water. It served to kill a variety of organisms, including cholera and typhoid germs. (In 1983, officials in Calcutta attributed a drastic drop in cholera deaths to the use of filtered and chlorinated water.) However, a 1980 report on "Drinking Water and Cancer," released by the President's Council on Environmental Quality, found "an association between rectal, colon and bladder cancer" and chlorinated water. The study did not take into account other factors, such as smoking and diet, and the Environmental Protection Agency (EPA) maintained the position that the benefits of chlorine outweighed the risks. However, cities were required to reduce the levels of chlorination by-products (trihalomethanes) to 100 parts per billion.

The same year, discussion of fluoride came into public consciousness as some studies indicated "crude or raw death rates in fluoridated cities was [sic] 15 percent higher each year than in non-fluoridated cities,"

Fear of contagion spread by flies called for drastic measures and arsenic was one method used to eliminate the house pest. However, the chemical was extremely poisonous and if placed within easy access it was possible children would ingest it and suffer dangerous, or worse—fatal, consequences. As noted in this ad, symptoms of arsenic poisoning were often mistaken for cholera infantum and inaccurately reported to health authorities, causing undue alarm and inaccurate statistics (*Kirklin [IN] Journal*, April 12, 1917).

due to generalized weakening of the body. David W. Dye, of the Schick Laboratories, argued that sodium fluoride was used in medical labs to study the cholera toxin. "Fluoride activates the enzyme adenyl cyclase to high levels, causing, in the same manner as cholera toxin, the profuse fluid and electrolyte loss from the blood stream into the intestine and hence the massive diarrhea."

Conversely, in 1984, Dr. Charles Daniel, a University of California-Santa Cruz biologist, reported that the toxin produced by cholera could renew growth in aging mouse cells. Toxin cells did not quit reproducing simply because they wore out as they aged, and the finding was considered a step closer to reversing the aging process. Cholera toxin was also used to encourage cells to multiply when researchers were growing skin in a test tube for burn victims. Daniel noted this was the first time scientists had been able to get healthy growth: "There are other things that stimulate cell growth, but only in a cancerous or precancerous state."[16]

33

Research Conducted During
the Seventh Pandemic

For the sake of our fellow citizens, we wish that the lessons of experience were as impressive and lasting as they are bitter. In that case, we might reasonably entertain the hope that the ravages which the cholera is making among us would in the end be productive of good both to those who now escape from the scourge and to future generations.[1]

In 1961, during a cholera epidemic in Manila, Robert A. Phillips, of the U.S. Navy (see also chapter 31), and Craig Wallace addressed the problem of oral rehydration, realizing that most patients would never have access to IV therapy. They discovered that victims were able to orally absorb potassium and bicarbonate but not sodium or chloride. They replaced some sodium with glucose, creating an isotonic solution with lower electrolyte levels, and discovered sodium and water absorption increased in direct proportion to the concentration of glucose, stopping diarrhea as long as the solution was administered. In 1962, together with Dr. Graham Bull of the British Postgraduate Medical School, the researchers tried an "oral electrolyte cocktail" on 30 patients; 25 recovered but five died of pulmonary edema. It was subsequently learned the cocktail had been made hypertonic because the glucose had been given in addition to the normal saline instead of replacing it. The glucose apparently pumped the excess sodium load into the patients, causing fluid overload. This setback halted progress toward oral therapy.

In the fall of 1961, Drs. Robert L. Martin and Burton Vaughan joined NAMRU-2 in the Philippines. After giving small amounts of several radioactive tracers to 12 patients, they collected 400 samples. In a two-year period, about 2,200 individual radioactive assays were completed: 1,200 for tritium radioactivity; 200 for chlorine and several hundred for carbon. Investigators found a considerable similarity between the gastrointestinal injury of cholera and acute gastrointestinal injury by radiation.

In 1963, warring against cholera in Taipei, Phillips remarked of his "cocktail," "We developed a cure which we couldn't use because of its side effects such as vomiting and fever." However, he added, "Now, with the use of antibiotics as a first step, we have come across a cure without those side effects." The method was to administer streptomycin before the cocktail, leading him to conclude, "If a cholera patient is living and not in unreversible shock when he arrives in hospital, he has no need to die of that disease."

In 1963, Richard Finkelstein isolated the cholera exotoxin that he called cholerogen. The same year, at the Thailand-SEATO Medical Research Laboratory, he and C. Benyajati gave an infusion of cholerogen to two healthy human volunteers. A dose four times that producing diarrhea in rabbits produced 18 liters of diarrhea. Finkelstein later began the work of purifying the cholera toxin, finishing it at the Southwestern Medical School, Dallas, with Joseph LoSpalluto. They demonstrated there were two components (A and B); both were susceptible to immune precipitation but only one of them was toxic. The cholera AB toxin became a standard model for studies of bacterial exotoxins.[2]

In 1965, Norbert Hirschorn was given access to Phillips' trial in Manila. He concluded a truly isotonic solution would avoid the hypernatremia seen in 1962. Hirschorn's work demonstrated that glucose and galactose stimulated sodium and water absorption, but fructose and maltose did not, demonstrating the existence of glucose- and galactose-mediated sodium pumps that could be used to counteract the cholera-induced sodium and water losses. Subsequent research developed oral rehydration packets (see below), allowing cholera to be treated locally and inexpensively. In 1967, Dr. Phillips, who received his medical degree from Washington University, St. Louis, was awarded the Albert Lasker Research Award, one of the most prestigious medical prizes in the U.S.[3]

It should not be surprising that in 1964, newspapers ran a story with phrases such as "Effectiveness of Vaccination Questioned" and "still controversial cholera vaccine," reinvigorating the old argument that cholera rarely struck the affluent and when it did, large numbers of this group tended to seek vaccination. Because few wealthy individuals would actually contract the disease, success rates were skewed, indicating high (although meaningless) success rates. Opponents charged that no "adequately controlled field studies have ever shown a clear benefit from either [cholera or typhoid fever vaccines]."

Under international agreement, the law required cholera shots for those arriving from infested areas. In order to justify this requirement, a laboratory established by SEATO at Dacca was chosen to initiate a pilot study in preparation for a large-scale field study. Dr. Abram S. Benenson, director of the laboratory, announced 13,900 individuals would be involved, half receiving the cholera vaccine while the remainder received a vaccine not known to be effective against the disease. Benenson also hoped a new oral vaccine developed at Jefferson Medical College (already being tried on medical student volunteers) and another developed at Dacca made of "living but toned-down bacteria" would afford long-lasting immunity.[4]

As Dr. Robert Phillips described it, the normal preventative inoculation for cholera was "just a little more effective than distilled water." With that in mind, the final thirty years of the century were consumed by research into the development of more effective vaccines and treatments. One approach was based on new evidence that the "vibrio comma" bacteria did not cause cholera, but rather the disease was brought on by poisonous toxins produced by the bacteria while growing in the human intestine. A 1969 report made to the joint United States-Japan Cooperative Medical Sciences Program by Dr. Charles C.J. Carpenter detailed the combined efforts of the Johns Hopkins Medical School in Baltimore, Downstate Medical Center, New York City, the University of Chicago, the University of Texas at Dallas and the National Institutes of Health to produce a new preventative. After achieving 90 percent effectiveness in dog trials, Carpenter indicated human testing was being done on convicts at prisons in Jessup, Maryland, and Galveston, Texas.

Undesirable results consisting of sore arms from injections using only $\frac{1}{25}$ the dose needed for practical use aborted the testing. In 1971, Dr. John R. Seal, director of the U.S. Health Service's National Institute of Allergy and Infectious Diseases and a key official in the United States-Japan cooperative, described a new, more stable anti-cholera toxoid developed as an outgrowth of the first trial. Composed of "toned-down versions of such toxin" to stimulate the production of an anti-toxin to fight and kill the bacteria, it was proposed to begin human testing of the method in some cholera-infested area of the globe.

Three years later, emphasis turned to the development of an oral vaccine. Dr. W. Allan Walker, principal investigator at Massachusetts General Hospital, reported in the journal

Proceedings of the National Academy of Sciences (*PNAS*) that antibodies in the intestine could prevent the toxin release by cholera bacteria from attaching itself to the intestinal cell wall. Stopping the attachment of this toxin would prevent the diarrhea and dehydration that led to death from cholera.[5]

After three years of joint research (see chapter 31), Drs. Willard F. Verwey and Yoshikazu Watanabe announced a new vaccine that offered hope of greater protection against cholera and the El Tor strain of paracholera, endemic in the Far East. Extracted from El Tor vibrio cultures, the vaccine went through the first phase of human testing without creating significant toxic reactions and all subjects produced substantial amounts of anti-cholera immune substances in their blood. After being directed against one (Agawa) of the two types of cholera organisms, an NIH grant was awarded to support research from the second type (Inaba) of cholera organism. The new agent was of "purified material, free of many of the toxic substances which are in the usual cholera vaccine, and laboratory experiments have proved it to be much stronger in its immunizing effect and less toxic." An additional grant to both coinvestigators was awarded from the National Institute of Allergy and Infectious Diseases of the U.S. Public Health Service in 1966 to continue their cholera immunization studies.[6]

Significantly, the work of Dr. Dilip Mahalanabis proved another point that has global implications in the fight against cholera. Working in a refugee camp in Bangaon, India, in 1971, he was overwhelmed by the number of cholera deaths. Having inadequate IV supplies, he made the decision to allow nonspecialists to administer oral rehydration salts (ORS). Coining the term "oral saline," he distributed pamphlets describing how the solution would work as well as IV therapy, a treatment already accepted by the local population. Quickly instructing previously untrained people, including family members and volunteers (an idea scoffed at by the medical fraternity), to administer ORS, within two to three weeks it became apparent that the system worked. The successful plan led to international acceptance.[7]

The value of ORS was proven during the Bangladesh Liberation war in 1971. When cholera broke out in Bangladesh refugee camps in May, several thousand persons were treated with a "simple, cheap home remedy" of drinking large amounts of water with a mixture of salt, baking soda and glucose. The death rate was about 10 percent, compared to 50 percent if the disease went untreated and 25 percent of those treated in hospitals. Among the last 600 treated, only six (1 percent) died. In 1979, WHO globally introduced ORS. It rapidly became the cornerstone of programs for the control of diarrheal diseases. Its use has reduced the annual number of deaths attributed to dehydration among children less than 5 years old from 4.6 million in 1980 to 1.5 million in 2000. ORS does not influence the infection process, however, and for those suffering from severe cases, IV therapy is still required.

In 1987, experts at the National Academy of Sciences found that the substitution of rice mixtures or rice and chicken soup was even more effective than the salt-and-sugar formulas for the treatment of diarrhea. On a slightly different note, habitual marijuana smokers were found to be more prone to cholera and food poisoning due to lower stomach acidity.[8]

After the 44th World Health Assembly passed resolution WHA44.6, the WHO Global Task Force on Cholera Control was begun in 1992. Its aim was to reduce mortality and morbidity and to address social and economic consequences of the disease. Priority activities include the following:

1. Encouraging improved surveillance to identify high risk areas;
2. Providing support for preparedness and response;
3. Gaining evidence on the use of Oral Cholera Vaccines;

4. Linking health and environment management to improve access to safe water and diminish waterborne diseases.[9]

In order to confirm the presence of cholera, stools from victims are sent to the laboratory to identify the presence of *V. cholerae*. A new, rapid diagnostic test (RDT) increases the process by allowing analysis at the bedside. This permits early warning and detection of first cases. A case is confirmed when *Vibrio cholerae* O1 or O139 is isolated from any patient with diarrhea.

WHO guidelines call for suspecting a case of cholera when:

1. In an area where the disease is not known to be present, a patient aged 5 years or older suddenly develops severe dehydration or dies from acute watery diarrhea;
2. In an area where there is a cholera epidemic, a patient aged 5 years or older develops acute watery diarrhea with or without vomiting.

Once *Vibrio cholerae* has been confirmed, the WHO definition of cholera is sufficient to diagnose cases. Further lab testing is required only for antimicrobial testing and to confirm the end of an outbreak.[10]

Research in 1995 and 1996 studied the emergence of *V. cholerae* O139 as the new serogroup associated with cholera, deducing its evolution as a result of horizontal gene transfer between O1 and non-O1 strains. The existence of cholera entertoxin (CT), first suggested by Koch in 1884 and demonstrated by De and Dutta, is important from the perspective of a serogroup acquiring the potential to cause epidemics.[11]

One of the most significant achievements in the fight against cholera came in 2000, when scientists announced they had unlocked the genetic blueprint of the cholera genome. The research team from the Institute for Genomic Research in Rockville, Maryland, discovered Vibrio cholerae has two round chromosomes with 3,885 genes. They are formed from approximately 4 million chemical building blocks known as "base pairs," about 3 million in the larger chromosome and 1 million in the smaller. The project cost $793,712, or about 20 cents per base pair. The researchers identified the genes by chemically breaking up strands of the cholera DNA. They analyzed the fragments separately and later discovered how to reassemble them in order.[12]

Cholera Control

Unlike other *Vibrio* species, *V. cholerae* was believed to be an organism of the human gut, incapable of surviving more than a few days outside that environment, as it was known to disappear from water after an epidemic subsided. Contaminated water supplies were implicated in the first six pandemics and properly treated water in the present day has eliminated that as a risk factor. However, in China, the Russian Federation, Latin America and other developing countries where treatment is inadequate, cholera is likely to appear; an epidemic in Latin America was exacerbated by failure to chlorinate the drinking supply, in part due to concerns over the carcinogenic effect of chlorination by-products.

Techniques such as immunofluorescence, microscopy, DNA hybridization, PCR and improved culture methods suggest that *V. cholerae* can survive longer in the environment than other fecal organisms or that it is an environmental organism in its own right. Research has revealed *V. cholerae* is widely distributed in temperate and tropical aquatic environments and has been found with a wide variety of aquatic life, including freshwater filamentous green algae,

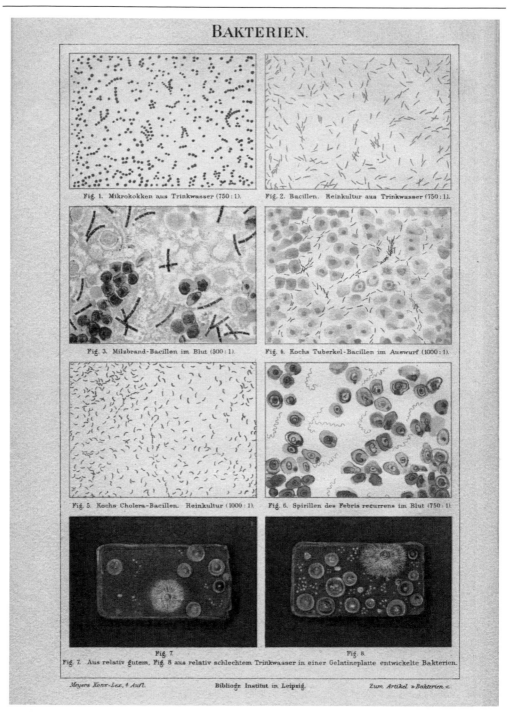

Figure 1: Mikrokokken aus Trinkwasser (750:1); Figure 2: Bacillen, Reinkultur aus Trinkwasser (750:1); Figure 3: Milzbrand-Bacillen im Blut (500:1); Figure 4: Kochs Tuberkel-Bacillen im Auswurf (1000:1); Figure 5: Kochs Cholera-Bacillen, Reinkultr (1000:1); Figure 6: Spirillen des Febris recurrens im Blut (750:1); Figure 7: Aus relativ gutem; Figure 8: Aus relativ schlechtem Trinkwasser in ether Gelatineplatte entwickelte Bakterien (1894 Bacteria Anthrax, Cholera and more chromolithography print in the authors' collection).

oysters, blue crabs and water hyacinths. It is also highly adaptable, undergoing major physical and metabolic changes while maintaining its virulence. It is also capable of assuming a dormant state in response to nutritional deprivation, elevated salinity or reduced temperatures, while surviving for extended periods in warm water.

Although it has been isolated from surface waters, no study has demonstrated water as a reservoir of toxic *V. cholerae* in the absence of a person with cholera using that water: "The overall body of evidence suggests that faecal-oral transmission is of primary importance, and long experience has shown basic water-supply and sanitation measures to be effective in controlling secondary spread of the disease.... It is also likely that environmental survival during inter-epidemic periods accounts for sudden multi-point outbreaks of cholera as occur, for example, in the Ganges delta area."

Many of the water treatments of the mid– to late 1800s have been confirmed by modern science, including slow sand filtration, chemical disinfectants, ultraviolet light and iodine. Boiling is also effective, as are chlorine-releasing agents. Individuals with reduced gastric acidity and blood group O are more susceptible to cholera infection.[13] On the subject of water filtration, it is interesting to note that a 2002 study of rural villages in Bangladesh, led by Professor Rita R. Colwell of the University of Maryland, College Park, determined that forcing water through the cloth of old saris could reduce cholera cases by about half and might also reduce other gastrointestinal illnesses. The sari cloth proved a cheaper and more effective filter than modern nylon mesh by trapping copepod, a type of zoological plankton commonly found in standing water on which cholera bacteria attached.[14]

The Trail to Cholera Immunity

Levine and Pierce wrote in chapter 14 of the text "Immunity and Vaccine Development" (*Cholera*, 1992) that "cholera is now recognized as one of the most striking examples wherein an initial clinical infection gives rise to a high level of enduring protection." Using this as the yardstick of what future vaccines must achieve, they cited research indicating that protective mechanisms within the body interfere with bacterial survival or growth within the small intestine; or, if the cholera toxin is moved to the large intestine by peristalsis, the vibrios may be unable to survive the unfavorable environment created by indigenous bowel microflora. They concluded that immunity was achieved through "the existence of both antibacterial and antitoxic immunity," suggesting a synergistic interplay between the mechanisms.[15]

Beginning in the early 1960s, field trials of killed whole-cell vaccines achieved moderate protection levels of a few months but were age-related (being lowest in young children), indicating the vaccine worked best "in immunologically primed populations by boosting underlying immunity." Toxoid and oral vaccines were also tested, some achieving 51 percent efficiency for at least 36 months. However, one drawback to oral vaccines of purified B subunit and killed vibrios, or killed vibrios alone, is that multiple doses are required "to prime the intestinal immune system," a relatively high cost of manufacture of the combined vaccine and the short-lived protection in young children.[16]

In 1995, a study done by the Army Medical Research Institute of Infectious Diseases (USAMRIID) prepared for Stage I of a study on a substance called LT (R192G), which they hoped would become the first oral adjuvant ever used in vaccines. In this case, the adjuvant is derived from a form of e. coli and is added to killed viruses that, it was hoped, would provide immunity to different forms of diarrhea.[17] By July 1996, the oral vaccine was being tested in Peru and had already passed Phase I and Phase II trials for safety and efficacy.[18]

After two years of community education, Phase III of a clinical trial of a bivalent, oral cholera vaccine was conducted in Kolkata in eastern India during September 2006. Initial reports indicated 20 episodes of cholera in the 52,212 people receiving vaccine and 68 episodes in 55,562 who received a placebo. Further data revealed 68 percent protection of all age groups two years after vaccination. Children aged five to 15 years had 88 percent protection.

Although by 2006, oral cholera vaccines had been available for more than two decades, they had never been extensively adopted because of high cost, limited availability and the need for two doses.[19] The development of live oral vaccines is presently taking three approaches: the use of recombinant DNA to delete from pathogenic *V. cholerae* 01 the genes encoding critical virulence properties; auxotrophic strains of *V. cholerae* being prepared to cripple the ability to proliferate in the human intestine; and the cloning of genes which encode putative protective antigens of *V. cholerae*.[20]

Japanese researchers took a different approach in 2007. They developed a type of rice that could carry a vaccine for cholera that they hoped would ease delivery of vaccines in developing countries that lacked refrigeration to store regular vaccines. Led by Hiroshi Kiyono, division of mucosal immunology at the University of Tokyo, a major advantage of this technique was that it caused immune reactions both systemwide in the body and in the mucosal tissues, such as the mouth, nose and genital tract.[21]

In March 2010, WHO updated its position paper (first published in 1991) on cholera vaccines, suggesting that they should be used in conjunction with other prevention and control strategies in areas where the disease is endemic. Use of vaccines should also be considered in areas at risk for outbreaks, as they have demonstrated protection of greater than 50 percent lasting two years.[22] An internationally licensed oral vaccine (OCV) is currently available for travelers. It is administered in two doses, 10–15 days apart. On a wider scale, WHO warns, however, that OCV should be used only "as an additional public health tool" and should not replace sanitary measures. Nor is OCV recommended if an epidemic has already begun due to its two-dose regimen and the time required to reach protective efficacy, its high cost and the heavy logistics associated with its use. Parenteral cholera vaccine has never been recommended by WHO due to low protection and the high occurrence of severe reactions.[23]

34

The Resurgence of King Cholera

Scientists err on cholera prediction: In 1922, scientists predicted the death of a disease. Cholera, they declared, was no longer to be feared as one of the most devastating killers in history. Scientists could not have been more wrong. Now, almost half a century later, a cholera pandemic is sweeping from Korea to the Celebes, across India to Egypt, and even into a corner of Europe where the Soviet Union has quarantined several towns on the Black and Caspian Seas.[1]

While it is tempting to think of cholera as a historical disease rather than one with dire contemporary implications, the tragic fact is that the incidence of cholera has grown rather than diminished. The world is currently embroiled in the Seventh Cholera Pandemic that began in 1961, with the El Tor biotype being the causative agent. (The classical biotype has been displaced worldwide except in Bangladesh, where it caused an epidemic in 1982 lasting several years; as of 1991, it is currently believed to be extinct.) The El Tor cholera began in South Asia, reaching Africa a decade later and appearing in the Americas by 1991. The disease remains endemic in many countries.

In 1994, cholera cases were reported from 94 countries.[2] Between 2000 and 2008 a total of 838,315 cholera cases globally were reported to WHO, a 24 percent increase compared with 676,651 cases reported between 2000 and 20004.[3] By the year 2011, there were 589,854 cases reported from 58 countries, with 7,816 deaths, although these totals are probably low due to under reporting. The true burden of the disease is estimated to be 3–5 million cases and 100,000–120,000 deaths *annually*.[4]

Particularly disturbing was the epidemic emergence of El Tor in Latin America in January 1991 after a 100-year absence from the region, and the unprecedented appearance in late 1992 in southern India of an epidemic strain of *V. cholerae* non-O1 (*V. cholerae* O139 Bengal).

The Alteration and Spread of Cholera

A cholera epidemic broke out in Madras, southern India, in October 1992. The causative organism was *V. cholerae* non-O1 (O139 serogroup). Within months, O139 strains were seen in Calcutta and Bangladesh. The O139 serogroup has spread rapidly into several Southeast Asian countries, but by 1994, a dramatic decline in O139 was observed, being replaced by strains of the O1 serogroup but differing from the O1 circulating before the emergence of O139. In August 1996, a resurgence of O139 with an altered antibogram was identified in Calcutta and other parts of India.

A total of 50,921 cases and 1,145 deaths were reported in 18 countries in Asia in 1995, with the case-fatality rate increasing from 1.3 percent in 1994 to 2.2 percent in 1995. The ability of *V. cholerae* to react to change offers significant difficulties to medical personnel because new serogroups have the advantage of attacking in the absence of preexisting immunity.

From 1970, *V. cholerae* had spread through most of Africa with a case-fatality rate between 4 percent and 12 percent. From 1991 to 1996, the number of cases remained high, ranging between 70,000 and 160,000, the worst year being 1994, when 42 percent of all cholera deaths were registered. The civil war in Rwanda displaced two million people in 1994, ultimately causing 12,000 deaths among refugees staying in makeshift camps in Goma and Zaire. Studies at Goma indicated the epidemic there was caused by a multi-drug–resistant *V. cholerae* O1 biotype El Tor. In 1996, as people returned home, 8,916 cases of diarrheal diseases were reported, the low mortality attributed to rapid and effective response by health officials. As of December 1996, twenty-six countries had reported cholera, with Nigeria, Senegal and Somalia having more than 1,000 cases each with very high case-fatality rates.

In 1991, cholera appeared in Latin America, the last remaining area of underdeveloped nations to have been untouched by the seventh pandemic. Enigmatic in origin, the epidemic began in three areas of Peru along the Pacific coast. Between 1991 and 1992 there were 750,000 cases with 6,500 deaths. Following trade routes, a year after its first appearance cholera had spread into the interior of Peru, Ecuador, Colombia, Brazil, Chile and central Mexico. Bolivia alone registered 21,567 cases and 3,210 deaths in 1992.[5]

Exposing inadequate sanitation and health care systems in Latin America, the "disease of poverty" threatened to destroy fragile economies as it reached into Central America and Mexico. Tourists shunned areas where cholera was suspected or confirmed and avoided eating seafood. To allay fears, at Ciudad Juarez, Mexico, in 1992, the threatened restaurant industry that garnered $250 million in sales annually installed water purifiers and required employees to take cholera-prevention classes. Similar precautions were taken by the El Paso Restaurant Association to preserve their estimated $370 million yearly revenue.[6]

As the situation worsened in Latin America, reports across the southern areas of the former Soviet Union indicated the appearance and spread of cholera in 1993. A year later, case numbers reached 609, with the disease also reported in the republics of Kalmykia and Chechnya and in the Crimea's capital of Simferopol. The old familiar story of civil war added to the misery of Somalis in 1994, as 3,600 were struck by cholera.[7]

By 1995, the CDC announced that cholera had its widest distribution in its history. Tragically, it had plenty of company. At least 30 previously unknown diseases were identified between 1973 and 1996, including the Ebola virus, a contagious hemorrhagic fever that appeared in 1977 and in 1995 destroyed thousands in Zaire. As a reminder that the "old" diseases were still potent forces with which to contend, sleeping sickness, meningitis, HIV and malaria were ever-present.[8]

January 1–November 15, 1995 Cholera Cases

Mexico	13,996	Ecuador	1,761	Argentina	157
Nicaragua	6,489	Guatemala	1,327	Costa Rica	23
Brazil	3,660	Colombia	1,163	Belize	19
El Salvador	2,780	Honduras	986		
Peru	2,558	Bolivia	718		

Cholera cases were up nearly 10,000 in Mexico from 1994. Between 1991 and mid–November 1995, cholera destroyed almost 10,000 lives. The most deaths occurred in Brazil, where 4,002 perished over that short span.[9]

Natural and unnatural disasters also added to the prevalence of cholera. In 1996, after a cyclone struck India, 5 million people were affected. The problems of lack of food, little sanitation and lack of medical supplies were compounded by the appearance of cholera, causing international concern, while a humanitarian crisis developed in Zaire as cholera set in among camps of refugees huddled together as the result of the ongoing war. On October 8–9, 1977, hurricane Pauline pummeled hundreds of miles of the Mexican coast, creating an instant cholera warning. More of the same grim news was reported along East Africa in December as heavy rains fueled cholera attacks. WHO reported 61,534 cases, with 2,687 deaths since January, but most came in the last several months of the year. For 1997, WHO reported a case fatality rate of 20 percent (up from a low of 3 percent) in Ethiopia, Kenya, Somalia, Sudan, United Republic of Tanzania and Uganda. Hurricane Mitch caused the worst disaster in memory in Nicaragua during November 1998. Touring the ravaged country, former President Jimmy Carter and his wife, Rosalynn, feared cholera and dengue would follow and asked the World Bank and International Monetary Fund to forgive the country's foreign debt.[10]

Cholera Surges into the 2000s

The first thirteen years of the new century brought no relief from staggeringly depressing headlines: "Cholera claims 390 in two weeks" (2000); "More than 100,000 hit by cholera" (2001); "South African judge acquits 'Dr. Death' of targeting blacks" (2002); "Cholera among many health concerns in Iraq" (2003); "Great Lakes system is under assault" (2004); "Cholera epidemic infecting thousands" (2005); "Aid worker says epidemic has killed 1,300" (2006); "Suspected cholera outbreak kills 680" (2007); "Zimbabwe faces water and cholera crisis, epidemic" (2008); "UN reports jump in cholera cases" (2009); "The tragedy after the tragedy: Cholera ravages an already ravaged Haiti" (2010); "Haiti cholera strain from South Asia" (2011); "UN concerned with increase in cholera cases" (2012). A brief time line of cholera in the 21st century follows:

2000: In March, 500 new cases of cholera appeared in Madagascar; in April, cholera was reported out of control in southwestern Somalia, where 390 people died over a two-week period; in October, a Vietnam flood was worsened by cholera and crocodiles.

2001: In January, cholera struck more than 15,000 people along the coast of South Africa; by June, the number reached 100,000, "with no end in sight."

2002: In July, the trial of Wouter Basson, the so-called Dr. Death, was held at Johannesburg; the prosecution listed the charge that he stockpiled cholera, HIV and anthrax for use against "enemies."

2003: In March, extensive cholera-causing bacteria were identified at five South Florida beaches; in June, nearly two months after the United States' war to topple Saddam Hussein's government, widespread health problems, including cholera, plagued Iraq; by August, WHO had registered 2,460 cases of cholera in Liberia but believed the number to be a "serious underestimate."

2004: In June, a report confirmed that a serious onslaught of foreign fish, mussels and other creatures had invaded the Great Lakes, prompting experts to issue warnings about the risks from botulism and cholera.

2005: Further studies on the Great Lakes indicated that of 42 ships inspected two-thirds carried deadly organisms in their ballast water, including cholera bacteria; cholera infected

31,259 people in nine west African countries (Guinea-Bissau, Liberia, Mauritania, Guinea, Senegal, Burkina Faso, Mali, Ivory Coast and Niger) between June and September, with 488 deaths in what the United Nations called an "unusually high incidence" of the disease.

2006: By May, a three-month cholera epidemic claimed 1,300 lives in Angola and infected 35,000 more.

2007: By February, 680 people died of cholera in Ethiopia, infecting 60,000 more; in September, 16,000 were reported with symptoms of cholera in Iraq.

2008: In November, a sprawling refugee camp in Goma, the provincial capital of the Congo, was struck by a cholera outbreak, while dozens died of the disease in the eastern portion of the country. Between August and December 1, the government of Zimbabwe reported 473 cholera deaths and 11,700 infected people, while the UN indicated a 4 percent death toll.

2009: By January, the death toll from cholera in Zimbabwe reached 2,225, with 42,675 infected and 1,550 new cases being reported every day.

2010: In two months, the worst cholera epidemic in 19 years killed 800 Nigerians and quickly spread to Cameroon, Chad and Niger. After the massive earthquake in Haiti, where cholera had not been present in decades, the disease spread rapidly through Port-au-Prince, where 1.3 million earthquake survivors had gathered. By October, 250 deaths were reported, with 3,000 sickened. A month later, the death toll from cholera reached 1,000, with over 10,000 hospitalized with acute diarrhea. In December, as mortality figures leaped to 2,000, DNA analysis indicated the epidemic could be traced to South Asia, introduced by humans rather than having arrived on ocean currents or arising within Haiti. The terror created by cholera led to charges that at least 45 people had been killed across Haiti due to accusations they used black magic or voodoo to spread the disease.

2011: The cholera death toll in Haiti reached 5,000 in May, with 250,000 sickened. The UN confirmed "the evidence overwhelmingly supports the conclusion that the source of Haiti cholera outbreak was due to contamination of the Meye Tributary of the Artibonite River with a pathogenic strain of current South Asian type Vibrio cholerae as a result of human activity." In August, the UN reported a high risk for cholera in famine-hit Somalia as 4,272 cases of acute watery diarrhea were registered.

2012: After a steady decline in cholera cases since June 2011, the UN reported a sudden spike in cases in April 2012 at Port-au-Prince due to governmental instability.[11]

Reasons for Failure to Control Cholera

1. Inadequate surveillance of outbreaks;
2. Reliance on ineffective quarantines and control measures;
3. Failure to report early outbreaks, resulting in delays in treatment and containment;
4. Inadequate access to treatment;
5. Inappropriate treatment;
6. Drought and an overall failure to improve hygiene;
7. Reliance on traditional rituals;
8. Shortage of supplies;
9. No simple long-term vaccination.

Failing to contain the spread of cholera through sanctions, WHO adopted the "Diarrheal Disease Control" plan. This focused on treating outbreaks where they were found on the premise that early detection and treatment would lessen the chances of its being transported beyond the area of contagion. Objectives included the following:

1. Oral rehydration therapy;
2. Personal and domestic hygiene;
3. Development of waste management facilities;
4. Frequent hand washing;
5. Food safety.

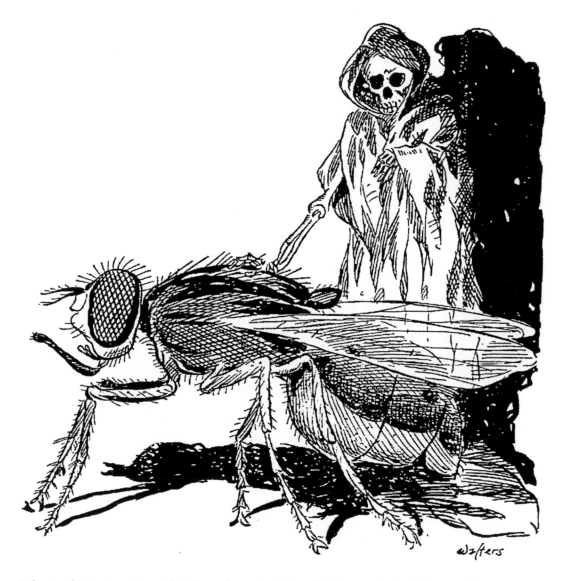

"The Death Carrying House Fly." Throughout the 19th and 20th centuries the "filthy pest" known as the house fly was often charged with spreading cholera, typhoid, tuberculosis, infectious blood poison and even leprosy. Numerous warnings were issued urging people to clean their premises and "swat the fly." Recent data suggests the fly had little to do with the spread of cholera, but the fly's massive presence certainly indicated the need for cleanliness (*Grand Rapids* (WI) *Tribune*, March 29, 1917).

Coupled with the long history of how improved sanitation efforts controlled cholera outbreaks, disinfectants continue to play a major role in containing it. Household bleach (diluted to 1 percent chlorine) and 2 percent tincture of iodine (2 drops to 1 liter of water) are useful and inexpensive agents. Sick rooms should be cleaned with a 2 percent chlorine solution and soiled clothes properly discarded. Items such as rags, long feared as a source of contamination, may be rendered safe by a thorough drying in the sun. While flies, often a harbinger of disease, indicate poor sanitation, it is likely they play only a small role in transmission.

Food, also cited as a predisposing cause of cholera, poses a threat primarily through contamination. Vibrios survive no more than 1–2 days on dry surfaces. Limiting danger from such items as potatoes is simple, as the vibrios are killed by thorough cooking, but moist vegetables eaten raw, such as lettuce, must be individually washed or chemically treated. Seafood, identified by early researchers as a causative, is of particular concern and should be thoroughly cooked and all food utensils, especially those of wood, should be carefully cleaned and dried.

Between 1973 and 1988, there were 38 confirmed cholera cases in the United States associated with the consumption of seafood from coastal waters in the Gulf of Mexico, while shellfish accounted for the spread of cholera from Latin America to the United States five times during 1991. Complicating matters, toxigenic *V. cholerae* strains were isolated from commercial oyster beds in Mobile Bay, Alabama. Ballast, bilge and sewage water from several ships from Latin America going to the Gulf of Mexico revealed the same toxigenic strains of *V. cholerae* O1 as those found in the contaminated oyster beds in the Gulf of Mexico. This supports the theory that ships were responsible for the initial introduction of this strain into the gulf.

Addressing one of the oldest concerns, WHO authorities suggested the burial of cholera victims within a short period of time, with interments being held close by. They urged the elimination of ritual feasting by mourners and warned that bodies should be handled as little as possible.[12]

In 1948, the International Health (formerly "Sanitary") Regulations (IHR) were created, ultimately binding 194 countries, including all member states of WHO, to assist the global community in preventing and responding to acute public health risks that had the potential to cross borders. The revised IHR (June 15, 2007) defined the rights and obligations of countries and established procedures WHO must follow in its work to uphold global public health.[13] Unfortunately, just as it had in the 1800s, this proved difficult to implement. Countries feared sanctions on commerce and those lacking the financial means had ineffective reporting systems. The first Caribbean conference on "Epidemiological Surveillance" was held in Jamaica in 1974. Noting the climate and social conditions in the Caribbean were different from other geographic areas, delegates placed emphasis on collaboration and the development of a surveillance program leading to the control and prevention of communicable diseases.[14]

Requiring cholera vaccination certificates for international travelers proved equally ineffective and in 1973, the 26th World Health Assembly abolished the requirement. Although some nations persisted in the demand, at present (2013) no country requires proof of cholera vaccination as a condition of entry. Furthermore, authorities acknowledged that quarantines and embargoes of people and merchandise were ineffective, and import restrictions based solely on the fact that cholera existed as an epidemic or was endemic to a country were declared unjustified.[15]

That stated, the historical concern that "carriers" spread cholera has proven accurate. Approximately 75 percent of individuals infected with cholera do not develop any symptoms, although bacteria are present in their feces for 7–14 days after infection. This creates the potential for them to contaminate the environment and infect others. Among those who develop symptoms, 80 percent suffer mild to moderate cases, while 20 percent develop acute watery diarrhea with severe dehydration that can lead to death if left untreated. People with low immunity from malnourishment or HIV are at greater risk of death if infected. In 1963, the fear of carriers achieved international attention when it was made public that Emperor Hirohito and Empress Nagako of Japan were vaccinated against cholera. They were scheduled to visit Yamaguchi, where a carrier had recently been discovered. This was the emperor's second cholera vaccination, the first coming more than 38 years before.[16]

On a less positive subject but one of international consequence (if not horror), after the mass suicide of 408 American cultists at the People's Temple, Jonestown, Guyana, in 1978, U.S. grave-registration teams were forced to wear protective gear during their work as a preventative against the growing threat of cholera.[17]

Advancements have ultimately been achieved by blending the old and the new, the theories of the individual with the efforts of the community. Ironically, manifestations of cholera have remained nearly identical over the centuries: the incubation period remains from 2 hours to 5 days. Modern physicians use the same basic observations to identify the earliest stages: excessive thirst, watery stools, loss of turgor and cold skin temperature. What have evolved are the explanations of how cholera kills: depletion of salts and water through diarrhea leading to hypovolemic shock and acidosis caused by loss of bicarbonate ions.

Up to 80 percent of cases can be successfully treated with oral rehydration salts. Clinical management of cholera in the modern era consists of rapid replacement of water and salts (by IV therapy in acute cases), maintenance of normal hydration until diarrhea stops, resumption of a normal diet to minimize nutritional deficiencies and the reduction of diarrhea through antibiotics, primarily tetracycline. The use of prophylactic antibiotics, however, is tempered by the concern of creating antibiotic-resistant strains. Erasing the standard wisdom of the 19th century, the use of opiates is now considered useless and possibly harmful. The use of antisecretory drugs may prove useful but none are currently used in clinical management.

Concern over diet obsessed physicians of the 18th and 19th centuries and hundreds of papers were published on the merits or detriments of certain foods. Those doctors prescribing carbohydrates were on the right path, as modern studies indicate these are well absorbed (80–85 percent) during acute attacks, while absorption of proteins and fats are reduced.

Beginning in the 1970s, clinicians advocated early feeding of cholera patients as part of the treatment. Studies subsequently confirmed that food does not interfere with recovery and can be absorbed even during episodes of the disease. Breastfeeding of infants and young children should be continued, adding additional fluids to their diet if necessary.

The work of De and Chatterje demonstrated that "the cholera toxin impairs intestinal permeability without disrupting the intestinal mucosa, altering intestinal motility, or producing an inflammatory response." This discovery led to the development of an inexpensive and effective oral rehydration treatment (ORT) of water, glucose and salts that reduced fatality from 30 percent in 1980 to 3.6 percent in 2000. According to the *Lancet* (2: 300–1, 1978), "the discovery that sodium transport and glucose transport are coupled in the small intestines, so that glucose accelerates absorption of salt and water, was potentially the most important medical advance of this century." The adequacy of fluid replacement is assessed by six simple factors:

1. Return of pulse to normal;
2. Return of normal skin turgor;
3. Return of a comfort level and the disappearance of cyanosis;
4. Return of normal fullness to neck veins;

5. Weight gain;
6. Return of urine output.[18]

Bioterrorism

The threat of germ warfare has never been far from world consciousness. As recently as 1949, Russia indicted 12 Japanese army men on charges they prepared and used bacteriological weapons against the Chinese in World War II. The indictment cited testimony from one of the defendants, Maj. Gen. Kawasima Kiosi, a Japanese army surgeon, that Emperor Hirohito issued secret orders in 1935 for the establishment of special biological units. During the war, it was alleged the Japanese intended to spread cholera, typhus, the black plague, gangrene and typhoid via contaminated lice and special guns and planes, and had actually experimented on living humans, including Soviet citizens.[19]

This debate was exacerbated in 1982, with the deathbed confession of a Japanese physician who admitted engaging "in a medical science designed to kill people." Among the charges was the launching of 9,300 military balloons carrying explosives, rats and plague-spreading fleas in ceramic pots. The physician was a member of the notorious Unit 731 that used human guinea pigs at its research center in northeastern China in the development of chemical and biological weapons. Chinese, Koreans, Mongolians, Russians and possibly some Americans were injected with typhus, cholera and other germs.[20]

On December 29, 1950, Ilya Ehrenbourg wrote an article in the official Russian Cominform publication stating the Americans had "atom bombs, plague fleas and the bacteria of hundreds of other diseases" to use in their defense programs. In March 1951, the same organ printed a cable from China, reporting "yet another monstrous crime by the American invaders of Korea." Noting that the U.S. had been a signatory of the Geneva Protocol of June 17, 1925, which prohibited the use of poison gas and bacteriological weapons," it charged "the butcher hordes [Americans] have cynically and shamefully violated this agreement" by cooperating with Japanese militarists who, in the war, "sprayed from planes the bacteria of cholera, typhus, anthrax and other epidemic diseases."

Linking charges from 1940, when it was alleged the "Japanese invaders" spread bubonic plague to citizens in Chekiang Province, China, "Red radio" in Peiping and Pyongyang hurled fresh accusations against the Allies in February 1952, charging them with using germ warfare in Korea to introduce cholera and the plague. Ignoring Chinese warnings that it planned on organizing "anti-epidemic teams to send to Korea to fight the disease spread by the American aggressors," a UN spokesman called the germ warfare charges "false and ridiculous." Other sources suggested the charges were either a stalling tactic linked to truce negotiations or a propaganda attempt to blame the UN for deadly epidemics the Communists were unable to check. All UN soldiers in Korea and accredited correspondents routinely received preventative immunization against cholera, but none were given for plague as it was presumed immunization would be available "if ever needed." Public health officials in Washington immediately announced there was no epidemic of plague or cholera in Korea.

By April, the Soviet Union brought charges before the United Nations that General Ridgway's troops were using germ warfare in North Korea and Manchuria. Reporters around the country demanded proof be submitted, fearing "the Reds will continue to circulate the diabolical lie and ignorant people behind the Iron Curtain will believe it." Additional charges by the Russians included that of collusion between a former officer in the Japanese army, named

Shiro Ishii, and the U.S. military, who worked together to produce some of the germs used against North Korea.

Accusations of biological atrocities raised its ugly head again in 1961, when cholera raged through China's southeast Kwangtung Province. Communists reportedly held mass meetings "raising the germ warfare charges as they did in the Korean War." Evidence that the Soviets were violating international treaties surfaced in 1986, when a report prepared by the Defense Intelligence Agency cited the accidental release of dry anthrax spores at Sverdlovsk in 1979. The report also charged the Soviets with using plague, cholera and tularemia for biological weapons in addition to anthrax. Further proof that the fear of war remained in the minds of Americans, reports from the American Association for the Advancement of Science in 1982 indicated that even if the United States survived a nuclear attack, the country would be plagued with "ancient diseases such as cholera and plague."[21]

At the annual G2 Health Ministers Forum, Switzerland, January 2003, delegates discussed dangers from bioterrorism. While stating that these mainly affect combatants, it was noted "we have over the past two decades seen a willingness to use biological and chemical agents to target civilians."

As early as 1970, WHO issued a guidance manual describing how countries should construct a preparedness program and respond to such an attack. The manual was revised and updated in 2002. Primarily, response to the deliberate release of a biological or chemical agent remains the same as during an accidental outbreak. In the case of cholera, that entails the following:

1. Proper and timely case management in treatment centers;
2. Specific training including avoidance of nosocomial infections;
3. Sufficient medical supplies;
4. Improved access to water, effective sanitation and waste control;
5. Enhanced hygiene and food safety practices;
6. Improved communication and public information.

Measures that have proven ineffective, costly and counterproductive include routine treatment with antibiotics; restrictions on travel and trade; and quarantines.

Since 1992, WHO has had official relations with the International Committee on Military Medicine (ICMM), acknowledging that the military can be a key to epidemic alert and response. (Military research for the protection of soldiers has also added to the key core of knowledge on cholera. Five of the most significant contributions include the work of Robert Phillips and Craig Wallace that isolated electrolyte solutions containing glucose for oral administration; the refinement by Phillips and Raymond Watten of IV therapy using isotonic saline solutions plus bicarbonate and potassium; the refutation of the desquamation theory of cholera pathogenesis by W.R. Beisel, E.J. Gangarosa and Robert Gordon; isolation of cholera toxin by Richard Finkelstein; and the development and testing of improved vaccines by David Taylor, Jose Sanchez and colleagues.) Additionally, member states of the World Health Assembly "have agreed to treat any deliberate use [of bioterrorism] as a global public health threat, and to respond to such a threat by sharing expertise, supplies and resources in order rapidly to contain the event and mitigate its effects." Addressing an important concern when contemplating large numbers of casualties, WHO also stressed that while "epidemics have never arisen from dead bodies," populations are often suddenly displaced and relocated to camps, causing mortality rates to jump 60 times over normal situations.[22]

Within recent memory, a panel probing South Africa's human rights abuses in 1998 revealed "a world of science gone wrong." Among the revelations at the trial of Wouter Basson was that one researcher, Andre Immelman, kept freeze-dried supplies of cholera and anthrax in amounts great enough to cause major epidemics.[23]

From a different perspective, in 2008, Sikhanyiso Ndlovu, health minister of Zimbabwe, announced, "Cholera is a calculated, racist, terrorist attack on Zimbabwe by the unrepentant former colonial power [Great Britain], which has enlisted support from its American and Western allies so that they [can] invade the country." Member nations of the Global Task Force on Cholera Control (including Great Britain and the U.S.) determined the epidemic to be caused by the breakdown of water and sewage systems and health systems.[24]

Cholera will not go away, nor will the present and future course of cholera be free of unforeseen consequences. Following an earthquake on January 12, 2010, cholera broke out in Haiti. As a consequence of this complicated tragedy, more than 316,000 people died, over 8,000 from cholera. According to a study conducted the same year by scientists at Pacific Biosciences, California, the Haitian strain was almost identical to types found in South Asia, differing greatly from those in Latin America. This suggested human transmission into Haiti.

The Institute for Justice and Democracy in Haiti believes those humans were part of the peacekeeping battalion from Nepal, sent by the United Nations. The institute alleges a local contractor failed to properly sanitize the waste of a UN base, causing cholera to leak into a tributary of one of Haiti's biggest rivers. The institute has threatened to sue the UN if that body does not agree to compensate Haitian victims. For its part, the United Nation's secretary-general issued a statement expressing profound sympathy for the people of Haiti and asked the international community to work together for a better tomorrow.[25]

35

From Snow to Koch to DNA
The Next-to-Last Chapter

Over the centuries, it has been speculated that cholera originated in the air or the water or the soil. Some modern research suggests it came from the sea, first infecting shellfish and then, through their consumption, humans. Others suggest the true origin may be within the human body itself. The main reservoirs of *V. cholerae* remain aquatic sources—such as brackish water and estuaries often containing algal blooms—and human beings. More frighteningly, recent studies indicate that global warming creates a favorable environment for the bacteria. New variant strains have been discovered in several parts of Asia and Africa, suggesting the possibility of more severe cases with higher fatalities.[1]

Sanitation experts, biologists, bacteriologists, theologians and physicians have all contributed to the debate on the eternal "why?" The answer remains elusive. It is perhaps fitting, then, that we end this text with a paragraph written in 1854 that places the ultimate solution within the realm of the "Final Frontier":

> Asiatic Cholera was introduced on the Ganges in 1816, by an unknown cause, the most probable of which [was] animalcula; probably introduced into our atmosphere by some of those aetherial globes which circulates through the aetherial space, constituting comets of various magnitudes, and sometimes falling into the atmosphere of the planets, and imparting new qualities to them. These animalcula breed whenever they find elements congenial to their existence.[2]

Ultimately, we expand the vastness of space to include the inner workings of microscopic beings, as well as the extraterrestrial existence of life beyond our ken.

Glossary

(All definitions are from the 18th and 19th centuries unless otherwise specified. Definitions are taken from the Lexicon *or* The Dispensatory of the United States *unless footnoted.)*

&c.   A common abbreviation used in the 18th and 19th centuries equivalent to the modern abbreviation "etc."

Accoucheur   One who assists at a birth; obstetrician.

Acidosis   An increase in the acidity of blood, typically seen in renal disease and diabetic acidosis.

Adjuvant   Any material that, in combination with a drug, enhances its effectiveness.[1]

Agar   A dried mucilaginous product obtained from certain species of algae, especially of the genus *Gelidium*. Because it is unaffected by bacterial enzymes, it is widely used as a solidifying agent for bacterial culture media.[2]

Alum   (Alumen) a salt; either of two colorless, crystalline aluminum-containing compounds used as an emetic, an astringent, in purifying water and in tanning and dyeing.

Amarus   *(sal catharticum amarum)* A component of medical bitters.

Amenorrhoea   A partial or total obstruction of the menses in women from other causes than pregnancy and old age.

Ammonia   A colorless, gaseous compound of nitrogen and hydrogen, usually diluted with distilled water. When mixed with tincture of camphor and spirit of rosemary it was called *Linimentum Ammoniae Compositum*. It possesses caustic properties.

Angina pectoris   A sharp pain or pressure in the chest caused by inadequate blood flow and oxygen to the heart muscle.

Animalculae   A term referencing a microscopic animal.

Anodyne   Something that relieves pain; a soothing agent.

Anti-cholera   A term used liberally to denote anything from nostrums and notions to wines and liquors supposedly possessing protection from cholera.

Antigen   A toxin or an enzyme capable of stimulating an immune response; a protein marker on the surface of cells that identifies the cell as *self* or *non-self*, identifies the type of cell and stimulates the production of antibodies.[3]

Apoplexy   To strike or knock down: a sudden abolition, in some degree, of the power of sense and motion, the patient lying in a sleep-like state. Typically seen in the elderly and the corpulent and brought on by a compression of the brain from accumulation of blood in the vessels of the head.

Aquafortis   A weak and impure nitric acid.

Arsenicum   Arsenic. Given internally in liquid form to treat fevers.

301

Arterialisation   (Arteriotomy) The opening of an artery, frequently performed on the temporal artery.

Assafetida   The juice of the root of the Ferula Assafoetida plant, native of Persia. It was a moderate stimulant, powerful antispasmodic, efficient expectorant and feeble laxative. Notwithstanding its repulsive odor, it was often used as a condiment in Persia and India.

Asthenia   Extreme debility.

Atony   Weakness or a defect of muscular power.

Aurist   A specialist in the ear, or organ of hearing.

Bacteria   Used in the same sense as "microbe" primarily by English writers. Most authorities considered these terms to refer to members of the vegetable kingdom (a cell without nuclei) allied to fungi or the ferments. In 1892 four shapes had been identified: oval-shaped (micrococcus); rod-shaped (bacterium); bent-rod (vibrio); corkscrew (spirillum).[4]

Bark   Quinine.

Basilic vein   (Basilica vena) The large vein that runs in the internal part of the arm used in bloodletting.

Bee cholera honey   Honey obtained from hives believed to have been destroyed by cholera. It was said to be dangerous to life (Midwestern U.S., mid–19th century).

Bicarbonate of soda   Prepared by saturating carbonate of soda with carbolic acid gas and then evaporating it into a white powder.

Bitters   (Amarus) The principal bitters used in medicine were the pure bitters, styptic bitters and aromatic bitters. Gentian, a bitter herb, was often a primary ingredient, along with quinine (cinchona bark). Bitters were prepared by infusion or distillation and included aromatic herbs and fruit for flavor; tonics were used to settle the stomach and for seasickness. The recipe for "Drake's Plantation Bitters" (1864) included pure St. Croix rum, Callsayn bark, roots and herbs and was taken "without regard to age or time of day."

Blister   (*Vesicatorium; Epispasticum*) A topical application, *Emplastrum vesicatorium,* which, when put on the skin, raises the cuticle in the form of a vesicle, filled with a serous fluid. The principle was that when a morbid action existed, it might be removed by inducing an action of a different kind in the same or neighboring part. A similar principle existed for pain: exciting one pain often relieved another (see sinapisms).

Bloodletting   This term includes every artificial discharge of blood made with a view to cure or prevent a disease. Bloodletting was categorized as either general or topical. The former includes *arteriotomy* and *venaesection,* while the latter includes the application of leeches, cupping-glasses and scarification.

Blue cholera   Another name for the "cold" of first stage of cholera, believed to be succeeded by a typhoid fever.

Brain fever   The delirium accompanying acute typhus.

Cajeput, oil of   A pungent essential oil obtained from plants of the genus *Melaleuca,* used primarily as a topical skin application and as an expectorant.

Calabar bean   The bean contains a chemical that affects signals between muscles and nerves; it was used in the treatment of eye disorders, constipation, epilepsy, cholera and tetanus.

Calomel   A chloride of mercury used as a purgative and as a fungicide. It was commonly administered as a laxative in the 19th century. Repeated or large doses resulted in mercury poisoning, symptoms of which include nausea and vomiting, abdominal pain, renal failure, gingivitis, behavioral and cognitive deficits, seizures, paralysis, pneumonitis and death.

Cameline, oil of A pungent yellow, semidrying oil obtained from the seed of the gold of pleasure. Also known as camelina, false flax, wild flax, linseed dodder, German sesame and Siberian oilseed. The family of *Camelina sativa* includes mustard, cabbage, rapeseed, broccoli, cauliflower, kale and brussels sprouts. It is native to Northern Europe and Central Asia and is traditionally used to produce vegetable oil and oil for lamps. Camelina has exceptionally high levels of omega–3 fatty acids.

Camphor (*Camphura:* Arabian. Called by the ancients "asphaltum, or Jew's pitch) Laurus camphora: the systematic name of the camphire tree. It was employed in fevers of all kinds, particularly in nervous fevers attended with delirium and in putrid fevers when bark (quinine) and other acids were contraindicated. It was also used in spasmodic and convulsive afflictions, including epilepsy; in chronic diseases such as rheumatism, arthritis and mania; and also externally to dissipate inflammation. The *United States Dispensatory* noted that in "immoderate doses it occasions nausea, vomiting, vertigo, delirium, insensibility, coma and convulsions, which may end in death."

Camphorein A cholera remedy developed in Vienna during the 1870s composed of chlorine gas passed through turpentine, used as an inhalant.

Carbo (*vegetabilis* coal) In medicine and chemistry, the term was commonly meant to mean charcoal.

Carbo Animalis Impure animal charcoal obtained commonly from bones; used in pharmacy for decolorizing vegetable principles, such as quinia and morphia. In most pharmaceutical purposes animal charcoal was purified my muriatic acid from phosphate and carbonate of lime, except for sulphate of quinia where it was used without purification.

Carbo ligni Vegetable charcoal. Powdered charcoal was considered antiseptic and absorbent and used in dyspepsia, dysentery and as a remedy in obstinate constipation. It was also used as a tooth powder. For domestic economy and on long sea voyages, meat imbedded in animal charcoal was kept perfectly sweet for months and water intended for long voyages was equally preserved by its addition.

Carbon See above.

Carbonate of lime Chalk, limestone, marble; an antacid and absorbent well suited to remove acidity of the stomach, more especially when accompanied with diarrhea. For exhibition, it is generally joined with sugar and aromatics, in the form of a mixture.

Carbonate of magnesia Magnesia; used as a cathartic. When sold in shops, it was usually adulterated with chalk.

Carbonate of soda Mineral alkali. In commerce it was called *barilla* or soda and contained a mixture of earthy bodies and common salt. Found abundantly in nature, particularly collected after the desiccation of temporary lakes; known from time immemorial as *nitrum, natron* or *natrum.*

Carbonic acid (Formerly called "fixed air") A colorless gas of a slightly pungent odor and acidic taste; carbonic acid water is diaphoretic, diuretic and anti-emetic. It was also used to allay thirst, lessen nausea and gastric distress and promote secretion of urine and used in the administration of magnesia and saline cathartics.

Carminative Expelling gas from the alimentary canal.

Castor oil *(Ricinus)* Oil extracted from the seeds of Ricinus communis plant, commonly known as oleum, ricini, palma christi or castor-oil. It is used as a quick but gentle purgative.

Catarrh (Catarrhus) An increased secretion of mucus from the membranes of the nose, fauces and bronchia; in mild form known as a cold and in severe cases as influenza.

Ceinture A belt or sash for the waist.

Cell Signified a mass of homogeneous, jelly-like material, called protoplasm, enclosed in a thin membrane or bladder, called the "cell wall." Imbedded in the substance of the protoplasm is a small body of a different composition called the "nucleus" (1892).[5]

Charcoal Powdered charcoal is antiseptic and absorbent, employed in dyspepsia; in dysentery it had the effect of correcting the fetor of stools and was used as a remedy for constipation. Also used as a preservative of meat. Water intended for long voyages was preserved by the addition of this powder.

Chlorate of lime (Hyperoxymuriate of lime; Salt of lime) This salt is obtained by passing a current of chlorine gas through a solution of lime in hot water, forming chloride of calcium and chlorate of lime. It has a sharp, bitter taste (see "Carbonate of lime").

Chloride A compound of chlorine with different bodies, used as a disinfectant.

Chlorine (1) A very poisonous gas; an active bleaching agent and germicide, used extensively to disinfect water and treat sewage. Chlorine water was used medically as a stimulant and antiseptic or diluted as a gargle for sore throat; (2) A mild form of cholera; spelled "cholerine" in France.

Chlorine gas "An ingredient in common salt," used for the purification of the atmosphere to prevent cholera and plague (1848).

Cholera An acute infection involving the entire small intestine, marked by profuse, watery, secretary diarrhea. The causative organism is *Vibrio cholerae.* Transmission is through water and food contaminated with excreta of infected persons (2001 definition). Through much of the 1800s practitioners believed cholera was caused by miasma or the electrical condition of the atmosphere.

Cholera, American Peculiar to the United States, considered milder than Asiatic cholera; appeared in the 1870s.

Cholera, Asiatic Cholera of the type found in Asia; considered to have its origins in a deteriorated state of the atmosphere, possibly containing animalculae carried by the wind; contagious (1832). Also known as "Cholera Asphyxia" or "Pulseless Cholera" or more commonly as "malignant cholera"; the most deadly form of the disease.

Cholera, common A widely used generic term used to refer to Cholera Morbus; also, "cholera disease."

Cholera, English Used in Great Britain to designate a milder form of cholera than that called Asiatic cholera; also known as "common cholera" or "cholera morbus."

Cholera, epidemic Widespread cholera; often used as a synonym for the single word, "cholera"; some authorities used the term "epidemic cholera" to refer to a compound malady seen in conjunction with, or actually being, typhus.

Cholera, Indian Cholera of the type found in India; contagious only under conditions of filth and lack of air, food and clothing (1832).

Cholera *accidentalis* Cholera that occurs after the use of food that digests slowly and irritates; one of two species of the genus (1842).

Cholera Banks Rocky shoals 10 fathoms deep, situated 10 miles southeast of Ambrose Light, a lightship located at the entrance of New York Harbor, nine miles east of Sandy Hook.[6]

Cholera bombshells Watermelons, so called because that fruit was believed to cause the disease (U.S., mid- and late–19th century).

Cholera carrier A healthy individual carrying the comma bacillus.

Cholera infantum Cholera in infants. An 1876 discussion on the topic noted that it rarely attacked infants before teething began and still more rarely after the process of dentition had been completed, so that nearly all cases of cholera infantum occurred between the onset and end of detention. Teething was believed to weaken the body, especially the stomach and intestines, impairing digestion and assimilation.[7] By the 20th century, the term no longer meant "cholera" in the scientific sense, but a severe form of infant diarrhea caused by bacteria in milk.[8]

Cholera mitior Characterized by languor or lassitude with spasms of the digestive system, but where respiration was not interrupted. When vital organs were affected, it transformed into cholera asphyxia (1848).

Cholera morbus Early uses of the term did not necessarily indicate a specific disease but one of the "humors" present in the human body, as an excess of the "bilious humor" made a person "choleric." When Asiatic cholera was introduced to England, the word "cholera" was transformed to it. In the 19th century, the meaning varied widely to include noncontagious and occasionally contagious gastrointestinal diseases that were, or resembled, cholera. Throughout the 1800s there was little consensus as to the use of the phrase: although generally considered milder than Asiatic cholera, in the U.S. particularly, it was not uncommon to see it described as "appallingly fatal." In the U.S. it was occasionally interchangeable with "English cholera" and was also called "spasmodic cholera." In the 20th century, the term was associated with food poisoning, or GI symptoms brought on by overeating or the consumption of cucumbers and watermelons.

Cholera nostra Literally, "our own private cholera."

Cholera-phobia 1830s English term for those who believed cholera actually existed as a health threat, as opposed to those who denied the disease either existed or posed a danger to the population.

Cholera pills Originating in British India, these consisted of 1 part opium, 2 of black pepper and 3 of assafaetida, administered with calomel and quinine. Used during the mid–late 1800s.

Cholera promoter Cucumbers (U.S., 1870s).

Cholera sobriquets "Stalking Monster" (Indiana, 1870s); the "Scourge" (Midwestern U.S., 1870s); "Prevailing" (Southern U.S., 1870s); "Summer trouble" (Southern U.S., 1870s).

Cholera *spontanea* Cholera which happens in hot seasons without any manifest cause; one of two species of the genus (1842).

Cholera *vulgaris* Another term for common cholera.

Cholrine Cholera matter.

Chyle The milk-like liquor observed in the lacteal vessels of the mesentery some hours after the patient has eaten.

Clyster   Enema.

Cocculus Indicus   (Cocculus) Indian cockle. Used by Arabian physicians; its shell is emetic, but it was chiefly used as a stupefying poison for fish, making them easier to catch.

Colchicum seed   The pharmacopoeial name of the meadow-saffron. Used in small doses as a cathartic and diuretic and in the treatment of inflammatory diseases such as gout and rheumatism; the expressed juice is also used to kill vermin in the heads of children.

Cold cholera   The first stage of cholera, where the patient suffers from a rapid change in body heat and diarrhea; bleeding was typically prescribed. The cold stage was followed by the second stage—acute internal inflammation.

Coleus Aromaticus   (Indian borage or Ajwain patta) The leaves of this plant are used as seasoning but more commonly as a medicinal herb due to its strong antioxidant property and therapeutic value. Juice from the leaves was traditionally used in India for diarrhea. In 1957 a physician at Calcutta claimed success in curing cholera with it.

Colic   (Spelled "cholic" early in the 19th century) Colica; commonly used to refer to all pains in the abdomen.

Collywobbles   Cholera; used in the United States in the late 1800s and early to mid–1900s.

Colocynth, extract   A powerful cathartic made from a Mediterranean and African herbaceous vine related to the watermelon.

Colombo root   (Calumba) A root imported from Colomba, Ceylon. As an antiseptic, it was a corrector of putrid bile and restrained alimentary fermentation, strengthening digestion. It was used as a tincture or as a powder.

Continued fever   An medical expression meaning typhus.

Copper, powder of   A virulent poison; the symptoms produced are exactly those of arsenic, only the taste of copper is strongly felt. Sugar, in the form of syrup, was said to be the antidote to copper poisoning.

Coruscations   Lightning.

Crassamentum   Blood clot; coagulation.

Cupping   Topical bleeding; performed with a scarificator and a cupping glass, the air within the glass rarefied by the flame of a little lamp containing spirit of wine and a thick wick. The larger the glass, the less pain the patient feels and the more freely the blood flows. When the mouth of the glass is placed over the scarificator, the rarefied air in it becomes condensed as it cools, the glass is forced down on the skin and a considerable suction takes place.

Cuprum   So called from the island of Cyprus whence it was formerly brought; copper. Described by the *United States Dispensatory*: "its combination produces nausea and vomiting, violent pain in the stomach and bowels, frequent and bloody stools, small, irregular and frequent pulses, faintings, burning thirst, difficult breathing, violent headache, cramps, convulsions and finally death."

Cwt.   The abbreviation for hundredweight.

the Damp   The smell or noxious air emanating from a well.

Dejectio   (Dejections) A discharge of any excrementitious matter; generally applied to the feces, hence *dejectio alvina*.

Dejectoria   (To cast out) Purging medicines.

Dengue   An acute infectious disease characterized by acute headache, joint pain and rash transmitted by Aedes mosquitoes.[9]

Dielectrics   A nonconductor of direct electric current.

Diphtheria   An infectious bacterial disease; symptoms include the formation of a membrane over the tonsils, uvula, soft palate and posterior pharynx. The word "diphtheria" came into general use around 1859; before that is was diagnosed as sore throat, croup or scarlatina and was thought to be caused by heat and stagnant air.

Disinfectants   Substances that disinfected the air to considerable distances. The best volatile disinfectants were turpentine, chlorine, iodine, bromine and sulphurous acid. Sulphate of iron was considered the best fixed disinfectant and germicide and carbolic acid the best volatile one.[10]

Do.   Ditto.

Drachm   Dram; one-eighth of a fluid ounce.

Dropsy   (Hydrops) A collection of serous fluid in the cellular membrane; in the viscera and the circumscribed cavities of the body. When diffused through the cellular membrane either generally or partially, it is called *anasarca;* when deposited in the cavity of the cranium, it is called *hydrocephalus;* when in the abdomen, it is called *ascites.* It was believed to be caused by a family disposition, excessive and long-continuing evacuations and a free use of spirituous liquors, preceding diseases such as jaundice, diarrhea, gout, scarlet fever, exposure for a length of time to a moist atmosphere, topical weakness and general debility.

Dysentery   (Dysenteria; contagious pyrexia) Symptoms include frequent gripping stools, tenemus, stools chiefly mucus sometimes mixed with blood. Dysentery occurs chiefly in the summer, occasioned by the use of unwholesome and putrid food and by noxious exhalations and vapors. A peculiar disposition in the atmosphere often seems to predispose or give rise to dysentery, in which case it prevails epidemically. It appears where a number of people are gathered together and not infrequently spreads with great rapidity (1842). The modern definition (2001) describes it as being caused by bacterial, viral, protozoan or parasitic infections, most commonly in places with inadequate sanitation where food and water are contaminated with pathogens.

Dyspepsia   Indigestion.

Eccoprotic   An opening medicine (cathartic), the operation of which is very gentle, such as manna and senna.

Electrolytes   An ionized salt in blood, tissue fluids and cells; they include sodium, potassium and chloride.[11]

Endemic   Referring to a disease that occurs continuously or is ever-present in sections of the population, as opposed to an epidemic that has a fixed beginning and end.

Erisipelatous   (Erysipelas) A skin lesion that appears as a red, swollen, hardened and painful rash, accompanied with high fever, shaking, chills, fatigue, headache and vomiting.

Ether   (Aether; sulphuric aether) A volatile liquor obtained by distillation from a mixture of alcohol and a concentrated acid; when taken internally, the properties were antispasmodic, cordial and stimulant. Applied externally, it was used for pain relief in toothache and headache.

Exhibition, for   When prepared for a patient, as in a medication. See "carbonate of lime" for an example of usage.

Extramural interments   Burials outside a city, specifically in reference to London.

Fauces   A cavity behind the tongue, palatine arch, uvula and tonsils, from which the pharynx and larynx proceed.

Fibrine   (Fibrin) Fine interlacing filaments that entangle red and white blood cells and platelets, the whole forming a clot.[12]

Flux   Dysenteria.

Fomes, fomite   Any substance that adheres to and transmits infectious material.[13]

Fomites   Articles of commerce or clothing imbued with infectious matter.

Friction   Strenuous rubbing to increase circulation.

Friotion   Friction.

Fusee   A large-headed match capable of standing straight in a strong wind.

Germicide   A substance that is not volatile, gives off no smell and kills germs only on the spot where it is placed. The best and most powerful (1885) were corrosive sublimate, chromic acid, acetic acid, alum, pyrogallic acid, tannin, sulphate of copper, permanganate of potash, boric, salicyllic, benzoic and picric acids, nitrate of lead and chloride of zinc. Strong mineral acids like nitric, muriatic and sulphuric were volatile or fuming, but no so when diluted with water. If corrosive sublimate failed to completely destroy cholera germs, they could be chemically destroyed by strong acids.[14]

Ghost stories   Reports of false deaths.

Ginger   (Zingiber) Cultivated in India and the West Indies. When the roots were scalded in boiling water and rapidly dried the product was called *black ginger* and imported almost exclusively from Calcutta. Ginger grown in Jamaica was prepared by stripping off the epidermis and drying the roots in the sun; this was called *white ginger* and was highly valued. It was used as a stimulant and carminative, given in dyspepsia, flatulent colic; imparted an agreeable and warming operation in bitter tonics. Externally applied it was a rubefacient. "F. Brown's Essence of Jamaica Ginger" was sold by Scribner & Devol in 1856 as being efficacious in epidemic and summer cholera.

Glands of Peyer   The small glands situated under the villous coat of the intestines.

Gruel   A watery or liquid food usually consisting of oat, wheat, rye or rice flour boiled in water or milk; a thinner version of porridge.

Hartshorn   (*Cornu cervi*) The horns of stags; when shavings were boiled they imparted to the water a nutritious jelly. The recipe included half a pound of hartshorn shavings in 6 pints of water; to the strained liquor add lemon or Seville orange juice, 4 ounces of mountain wine and half a pound of sugar. The medical use was limited to nutritive and demulcent (soothing) value similar to calfsfoot jelly.

Humor   (Humour) The general term for any fluid of the body except the blood.

Hyoscyamus   The pharmacopoeial name of henbane; also known as mandrake and nightshade. Although now known to be a deadly toxin, it was occasionally used as a "magic" potion to induce hallucinations. During the 19th century henbane was used in various and spasmodic diseases such as epilepsy, hysteria, palpitation, headache, paralysis, mania and scirrhus. Henbane was sometimes given as a substitute for opium as it was free from the constipating quality of that treatment. It was given in the form of inspissated juice of the fresh leaves in a dose between 1–2 grains that required a gradual increase to be effective.

Hypocondriasis A languor, listlessness or want of resolution and activity, with respect to all undertakings; sadness and fear from uncertain causes, with a melancholic temperament.

Hypotension Seriously low blood pressure.

Influenza (*La gripe*; *cararrhus a contagione*) The Italian word for influence, so named because it was supposed to be produced by a peculiar influence of the stars. An infectious disease, the flu is spread by airborne transmission, causing chills, fever, sore throat, muscle pains and weakness and can lead to pneumonia. It was a dreaded and deadly disease throughout the 18th and 19th centuries. Authorities in the 1830s differentiated influenza from cholera by the observation that the latter chiefly affected the lower classes while the former was more general and indiscriminate.[15] During the 19th century, influenza was also believed to be a precursor of cholera.

Injection In the early and mid–19th century the word referred to an enema.

Injection, saline By late 1831, injections of saline into a patient's veins were being experimented with on cholera victims with guarded success.

Inspissated A substance thickened, dried or made less fluid by evaporation.

Intermittent/s Suspending activity at intervals; symptoms that recur.

Jatropha (Tapioca) Used as a diet for the sick and convalescent.

Kaolin A type of earth or mud, a product of the erosion of igneous rock; chemically known as aluminum silicate. Used in China through the 20th century in the treatment of cholera and ulcers.

Kill Johns Apricots, so called because they brought on diarrhea, especially among soldiers in the Eastern Theatre of the Crimean War (British).

King Cholera Commonly used 19th century sobriquet for the terrifying and seemingly all-powerful disease.

Kioh-kin-tiau The Chinese word meaning "the disease which contracts the tendons of the leg," referring to cholera.

Kreosote/creasote A volatile oil discovered in 1830 as a byproduct of the distillation of wood. It is an irritant, narcotic, styptic and antiseptic. Internally, it was used to treat diabetes mellitus, epilepsy, hysteria, chronic catarrh, haemoptysis and pulmonary consumption. Externally, it was used as an application on eruptions, wounds and ulcers and as an injection and gargle. Its most remarkable power was in preserving meat. Excessive doses were poisonous, causing giddiness, blurred vision, depressed action of the heart and coma. There was no known antidote for creasote poisoning.

l. An abbreviation used in the early 1800s in England before the symbol £ (pounds) came into general usage. Also used without the italics.

Laudanum Tincture of opium.

Lazaretto An isolation hospital for people with infectious diseases.

Lead, sugar of A crystallizable salt, called "sugar" from its sweet taste. An acetate, it was usually crystallized in needles, which have a silky appearance and were used as a coagulator of mucus. Acetate of lead in solution was also used as external applications to inflamed surfaces and scrofulous sores and as eye washes. In extreme cases of hemorrhage from the lungs and bowels it was used in minute doses as a corrugant or astringent. Epsom or Glauber salts were used as a counter-poison for a dangerous dose of sugar of lead.

Magisterium bismuthi   Used as a specific in gastric catarrh and ulcer with some astringent properties. When taken internally, it formed a continuous sheet over any ulceration, which it protected from mechanical injury from food and the action of gastric juice. It was used to treat diarrhea because of its astringent and protective action on the intestine.

Manna   *(Fraxinus; Fraxinus ornus; Fraxinus Excelsior)* The condensed juice of the flowering ash tree, possessing diuretic qualities, used in the cure of intermittents.

Marasmus   Consumption of the bowels.

Mesenteric glands   (Mesentery: a membrane in the cavity of the abdomen attached to the vertebrae of the loins and to which the intestines adhere) The glands were situated in the cellular membrane of the mesentery. The chyle from the intestines passes through these glands to the thoracic duct.

Microbe   A small living thing, either animal or vegetable (1892).[16]

Micro-organism   A minute animal or vegetable body. But it was not used in quite so restricted a sense as "microbe" or "bacteria."[17]

Milk sickness   A common expression in the Midwest, particularly in Kentucky, Indiana and Ohio; the complaint was attributed to drinking the milk or eating the meat of cattle "affected in a peculiar manner." Its symptoms were described as precisely those of Asiatic cholera. In 1838 the governor of Kentucky offered a $1,000 reward for the discovery of the disease that it might be prevented.[18]

Mithridate/mindereri draughts   (Mithridatium: the electuary (*confectio*: confection). According to the *London Pharmacopedia,* anything made from sugar, from Mithridates, king of Pontus and Bithynia, who used a composition of 20 leaves of rue, 2 walnuts, 2 figs and a little salt to guard against the effects of poison.

Moonshine speculations   A humbug scheme; an impracticable idea or unfeasible project (United States, 1850s).

Morbid anatomist   A physician who specialized in post mortem examinations.

Mordechie   Arabic word meaning "the death blow," used in reference to the fatal outcome from Asiatic cholera; also corrupted into the French *mort de chien* (dog's death) signifying the same thing (19th century).[19]

Moukden   A Chinese cholera god represented by five heads: a central human head surrounded by those of horse, ass, ox and sheep, able to inflict or recall the disease.[20]

Moxa   (*Artemisia Chinensis*) A Japanese word for a method of prevention and treatment for various diseases. Dried leaves of the young Mugwort tree were rendered into powder and a small cone of this substance was placed on premoistened skin. The powder was set on fire and allowed to burn down, producing a small dark-colored spot. Garlic was then placed over the wound to promote ulceration. In England, the word "moxa" was used to indicate a similar method but one in which were substituted rolls of cotton soaked in oil of turpentine or spirit of wine for Mugwort leaves.

Mulligatawny soup   (mulligatany) A spicy meat soup originating in India occasionally prescribed for cholera patients.

Mulligrubs   A despondent, sullen or ill-tempered mood; a gripping of the intestines; colic.

Muriatic acid   Obtained by the action of sulphuric acid on chloride of sodium or common salt. It is a refrigerant and an antiseptic; distilled with water, it was given for fevers and for some forms of syphilis and to counteract phosphatic deposits in urine. It was also used as a gargle for sore throats. When swallowed, it was highly irritating and corrosive.

Mustard seed   (White) Ground into powder and used as an emetic or diluted in water and administered as an enema.

Naphtha   (Naphthalene) A colorless to reddish-brown volatile aromatic liquid, similar to gasoline. Petroleum or pitch; ancient references refer to it as a "miraculous flammable liquid." It was found on the shores of the Caspian Sea, in Sicily and Italy. The fluid was used as an external application for removing old pains, nervous disorders such as cramps, contraction of the limbs and paralytic afflictions.

Nitric acid   In medicine, it was used as a tonic and as a substitute for mercurial preparations in syphilis and afflictions of the liver; in the form of vapor it was used to combat contagion.

Nitrous acid   (*Acidum nitrosum*) Fuming nitrous acid. The acid is best obtained by exposing nitrate of lead to heat in a glass retort. Pure nitrous acid comes over in the form of an orange-colored liquid. When mixed with water, it is decomposed and nitrous gas is disengaged, occasioning effervescence.

Nitrous oxyde   (Nitrous oxide; "Oxygen gas") When inhaled, it elicits an irresistible propensity to laughter, a rapid flow of vivid ideas and the pleasantest period of intoxication, without any subsequent languor, but is more generally followed by vigor and a pleasurable disposition to exertion, which gradually subsides.

Noncontagionist   Person/s who believed cholera was caused by aspects unique to a specific place or environment: atmosphere, miasmas or abrupt changes in temperature; also "anti-contagionist," or "anti-contagionism."

Nosocomial   An infection acquired in a hospital or other health care setting.[21]

Nosology   The doctrine of the names of diseases.

Occulist   (Oculist) One who treats diseases of the eye.

Oil doctors   (British, circa 1854) Medical men who prescribed castor oil to treat cholera.

Ordure   Excrement.

Parenteral   Any medical route other than the alimentary canal (oral), such as IV, subcutaneous and IM.[22]

Pathogen   A microorganism capable of producing a disease.

Penny-a-line   A familiar term for reporters.

Pennyroyal   A plant in the mint family used in cooking by early Greeks and Romans. In the 18th century it was used to eradicate pests and treat rattlesnake bites. Although oil of pennyroyal is highly toxic, dried leaves were used to settle upset stomachs and relieve flatulence. Fresh or dried leaves were also used to treat colds, influenza, and abdominal cramps and to induce sweating.

Peppermint, oil of   (*Mentha piperita*) The stomachic, anti-spasmodic and carminative properties of peppermint render it useful in flatulent colics, hysterical afflictions, retchings and other dyspeptic symptoms, acting as a cordial; used as an essential oil, a simple water and as a spirit.

Pernicious fever   Generically, a fatal or harmful fever; a term used in the 18th century to cover a variety of fevers, especially malarial and cholera.

Peruvian bark   Quinine: Containing cinchona bark used in the treatment of malaria.

Physic   The profession of medicine; also used in reference to a cathartic.

Poodeena   (India) mint; used in combination with onion juice and black pepper to cure severe cases of cholera.

Popliteal   A small triangular muscle lying across the back part of the knee joint.

Potash   (Pot-ash) Potassa: Potassium or any of its various compounds; vegetable alkali.

Potassium, bromide of   (*Potassii Bromidum*) A salt widely used as an anticonvulsant and sedative after its introduction in 1857. It was originally used to treat epilepsy. In irritable condition of the bowels it was apt to cause diarrhea, often requiring treatment by opium. In the 20th century bromide compounds were used to treat headaches (Bromo-Seltzer) until 1975.

Praecordia   The forepart of the region of the thorax.

Prussic acid   (Acidum Hydrocyanicum) A mixture of cayanuret of silver, 50.5 grains, muriatic acid 41 grains, distilled water 1 ounce; after shaking, pour off the insoluble matter. A deadly poison; in a diluted state it was used as an anodyne and antispasmodic. The *London Medical Times* (1849) reported it was used in extreme cases of collapse in cholera patients.

Ptyalism   Increased secretion of saliva from the mouth.

Pulse   (Food) Legumes.

Purl   An alcoholic drink consisting of half a pint of hot beer, a glass of gin and about an ounce of sugar.

Purpura   A disease consisting of small, distinct, purple specks and patches, attended with general debility but not always fever, caused by an extravasation of the vessels under the cuticle. Purpura was divided into five distinct species: *haemorrhagica* was considered the most severe, producing whip-like marks, violent bruises and spots on the tongue, gums and palate, producing copious bleeding. It was sometimes seen as sequels to smallpox and measles and in those who were ill-fed.

Putrid fever   (*Typhus gravior*) The most malignant species of typhus.

Pyaemia   Septicema.

Pyretic   Of or concerning fevers.

Pyroligenous acid   (Also spelled "pyroligneous") *Acidum Pyroligneum.* Diluted acetic acid, obtained by the destructive distillation of wood. An acetic acid of medium strength employed in forming several acetates. It was useful in preserving fish, beef, pulpy fruits, bulbs and fresh leaves. The crude acid in a diluted state was used as an application to gangrene and ulcers, acting as an antiseptic and stimulant.

Quassia   A secret remedy in treating malignant endemic fevers; bitterwood; a prepared form of the heartwood or any of these trees. It was said to have been introduced by a Negro of Surinam named Quassia, who presented it to a Swede named Rolander. It was used as simple bitters adapted to dyspepsia and to aid the debilitated state of the digestive organs, and given with advantage in malignant fevers. Used by brewers in England (1850s) to impart bitterness to their liquors.

Quincies   1. Diseases of the mouth; 2. (*Pyrus cydonia)* Quince tree. The London College (1760s) directed that seeds of this tree be made into a decoction for afflictions and excoriations of the mouth and fauces.

Quinine   (Also referred to as "bark"; *Cinchonina*) Typically Peruvian bark, used to treat fever.

Considered the most valuable remedy in continual fevers connected with debility in such diseases as typhus, confluent smallpox, dyspepsia, rickets and dropsy, the powder was given orally or as an enema (see "bitters").

Rhubarb (Rheum) from Rah, a river in Russia (Wolga) from the banks of which it was first brought. *Rheum palmatum:* the pharmacopoeial name of the officinal rhubarb, introduced in 1732. Used as a gentle purgative.

Rickets (*Rachitis*) A disease of children between 9 months and 2 years, characterized by a large head, prominent forehead, protruded sternum, flattened ribs, big belly and emaciated limbs; stools are frequent and loose, with a slow fever followed by cough and difficulty in respiration. Treatment consisted of a system of invigoration, tonic medicines and the consumption of chalybeates (a tonic containing salts of iron). Ricketts is now known to be caused by a deficiency of vitamin D and an inadequate calcium supply and is treated by supplying those essential nutrients.

Rusk Dry, or twice-baked, bread.

Sago (*Cycas circinalis*) The systematic name of the palm tree which affords a sago; a dry fecula obtained from the pitch of this palm; It was much recommended in febrile, phthisical and calculous disorders. To make it palatable, lemon juice, sugar and wine were added to the pitch after it was softened by boiling.

Salts of lime Combinations of the different acids with the salifiable base lime.

Sari A garment of southern Asian women consisting of a long cloth draped around the body and head or shoulder.

Sarsaparilla Around the middle of the 16th century it was introduced into Europe as a remedy for venereal complaint; it fell into disuse until the 1700s when it was again used for the treatment of syphilis and to restore the system after mercury overdose or the ravages of cholera. When imported from China and Japan it was commonly known as China root; species of Smilax grown in the United States were found to contain no useful medical properties and preparations sold in the U.S. in the 1800s were typically inert from age or having been obtained from inferior species.

Savoyard A person from Savoy, a former duchy of southeast France, western Switzerland and northwest Italy. In 1720 the duke of Savoy gained the title "king of Sardinia."

Scarificator An instrument containing a number of lancets, sometimes as many as 20, which are so contrived that when the instrument is applied to any part of the surface of the body and a spring is pressed, they suddenly spring out and make the necessary punctures; used in cupping. The instrument is so constructed that the depth to which the lancets penetrate is at the option of the operator.

Scavenging In 19th century England the term referred to the removal of visible filth from privies, dust bins, stables, cowsheds and pigsties.

Scirrhus Known by a hard tumor of a glandular part, indolent and accompanied by little or no discoloration of the skin until it becomes malignant as a cancerous disease.

Scruple A weight of 20 grains.

Scurvy (*Scorbutus*) A disease characterized by extreme debility, pale complexion, spongy gums, livid spots on the skin, foul ulcers, fetid urine and extremely offensive stools. A disease of sailors and those shut away and due to a deprivation of fresh provisions and eating a diet of salted or putrescent food. Prevention and cure lay in a proper diet of fresh vegetables, primarily those which contain a native acid as oranges, lemons, limes, vinegar, sour crout and fermenting liquors such as spruce beer and cider.

Secale cornutum   Ergot. As described in the *United States Dispensatory,* it produced irritation of the stomach and bowels, great muscular prostration, loss of sensation and sometimes spasms; its symptoms were similar to those of arsenic. The *Lexicon* noted it was a dangerous medicine as its effect was not controllable.

Seidlitz powder   Comprising tartaric acid, sodium bicarbonate and potassium sodium tartrate, dissolved in water and used as a cathartic.

Seltzer water   From Neider Seltzer, a German town about 10 miles from Frankfurt, on the Mayne, where a saline mineral water rises which is slightly alkaline, highly acidulated with carbonic acid. It was used to relieve some symptoms that indicate a morbid affliction of the lungs, in slow hectic fever, foulness of the stomach, bilious vomiting, acidity, heartburn and bloody and offensive stools.

Septic acid   Nitric acid.

Septon   A principle in medicine believed to be the essence of infection; air deficient in oxygen containing poisonous emanations.

Serogroup   An unofficial designation denoting a group of bacteria containing a common antigen, possibly containing one or more serotype, or genus (21st century definition).

Ship fever   A generic expression used along the western waterways of the U.S. referring to a disease similar to (or identical with) malignant cholera, generally used to identify fatalities among immigrants.

Silver, nitrate of   *(Argentum).* Composed of nitrate of silver, hydrocyanic acid and distilled water. Externally, it was used as a vesicant, stimulant and escharotic and used as a mouthwash for healing ulcers produced by mercury. In the solid state it was used to destroy strictures of the urethra, warts, fungous flesh and surfaces of ulcers. It was also used to cauterize pustules in smallpox. Used in overdose, it was a corrosive poison.

Sinapisms   (Sinapismus) A mustard plaster; a mixture of mustard and vinegar in the form of a poultice applied to the calves of the legs or soles of the feet as a stimulant and employed in low fevers to supersede the use of a blister.

Sloe-juice   (Prunus Spinosa) Derived from the sloe tree; used as an astringent gargle and much used in hemorrhages, or large blood flows.

Slow fever   Low-grade fever.

Sneaks   A class of thieves who went around England hawking quack medicines, pens and pencils and who were also known to commit numerous robberies in gentlemen's houses.

Soda, carbonate of   See carbonate of soda.

Spasmodic cholera   Indian cholera; cholera exhibiting the symptoms of that seen in India.

Speckled disease   Smallpox.

Spotted fever   A vague name for fevers in the 19th century; in modern times it references a tick-borne disease characterized by fever, headache, abdominal pain, vomiting and muscle pain; a red rash may also appear on the skin. Typhus and similar diseases are caused by the Rickettsia bacteria.

Stella; stellaria   Star-like appearance; criss-crossed.

Summer complaint   A nonspecific term used to refer to nonfatal cholera morbus and occasionally to cholera infantum.

Sweating sickness   (*sudor anglicus*) A mysterious, highly virulent disease that first appeared in England in 1485, later spreading to continental Europe. It was characterized by a sense of apprehension, followed by cold shivers, giddiness, headache, severe pains in neck and limbs, followed by great exhaustion. A sweating stage followed that included fever, headache, delirium, tachycardia and intense thirst. Mortality was high. The final outbreak was seen in 1551. Symptoms were similar to cholera and it may have been caused by poor sanitation, sewage and contaminated drinking water. It was believed to have caused the death of Arthur, Prince of Wales, brother of Henry VIII of England. In 1894 it was believed to have been caused by a fungoid infection in wheat.

Synapism   Usually a blister made of mustard; any irritant including turpentine cloths or garlic; occasionally used on the principal of counter irritation when a synapism was applied to one part of the body and a blister on another. For example, a synapism was applied to the epigastric region, followed by a stimulating enema to produce copious evcuations.

Tartana   A small fishing vessel.

Tartar emetic   The residue left from grapes on hogsheads of wine. After crystallization it forms a white powder used as a diuretic in inflammatory and bilious fevers, diarrheas and dyspepsia. Poisoning by tartar emetic was believed to cause symptoms similar to cholera.

Tartrate   A salt of tartaric acid.

Tea (black)   Popular in the Southern U.S. during the 1850s for use in treating cholera because it was believed to contain iron.

Tea (green)   Believed to be strongly impregnated with copper, its use was discouraged during cholera season.

Telluric   From the Latin *tellus,* meaning of, or relating to, the earth, as in natural forces or currents.

Tenesmus   A continual inclination to go to stool without a discharge.

Thebaic tincture   A mixture containing Egyptian poppies.

Thrush   Spreading ulcers in the mouth.

Turpentine, oil of   Used in frictions.

Typhus   A species of continued fever characterized by a great debility, a tendency of the fluids to putrefaction and the ordinary symptoms of fever. Victims suffered smallness of pulse (bradycardia); in the more advanced stage purple spots emerged on various parts of the body along with fetid stools and rapid pulse (tachycardia). During the mid–19th century it was considered contagious, transmitted by person-to-person contact or from effluvia arising from decomposing vegetable or animal matter.

Typhus, sinking   (*Typhus syncopalis* or *synocha*) Improperly called spotted fever. Inflammatory or continuous fever characterized by fever, frequent, hard pulse and high-colored urine; senses not impaired. In the mid–19th century it was believed to be caused by a sudden transition from heat to cold, swallowing cold liquors when the body was much heated by exercise, intemperance, violent passions of the mind, or suppression of habitual evacuations.

U.C.   Upper Canada.

Venesection   Phlebotomy; cutting of a vein, as in bloodletting.

Veratrum album   White hellebore. A violent emetic and cathartic capable of producing dangerous and fatal effects when incautiously administered. In small doses it was a general stimulant to the secretions. It was also used as a cure for gouty and rheumatic afflictions.

Veratrum nigrum   *(Helleborus niger)* Black hellebore, or Christmas rose. It was administered in large doses as a cathartic; it was also recommended in dropsies and some cutaneous diseases. The *United States Dispensatory* described it as a "violent emetic and cathartic—even in small doses it sometimes occasions severe vomiting, hypercatharsis with bloody stools and alarming symptoms of general prostration."

Vesication   A small skin ulcer.

Vis medicatrix naturae   The medical philosophy, based on the teachings of Hippocrates, purporting that "nature is the best physician," or the tendency for a body to heal itself.

Washerwoman's hands and feet   Descriptive phrase used to describe the swollen and reddened hands and feet of cholera victims in the final stages of the disease.

Widow Trueby's water   An anti-infection fluid used in the early 1700s made from the distillation of poppies.

Wood vinegar   From Pliny: used in the preservation of Egyptian mummies.

W.T.   Wisconsin Territory.

Yellow fever   An acute, infectious disease transmitted by a mosquito, characterized by high fever, headache, muscle aches, nausea, vomiting and gastrointestinal disturbances such as diarrhea. The cause was not known in the 19th century.

Zoophytes   Any of numerous invertebrate animals resembling plants in appearance or mode of growth. Used in reference to a fungoid in the 19th century.

Zymotic   From the Greek word signifying fermentation; includes the whole series of epidemics and contagions. "The origin of these may be traced to the propagation of certain living molecular atoms, not as yet scientifically classed and understood, which, entering into man's body, transmute his tissues into their own substance, 'so that he can no longer live his own life.' The process is analogous to fermentation, and each zymotic atom is the little leaven that leavens the whole lump."[23]

Appendix I

Cures for Cholera
Throughout the Ages

One word about remedies. We would say to the public, trust none of them, try none of them.[1]

The above quotation continues: "Out of one hundred and one nostrums and courses of treatment recommended by every good natured noodle that fancies he has been cured of cholera because he took certain remedies, there is but one ingredient of any potency in the disease, and that is opium." The point here is not that opium was a cure for cholera: it was not. The true significance is that *everyone* (even when they were advising against it) had a "cure" for cholera.

As this malignant disease swept across the globe, eventually touching every sunlit plain and dark corner, people were desperate for help. They sought relief from the writings of ancient physicians and the gossip of housewives; they bought well-advertised brand names puffed with testimonials by the famous and the nondescript; foods that were shunned by some nationalities were advocated by others; books, pamphlets, placards and newspapers were scoured for magic potions. Sufferers of all centuries and generations rubbed themselves with liniments and wrapped themselves with mustard plasters and flannel. They purged with mercuric poisons, doped themselves with narcotics, knocked themselves silly with chloroform and ether, held camphor to their noses, sought divine intervention, cursed devils and resorted to superstitions.

No one knew what caused cholera and for most of the 17th, 18th and 19th centuries, experts could not even agree on nomenclature. The malady was Cholera morbus, India cholera, Asiatic cholera, English cholera or not even cholera, at all, but some mysterious disease beyond any realm "dreamt of in your philosophy." The new concept of "sanitation" became a buzz word: swamps were drained, sewers dug, "extramural" burials took the place of graves; living at higher elevations was a preventative, "sweet water" was an indication of purity, and noxious odors were harbingers of death. When all else failed, the wise recommended doing nothing at all, and the literate turned to the only known universal "cure": humor.

One particularly pithy notice came in 1836:

> *Cholera.*—The Lowell Courier, of a late date, states that a man in that town, after drinking in the course of half day about twelve glasses of gin was attacked by the cholera, and in a few hours was a corpse! We are at a loss whether to record this as a case of *cholera, suicide or poisoning.*[2]

If there were no answer for what to call it or how to make it go away, the manner in which to catch cholera was hardly debatable, as those on both sides of the Atlantic had some pretty specific instructions:

Recipe for the Cholera.—Major Noah, in his last Star, gives the following directions for manufacturing a genuine case of Cholera. "Eat two cucumbers, dressed or raw as you prefer—then take a quart of blackberries, four green corn, four young potatoes mashed,—a lobster, or a crab—some ice water, and wash the whole down with a quart of buttermilk, and you will shortly have a touch of the real thing."[3]

A RECEIPT TO GET THE CHOLERA MORBUS

Take some thousands of Cats that have long ceased malrowing,
Take ditto of Dogs who have done bow-wowing,
Take ditto of Hogs quite dead for some weeks,
Take ditto of Pigs who have finished their squeaks,
Take ditto of Rats who no longer are gnawing,
Take ditto of Crows who have ended their cawing,
And into a river on black mud that rests,
Deposit these horrible putrescent pests,
And all kinds of decomposed stuff that you're able,
The refuse of garden, of sink-hole and stable,
And let it go forth with a taste that endures,
From those outlets of filth that are called common sewers,
When these are all mixed, take a filter and a rain,
Bearing this well in mind that the taste will remain,
And the more that you filter, the more that you strain,
You filter through decomposition again,
And double and trebly you add to the savour,
The pureness and brightness and exquisite flavour;
Then let it be drank by youth or adult,
And the cholera morbus will be the result.[4]

With that settled, some exasperated finger wagging elicited a smile.

CHOLERIC WRITING.—The cholera has produced a host of writers, from whom much information and amusement is to be derived. In the *Times* a few days ago, we had the letter of a Mr. Thomas Single, Churchwarden of Mile End, which is a model of composition. "*False* reports," quoth the Churchwarden, "ought to be corrected by those who make them, if *truth* be their object"; that is to say, those who tell lies are under a most urgent obligation of being scrupulous as to their veracity.

"The case of cholera," continues our author, "at Stepney, reported by the Central Board, proved to be, on examination by a dozen doctors, *all* of whom agreed, *except the two* who are paid to hunt for cases—

This court of unanimity is, however, not quite original. We remember a precedent in Galway, under the reign of Dick Martin himself, when, at a country meeting, "It was resolved unanimously, with only two dissentient voices of no importance." But to proceed—

"The case of cholera proved to be—no cholera whatever, and that the young man died from inflammation and stoppage in his bowels."

Here is an ingenious case of cholera! It not only proves itself not to be itself—but also testifies that a person, whose sex it determines, and whose age it fixes, died from disordered intestines.

This is, indeed, *choleric* composition. Perhaps when Mr. Single penned it he saw *double*.[5]

Although frequent missives during the Second Cholera Pandemic (1829–1849) decried the Jews, who were "known for their want of cleanliness and their mode of life," Mr. River, commissioner of the district of Bochnia and a member of the sanitary establishment there, found great value in a cure they used there against the cholera morbus. In a letter to friends, dated Vienna, August 9, 1832, he observed, "The Jews of Weizniz have been eminently judicious in their treatment of the cholera; for in that town, out of 240 individuals who have been attacked by it, every one of them has been saved, with the exception of two persons who refused to submit to it."

The remedy they used consisted of mixing a pint of strong spirits of wine with half a pint of good white wine vinegar. To this was added 1 ounce of powdered camphor, 1 ounce of flour of mustard or bruised mustard seed, a quarter of an ounce of ground pepper, a full teaspoonful of bruised garlic and half an ounce of powdered cantharides. It was to be mixed well and exposed to the sun for 12 hours, with care being taken to shake it repeatedly. As soon as a person was attacked, they were to be put to bed under warm coverlets and hands and feet rubbed powerfully and uninterruptedly with warmed lotion. During this operation, the patient was to take a glass of strong drink, composed of 2 parts of chamomile flowers and 1 part balm mint:

> Persevere in this course, and at the end of 15 minutes at the utmost (the patient's head and body being kept well covered beneath the bed-clothes), he will break out into a profuse perspiration. The patient must be kept in this state between two and three hours, but care must be taken that he does not fall asleep. After this, remove the extra covering from the bed, and he will drop into a slumber, which will last between 6 and 8 hours, and be accompanied by a gentle perspiration. When he awakes, he will find himself weak, but the disease will have entirely left him and he will require nothing further but rest and a moderate diet to restore him to perfect health.
>
> Especial attention must be paid that after the rubbing, the patient does not so much as lift a finger above the bed-clothes, for the slightest chill, while the perspiration is upon him, would be his death. When the cramps in the stomach come on, very hot dry bandages of bran and ashes were applied to the pit of the stomach, and when necessary, a bladder of hot water to the region of the navel. The great point is to produce strong perspiration and to restore the circulation of the blood, which, at the beginning of the attack, is drawn from the surface of the body, and thrown with frightful virulence on its inward parts.

The writer added his testimonial by stating that he was an eyewitness to its good effects, having used it to save the lives of three of his servants.[6] Either the above remedy worked or matters changed considerably, for in 1876 one article noted "The Jews are the healthiest and longest-lived people on earth. Their immunity from diseases of all forms is remarkable.... It is declared that the cholera never chose one of them for its victim."[7]

The idea that sweating was important to the cure of cholera was also promoted by Dr. Beach, physician to the 10th Ward, New York. In his dissertation in the *American Practice of Medicine* (vol. 2) he wrote of his practice during the cholera epidemic of 1832: "In a word, the leading indication in the cure of cholera, either in the confirmed or collapsed stage, is to *establish reaction,* or in other words, to *promote perspiration.*"[8] Unfortunately, hydration, not dehydration, was the answer, but this practice persisted for many decades.

When cholera struck France in early 1832, the minister of Commerce and Public Works, Count D'Argout, issued a proclamation outlining numerous preventative measures (see chapter 10). As chloric solutions were universally recommended as a useful precaution against infection, the following receipt was provided:

> Take one ounce of dry chlorate lime, and one quart of water; pour a sufficient quantity of water on the powder to make it into a paste, and then dilute it with the remainder. Strain off the solution and keep it in glass or earthern vessels well stopped. A portion of this solution should be poured in a shallow earthen bowl and placed in every room in the house. The chlorate of soda is nearly as good, used in the same manner, in the proportion of one ounce of chlorate to ten or twenty ounces of water. No family should be without these preparations.[9]

Interestingly, fear of cholera on the Continent created a considerable demand for colonial produce—sugar and coffee. Both were consumed as an antidote although most medical authorities advocated against the use of these items, prompting one newspaper to run the disclaimer that excessive use of sugar and coffee "must pre-dispose to the disease."[10] A cure of a more jovial sort was suggested by the Englishman Dr. Blick. He stated that while a "heavy feeling" would predispose the body to infection, "the stimulus of constant intoxication, by promoting counter-irritation, would be a preventative!" At the same time, the French physician M. Magendie treated his cholera patients chiefly by having them drink freely of "*punch and hot wine.*"[11]

When cholera reached North America in 1832, nearly all treatments there were based on European methods and recipes. The "No. 1 powder" consisted of carbonate of soda, half a drachm; common salt, 20 grains and oxymuriate of potach, 7 grains, administered every hour in half a tumbler of water. Common Seidlitz powder or effervescent soda was given to calm the stomach. Extreme thirst was quenched with soda water or seltzer, in quantities not exceeding a wine glassful at a time.[12]

Water for drinking was to be filtered; if consumed "pure," it should be whetted with vinegar or brandy; reddened water (water with red wine) was also considered beneficial. Aromatic water, containing a stimulant infusion of peppermint or chamomile (a pinch of mint or 6 heads of chamomile to a half pint of boiling water, cooled and added to a pint of cold water) was also acceptable. However, ice cream and ice milk were especially to be avoided! The recipe for rubbing liniment included half a pint of brandy, 2 gills of strong vinegar, ½ ounce of mustard flour, 2 drachms each of camphor and pepper, 2 cloves of pounded "garlick." The whole was to be placed in a glass bottle, well stopped and allowed to infuse for three days, either in sun or some warm place.[13]

Equally strong was the philosophy that if small doses of medicine helped, larger ones were better. A report from the *Rockingham (VA) Register* (August 24, 1833) provided a perfect example (italics and exclamation points in the original):

> A Mr. Holloway, of Russelville, Ky., supposing that he was attacked by the Cholera, took, in the course of a few minutes, 150 grains of calomel, 4 cups of red pepper, one cup tincture of camphor, a table spoonsfull spirits of turpentine, one quart of whisky! and two table spoonsfull of a stimulus composed of myrrh, camphor, oil of peppermint and opium!!—*and survived the treatment!!!*

The editor noted, "We hope his example will not be followed without consulting a Physician!" There was, however, no mention of whether Holloway cured his cholera.

Due to the fact many diseases in the 19th century were believed to originate from a miasmic effect, burning fires in the house and along the streets was believed to drive off bad air. On a similar vein, Mr. Brooks, the eminent anatomist, recommended the firing of guns as a preventative of cholera.[14] In June 1832, the 47th Regiment fired blank cartridges through the streets of Newry where cholera raged: "This experiment was advised by medical men."[15] The following month a Paris journal advocated explosions of gunpowder and large fires in open spaces, the fires composed of tar barrels, coals and the like to render the atmosphere "innoxious." The editor added, "We are not aware that the Medical Board has ever recommended the adoption of such means; they preferred scientific jargon and mystification to common sense."[16] This technique was also used in epidemics of typhus and yellow fever in Europe and the United States.

There was also hope for immunity. One news report indicated that of the several hundred Poles living in Paris, none had contracted cholera. Since they resided in their homeland when the scourge ravaged that country, "May it be concluded that they thus became accustomed to the morbific miasmata, and that the epidemic which desolates us has, in consequence, no effect on their bodily systems. This circumstance is not unworthy of serious examination."[17]

Testimonials for numerous concoctions supposedly providing "sure cures" for cholera filled the English newspapers during the 19th century. While it is probable these medicines or treatments were wholeheartedly believed in by those espousing them, most were ineffectual at best and harmful at worst. Physicians or their friends typically wrote to the newspapers, sharing their exotic secrets. Occasionally, they sent recipes to ambassadors or men in authority, hoping to use their influence to promote a specific method. In 1832, a "sensible English physician" related his discovery to M. de Montbel, the ex–French minister. Writing from Vienna, the doctor described Dr. Queen's remedy as employing *camphor* in the first stage, *veratrum nigrum* in the second and *powders of copper* in the third stage. By these means he cured 34 out of 37 patients.[18]

Science was often confused with superstition, and in 1832 the clerk of a church near Stockport, in reading the Order in Council, recommended inhabitants to "whitewash *themselves,* as a preventative against cholera." The editor for the *Age* (July 1, 1832) parenthetically added, "Many persons are much *indebted* to this *whitewashing,* as a remedy for long *confinement* on many *accounts.*"

Denying the presence of disease was another way to "cure" it. A pamphlet by Mr. W.S. Prior, "A Fatal Blow to the Cholera Morbus," asserted that there was no such thing as "blueness or cramps," as these would indicate mortification of a body part and mortification of the whole body meant death. Calling Prior "neither more nor less than a 'Quack,'" one reviewer noted, "according to Mr. Prior's opinion, every poor devil who has had cramps must have for several days previously been dead. A *duck* were Mr. Prior's most suitable critic."[19]

In France it was noted that physicians were "sufficiently agreed" that at the outset of cholera symptoms, venesection (cutting a vein) was used "in order to give force to the circulation; they then favour a re-action, by means of stimulants employed internally, and especially externally; and blood-letting is again resorted to during that period."[20]

On the American side, a New York physician prescribed marshmallow tea; unfortunately, he was misunderstood (misunderstanding being a more dangerous "malady" than cholera, down to the present day) and the patient was given boiled muskmelon. The cholera was "cured" by the death of the victim.[21] On the subject of musk, albeit in another form, a physician found musk to be a decisive cure. He administered 15 grains of musk rubbed into a lump of sugar and dissolved in a glass of water, finding it relieved cramps, purging and vomiting.[22] Sweetened, grated ginger, boiled and strained, was also believed to have the same effect, while Dr. Jennison, of Cambridge, prescribed rigid fasting for 48–60 hours for persons afflicted with the bowel complaints that generally proceed cholera. Dr. Marshal Spring added that any disease could be overcome by abstinence, and Dr. Makie, a New York physician, recommended the "free and thorough use of the stomach pump for the cure of cholera."[23]

In 1852 it was "fully ascertained, says the report of a French medical commission," that cholera had never proven epidemic where rainwater was exclusively used. Galveston, Texas, was held as an example of the truth of the statement.[24] Fourteen years later, Dr. F. Sims of that city added his own compelling argument:

> It is simply the constant use as a beverage of PURE WATER; and the *abstinence* from liquids holding in solution lime, magnesia, or their compounds. But it is too simple and cheap to believe in.... If it was recommended by the "retired clergyman," "sold by all druggists," and warranted equal, if not superior to the celebrated "Astrologico-magnetic, Univer-celestial pills for the cure of all diseases," it might command a larger share of public confidence.[25]

By 1871, "the book" used by ships' captains included this sure cure: A tablespoon of salt and a tablespoon of red pepper in a half-pint of hot water. The medicine was said to act quickly as an emetic, bringing up very offensive matter that "sticks like glue." Walles Lewis, an English physician, suggested an "orangeade," made by a concentrated compound infusion of "orange peel, 3 ounces; simple syrup, 12 ounces; boiled, filtered water, 4 gallons. Mix well and add 3 ounces of diluted sulphuric acid, taken a wine-glassful at a time." Parenthetically, in 1885, Dr. John C. Peters of New York warned "much mischief has been caused by a popular medicine largely composed of red pepper, ginger and brandy, and which ... is among the most injurious that could be selected in cases of real cholera."[26] Underscoring the danger of nostrums, the *Journal of Chemistry* (1881) offered a simple explanation that stands as well today as it did then.

Every Man His Own Doctor

Many a man who, if his horse or cow is sick, sends at once for the veterinary practitioner, will run the risk of prescribing for ailments of his own that are on the face of them quite as serious and as much in need of professional treatment.

He will take the advice of an ignorant neighbor as to what is "good for" an illness, when he would laugh at the idea of going to the same person for counsel in any other business or concern whatever. In the days of our grandmothers, when the household materia medica consisted of "roots and yarbs," with a few simple drugs like epsom salts, this domestic or "lay" prescribing was less dangerous than in these latter days when concentrated and powerful agents have become so common and familiar.

The household remedies of the olden time were rarely liable to do much harm, even if they did no good. The cure was generally in reality left to nature, though the "roots and yarbs" got the credit of it. But most of the drugs of our day are not of this inert or negative character, and the danger in their use by the ignorant is a real or serious danger.

The most powerful medicines that unprofessional people of a former generation ventured to fool with bore about the same relation to those in vogue that gunpowder does to nitro-glycerine; yet the latter are used even more recklessly than the former ever were. A little knowledge is not always a dangerous thing, but when it leads a man to think he can "doctor" himself, in ailments of any serious nature, the old and often-abused proverb is indisputably true.[27]

Metals and Galvanic Electricity

In an era where grand conclusions were drawn from extremely small samplings, an 1834 article began this way: "It is announced that a certain cure for the Cholera is now known." After that grandiose statement, which, it would have been supposed, merited headlines in bold, 72-point type, two sentences sufficed to announce that Dr. McCaig of Toronto gave "sugar of lead in doses of five and even twenty grains in solution with water. He tried the experiment on *two persons* who were in the last stages of the disorder, and cured them. This treatment is becoming general at Toronto."[28]

Typical of the times, a correspondent from Paris wrote that "for a great length of time a most unwholesome north-east wind has prevailed, which blows into the mouth a peculiar taste of copper; this is the dreadful malaria that destroys, and the poor ignorant people imagine themselves *poisoned!!*"[29] Another explanation for the taste of copper came from M. Cagnard Latour, of the Paris Academy of Sciences. After a "stone *fell from the clouds*" into a courtyard, he determined it contained a portion of copper. From this he drew the conclusion that the air of Paris was "infected with miasmatic copper emanations, which we swallow, and which, being taken into the blood, affect the intestines, and produce the cholera morbus. This speculation forms the substance of a grave memoir presented to an eminent scientific body." Copper was also alleged to have come from beef, analyzed by order of the London Board of Health.[30]

According to the popular statement, what goes around comes around. During the French cholera epidemics of 1832 and 1849, Dr. Burg made the observation that every coppersmith retained perfect health and that in the copper foundries, 200,000 workmen scarcely fell victim. He "attributed the immunity to the action—electric or otherwise—of the copper," and inferred that if persons would surround themselves in rooms where 15–20 sheets of copper were placed, or wore metallic belts of flat copper and steel, with cardboard between them to prevent immediate contact, they would be secure against the malady. His alleged discovery was based on a "a diminution of the electricity of the atmosphere as compared with normal periods."

Burg's theory had far-reaching effects: after it was publicized in England in 1853, many citizens of New Orleans provided themselves with pieces of copper, which they carried as a protection. The same year, M.D. Gottengensis wrote to the *New York Daily Times,* recommending cholera be treated with sulphate of copper. He explained that salts of copper in large doses were speedily emetic; second, in small and oft-repeated doses they were "powerfully *tonic* and *styptic,* thereby counteracting the relaxation of the intestinal canal, which permits the infiltration of the fluid contents, producing the characteristic *rice-water dejections."* He tipped his cap to the editors by concluding, "I am pleased to find you desirous to inform the public on medical matters; nothing would more tend to eradicate quackery."[31]

A resurgence of the copper cure came in 1869 when homeopathic physicians promoted it as "the best medicine as a *preventative."* Using Dr. Burg's study that deaths among copper workers amounted to only 3:10,000, the French chemist M. Dumas presented the findings to the Academie des Sciences in Paris as an illustration of the law *similia similibus curantur.* In 1870 a subsequent report found that coppersmiths were exempt from cholera because they breathed sulphurous acid that prevented fermentation and thus destroyed cholera germs. The *Scientific American* noted, "This is the more remarkable when we consider that the salts of copper are all virulent poisons, and would seem to be another instance of the mutual destruction of deleterious influences."[32]

"Nearly 100 years since," wrote William Hooper Halse, professor of medical galvanism, in 1849, Mr. Wesley had expressed sentiments exactly similar to his own: that, "the ELECTRIC or GALVANIC FLUID is itself identical with the NERVOUS FLUID, and that a deficiency, or an irregular distribution of it to the various parts of the system, is the cause of most diseases." He added that Dr. Arnott, in *Elements of Physics,* stated, "Galvanism can excite the muscles to their usual actions; it affects the secretions and the digestive functions, and the breathing in Asthma."

According to this belief, cholera was most prevalent when the atmosphere was deficient of this electric fluid, "and that those whose bodies have not a full supply of it, are most likely to fall victims to the disease; whilst, on the contrary, those whose bodies are saturated with it, escape the ravages of the disease." Halse regretfully added, "We must not, however, expect the generality of the Medical Profession to recommend this simple agent, for the drug system, although it is to their patients Death, is to them Life."[33]

In June 1855 two Italian physicians, Dr. Rossi of Florence and Dr. Concata of Padua, made near simultaneous announcements that several cholera victims had been restored to health by means of electromagnetic current. Both concluded the disease resulted from some electro- or animal-magnetic disturbance for which galvanism was the proper remedy.[34]

Parboiling, Ice and Frictions

Steam baths were often favored as a means of curing cholera. The Cholera Hospital, Calton, was fitted with a special bed frame of tin tubes on which a thin cotton mattress was laid.

Using steam from a boiler, in a few minutes the temperature of the bed could be raised to 212° and the patient put into a profuse perspiration. Steam baths, warm baths and cold baths were also at hand if the doctor changed his prescription. Significantly, a disinfecting room for clothes and furniture was also provided, where the items were exposed to a high atmospheric temperature. The cost, it was observed, "is insignificant, compared to the advantages that may result from them."[35]

The use of water—its benefits, dangers and temperatures—was argued well beyond the mid–point of the 19th century. The *Journal of Health* advocated attention to the skin and stomach to avoid cholera. For the skin, it promoted daily frictions with a coarse towel and tepid or warm baths "twice, or at the least, once a week, or in lieu of this, daily sponging the surface with salt and water with the chill taken off it."[36] Professor Oertel, of Ansbach, Germany suggested "the most severe fasting—much drinking of cold water—much washing with cold water. In short, a complete inundation of the whole human body with cold water, both inwardly and outwardly!! ... If there exists the remedy against the effects of this fatal disease, it is positive and singly *cold fresh water!*—courageously, properly and perseveringly applied. Therefore, on such constitutions that apply cold water plentifully, both inwardly and outwardly, the Cholera will and can have no effect."[37]

An American took this one step further, avowing "pouring cold water in a continued stream upon the head, is one of the most effectual remedies in most cases of nervous or convulsive diseases," including histeria [*sic*], epilepsy, delirium tremens and catalepsy, as well as in convulsions of children from teething.[38] Under the heading "Abatement of Cholera," from the *Cincinnati Republican,* the question of ice was discussed, noting "some have a prejudice against meddling with it at all." Readers were assured that large draughts of excessively cold ice water were sometimes pernicious, but there was no objection "to the prudent and regulated use of that article. Ice creams, also, are safe and beneficial. They should always, however, be dissolved in the mouth. It is a mistake that ice, iced drinks, and ice cream should not be taken when the body is surrounded with a hot atmosphere. Then is the proper time."[39] Dr. R.W. Dudley, of Lexington, Kentucky, had a slightly different take: "Dashing buckets of cold water upon the entire surface was effectually tried in cases of collapse, without any of those pleasing results, so warmly urged upon the attention of the medical community by the advocates of that practice."[40]

Water Cure Establishments became popular again in the late 1860s. Promoting the "Roman or Turkish bath," numerous medical authorities, including Dr. Thudichum, promised treatments would control fatal symptoms of cholera, typhus, yellow fever and kidney disease.[41]

Under the Influence

James Hill, M.D., Resident Surgeon, Peckham House Asylum, was an early proponent of using chloroform to treat cholera patients. First suggested by assistant surgeon Francis Ferguson in 1848, the idea was to administer chloroform by inhalation for the purpose of tranquilizing the nervous system to stop vomiting and cramps. Out of 17 cases, five died, eight recovered and four remained under treatment.[42] Hill's letter eventually made it across the Atlantic, where the *Hillsdale Whig* published it March 27, 1849.

The most famous patient "cured" by ether was the author Alexandre Dumas. According to his own testimony, on April 15, 1832, he contracted "Asiatic, European, epidemic or contagious cholera" and was near death when his housekeeper brought him a glass filled with pure ether and a lump of sugar. He wrote, "To describe the convulsions caused by this diabolical liquid, as it traversed my torso, would be impossible, for I lost all consciousness almost immediately." After waking, he believed himself "dead or in hell," but after Dumas broke out into copious perspiration, a physician declared him cured.[43]

The use of chloroform and ether to treat cholera would prove to be of significance. Although the idea ultimately was determined to be false, the concept may have been one precipitating factor in Dr. John Snow's interest in tracing the path of disease. By 1854, when an epidemic devastated Soho, he had already earned a reputation as England's most eminent anesthesiologist, having had the honor to practice on Queen Victoria herself, with Dr. Ferguson assisting.

From his study of gas diffusion (discovered and analyzed by the Scottish chemist Thomas Graham), Snow first supported the theory that miasma, or poisons floating in the air, was so massively dispersed that it posed no health risk. Pertaining to cholera he was correct, but he erred on a larger scale, as industrial fumes were carcinogenic. Moving beyond that issue, as the respiratory system was relatively unaffected by cholera, he reevaluated the alimentary canal as the primary source of trouble. That suggested cholera was ingested, not inhaled, and his subsequent investigations mapping the local water supply around Golden Square led to the proof that would eventually immortalize him.[44]

M. Bruno Taron, surgeon-major of the Ottoman army and physician at Marseilles, claimed to have cured his own bout of cholera by inhaling freely of sulphuric ether, which he attributed to the power of ether over the nervous centers. As trials of this nature were common in the East, it was supposed "academies of medicine will doubtless gather positive information on this subject, and order new trials with all conditions which may render them decisive for science."[45]

Of lesser consequence, cholera played a small, ancillary role in the marketing of alcohol. In Britain, the Forbes Mackenzie Act dictated the closure of pubs on Sunday but it did not take long for druggists to supply the craving. As long as they sold whisky scented with camphor and tinted with burnt sugar, this "Sunday dram trade" was legal and enormously lucrative. Single doses were poured out of a medicine glass, while bottles were carefully labeled "cholera mixture." This trade was augmented by a liquid known as "finish"—a compound of methylated spirits and French polish used by furniture polishers. Known for its superior cheapness and strength, the Sunday dram quickly came in vogue. Undercover detectives vied for the opportunity of catching "druggist-shebeeners" selling whisky, until one druggist recognized the official and added croton oil to his purchase. The detective soon found he had consumed "cholera mixture with a vengeance" and thereafter fewer volunteers were found.[46]

Wine importers were also quick to promote their product. In 1865, a pint of claret was promoted as containing 10 grains of iron, a "full medical dose," while, "when properly administered," it was said to cure the most obstinate cases of cholera. Beer manufacturers in the United States, long maintaining their brew was health food (supported by the idea English and German ladies were healthy and pretty in consequence of their beer drinking), made the case that during the 1832 New York cholera epidemic and the English epidemic of 1849, none of the brewers died of it. It was also noted that mortality in New England was greater than in the middle and western states because of their "ultra temperance laws."[47]

The Medicine Chest

During the 1840s as the Second Cholera Pandemic raged, newspapers were filled with sure cures. In a carefully worded advertisement meant to convey approbation, Dr. Jaques Lemae offered "in conformity with the instructions issued by the Government General Board of Health," the "Asiatic Cholera Tincture" for an infallible remedy when taken in accordance with the directions of the seller, who incidentally supplied the government instructions with every bottle. He also sold the "Anti-Cholera Fumigations" for purifying the air of sick chambers. Money orders were to be sent to him at the impressive address of "Asiatic Cholera Tincture Depot."[48]

The Wholesale Herbary offered Grimstone's celebrated Herb Tobacco (prepared from medicinal herbs only) for the cure of colds, asthma and all pulmonary diseases. It also prevented the spread of infection by fumigation, especially useful against cholera.[49]

The celebrated French chemist M. Dumas was involved in a study involving the trichlorure of carbon, employed in Berlin as an "infallible remedy" for cholera,[50] while in the village of Hukeems, in Berar, the leaves of poodeena (mint), onion juice and black pepper were used.[51] More significant, another writer suggested "eating freely of common salt." The writer believed the beneficial effect probably depended "upon salt stimulating the digestive organs to produce a perfect digestion and assimilation of food," and to maintain "a more than usual saline condition of the blood; for it is well known that one of the earliest effects of cholera is to deprive the blood of its saline materials."[52] For preventing cholera, Dr. Searl suggested "Calomel, Socotrine aloes, and Castile soap," of each 20 grains, made into 12 pills." These increased the secretion of bile, thereby tending to purify the blood, open the bowels and excite all the functions.[53]

For a trifling expense, the "Patent Bed Feather Alkali Washing Factory" offered to rid beds and mattresses from all impurities in preparation against cholera.[54]

Pocket Medicine Boxes

In 1848 the Irish Central Board of Health published what they considered necessary components of the "pocket medicine-boxes" for hospitals to use in the treatment of cholera:

1. Powders—Carbonate of ammonia, in waxed papers, each paper containing 40 grains, to be dissolved in half a pint of water, giving 2 tablespoons every hour;
2. Powders—Compound powder of chalk with opium in packets containing 10 grains, giving one powder every half hour until looseness stops;
3. Pills of powdered opium, each containing ¼ of a grain of opium and 2 grains of powdered ginger, mixed with oil of peppermint, one pill given every half hour until looseness stops;
4. Pills of mercury and opium, each containing ¼ grain of calomel, 2 grains of hydrargyrum c. crota (mercury with chalk) and ¼ grain of opium, mixed with oil of caraway (which served to distinguish them from plain opium pills), given every half hour;
5. Bottles (1 or 2 ounce phials with cork stoppers) of:
    a. Tincture of opium (laudanum)
    b. Hoffman's liquor
    c. Tincture of rhatany
    d. Creosote

It was also recommended that a small jar of strong brown mustard be kept on hand.[55]

Creosote, mentioned above, is an oily liquid obtained by distillation of coal tar, used primarily in preserving wood. At mid–century it was considered by some "the most powerful of all antiseptics." In 1849, Henry Stephens published a treatise, the chief object of which was to promote his cure by showing "that the means of preserving organised bodies from decay, pointed to the only true curative principle in the treatment of fevers generally, and more specifically cholera." Offering several testimonials, he then provided his formula:

Creosote	1 to 2 drams
Spirits of Wine	5 do.
Tincture of Opium	1½ oz.
Aromatic Spirit of Ammonia	4 oz.
Oil of Peppermint	1 dram
Oil of Cinnamon	1 do.
Distilled Water	24 oz.

After the ingredients were mixed, this made a quart imperial measure, of which 1–3 tablespoons might be taken and repeated according to the urgency of the case. Stephens suggested every person carry a vial of creosote and take 1–3 drops upon a lump of sugar occasionally as a great preventative.

Likely unconvinced by Stephens' claims, an editorial running in the same paper asked, "Being thankful for the cures or recoveries which undoubtedly take place under their hands, we, nevertheless, cannot help asking our doctors is there no guiding principle in the treatment of disease; but is medicine nothing better that a *sortes Virgilianae*—a great gallipot lottery in which chance determines the prizes and the blanks?"[56]

If creosote and physicians failed, a recipe from Dantzig suggested better results by using "a morsel of mineral coal the size of a walnut, a piece of ginger of the same size, four or five laurel berries peeled, and two tablespoons of common tansy (*rheinfarrenkraut*); the whole pulverized and mixed with hot tea, or even water, and swallowed warm, much tea to be drank afterwards."[57] A different authority from Kioffa, Russia, administered 1½ glasses of spirits of wine and water with 4–5 teaspoonfuls of powdered charcoal and 3 drops of oil of mint; afterward the patient was to take violent exercise until perspiring strongly. As an antidote for himself, every morning the author consumed 1 teaspoonful of charcoal mixed in a fresh egg. The charcoal used was from beech trees, but "any wood that is free from rosin will do."[58]

After observing the "total failure in all remedies hitherto proposed" to cure cholera, Dr. G.J. Berwick of the Bengal medical service became drawn to the resemblance between that disease and jungle fever "arising from malaria or marsh miasma." He determined that quinine exercised the same controlling power over cholera as it did over jungle fever "or any other disease arising from that peculiar atmospheric state which has been termed malaria." Using quinine at Dum-Dum, where he had charge of a body of European artillery, he found it allayed the irritability of the stomach, quieted the spasmodic muscular action, and neutralized the "morbific poison, the cause of the disease."[59]

A homeopathic medicine chest would look significantly different than one kept by "regular" physicians. In 1865 homeopathic medicines for the treatment of cholera included the following:

Tincture of Camphor
Tincture of Arsenicum, 3rd decimal
Trituration of Cuprum Aceticum, 1st centesimal
Tincture of Ipecacuanha, 1st centesimal
Tincture of Mercurius Corros, 3rd decimal

Tincture of Veratrum, 1st centesimal
Trituration of Carbo-Vegetabilis, 3rd decimal
Tincture of Iris Versicolor, 1st centesimal

Water used to mix the preparations was to be as pure as possible; where distilled water was not available, filtered water or water that had been boiled and allowed to grow cold was used. Twenty drops of the tincture or 12 grains of the trituration was the usual dose. In the case of diarrhea, 1 teaspoonful was required; in Asiatic cholera, a desert spoonful. In severe cases, a tablespoonful served. In cholera, the dose was given every 10–15 minutes until improvement. As a preventative, 1 grain of cupeum acet. was suggested every night and morning. A solution of sulphate of copper was also used as a fomentation, applied on flannel and placed on the abdomen and spine.[60]

In 1866 Dr. Rubini of Naples announced the cure of 592 cases of cholera by the saturated spirits of camphor. (Ordinary spirits of camphor consisted of 1 part camphor to 9 parts wine; Rubini used a mixture of equal camphor and wine. By comparison, the homeopathic preparation was made by mixing 1 part camphor to 5 of spirits of wine.) Subsequent research by Dr. Quin did not duplicate the positive results, leading to the disclaimer that the treatment had to be started from the commencement of the disease.[61]

Equipment and supplies for a 21st century cholera field treatment center are simplified considerably:

Rehydration supplies:
    240 liters of lactated Ringers
    Disposable syringes and needles
    Nasogastric tubes
    1,300 packets of Oral Rehydration Solution (ORS) for 1 liter each
Antibiotics:
    3,200 capsules of tetracycline 250mg capsules
    600 doxycycline 100mg capsules
Other supplies:
    Water dispensers for making ORS in bulk
    20 liter bottles, 40 tumblers
    Kidney pans, spirit lamps
    Disinfectant, soap, bleaching powder.[62]

Curatives, Restoratives, Solemn Truths and a Coroner's Inquest

Absolute proof in the belief of cholera cures came from England, where a bottle of "cholera mixture" was kept against emergencies in the front lodge of the Bank of England from the 1833 epidemic through at least 1932.[63]

Brandreth's Pills were some of the most advertised of all the anti-cholera nostrums. In 1848, under the title "Twelve-Fold in Ten Years," its creator claimed, "Can any other medicine be pointed out that has sustained its reputation—that has increased in the confidence of the public in an equal proportion?" Using the preposterous claim "no malady—no, not even Cholera, would be of a dangerous character" were these pills "vigorously resorted to when the first symptoms were perceived," the advert continued: when "over two millions of our citizens have approved," they became "no longer a private, but a public medicine."

Close behind were "Morison's Pills," first appearing in the 1820s. Manufactured and promoted by the Society of Hygeists at the British College of Health (see chapter 7), the pills were said to work by cleansing the system. By 1866 the society used quotes from Dr. George Johnson, the famous "Caster Oil Man," who advocated "purging and vomiting" as the only means of curing cholera. At the same time, the society accused Johnson of plagiarizing James Morison's "Hygeian system" as his own. (To put the Society of Hygeists in context, they also believed that smallpox could be cured only by vegetable purgation and they delighted in the fact that the newly formed Anti-Vaccination League would number the days of vaccination.)

Affixing the name of a physician to a "medicine" or a testimonial was a common way of supplying instant credence. In 1835, advertisements for "Dr. D. Jayne's Carminative Balsam" supplied the names of doctors from New Jersey, Connecticut, Maryland, Virginia and Pennsylvania. Having already been three or four years before the public, the maker vowed its product, "put up in round brass moulded vials" of 2 and 4 ounces each, had repeatedly effected cures when every other means failed and promised the "medicine" would suppress cramps attending malignant cholera in from one to three minutes. Dr. G.C. Vaughn's "Vegetable Lithontriptic Mixture" was not only promoted by using a long, indigestible word in its title, it also was marketed as being the "Great American Remedy," associated with the Western New York College of Health, which may or may not have been an institution of higher learning.

To the 19th century pitchman, all that mattered were sales: if stretching the truth, or stating an outright lie, sold product, nothing else mattered. No statement was too brash to use. In 1849, bold, capital letters proclaimed, "CHOLERA PREVENTED by the CONSTANT USE of the PYRETIC SALTS," which "received the recommendation of the physicians to the Cholera Hospital." In England, where titles were tantamount to respectability, "Sir William Burnett's Patent Disinfecting Fluid" for the prevention of cholera and contagious diseases was offered as the "Cheapest, and the Most Healthful" deodorizer and purifying agent.

Once a brand had been established, the public was encouraged to "ask for it by name." The makers of the "Rev. R. Hibbard's Vegetable Anti-Billious Family Pills" (note the use of the nearly failsafe "reverend" and "family") urged buyers to beware that a "spurious article is not imposed upon you." Protecting a brand name reached a ludicrous point in 1834 when Lewis Wickey asserted that a "fellow" named David Tschudy claimed to have purchased the receipt (recipe) for "Wickey's Cholera Medicine" and was selling it without Wickey's permission. The latter responded by stating Wickey was "entirely mistaken." In response to these published letters, George W. Hays (presumably another agent) sarcastically noted Wickey, "who is nicknamed Dr ... is an illiterate quack—He can tell you the price and quality of a Glass of Brandy or wine, but as to common decency he is ignorant." After further elucidation that Wickey was "a sap headed ninnyhammer," Hays added that no one had ever heard of Tschudy and he certainly did not sell the cholera medicine.

Immediately under the above was another ad for "Cholera Medicine," sold by J.G. Beard, being an agent for Dr. P. Fabracy, "who has purchased the receipt of the inventor, Dr. Louis [*sic*] Wickey."

Amid the name-calling and miraculous claims lay a dark side to these popular over-the-counter mixtures. In 1854 a coroner's inquest was held on the death of Miss Anne Colyer, who had taken "Waterton's Cholera Specifics" as a cure for cholera. Mr. Rodgers, lecturer on chemistry at St. George's School of Medicine, London, analyzed the medicine and found it contained "a large quantity of ammonia, so strong it destroyed the cork in the phial." The jury returned after half an hour with a verdict of death by cholera, "accelerated by the use of Waterton's medicines."[64]

The "Diet Table" During the Prevalence of Epidemic Cholera

The role of diet, either in causing or curing cholera, was a continuing theme throughout the 19th century. In 1832, one author explained the greater severity of cholera in France than in England by suggesting the food of the poor in Paris consisted of "*haricots* (horsebeans), lentils, and other pulse [legumes]—sallad (composed of every species of green trash, haricots, and often of cold potatoes, sliced in salt and vinegar)—a few of them able to add to their haricots grease lard, or pan of pork." This diet, along with "great dram-drinking," predisposed the human frame to disease.[65] Added to the list of dangerous foods were unripe and unwholesome fruits that brought on "peculiar and temporary" disturbances.[66] On the other side of the spectrum, physicians at Constantinople recommended figs as a preventative of cholera. They were said to exercise a healing influence on diseases that manifested themselves in a derangement of the digestive functions and "commonly precede an attack of the cholera," while in Berar, the leaves of poodeena (mint), onion juice and black pepper were employed as a curative in severe cases. Slightly more palatable was wine and jelly made from English black currents, said to arrest early stages of cholera.[67]

As early as 1834, an enlightened London medical correspondent wrote the following:

> The causes which especially predispose to an attack of cholera are a weakened state of the lining of the stomach and alimentary canal.—This state is so decidedly obviated by eating freely of common salt with our meals that I believe full two-thirds of the cases which occur, might be prevented by having recourse to this simple preservative remedy. The quantity taken should be exactly what the stomach will bear without after inconvenience; from one-quarter to one-third of an ounce during the day is sufficient.

He added that it was "absurd" to suppose fresh fish, vegetables and ripe fruit predisposed a person to cholera. When taken in moderation, they lessened "the susceptibility to all disorders."[68] Although the use of salt/saline was vital to the simple rehydration process that would eventually be used as a cure, those advocating its use never succeeded in convincing medical authorities or the public. It would not be until the 20th century that its importance was recognized and it was universally administered. That left nearly 100 years for doctors and laymen to argue over the benefits and dangers of that four-letter word, "food."

In 1848, Dr. Toogood Downing recommended the following selection of food to sustain a proper constitution during the visitation of cholera in England presumably, his meal plan was meant for those with discretionary spending:

> BREAKFAST: Bread, baked previous day; toasted bread, biscuit; rusk, with butter; an egg, boiled 3½ minutes; mutton chop; cold chicken. To drink: tea, coffee, milk, water.
>
> DINNER: Mutton, boiled or roasted; roast beef; eggs, boiled or poached; boiled or roast fowl; tripe; rabbit; minced veal; sago; tapioca; arrowroot; semolina; rice; rice-milk; bread; biscuit; light puddings; mealy potatoes. To drink: toast-and-water; weak brandy-and-water; bitter ale; sherry-and-water; porter; stout.
>
> TEA: Bread and butter; dry toast; rusk; plain seed-cake; biscuit. To drink: coffee, black tea.
>
> LUNCHEON or SUPPER: A few oysters or a small mutton chop with bread.

A few glasses of good wine, port, sherry, or Madeira, spiced negus, warm brandy or rum and water might be taken during the day with discretion. Light meals should be eaten every fourth or fifth hour and much fat should be avoided. Care should be taken to properly masticate food and rest was suggested after meals.[69]

DWELLINGS OF THE INDUSTRIOUS CLASSES

If prevention were the best cure, Dr. Southwood Smith (a member of the General Board of Health, London) provided proofs in his 22-page, 1845 pamphlet, *Results of Sanitary Improvement; Illustrated by the Operation of the Metropolitan Societies for Improving the Dwellings of the Industrious Classes, the Working of the Common Lodging-Houses Act, &c.* The idea had its origins in the early 1840s, when several philanthropic gentlemen formed an association for the purpose of testing their convictions by experiment. Their plan was to erect a large building, properly divided into suites or apartments capable of accommodating a number of families with the following sanitary conditions:

1. The thorough subsoil drainage of the site;
2. The free admission of air and light to every inhabited room;
3. The abolition of the cesspool and the substitution of the watercloset, involving complete house drainage.
4. An abundant supply of pure water;
5. Means for the immediate removal of all solid house refuse not capable of suspension in water or of being carried off by water.

The Metropolitan buildings, Old Pancras Road, were constructed and the apartments let primarily to artisans or the better-paid laborers. Dr. Smith's results indicated the following:

1. In 1850, total population was 560, with 7 deaths;
2. In 1851, total population was 600, with 9 deaths;
3. In 1852, total population was 680, with 9 deaths;
4. In March 1853 at full occupancy (1,343, of which 490 were under 10 years), there were 10 deaths, five of whom were under 10 years.

By comparison, in 1853 at the Potteries (in the poor quarter), the population was approximately 1,263, with 384 children under the age of 10. Total death from all causes was 51, of which 42 were children under age 10. Deaths for the whole of London were three times that of the metropolitan buildings, while at the Potteries, mortality was nearly six times greater. Among children under 10, deaths in London were 4½ times greater and at the Potteries 10 times more numerous. While deaths in the general population of London averaged 12 percent from typhus and cholera, not a single case was reported at the "Model Dwellings."

Just as significant to Dr. Smith, he maintained that while "natural life has been prolonged, moral health has also been promoted," affirming "the intemperate have become sober, and the disorderly well-conducted, since taking up their abode in these healthy and peaceful dwellings."

In addition to proving their theory that sanitary measures promoted health and well-being, there lay a pecuniary motive, amply demonstrated by the fact "an interest [in the Metropolitan] of about 5 per cent. may be certainly counted upon.... No inconsiderable portion of Railway property is far less secure and profitable than these buildings." One editorialist noted "the establishment of a society, with a subscribed capital of £45,000, for the erection of suburban villas and villages for working men, is another proof that the most truly benevolent work of the day is engaging the head of the capitalist as well as the heart of the philanthropist."

Not everyone applauded Smith's efforts. One editorialist questioned the viability of such a project, stating that unless it paid 7½ percent on investments, other builders would not be tempted to follow suit, and even if they did, the 4–5 shillings per week rent was well beyond the means of the average laborer. A different slant was taken by another writer, who noted that those who dwelt in the Metropolitan were people likely to live wholesomely, while those who lived in the Potteries and Jacob's Island were allowed to wallow in their mire, "so long as the General Board of Health allow such places to exist."[70]

By 1873, New York authorities advocated direct ventilation in houses as a means of warding off cholera by diminishing the evil effects of defective pipes and untrapped sewers, noting "fresh air is one of the best preventatives against its attacks."[71]

Homeopathy vs. Allopathy

Although not the originator of homeopathy, Dr. Samuel Hahnemann popularized the idea in the early 1800s. His theory held that a sick person could be cured if given minute doses of a substance that caused similar symptoms in a healthy one. He called this "the law of similia," and his method of healing "homeopathy," from the Greek *homoios* (like) and *pathos* (suffering). He likewise originated the word "allopathy" (meaning the opposite of suffering; commonly spelled "alopathy" in the mid–1800s) for the conventional system of medicine. The *Taber's* defines "allopathy" as "a system of treating disease by inducing a pathological reaction that is antagonistic to the disease being treated" and notes it is erroneously used to differentiate it from homeopathy. Homeopathy is defined as being based on the idea that very dilute doses of medicine that produce symptoms of a disease in healthy people will cure that disease in affected patients. It differed from traditional medicine in that it emphasized stimulating the body to heal itself.[72]

From the beginning, proponents of both sides waged verbal and print war on the other, citing and interpreting statistics to favor their causes. Typical of the times was an article in the *New York Tribune*:

> The number of deaths from cholera, in England, under homeopathic treatment, have been from 5 to 12 per cent, while the deaths from the same disease under alopathic treatment have been from 50 to 60 per cent. Should these be facts, it is time for an examination of the subject. If so much greater number recovered by administering next to nothing, certainly all would have recovered if they had administered nothing. Viva la humbug![73]

Describing homeopathy in 1849, one writer reported there were 3,000 practitioners in the United States, most of whom were graduates of the "old school" before converting to the new system. During cholera visitations, homeopathic physicians promoted diet as being of critical importance, urging the consumption of roast beef, mutton and beefsteak, good potatoes, boiled or roasted; no other vegetables and no fruits or pastries.[74] This strict regime of diet resulted in several prosecutions, one of which was presented under headlines: "Death From Starvation Under Homeopathic Treatment," "Verdict of Manslaughter Against a Homeopathic Surgeon" and "Alleged Death from Homeopathic Treatment." Originating in England, the coroner's inquest determined that the cholera patient Richard Pearce was given only beef tea and arrowroot, and "pills too tiny to see without glasses." After an exhaustive examination and conflicting testimony on whether the man died of "exhaustion" from lack of food or from cholera, the jury concluded Charles Thomas Pearce "did improperly and unskillfully treat and manage the said Richard Pearce for the cure of a natural disease," concluding C.T. Pearce was guilty of manslaughter. He was consigned to Newgate Prison.[75]

Around the same time, it was reported that 22 homeopathic physicians in New York and Brooklyn had treated 162 cholera cases with only 23 fatalities, causing the *London Spectator* to agonize over claims and cures, asking, "Calomel, or saline solutions, or infinitesimal doses of white hellebore—to which of these shall we have recourse under the visitation of this terrible epidemic?"[76]

An article appearing in August 1849 in the *Cincinnati Methodist Expositor* (reprinted in the *Daily Times,* August 13, 1849) brought into question the published data of two homeopathic physicians, J.H. Pulte (also spelled Pulti) and B. Ehrmann. Sarcastically noting their claims brought on "the loudest blast of the trumpet since the falling of the walls of Jerico," an extract of their report stated that the doctors had treated 1,116 cholera patients between May 1 and August 1, of which 638 exhibited vomiting, diarrhea and cramps; of these, 60–70 were in a deep state of collapse. The others were prevented from running into a higher state of disease by early application of proper homeopathic medicines. A great many of the collapsed cases were cured, success depending on which medicines were used in the early stages. Of those improperly treated by opiates (by allopaths), success proved difficult. Besides the cholera cases, they treated 1,350 cases of diarrhea and dysentery and lost none.

The homeopathic treatment consisted of camphora, the tincture of which was prepared in the proportion of 1 part of the gum to 6 parts alcohol, as prescribed by Dr. Hannemann in 1829. One or two drops were given every five minutes until profuse perspiration ensued. If the disease progressed into the second stage, veratrum, cuprum, secale cornutum (ergot) were administered; in the case of collapse, carbo (vegetabilis coal) and arsenicum (the latter two in the 30th dilution), were added.

The authors of the *Expositor* (a religious journal) objected to the physicians' conclusions on two grounds: first, that it was "undignified and unprofessional to appear in the public prints in praise of one's self," and second, it was "immoral," in that the doctors used strong doses of camphor, making them allopaths. An equally lengthy rejoinder by a homeopathic physician in Janesville, Wisconsin, detailed Pulti and Ehrmann's two acknowledged deaths, denied that seven other deaths were caused by their treatments and defended the use of camphor as a homeopathic medicine.[77]

The Air We Breathe

Contamination by atmospheric dust was first propounded in the late 17th century by Bishop Berkeley, who noted "the whole atmosphere seems alive. There is everywhere acid to corrode and seed to engender. Iron will ruse and mould will grow in all places." By 1846, Robert Angus Smith demonstrated that breath was laden with organic matter and if condensed and preserved for a week, it became the abode of small animals capable of detection by microscope. Louis Pasteur's experiments on spontaneous generation proved that carefully filtered air allowed no organisms to appear in vegetable solutions, but this was used as proof that organisms "owed their origin to germs floating in the air."[78]

This idea perpetuated the notion that cholera was caused or spread, perhaps both, by airborne contagion. One lingering belief held that when the air was deficient of ozone, the disease was likely to appear. This idea obtained considerable traction in the mid–19th century, and the newspapers were filled with theories and dire warnings. It was not without its detractors, however. After a heavy rain has just passed, one writer for the *Cincinnati Enquirer* noted, "If there was any *ozone* in the atmosphere before, the storm of last night week must have entirely driven it away. But the epidemic still rages—decreasing one day and then mounting still higher the next.[79]

The ozone discussion persisting into 1865, M. Allnutt proposed a solution to the problem by adding ozone into the sick room where cholera patients rested. He suggested placing a small piece of phosphorus, half an inch long, in a quart bottle: "Half cover the phosphorus with water, then cork the bottle with a cork in which is cut a notch, to allow the vapour slowly to exude. Care must be taken not to allow this phosphorous vapour to act too long, as an overdose of ozonized air is hurtful to animal life. One hour is long enough to ozonize the air of a large bedroom."[80]

Microscopic analysis in 1872 "proved" that animal or vegetable life in the air caused disease. Dr. Salisbury took atmospheric samples from a Southern bayou to Chicago, where he released it into a man's chamber; within days the individual contracted chills and fever and "living things" were found on his tongue. It was expected this discovery would confirm cholera originated from the atmosphere.[81] In an article entitled, "How to Keep Off Pestilence," the *New York Times* (April 4, 1872) noted that a large number of maladies fell under the generic name of "foul air diseases," including scarlet fever, diphtheria, typhoid, cholera and smallpox. In a warning to those New Yorkers who felt protected by their money, the author cautioned, "The wealthy lady of Fifth-avenue, and the carefully-nurtured children on Park-avenue, must breathe every morning the germs which have just come from the fever-nests of the Five Points or the cholera-heaps of Mackerelville." In line with this, articles appearing in various newspapers around the world throughout the 19th century reported the supposed connection between the absence of birds and epidemic diseases in the air. A typical report from London asserted that birds left affected districts and did not return until the first decrease in the disease.[82]

At times, "the air we breathe" fell into the category of "remedy." During cholera epidemics at Vienna in the 1870s, a substance called "camphorein" was prepared by passing chlorine gas into pure turpentine oil until saturated; this produced a thick, heavy, oily brown fluid with a strong smell of chlorine. It was freed from muriatic acid by washing with water and given to patients to inhale, reportedly with great success.[83]

Sanitation and Disinfection

The use of disinfectants, by whatever name, existed for centuries before it became a recognized science in the 19th century. Ancients burned pitch and sulphur to cleanse the atmosphere, sprinkled vinegar in sick rooms and employed odoriferous substances to mask smells in the belief they minimized or eliminated danger. The first major step toward modern sanitation came in 1773 when Guyton Morveau fumigated hospitals with muriatic (hydrochloric) acid. Dr. Carmichael Smyth followed in 1802 when he received a £5,000 grant from Parliament to perform the same service with nitrous fumes. Chlorine superseded both, while carbolic acid was used in sewers.

Unfortunately, authorities such as Robert Angus Smith supported the German physician Pettenkofer's theory that soil had powerful disinfecting powers, enabling it to absorb germs while remaining pure. Only areas with porous or permeable soil, weakened by the recession of ground water, were capable of sustaining epidemics. Pettenkofer's idea was so persuasive it delayed acceptance of the water-borne hypothesis advocated by Drs. Snow and Budd.[84]

Sanitary reform took a huge step forward with the establishment of the New York Board of Health in 1866. The new board's immediate challenge was the cholera epidemic then raging in the city that "threatened a dire visitation [and] was effectually battled against, dislodged, and finally stamped out" by a combination of modalities: science, sanitation and statistics. Inspectors clearly traced the source of cholera, streets and sewers were cleaned and an accurate system for the registration of deaths, marriages and births was instituted. The cost for all this amounted to $250,000, "far below the amount squandered under the old disgraceful *regime.*"

In their first annual report, "Epidemic Cholera in the Metropolitan Sanitary District during the year 1866," the Board of Health set out its accomplishments. Having replaced "pot-house politicians" (one of whom described hygiene as something that "smelt bad"), the new commissioners greatly mitigated the distress of the city. Among their achievements was the banishment of butchers and bone-boilers to the suburbs, the elimination of cattle-driving through the streets by daylight, and correction of defective sewage pipes, which greatly improved sanitary conditions for tenement and private dwellings.

Compared to the epidemic of 1854 where mortality from cholera and cholera morbus reached 2,810, in 1866 the death toll numbered only 1,435. Deaths from diarrhea, dysentery and cholera infantum in 1854 was 2,592, compared to 3,524 in 1866. The increase was attributed to population growth, the gradual increase in fatal diarrheal diseases and more accurate reporting.

In addition, the board of health embraced theories based on the work of the English authorities Farr, Simon and Budd, who dictated that excreta from the sick "were the only means of propagating and spreading the Asiatic Cholera." The liberal use of disinfectants was attributed to lower mortality and such efforts were promised to continue, "until every class of the population is surrounded by the safeguards of hygiene."

In reviewing the new board of health's accomplishments, the sanitary committee held one black mark against it: the failure to acquire land accommodation for passengers arriving on infected vessels. In defending any lack of progress on that front, board members argued they had made a gallant attempt to establish quarantine sites but faced dramatic opposition from inhabitants living near selected parcels. Complicating matters, "the General Government refused them either Sandy Hook or Bedloe's Island, and the Courts drove them from Seguine's Point." This forced the necessity of housing infected immigrants in narrow, cramped floating hulks. The two organizations did agree that if there was to be quarantine at all, it should be upon land.[85]

In a follow-up article, the *New-York Times* ran a comprehensive discussion on the subject of disinfection, noting the fact "we persistently create those sources of evil that we are compelled to destroy." The idea of using disinfectants to combat cholera was attributed to William Budd. His letter on the subject in 1849 greatly influenced European and Continental scientists as well as Dr. Elisha Harris of New York, who, in 1854 attempted to stamp out infectious diseases by the use of carbolic acid.

Carbolic acid was obtained from coal tar, either by distillation or chemical process, and could be produced in sufficient quantities for sanitary purposes for less than $2 a gallon. It did not exist in large amounts, however, as 100 gallons of tar contained about 2 gallons of acid. What was called in New York the "dead oil of coal-tar" was four times as rich in the disinfectant as the coal-tar itself. In 1866 the board of health was among the first body to apply disinfectants, scientifically and upon a large scale, for the purpose of controlling and preventing the spread of epidemic cholera.

Second to carbolic acid was sulphate of iron in a ratio of 1 pound of copperas to 1 gallon of water. This disinfectant was advocated by Pettenkofer, who also taught that cholera patients could be attended with perfect impunity if rooms were kept clean and soiled linen was washed with boiling soapsuds. Where disinfectants were needed around sewers, drains and foul places, a combination of both was even more effective. The use of chlorine (widely used on ships infected with yellow fever), however, was considered worthless as a disinfectant, although its value as a deodorant was not disputed.[86]

The main complaint by London hygienists came against such trades as tar distilling, soap making, blood baking, naphtha refining, bone boiling, butter making and animal charcoal makers who "proceed to do as much as possible to neutralise the good effects of sanitary reform." While making few inroads against those in commerce, some success was achieved when the East London Waterworks, responsible for the epidemic in 1866, determined to decrease the supply of water to East London on the philosophy of "better have scarce pure water, than plentiful impurity."[87]

The Definition of "Disinfectant" (1880)

A true disinfectant is anything which, when added in moderate proportion, will destroy the life of "bacteria" (microscopic beings belonging to the vegetable kingdom) and stop putrefactive decomposition; also, inferentially it will destroy the disease germs. A true disinfectant must be antiseptic; that is, it must possess the power to destroy or to render inert the products of the decomposition of organic matter, or the morbid action in the living body, through the agency of a reaction, in which the disinfectant itself undergoes chemical destruction.

To change smell by deodorizers is not to disinfect: the product of decomposition is still present but by overwhelming the nostrils, can no longer be detected.

Disinfectants are classified by physical condition: as in solids, lime, dry earth, ashes, etc; the fluids, such as mineral acids, and solutions of the salts of almost all metals; and the gaseous, as ozone, nitrous and sulphurous acids, Chlorine, bromine, iodine, etc. Imponderables such as heat and light are also included.[88]

Neuro-Physiology, Therapeutics and Imagination

Although Dr. John Chapman of London had tried his remedy on only one cholera patient, he felt free to write a pamphlet, "Diarrhoea and Cholera" (1865), announcing his theories and cure for the disease. Purporting to show that the fatal character of diarrhea was caused by "heat or motion and nervous irritation," he inferred that the malady was "essentially influenced by atmospheric temperature." Considering diarrhea and cholera essentially the same disease, he sited statistics to prove his point: "The largest total annual mortality from diarrhoea occurred in England in 1857, when the deaths from this cause numbered 21,189, the deaths from cholera being 1,150. In 1854, when the mortality from the latter disease was 20,097, the deaths from diarrhoea amounted to 20,052."

More interestingly, Chapman believed mental emotion was productive of diarrhea, stating "cholera is neither contagious nor infectious in any sense whatever except through the depressing influences of fear" and offering five examples of women who suffered from the malady after stress. The most amusing of his cases concerned a woman who complained diarrhea had been brought on by reading George Eliot's *Romola.* Her "preternatural excitability" was cured by the application of ice bags made of India rubber divided into cells and placed along the spine; ice taken internally, however, was, according to Chapman, to be strictly avoided.

The use of ice along the spinal cord was believed to modify the temperature of the spinal region, eliminating diarrhea that was caused by "the combined action of the hyperaemic spinal cord and sympathetic nervous centres, in the same manner as they induce phenomena ... in summer cases of diarrhoea, and of sea-sickness."

Ignoring the use of proven drugs (veratrum album, cuprum and jatropha), Chapman's method was based on Claude Bernard's discovery that one of the functions of the sympathetic nerve was to give tone to the arterial system of blood vessels, constricting them when the force was greatest and expanding them when the force was lessened. Chapman speculated that action of the spinal nerves on the glandular system was produced by heat and cold to the spine, leading to his treatment. In a review of his work, one author opined, "Dr. Chapman's is one of the most signal exceptions to the rule that physiological discovery has been barren of therapeutic suggestions."

Later the same year, Chapman tested his treatment in Southampton, claiming to have been successful in four out of six cases. In his 1871 pamphlet, "Cases of Diarrhoea and Cholera," he purported that noxious effluvia excited the "already hyperaesthetic brain and spinal cord" of those exposed to solar heat, exciting diarrhea and cholera. Considering the amount of press and praise Chapman received, this minute sampling was indicative of how desperate people were for a simple, immediate cure with scientific overtones.

Henry F. Roberts of Pittsburg held a similar idea. In 1872 he claimed Asiatic cholera was "a *disease of the nerves*, and not of the bowels at all" resulting from a derangement of the nervous system "by which the blood ceases to circulate in the capillary or small vessels on the surface of the body," producing no serious effects until it extended to the larger vessels.[89]

The idea that imagination played a large part in health was not unique to Chapman. Writing for the *Boston Post,* one columnist cited the physiological law advocated by Francois-Joseph-Victor Broussais (1772–1838): "When the thoughts are directed to a certain portion of the human organism it causes a determination of nervous influence, perhaps of the blood, to that part of the system." In other words, thoughts about cholera, mingled with fears, could invite the disease. Broussais' 1816 work, "The Examination of Medical Doctrines," purported that all disease originated as an irritation of the gastrointestinal tract that passed to other organs "sympathetically." Treatment was aimed at controlling inflammation through the administration of relaxants, bloodletting and leaches. His ideas became popular in Paris but fell out of favor in 1832 after his treatment of cholera patients ended disastrously.[90]

One story on the influence of fear occurred in a Paris hospital in 1853 when a nurse was assigned to watch a patient recently admitted with cholera. The nurse, known to be morbidly afraid of the disease, was not told of the diagnosis, but when a Sister stopped to inquire of the patient, she "happened to let out the secret." The nurse dropped to the floor in a swoon. After being revived, he developed diarrhea and died the following day.

One common story about the influence of imagination related how a family member died on the spot after viewing movement in the corpse of a recently deceased cholera victim. The action was explained by the "well known fact" that persons who died of cholera retained the warmth of the blood for a long time, frequently alarming bystanders by contraction of the muscles. Another oft-repeated story involved a prisoner who was promised a pardon if he would lie in the bed of a recently deceased cholera patient. The prisoner subsequently developed "a regular attack," owing to imagination.[91]

Religion and Cholera Cures

Religion, of course, had its own role to play, although not without contention. One writer, in commenting on the English cholera panic of 1854, began with a history lesson. He remarked that at the beginning of the 14th century when signs of the black plague appeared, the inhabitants of London, "instead of accurately examining the influences which affected their health, immediately ascribed their danger to the use of sea-coal." They petitioned the king to abolish that fuel and "from that time to this people have been quite as ready to reflect upon the mercy and wisdom of Providence as to believe in the slightest dereliction of duty on their part." He continued:

> Nothing can be more ridiculous or hypocritical than to talk of humbling ourselves, and repenting our sins, if only the cholera pass away from us, while we go up, like the beggarly deputation from Hammersmith, and pray the Commissioners not to make us pay a few farthings each for the sake of the public health. It is quite true that the epidemic which has afflicted us is the consequence of a national sin; but that sin is, not Protestantism, as the POPE says; nor preaching in surplices, as one party affirms; not going to war, as the lovers of peace declare; but stinginess combined with indolence; for from the union of these two prolific causes have sprung the whole brood—indecency, dirt, and nuisance, generating typhus, cholera, and putrid fever, which annually cut off thousands of victims.

More cuttingly, B.H. Cowper of the Evangelical Continental Society mentioned that while in Liege in 1859 there was a "cheap and easy remedy" offered for sale at booksellers in the form of a small handbill costing four cents. On it was printed, "Prayer to be stuck up on the inner door of one's house, in order to be preserved from cholera and every other misfortune." Below was an image of the Virgin Mary with a prayer for protection. Cowper concluded, "Can any superstition or idolatry go further than this?"

Intolerance was not limited to Protestants and Roman Catholics. In 1849 an "extraordinary case of neglect" was charged against the elders of "a sect called Latter day Saints" for their treatment of two sisters who came to them suffering from cholera. Rather than summon a doctor, the group joined in prayer, administered brandy and covered the sisters with hot flannels. After the sisters died, the elder "was not so spiritually minded" as to prefer a charge of 10s for arrears of rent and 12s for medicine, medical attendance and funeral charges.[92]

"Miracle mongers" were at work in Cadiz in 1854 at the hands of some Malays. Their technique consisted of using a form of massage on the victim's breast and abdomen until small round substances were found under the skin and crushed. The method was employed on the belief that little worms attached to the heart caused cholera. Once the worms were coaxed out and destroyed, the patient instantly recovered. The *American Medical Monthly* (November 1854) reported the Malays asked for no fees and the superstitious of the city flocked to them. Also on the subject of "seen and not believed" was the Chinese technique of sticking a pin under the tongue, below the roots of fingernails and in the pit of the stomach to cure cholera.[93]

In 1871, people living at Dawydkowo, near Moscow, combined superstition with more conventional religion by putting into action a new plan. Twelve virgins led by a widow and her bairn dragged a plow around the boundaries of their parish at the witching hour of midnight in hopes the furrow would keep cholera at bay. Orthodox clergy followed, blessing their efforts.[94]

"Like a thief in the night"

One of the most persistent beliefs in the 1800s was that elevation protected against cholera. Without putting together the idea that dwellings situated above and away from rivers were those least likely to receive water from contaminated low-lying sources, numerous authorities continued to purport that the disease had "never risen to any great height perpendicularly." Citing the fact that while Moscow, on the low banks of the Moskwa, was repeatedly invaded by cholera, the elevated Kremlin and monasteries with high walls in Italy, France and Spain uniformly escaped. Dr. T.S. Bell of Louisville argued that sleeping in the second story of any good residence was as important a preventative as any other. He also believed another common misconception that cholera acted "alone at night and upon sleeping persons." According to him, the "wakeful, moving individual" was in no peril from the disease that stole "like a thief in the night."[95]

Of more use for those who occasionally felt the urge to sleep, the London Metropolitan Free Drinking Fountains Association was formed to eliminate the need of drawing water from slimy water butts. By 1866, the association had already constructed 140 well-maintained fountains in London from which 8,000 persons a day were known to drink daily and which served over 300,000 during the summer.[96]

Advances and "Some Stupidities"

Under the heading "Some Stupidities," it was reported in 1869 that the ravages of cholera were due to the influence of smallpox vaccination on the system. In negating the supposition, the editor adroitly noted that those who formerly died of smallpox were now kept alive to take their chances with other diseases.

A professor at the Vienna University developed a different approach to saving cholera victims given up as lost. Using the "so called transfusion process," he infused 20 ounces of blood from healthy young men or women into their veins, finding "success was almost immediate." Faces assumed a more natural color, the pulse normalized and the patients became well in hours.[97]

On a similar topic, the *Pittsburgh Medical News,* July 21, 1870, reported that cholera patients exhibited a large excess of albumen in the blood and none in the urine. Noting that in every disease the blood and urine were simultaneously altered in composition, any deviation in one involved a corresponding deviation in the other. This led them to the conclusion that when the precise deviation was known, the nature of disease could be determined "with more nearly mathematical precision than is possible by any other method of diagnosis."[98]

In 1870 the concept of the "Earth Closet" came into vogue, prompting New Orleans to adopt it throughout the city on the premise that cholera and yellow fever were directly produced by the feculence for which no system of removal existed. "Destined to supercede cess-pools, privy-sewers and water-closets," the principle of the earth-closet system was that "*dry earth* is the best deodorizer and disinfectant of organic, fecal and offensive matter, absorbing and assimilating it. It has all the advantages of the water-closet, without its evils, at far less cost."

Based on the ideas of Pettenkofer that soil absorbed impurities, the earth closet was designed to eliminate water-borne waste that infected the air and carried poison into wells. It might be described as "kitty litter for people": a commode the size of an armchair and weighing 60–100 pounds was capable of being moved from room to room "without the least offensive odor." The earth, after being cleaned and dried, could be used repeatedly. The Earth Closet Company manufactured the item, having its northwest agent in Chicago. As proof of its success, the Riverside Company proposed to create an entire suburb of that city using the earth-closet and dispensing with sewerage except for surface water.[99]

One new invention that retained its usefulness was the hypodermic syringe. In 1872, Dr. Patterson, superintendent of the British seaman's hospital, Constantinople, treated cholera patients with injections of morphine. This eased cramping and sent the patients into a deep sleep during which they gradually regained color and warmth. Out of 42 patients treated, 22 recovered and 20 of the more severe cases died; of 10 patients treated in the ordinary way, only one recovered.

The following year, Dr. J. Joseph Williams, professor of physiology, Cumberland University, had better results injecting morphine and quinine under the skin. If violent sweating developed, he injected atropine. To aid digestion he gave diluted muriatic acid and sacharated popsin with water (artificial gastric juice) on the theory that if the bowels and stomach could be stabilized, nature would restore secretions and the healthful working of the whole system. Of 400 cases, he was said to have lost only one.

In 1876 Surgeon Major A.R. Hall, who served in the Medical Department of the English army in Bengal, recommended putting the sedative chloral hydrate under the skin by hypodermic syringe in order to control the "spasmodic contractions" of the heart. If a more powerful sedative was required, he used prussic acid, calabar bean or bromide of potassium; opium, a stimulating narcotic, was to be avoided. For patients in collapse, he encouraged them to drink cold water.[100]

The Rev. D.M. McClellan (1873) advised "quit dram-drinking, if you would not have the cholera," while Professor Mantegazza discovered that certain odorous flowers developed ozone in the atmosphere. He recommended strongly scented flowers such as sunflowers (popularly believed to prevent fever and ague) be planted around houses in order that the ozone they emitted exert a powerful oxidizing influence.[101]

The "best remedy" for cholera in its incipient stage was devised by the College of Physicians, Philadelphia, in 1866 and was still in use in 1873. The remedy consisted of 2 ounces each of laudanum and tincture of capsicum, half an ounce of essence of peppermint and two ounces of Hoffman's anodyne, 10–20 drops taken and repeated every 20 minutes.[102]

A discovery in 1851 by Schwade that the number and magnitude of sunspots varied regularly within a period of 10–11 years caused researchers to seek a correlation with meteorological events on Earth. In 1872 that seemed to come to fruition when B.G. Jenkins, of the Inner Temple, London, in conjunction with the Russian Imperial Academy of Sciences, presented a paper to the British Historical Society maintaining that "cosmic influences lies at the origin of cholera." Jenkins demonstrated that the "maxima and minima [of disease] coincide with the maxima and minima of solar agitations, auroras, banners, earth currents, magnetic storms and great electrical cyclones." He added:

> It is a well known and curious fact that the last year of every century—e.g., 1800—has a minimum of spots, and by various processes, different physicists in distant countries, working from photographic and other sun records, have reached the same result, that the period of time in which this minimum returns is about eleven years and a half. But the maximum year falls about five years after the minimum, and not midway in the period.

Jenkins concluded that the cholera period was equal to a period-and-a-half of sunspots. According to this reasoning, 1866 was a maximum year for cholera and the next would be in 1883. Contrary to popular belief, Jenkins purported that cholera originated in seven distinct and equidistant seats on, or near, the Tropic of Cancer, of which the Gangetic was the most important. The others were to the east of China, to the north of Mecca, on the west coast of Africa, to the north of the West Indies, to the west of lower California and among the Sandwich Islands. This explained how vessels, sailing in these cholera streams were suddenly struck by the disease. If this idea proved too complicated, advocates in 1880 promoted the idea that the United States government plant forest trees, as it was their belief cholera often passed a wooded district while "reveling" in a treeless one.[103]

On a slightly more humorous subject, a study done in 1885 seemed to prove that marriage for the male sex was a preventative against death by cholera. Published by the Municipality of Paris in the *Bulletin Hebdomadaire de Statistique Municipale,* its table presented the ratio of deaths by cholera per 100,000 during the late epidemic, from November 3 to November 29, 1884.

Ratio of Deaths (in years)	Single	Married
25–36	51	18
30–35	78	21
35–40	58	40
40–45	152	44
45–50	83	47
50–55	167	37
55–60	83	57
60–65	117	
65–70	89	46
70–75	455	

Female mortality from cholera was also lower among married women in the ratio of 379:561.[104]

Malignant Cholera vs. Cholera Morbus

In order to distinguish malignant (Asiatic) cholera from cholera morbus (sporadic cholera), a New York physician provided the following table:

Malignant Cholera

Usually preceded by a simple painless diarrhea; if sudden, commencing with a very profuse discharge from bowels with or without vomiting, accompanied by severe pain down the thighs and exhaustion.

Discharges consisted of watery or turbid fluid, with rice-like particles with a peculiar alkaline odor, free from foecal smell and devoid of bile.

Prostration and lowering of temperature very rapid; surface temperature 4–8° but internal heat increased. Cramps usually beginning in fingers and toes, extending to arms and legs. Urine suppressed early.

Purple hue to lips; indifference and apathy but mental faculties clear; excessive wakefulness. The "facies cholerica" not easily forgotten—features pinched and corpse-like, eyes encircled by a purple band, cornea flattened, arteries in neck pulseless.

Sporadic Cholera

Commences with incessant simultaneous vomiting and purging, the pain being of a gripping nature.

First discharges the contents of stomach and bowels, afterwards green or yellow; very offensive odor and impregnated with bile.

Prostration and lowering of temperature progressive resulting from the exhausting drain of discharges. Surface temperature not depressed and internal temperature normal. Cramps limited to abdomen and legs.

Expired air natural. Urine rarely suppressed. Pallor livid but never the peculiar blueness of true cholera. The mind clouded at the end; sleepiness from exhaustion.

In collapse, features pinched; the whole eyeball appears sunken but without flattening of the cornea; characteristic aspect of true cholera wanting.[105]

Battle Cries: Can We Be Protected Against Cholera?

As the world came slowly to acknowledge, if not accept, the germ theories of Pasteur and Koch, attention turned to protection. In 1884 Jaime Ferran of Catalan (described as a 33-year-old physician of short stature, square-built with swarthy features, a black beard turning gray and large eyes and who studied at Tortosa and Tarragona) attained worldwide interest with his claim of having developed a cholera vaccination using a graduated virus that offered immunity "for a certain time," provided five days were allowed for the vaccine to work.

As proof of his success, Ferran gave an account of his work at Alcira (in the province of Valencia) where nearly 9,100 out of a population of 16,000–22,000 submitted to inoculation. Results showed that the proportion of cholera cases among inoculated to noninoculated was 59:261, while deaths were cited as 10:120. Alcira, however, was an especially well-to-do town and deaths were chiefly among the poor; Ferran offered no proof that his wealthier patients who received the prophylactic were actually at risk. Moreover, the epidemic was not severe, with 320 out of 22,000 (published reports varied considerably) perishing between May 1 and June 26.

While the disease spread to Madrid and westward along the Mediterranean, stories of Ferran's success made him a worldwide hero. His name and theories became so popular physicians from Europe gathered at Valencia to investigate his methods. M. Brouardel, M. Gibier and Van Ermegem, the French and Belgian delegates sent to investigate the claims, asked Ferran what he meant by vaccinating "with virus containing cholera bacilli scientifically graduated and attenuated by his own methods." On these and other points Ferran refused to elucidate on what he called his "property." He further refused requests from the Pasteur Institute, Paris, to supply them with samples of his inoculation for study. Those who more closely observed his technique reported the vaccine was heavily contaminated with other microorganisms and that only a small portion of the bacteria were *V. cholerae*.

Notwithstanding, there were serious commercial as well as scientific considerations. While Ferran apparently inoculated the people of Alcira gratis, his disciples (often referred to as "puffers") charged as much as 12½ francs for one inoculation, making 8,000–10,000 francs daily. One intimate friend remarked, "There's millions in it." And, as reported, hundreds of doctors, journalists and statesmen, "hungry to share the millions, have a direct interest in spreading inoculation and tinkering statistics." The French report declared Ferran's operation "harmless," but "not very effectual," the sole worth being the sense of protection it conveyed to those receiving inoculation. In the final analysis, the same newspapers that lauded him eventually ran such headlines as "Fixed for a Quack."[106]

In 1891 Pasteur asked W.M. Haffkine to develop an immunizing agent against cholera. Haffkine prepared two modified *V. cholerae* strains that were tested in India in 1893 and 1894 (42,197 individuals) and 1895–1896 (30,000 individuals). However, the most important tests were conducted on small groups residing in prisons and on tea plantations, the testing believed to be the first attempts to determine efficacy by controlled field trials. Although statistical analysis indicated the vaccines were efficacious, there was difficulty in standardizing it and producing it in large quantities. Notwithstanding, the Haffkine vaccine was used during World War I.

The use of nonliving whole cell *V. cholerae* as oral vaccines was reported in 1893. In 1896, W. Kolle promoted the use of agar-grown, heat-inactivated whole *V. cholerae* organisms. This nonliving vaccine was easier to prepare and standardize and replaced Haffkine's vaccine. Kolle-type vaccines were first used on a large scale in 1902 during the Japanese cholera epidemic.[107]

Cholera Infantum

The year 1882 was a particularly bad one for cholera infantum. On July 16 New York City authorities reported 86 children had died of the disease within 24 hours; in Boston, 111 fatalities were recorded in the first three weeks of July; in Philadelphia, during the first week of August, 166 infants perished. Little by way of medical help was provided. One expert suggested the use of a spice poultice comprising cloves, allspice and cinnamon mixed in half a cup of cold water and thickened with flaxseed. It was to be applied over muslin and placed on the abdomen.

A discussion of cause was even more obscure. Although Pasteur and Koch's theories were widely published, many physicians continued to espouse their own ideas. One seriously suggested that the disease was caused by "some lesion of the brain." The Guernsey County Medical Association, Ohio, advocated the idea that "all diarrhetic diseases in children were alike in nature, only differing in degree." One physician stated the disease was the result of "vitiated secretions of the liver passing into the stomach" and prescribed castor oil. Another made the startling observation that cholera infantum prevailed only in the United States. His treatment consisted of mercurials to allay irritability and "leave the rest to Nature." He concluded the "cause of the disease cannot be assigned; though it must be something in the atmosphere."[108]

In 1914, Dr. Ellie Metchnikoff of the Pasteur Institute announced his finding that infantile cholera was contagious. Describing the disease as "not unlike Asiatic cholera," he noted it appeared as a very simple intestinal trouble, then almost immediately became fatal. Having seen flies in connection with Asiatic cholera, Metchnikoff stated that flies spread the disease and recommended "swatting" them whenever found.[109]

The 20th Century

The scientific discoveries of the 1800s progressed into the 20th century with a multifaceted emphasis on prevention, research and serums. Sanitation constituted much of the first prong, but attention was also directed toward dietary considerations. Among the most important was the public reeducation concerning milk. Koch first noted that milk was a suitable culture medium for the cholera bacillus in 1884 but he was not the first to do so. Professor Gaffky, in a report contained in the Cholera Commission of India, warned of the unsanitary condition of dairies, while in 1876 Dr. Payne, the health officer of Calcutta, offered similar observations. Diluting milk with water (among other noxious substances) was a common practice in most, if not all, countries, significantly adding to the danger of contamination. Studies made by Albert H. Buck, M.D., indicated that of 330 milk-borne epidemics, 243 were reported by English authors, 52 by Americans, 14 by Germans, 11 by Scandinavian and 5 each by French and Australian writers. Buck concluded the high number of English and American cases resulted from the consumption of raw milk, while on the Continent milk was rarely used without first being boiled.

More frequent articles were also appearing on the successful use of saline. At the Chinese Cholera Hospital in Shanghai, circa 1909, Drs. Cox, Thue and Christensen used warm intravenous saline therapy to raise the body temperature of those arriving in the "cold stage" of shock. Dr. Cox's apparatus automatically fed the reservoir, maintaining the correct temperature while filtering the solution through a Berkefeld filter. It was noted that hundreds, or more than a thousand ounces could be transfused while the patient remained in a state of shock but that the treatment had to be discontinued when the patient's temperature reached a certain point.

Interestingly, regarding a Cincinnati physician named Dr. John M. Scudder, who had used the injection of strong salt solution on cholera patients to good effect, one American newspaper wrote, "The truth is the world is filled with very modest physicians who have in trying times performed many deeds of heroism and effected many cures, but the world learns of the means slowly, not because of hesitancy but because of a natural modesty."

In 1909 Signor Salimbini, a staff member of the Pasteur Institute, developed a serum said to cure cholera from testing done on patients at St. Petersburg, where mortality was diminished by 23 percent. Another Pasteur researcher, Dr. Happkine, developed a vaccine by taking bacilli from the cholera subject and creating a culture. The culture was then injected under the skin and the patient was exposed to the epidemic. Local infection followed with a slight reaction and then immunity. In commenting on the above, Professor Metchnikoff, head of the Pasteur Institute, warned that neither serums nor vaccines should remove attention from elementary sanitary precautions such as boiling water. Cholera vaccines "must be used discreetly," he added. "Those who contract it deserve blame quite as much as pity."

In 1914 another discovery from the Pasteur Institute concerned the research of Drs. Frouin and Roudsky, who demonstrated that the salts of a rare earth, lanthanum and thorium possessed properties which both sterilized and destroyed virulent cultures of Asiatic cholera.[110] Professor Puntoni of the University of Rome announced findings indicating tobacco was powerless in the presence of influenza, typhoid and diphtheria germs. Using Tuscany cigars, Macedonian cigarettes and very strong chewing tobacco, he exposed germs to smoke, finding them just as robust after an hour as they were at the beginning. He also noted that no smoker or chewer could hope for protection against tuberculosis, as was then commonly believed. On the positive front, he determined tar, nicotine and formaldehyde in tobacco were effective as disinfectants against cholera and meningitis germs.[111]

The Old Is New Again

Perhaps the best way to end this appendix is to bring the idea of "cures" full circle. In 1986, the United States State Department of Health cited the manufacturer of a product called "Kinker's Cholera Balm." Taking a page—and a recipe—from the 1800s, the maker, Charles Mergenthaler, promised his product was effective in treating "pain in stomach and bowels, colic, cramps, cholera morbus, dysentary [sic], diarrhea and summer complaint." The red solution was found to contain ether, peppermint, cinnamon, camphor, red pepper and rhubarb.

Mergenthaler was given the option of ceasing production or revising the label statements, upgrading quality control and registering with the state as required by law. In the final, 21st century, analysis, a spokesman for the Department of Health concluded, "As with many unproven medications we take action against, there is no evidence that this product could be effective in treating any of those conditions. And while the product probably is not harmful, we get very concerned when a drug like this is claimed to be effective against serious diseases such as cholera, which can be fatal."[112]

In the 19th century this patent medicine man might have made a pretty penny. Two hundred years later, he could have been more successful selling the "10-cent cure" composed of salt, sugar, bicarbonate of soda and potassium[113] and calling it "Kinker's Oral Rehydration Balm."

Appendix II

Cholera Morbus Mortality
Statistics in the 19th Century
The Harvest of Death

The great master of the science of statistics has laid claim on behalf of his favourite study to a wider scope and more potent influence than men were for a long time willing to accord to mere aggregation and assortment of numerical statements. "Everything," says Quetelet, "which pertains to the human species belongs to the order of physical facts. The greater the number of individuals the more does the influence of the individual will disappear, leaving predominance to a series of general facts dependent on causes by which society exists, and is preserved." All civilised Governments have in some measure recognized these lofty preten-sions; and the value of statistical inquiries is everywhere acknowledged. There is no subject of investigation, probably, on which statistics are likely to let in so much and so useful light as the ebb and flow of human life, the causes of those sinister influences which culminate in death, and the methods by which disease may be averted.[1]

Improved international communication and a desire to compile and publish statistics in the 19th century offer an intriguing study of the prevalence and spread of disease. During the cholera epidemic in England (1831–1832), daily reports reveal a harrowing picture of how rap-idly new cases were reported and deaths accumulated. Numbers occasionally fluctuated wildly, even between newspapers of the same date citing the same sources. An inability to definitively separate cholera from similar diseases, the reluctance of some reporters to submit data, and, occasionally, local and national governments desiring to either augment or minimize the sever-ity of an epidemic skew these figures.

The most accurate and complete statistics came from London. Bills of Mortality were commenced in the reign of Queen Elizabeth, where thousands were killed by zymotic diseases, or those related to fermentation, encompassing epidemics and contagions. The bills appeared weekly from 1603 until a new system of registration was introduced and placed under the con-trol of the registrar-general. Thereafter, medical attendants certified the cause of nearly every death; 135 registrars copied the certificates for the week ending Saturday and sent abstracts to the office of the general registrar every Monday.[2]

Statistics from other countries were often compiled by eyewitnesses who tended to exag-gerate numbers according to personal observation and hearsay. Cholera may have seemed to be increasing to one correspondent and decreasing to another. State leadership, on average, tended to downplay outbreaks, accounting for the difference between official and private num-bers. That noted, even "ballpark" figures give the historian a fairly clear idea of the severity of the disease and the terrible toll it took on human life.

345

Analytical Table of Cholera
Prior to Its Appearance in England (1831)
(Published by a German Newspaper)

Locale	Census	Cases	Died	Of 1,000 Attacked percent Who Died
Moscow	350,000	8,576	4,690	54.6
St. Petersburg	360,000	9,247	4,757	51.4
Vienna	300,000	3,980	1,899	47.7
Berlin	240,000	2,220	1,401	63.1
Hamburgh	100,000	874	455	52.1
Prague	96,600	3,234	1,333	41.3
Breslaw	78,800	1,276	671	52.5
Koenigsberg	70,000	2,188	1,310	59.9
Magdeburg	36,600	576	346	60.0
Brunn	35,300	1,540	604	32.7
Stettin	24,300	366	250	69.9
Halle	23,800	303	152	50.3
Elbing	22,000	430	283	65.8
Hungary	8,750,000	435,330	188,000	43.23

In contrast to the above, other returns from St. Petersburg for the year 1831 indicated that 8,856 males and 4,296 females died of cholera, "or very nearly 53 out of every 1,000 souls." Contemporaries considered the disparity of male-female deaths, when "the number of male children born should almost treble that of females, to be 'ill-omened.'"[4] An 1832 London medical paper estimated the average annual mortality occasioned by cholera in India during "the late severity" at two million and a half. The whole number swept off since 1815 was put at eighteen million. In China, cholera was said to be even more fatal owing to the density of population.

In the town of Muscat, Arabia, the mortality amounted to one-third of the population, while in the cities of Busheer, Shiraz and Yerd (under a dry, pure atmosphere), it was one-sixth. In Bagdad and Bussorah (Mesopotamia), surrounded by a moist atmosphere, one-fourth or even one-third perished. At Erevan and Tauris, one-fifth of the population died, but at Erzeroum and Kars, in the mountains of Armenia, mortality was much diminished. In Syria, the proportion of deaths varied, averaging about one-tenth of the population. Females generally outlived their male counterparts, a fact attributed to "the female constitution, their sedentary habits and regimen."

During the epidemic of 1832, the longest prevalence of cholera in Russia was 114 days, the shortest 20, which took place about the close of autumn. In the Caucasus, 16,000 persons were victims, of whom 10,000 died. The entire number in the dominions of Russia was estimated at 100,000, of whom 60,000 perished.[5]

Statistics from the French Cholera Epidemic
Dating from the Commencement of the Disease, March 26, 1832

Date	Cases	Deaths
March 31	281	100
April 2	735	267
April 5	1,052	395
April 7	2,360	912
April 8	3,077	1,199
April 9	4,923	1,879
April 12	5,906	2,236
April 13	8,349	3,226[6]

It is often difficult to grasp the enormity of a disaster by lump sums. The following table demonstrates how cholera destroyed lives day by day and presents a far more horrific picture.

England and Scotland (1832)

Date	Total Cases from Commencement	Total Deaths	Date	Total Cases from Commencement	Total Deaths
June 1	10,601	3,977	July 7	15,785	5,833
June 4	10,695	4,029	July 11	16,952	6,312
June 5	10,756	4,047	July 12	17,308	6,454
June 7	10,850	4,079	July 13	17,578	6,548
June 9	10,997	4,145	July 14	17,883	6,658
June 11	11,088	4,197	July 15	18,375	6,884
June 12	11,152	4,215	July 17	18,554	6,946
June 13	11,311	4,267	July 18	19,174	7,134
June 14	11,398	4,310	July 19	19,641	7,302
June 16	11,594	4,375	July 20	20,010	7,448
June 18	11,823	4,161	July 23	20,874	7,815
June 20	12,000	4,517	July 24	21,099	7,909
June 21	12,127	4,551	July 25	21,417	8,027
June 22	12,257	4,603	July 26	21,864	8,169
June 23	12,370	4,656	July 30	22,781	8,535
June 25	12,744	4,777	July 31	22,960	8,595
June 26	12,874	4,906	August 1	23,307	8,745
June 27	13,115	4,974	August 2	23,698	8,899
June 28	13,430	4,969	August 3	24,088	9,057
June 29	13,596	5,059	August 4	24,434	9,201
July 1	13,825	5,141	August 6	25,056	9,491
July 2	14,355	5,323	August 9	26,685	10,103
July 3	14,541	5,403	August 30	43,872	16,230
July 5	15,164	5,624	September 22	55,711	20,177

Ireland (1832)

Date	Total Cases from Commencement	Total Deaths
May 25	5,836	1,744

Dublin

Date	Total Cases from Commencement	Total Deaths
May 1	501	187
June 3	3,167	884
June 7	3,214	888

Cork

Date	Total Cases from Commencement	Total Deaths
June 4	2,564	582
June 6	2,645	613[7]

Contagious Maladies: Putting Cholera in Context

London, being one of the most commercial cities in the world, was exposed more than any other to contagious disorders brought from distant parts. The following table represents the most dreadful years of mortality.

Statistics of London

Monarch	Year	Disease	Number who Died
Edward III	1348	Pestilence	57,000
Henry VII	1500	Pestilence	30,000
Henry VIII	1518	Contagious fever	30,000
Elizabeth I	1563	Pestilence	21,500
Elizabeth I	1593	Pestilence	17,899
James I	1603	Pestilence	30,758
Charles I	1625	Pestilence	35,417
Charles I	1636	Pestilence	10,400
Charles II	1665	Pestilence	68,596
George II	1729	Putrid fever	5,225
William IV	1834	Asiatic cholera	5,027

Official returns of London for the 1832–1834 cholera epidemic reached 10,545 cases; and throughout Great Britain, including the capital, cases numbered 74,464. The deaths amounted to 28,438, according to the calculations of Sir William Pym.

Population of London
(From Tables Prepared by M. Moreau Jomnes)

Monarch	Year	Population
Henry II	circa 1170	40,000
William III	circa 1700	674,000
George III	circa 1760	676,000
George III	1801	1,097,000
George III	1811	1,304,000
George IV	1821	1,574,000
William IV	1831	1,860,000

From 1744 to 1800, during the period of 56 years, deaths in London exceeded births by 267,000, or an average yearly loss of 4,800 persons. From 1801 to 1830, during a space of 30 years, births exceeded deaths by 102,975, or an average of 3,600 per annum.[8]

Mortality in Calcutta

A report by Samuel Brown, Equitable Office, Blackfriars, dated July 24, 1848, provided numerous tables comparing mortality in England and India, with an emphasis on how seasonal factors influenced the health of the populations. His purpose in separating cholera from other diseases stemmed from the fact its fearful character presented itself "to the mind of an European in the most striking light."

Population and Mortality in Calcutta:
Table Showing the Mode in which the Proportion of Deaths in Different Months Is Affected by Cholera
Proportion in Each Month to 100 Deaths

Month	Protestant Burial Ground 1796–1815	1819–1838 Since the Cholera	1832–1838 Hindoos	Mussulmans [Muslims]
January	7.47	6.47	3.76	4.26
February	5.48	4.3	4.08	6.73

Month	Protestant Burial Ground 1796–1815	1819–1838 Since the Cholera	1832–1838 Hindoos	Mussulmans [Muslims]
March	5.97	6.89	12.33	15.07
April	6.46	8.6	17.77	16.56
May	7.96	10.95	14.28	15.94
June	7.07	8.29	4.05	7.46
July	7.75	8.12	6.01	4.57
August	10.18	9.71	5.3	5.02
September	10.36	9.68	5.16	4.16
October	9.95	9.43	6.78	6.8
November	11.12	9.17	11.1	7.9
December	10.23	8.39	9.38	5.53

Presidency General Hospital, 1827–1838

Month	Cholera Patients Admitted	Died	Excluding Cholera Admitted	Died
January	3.49	2.96	10.14	8.41
February	1	1.34	6.47	6.61
March	6.97	9.14	5.45	5.41
April	33.37	33.6	7.81	5.56
May	17.18	10.22	8.45	7.28
June	3.99	1.61	8.17	6.23
July	3.99	1.61	8.17	10.88
August	4.61	4.84	7.59	8.56
September	1.25	1.31	7.41	10.8
October	6.1	7.26	8.44	10.21
November	7.35	8.6	12.9	8.71
December	3.99	3.76	10.45	11.34

Assuming the population returns of 1837, the deaths by cholera of Hindus, being 15,204 in seven years in a population of 157,473, were 1.47 percent per annum, and those of Muslims, being 2,911 in the same time, were not quite .7 percent per annum. It was observed that among the admissions to the Presidency General Hospital, which were principally of Europeans, 68.2 percent were admitted in the four months from March to June, inclusive, and that out of the total number of admissions by cholera, 31.6 percent died within these four months only.[9]

The Mysterious and Capricious Cholera

During the cholera epidemic of 1849, the *Cincinnati Gazette* offered an interesting look at the progression of the disease.

It appears here, there, everywhere, suddenly, and often giving no warning, without reference to lines of travel, regardless of natural water courses, wholly independent of the prevailing winds, and uncontrolled by the topographical character or geological formation of the districts within its general course. Spending itself where it lights first, either gently or ferociously, it disappears, and while neighboring points are standing in awe of its proximity, and daily expecting its desolating presence, it suddenly appears in altogether another region, a hundred or two or three hundred miles away. And again, two or three weeks or two or three months afterward, while those who seemed to have escaped are still warm in the congratulation of each other, and are beginning to talk and to write about the superior healthfulness of their towns, the destroyer retraces its steps, strikes at their best and their worst, their strong and their feeble alike, and carries mourning to nearly every household.[10]

Deaths for the Week, Cincinnati, 1849

July	Cholera	Other Deaths	Total
3	127	39	166
4	130	53	183
5	137	38	175
6	91	58	149
7	35	45	128 [sic]
8	74	80	104 [sic]
9	78	40	118
Total	722	301	1023

Of the above interments, 730 were in the foreign cemeteries and 63 were in the public ground, showing a dreadful mortality among the foreign population. The entire population of Cincinnati was estimated at 40,000.[11] Cincinnati was not alone in suffering large losses from the immigrant population. At St. Louis, it was believed that at least two-thirds of cholera victims were foreign born.

Deaths for Two Months, St. Louis, 1849

For the Week Ending	Cholera Deaths
May 7	135
May 14	273
May 21	192
May 28	186
June 4	144
June 11	283
June 18	510
June 25	763

This made a total of 2,486 cholera deaths. From June 25 until June 30, when the *St. Louis Union* published the statistics, it was estimated 130 died *per day,* bringing the two-month total to 3,136.[12]

A third city singled out for tragic losses among those who had come seeking a better life was New York. A sampling by the *Sun* of the nativity of cholera deaths for one typical week revealed the following:

Nativity	Cholera Deaths, 1849	Nativity	Cholera Deaths, 1849
New York	72	England	10
Massachusetts	2	Ireland	138
Rhode Island	1	Scotland	5
Connecticut	4	Wales	3
New Jersey	12	France	8
Pennsylvania	2	Germany	28
Delaware	1	Poland	1
Virginia	1	Denmark	1
Georgia	1	Portugal	2
Ohio	1	Unknown	17
Total U.S. Natives	**96**	**Total Foreign-born**	**311**

The chief cause of the dreadful mortality among the Irish and Germans was said to be the imprudent use of a vast amount of vegetables.[13]

Matters were approached from a different perspective in Alabama, where cholera was attributed to alcohol.

Cholera Deaths in Alabama from the Commencement
of the Disease to the Cessation of Daily Reports
June 1849

Intemperate	140
Free Drinkers	55
Moderate Drinkers	131
Strictly temperate	5
Members of Temperance Societies	2
Idiots	1
Unknown	2

It was recorded that the collector of the above facts was a "gentleman of intelligence, of integrity, and of warm benevolence."[14] Adding to the confusion were articles such as the one published in the *Alta California* (August 23, 1849) where one authority stated:

> The real truth is, that the Epidemic Cholera, as distinguished from common Cholera (*Cholera vulgaris* stupidly called Cholera *Morbus* or Cholera *disease*,) is a compound malady consisting of two distinct maladies united in this epidemic,—as in the Lung-fever (*pneumonitis typhoides*,) which occasionally visits New-England, and various portions of the Northern sections of the Union, in the same epidemic character.
>
> In each of these fatal epidemics, there is a topical affection of a mucuous membrane and the parts subjacent, coupled with a constitutional febrile affection of the whole system. In both, that affection is a *typhus fever*, (in the widest sense of that term)—a malady in which the vital energies are "below par."

1849: The Year of the Cholera

"The year 1849," began an article in the *Patriot* (London, December 31, 1849), "will be most memorable in our domestic annals, as the year of the Cholera." The epidemic actually began in the ports of London and Hull toward the end of September 1848 and by early October was reported in Edinburgh, Leith and Newhaven. The rate of mortality in London was only slightly affected until July 1849 and reached a climax in the week ending September 8, after which it rapidly declined.

Compared to the cholera year of 1832, when it was calculated 1 in 319 suffered from the disease, in 1848–1849 the number was 1 in 153. Although cholera "swept away thousands on thousands of all ranks," not every occupation suffered equally, as indicated by an account offered by Dr. Guy:

Occupations of 4,312 Males, Aged 15 and Above
During the Cholera Epidemic in London, 1848–1849

Labourers	756	Porters or messengers	99
Sailors and Greenwich pensioners	299	Tailors	80
Shoemakers	151	Painters and plumbers	73
Gentlemen of independent means	135	Cabinet-makers	70
Carpenters	111	Soldiers	62
Weavers	102	Coachmen and cabmen	57
Clerks or accountants	100	Coalporters and coalheavers	53

Bakers	52	Medical men	16
Carmen and carriers	52	Saddlers	15
Bricklayers	47	Builders	14
Engineers	44	Booksellers	14
Licensed victuallers	42	Carpenters and undertakers	14
Grooms and ostlers	37	Cheesemongers	13
Cabmen	35	Magistrates or lawyers	13
Sawyers	33	Stokers	13
Butchers	32	Oilmen	13
Coopers	28	Fruiterers	12
Watermen	27	Architects or engineers	11
Master marines	25	Fishmongers	11
Footmen and man-servants	25	Merchants	11
Policemen	24	Officers in the army and navy	11
Tanners	22	Custom-house officers	11
Plasterers	20	Railway guards	10
Grocers	20	Master shoemakers	8
Shipwrights	20	Excise officers	7
Travellers	19	Ballast heavers	7
Turners	18	Watchmen	7
Bargemen	18	Master tailors	6
Drapers	17	Drovers	6
Masons	17	Tobacconists	6
Coachmakers	16	Clergymen	6
Letter-carriers and postmen	16	Wine merchants	5

"Labourer," "gentleman" and "man-servant" were loose terms, but the statement that 1 in 67 labourers, 1 in 200 gentlemen and 1 in 1,572 manservants (including footmen) died of cholera "expresses something near the risk incurred by the three classes in the epidemic. The domestic manservants of London were 39,300 in 1841 and 25 died of cholera; the clergy, doctors and lawyers did not exceed 12,000, yet 35 persons belonging to the learned profession died of cholera in 1849."[15]

Comparison of Deaths in London by District, 1848–1850

District	Population 1841	Area in Square Miles	Deaths 1848	Deaths 1849	Deaths 1850
West	300,711	17.2	8,118	9,382	7,232
North	375,971	20.5	10,309	11,053	9,488
Central	373,653	2.8	9,658	10,843	8,256
East	392,444	8.8	13,009	14,841	10,337
South	501,190	66.2	15,496	22,318	13,266

Mortality by Disease in London, 1849

Zymotic diseases (excluding cholera)	14,208
Cholera	14,105
Dropsy, cancer and uncertain	2,329
Tubercular diseases	8,987
Diseases of the brain, spinal marrow, nerves and senses	6,242
Diseases of heart and blood vessels	1,931
Diseases of lungs and organs of respiration	8,242
Diseases of stomach, liver and digestion	3,139
Diseases of kidneys	585
Childbirth	466

Rheumatism, diseases of bones and joints	395
Diseases of skin and cellular tissue	75
Malformations	172
Premature birth and debility	1,256
Atrophy	1,332
Age	2,239
Sudden	713
Violence, privation, cold, intemperance	1,694

The year 1850 presented "a most pleasing contrast" with 1849, as cholera deaths dropped significantly, returning tubercular diseases and "diseases of the lungs and organs of respiration" to the spot as number one killer of Londoners.

Mortality by Disease in London, 1850

Zymotic Diseases		*Sporadic Diseases*	
Smallpox	498	Dropsy, cancer and uncertain	2,270
Measles	977	Tubercular diseases	8,539
Scarlatina	1,178	Diseases of the brain, spinal marrow, nerves and senses	5,965
Hooping-cough	1,572		
Croup	307	Diseases of heart and blood vessels	1,965
Thrush	146	Diseases of lungs and organs of respiration	7,822
Diarrhea	1,884	Diseases of stomach, liver and organs of	
Dysentery	182	digestion	2,955
Cholera	127	Diseases of the kidneys	614
Influenza	109	Childbirth, diseases of the uterus	467
Purpura and scurvy	43	Rheumatism, disease of the bones	411
Ague	18	Diseases of skin and cellular tissue	87
Remittent fever	87	Malformations	176
Infantile fever	44	Premature birth and debility	1,318
Typhus	1,923	Atrophy	1,118
Puerperal fever	199	Age	2,149
Rheumatic fever	67	Sudden	709
Erysipelas	344	Violence	1,511
Syphilis	122	Privation, cold and intemperance	285[16]
Noma or canker	17		
Hydrophobia	1		

The diminished rate in the increase of population between 1841 and 1851 was explained by the influenza epidemic of 1847 and the cholera epidemic of 1849.

Great Britain Population Statistics
Comparison of 1841 and 1851

	1841 Population	*1851 Population*
England and Wales	15,911,757	17,905,831
London	1,948,369	2,363,141

The *Medical Times* stated the rate of mortality in England and Wales (exclusive of London) for this 10-year period was 1 in every 3.91 of the corrected population, while that of London was 1 in 3.89, indicating a higher rate of mortality in the metropolis. This was explained by the supposition fewer births were registered in the city, skewing the numbers.[17]

If mortality was severe in England, the kingdom of Poland suffered horrific casualties between the first appearance of cholera until the 18th of December.

Cholera in Poland, 1848

Locale	Cases	Recovered	Died
Warsaw	4,086	2,445	1,623
Government of Warsaw (exclusive of the capital)	14,804	5,547	4,145
Government of Lublin	15,355	8,623	6,626
Government of Radon	4,607	1,920	2,380
Government of Plock	7,316	3,233	4,010
Government of Augustown	8,046	5,217	2,775[18]

"Which Is Worse—War or Cholera?"

In 1854, on the verge of what would become a year of horrific mortality from cholera, the above question was placed before the British public. During twenty-two years (1793 to 1815) of military and naval expenditure, official returns indicated that there were 19,796 deaths and 79,709 wounded, giving an annual average of 899 killed and 3,623 wounded. In all, nearly 120,000 soldiers were affected from campaigns, including deaths from disease, exposure and hardship. Compared to these were the returns from England and Wales arising out of the cholera epidemic in 1848 and 1849, a period of two years. Official mortality from cholera and diarrhea was placed at 72,180 out of 144,360 attacked; worse, the average annual deaths from *preventable* diseases, including typhus, was placed at 115,000, while 11,419 soldiers died by violence.

Comparing those killed in nine great battles, including Waterloo (4,740), with the number killed by cholera in London in 1848 and 1849 (14,139), there was "a difference of 9,399 in favour of war." It was also observed that 12–20 percent of medical men died from cholera and London missionaries "died as fast as those in foreign countries." Additionally, from the returns of 12 unions, 3,567 widows and orphans resulted from the epidemic, entailing an expenditure of £121,000 in only four years.

At Newcastle, during the epidemic of 1853, it was calculated that the disease cost the town £3,800 for medicine and burials; added to that was the expense (calculated at £50 a week for 8 years) to support the widows and destitute, equating to £24,600. In addition, there were 20 benefit societies in town: estimating an average loss of contributions at £500 each, that increased the loss by £10,000. "The subject," it was opined, "is a wide one."

Comparisons between expenditures on war and sanitation reappeared with some regularity. In 1886 Edward Chadwick presented some striking data indicating how much more European governments expended for the destruction of human life over that of preserving it. It cost $1,000,000 for the cost of a military ship; directed toward sanitary reform the same money would cover 66,000 houses. If this health effort reduced the death rate by 5:1,000, the saving of life in England would be 1,667 per annum. Spread across a decade, 16,667 lives could be saved and 333,333 cases of sickness avoided.[19]

In a fascinating adjunct to the subject of war, in 1876 Lord Napier of Magdala issued an order that British soldiers in India were exempted from the requirement of wearing their waistbelts as girdles to their white clothing. Historically, it was noted, it was "notorious that in all hot climates the wearing of a sash or belt round the loins, either above or under the clothing, is about one of the best preservatives that can be devised against cholera and dysentery; and it was this especial object that when the Zouaves were organized by the Duc d'Aumale a broad abdominal sash was included in their uniform. There is of course a great difference between a stiff, tightly-buckled girdle of tanned hide, and a broad, thick-folded ceinture of soft silken or woollen material; but the surcingling girdle is, nevertheless, of immense sanitary value in warm latitudes." It was hoped the medical officers would not allow the soldiers "to encounter the chill air of eventide without the protection of under-belts of flannel."[20] By 1885, however, these "cholera belts," as they were originally called, were reissued to British soldiers serving in Africa, although the name, bearing an unpleasant connotation, was changed to "flannel belts." Cholera belts or girdles, constructed of heavy wool for winter and light wool in summer, were still advocated as late as 1906. Every foreign resident of India was reputed to own several dozen that they never removed.[21]

Great Britain and the Cholera Epidemic of 1854

Date	Cholera Deaths	Diarrhea Deaths
July 15	5	46
July 22	26	58

(The eastern districts, especially Limehouse,
were the chief field of its earliest operations.)

Date	Cholera Deaths	Diarrhea Deaths
July 29	138	84

71 cases occurred on the south side of the river

August 5	399	—

290 on the south side

August 12	644	—

416 on the south side

August 19	729	192
August 26	847	214
September 2	1,287	—
September 9	2,050	276

(954 males, 1,096 females, 614 children
under age 15 and 1,128 over age 60)

September 16	1,549	—
September 23	1,284	—
September 30	754	165
October 7	411	98
October 14	249	102
October 21	163	78
October 28	66	46
November 4	31	35
November 11	23	—
November 30	0	—

By comparison, the cholera epidemic of 1849 began about the end of May, six weeks earlier than in 1854, and its progress was slower; but in the fourth week of August, it reached a higher rate of mortality than in 1854. The first seven weeks of 1849, deaths for each week were 9, 22, 42, 49, 124, 152, 339; the last week of August had 1,272 deaths. On September 16, 1854, a total of 7,669 cholera deaths had been recorded; in 1849 during the same period there were 11,825 deaths. In both years mortality was highest on nearly the same day in September. Total cholera deaths on September 23, 1854, reached 8,953, compared to the same period in 1849, when there were 12,664 deaths.[22]

The British loved statistics and those provided by Registrar-General William Farr were printed, reprinted, analyzed and reanalyzed. Coupled with firsthand accounts, they provide a grizzly picture of natural disaster. In a pamphlet published by Henry Whitehead, the 28-year-old curate of St. Luke's Church, Berwick Street, Whitehead sketched a scene of "unflinching and admirable courage":

> If a person were to start from the western end of Broad-street, and, after traversing its whole length on the south side from west to east, to return as far as the brewery, and then, going down Hopkin's-street and up New-street, to end by walking through Pulteney-court, he would pass successively 45 houses of which only six escaped without a death during the recent outburst of cholera in that neighbourhood. According to a calculation based upon the last census, these 45 houses contained a population of 1,000. Of that number 103 perished by the pestilence. The population of the whole district of St. Luke's is under 9,000; during the late cholera visitation there were 373 deaths. The pestilence did not settle down upon the district by slow degrees; it enveloped the inhabitants at once in its full horrors. Of the deaths, nearly all took place in the first fortnight, and at least 189 in the first four days.[23]

The Registrar-General broke the numbers down even further. In the meticulously compiled study for the week ending October 28, 1854, it was stated "the mortality of the fatal sub-districts, such as Berwick-street and Golden-square, from which the people fled or were carried, is understated.... In the Hanover-square sub-district, 9 in 10,000 people died of cholera: in the Golden-square sub-district 189 in 10,000."[24] The year-end summary provided by the Registrar-General provided further comparisons.

> The cholera in 1849 (15 months) was fatal to 14,593 persons; in the last epidemic, extending from August, 1853 to November, 1854 (16 months), 11,495 persons fell victims. Allowing for increase in population, the deaths to every 10,000 living give an average of 64 in the former and 46 in the latter. By cholera and diarrhoea together, the deaths were in—
>
> | 1848–49 | 68,431 | 81 in 10,000 |
> | 1853–54 | 15,762 | 63 in 10,000. |

Those living in the north and central metropolitan districts suffered a mortality of only 16 to 10,000, while the south had 93 to 10,000 cut off by cholera. Using Registrar-General Farr's theory that elevation of the soil "had a more constant relation with the mortality from cholera than any other known element," mortality was the inverse relation to elevation. Adding a touch of commerce, it was concluded that "for a person of average condition dwelling under 20 feet of elevation, the premium to insure 1,000*l.* would be 12*l.*; while for those living at from 100 to 350 feet elevation the life-office would be secure with a 2*l.* premium."[25]

In discussing elevation, a writer for the *Morning Chronicle* (November 4, 1854; italics added) differed from the registrar-general by astutely observing as follows:

> Local elevations, however, although it may produce a great effect upon the aggregate mortality among a population diffused over an extensive district, does not, in the smaller sub-divisions, appear to have any regular or invariable influence. The Berwick-street and Golden-square districts are respectively 65 and 68 feet above high-water mark; yet more than 450 deaths have occurred in those places, among a population not amounting to 25,000.... In several recent weekly reports, public attention has been called to the exceedingly large proportion of deaths in those dwelling-houses situate within the southern districts, which have been furnished by the Southwark Company with water taken from the Thames at Battersea.... *It is impossible to deny that a discovery of very considerable value has been*

made. We do not write in ignorance of the fact that observations were made on the subject during the visitation of 1849, but we are not aware that evidence so clear and cogent as that which seems now to have been collected has ever before been produced.

Tragically, the debate was far from over.

In the non-epidemic year of 1855, the numbers provide an interesting comparison.

London Cholera and Diarrhea Deaths in the Non-epidemic Year of 1855

Month	Cholera Deaths	Diarrhea Deaths
May 12	1	—
June 16	—	17
June 23	—	25
June 30	—	33
July 7	6	28
July 14	—	45
July 21	4	67 (59 were under the age of 3)
July 28	9	93
August 4	—	110
August 11	5	146 (126 were under the age of 3)
August 18	12	154 (141 were under the age of 3)
August 25	—	134 (111 were under the age of 3)
October 6	0	51
October 27	7	—

By September 2, deaths by diarrhea had decreased. It was noted that the increase in the second week of July correlated to a mean temperature of 64.5° (heat being considered a predisposing factor), higher than it had been in preceding weeks. Not surprisingly, infants were the principal victims.[26]

Cholera, certainly, was not the only danger to Londoners. In 1855, attention turned to "cold" as a major source of death. While it was noted "cold is less fatal than dirt in the air and water of London, through which the cholera, dysentery, and other matters that induce zymotic diseases are diffused," statistics were chilling. For the six coldest weeks (January 20—February 24) the mean temperature was 28.4°. A total of 1,604 died from cold. After deducting the average deaths at each age, age-specific deaths were broken down as follows:

London Deaths from Extreme Cold, 1855

Age	Deaths
Under age 20	419
Age 20–40	200
Age 40–60	392
Age 60–80	752
Age 80 and upwards	205

Comparison Between Cholera and Cold Mortality, 1854, per 10,000

Age	Cholera	Cold
Age 20–40	24	2
Age 40–60	39	9
Age 60–80	64	51
Age 80–100	90	207

Correlating the availability of cleanliness to health, the Committee for Promoting the Establishment of Baths and Washhouses for the Labouring Classes reported there were 13 baths and washhouses in London, at which 1,220,739 baths were administered, for a total of £17,062, and 421,010 linen washings of about 1,684,404 persons were performed for a total of £6,096. Twenty of the poorer districts were still without public baths and washhouses.[27]

Cholera Mortality in New York City, 1854

	Total Deaths	Cholera Deaths
July 29	1,139	241
August 5	1,148	362
August 12	1,050	278[28]

Franklin Street Hospital (New York), 1854

	Received	Died	Disch'd Cured	Remaining
To August 13	475	229	205	35
14	9	5	8	31
19	523	249	237	31
20	9	4	5	31
21	2	3	3	27
22	4	0	5	26
23	9	3	5	27
24	9	3	5	26
25	9	3	5	27

Mott Street Hospital

	Received	Died	Disch'd Cured	Remaining
To August 13	84	37	25	21
14	2	—	3	20
19	110	49	45	15
20	9	4	5	31
21	3	2	3	15
22	6	3	2	16
23	5	1	2	18
24	1	0	1	18
25	2	2	3	15

Blackwell's Island

	Received	Died	Disch'd Cured	Remaining
August 13	20	12	—	20[29]

Health Statistics from the Crimean War

The Crimean War was the first major conflict to be extensively covered by journalists, and their eyewitness accounts brought all the glory and the tragedy to readers around the globe. One detail filling nearly every column was statistics, although at least one newspaper entertained the idea "very exaggerated notions have been formed from the letters of the Correspondents in the daily papers, of the amount of sickness among out troops in Turkey."

By "official authority," for the week ending August 5, 1854, there were 1,862 soldiers in hospital, or 7.73 percent of the total strength of the army. Deaths during the week amounted to 205, of which 167 were attributed to cholera. Other sicknesses were fevers (579), diseases of the chest (69) and diseases of the stomach and bowels, exclusive of cholera (667). The

French troops under General Canrebert, performing arduous service amid the swampy ground and under a broiling sun, suffered greatly from malignant cholera; 60 men were lost in one day, "dying suddenly, as our troops die in India."[30]

The Study of Water: England, 1859–1863

The idea that impurities in water caused cholera gained strength after Dr. Snow's study on the outbreak in Golden Square in 1854 but was by no means universally accepted. However, more frequent scientific studies were conducted as the march toward complete recognition crawled slowly forward.

In 1858, Dr. Robert Dundas Thomson of St. Thomas' Hospital reported that Thames water sampled at London Bridge contained 88.8° of impurity and 10.24° of organic impurity, with 1 grain of carbonate of ammonia per gallon, derived from animal matter in the sewage. In July 1859 the amount of the same salt was .72 grains. The study noted the smell of the river was "distinguishable at even a greater distance than last year," but it subsided with the temperature. In the following tables, "Total Impurity" indicates the degree or grains of foreign matter in solution, while "Organic Impurity" indicates the degree or grains of which are vegetable or animal matter.

Study of Water in Glasgow and London, July 1859

District	Total Impurity per Gallon (grs. or degree)	Organic Impurity per Gallon (grs. or degree)
Distilled water	0.0	0.0
Loch Katrine, Glasgow	2.14	0.60
Thames at London Bridge	159.20	16.80
Aldgate Pump	49.12	13.94
THAMES COMPANIES		
West Middlesex	15.72	0.72
Grand Junction	15.40	1.20
Chelsea	15.48	0.92
Southwark	14.76	0.76
Lambeth	16.00	1.16
OTHER COMPANIES		
New River	14.60	1.16
East London	16.36	0.92
Kent	21.68	1.84[31]

Study of Water in Glasgow and London, March 1860

	Total Impurity	Organic Impurity
Loch Katrine, Glasgow	3.36	0.96
Well, Newton, Wisbeach	348.80	21.00
THAMES COMPANIES		
West Middlesex	20.40	1.84
Grand Junction	20.56	1.76
Chelsea	20.56	1.60
Southwark	20.56	1.48
Lambeth	19.68	1.68

District	Total Impurity per Gallon (grs. or degree)	Organic Impurity per Gallon (grs. or degree)
OTHER COMPANIES		
New River	20.72	2.00
East London	22.40	2.00
Kent	25.92	2.08

The shallow well at Newton was situated in a locality where cholera prevailed,[32] clearly indicating there was a long way to go in public sanitation.

**Study of Water in Glasgow and London,
September 1863**

Loch Katrine, Glasgow	2.35	.605
Manchester Water Supply	3.33	.680
Aldgate Pump, City	49.12	13.94
THAMES COMPANIES		
West Middlesex	16.04	1.16
Grand Junction	16.48	1.12
Chelsea	17.08	1.80
Southwark	17.00	1.88
Lambeth	16.64	1.60
OTHER COMPANIES		
New River	15.20	1.20
East London	19.36	1.52
Kent	27.44	3.68

Dr. Thomson noted that some of the waters for domestic purposes were purer, while others contained more foreign ingredients than previously. Of note, Sir Walter Scott celebrated the water of Loch Katrine in his poem "The Lady of the Lake."[33]

In 1909 a report from the director of Water Examination on Research Work dealing with the vitality of the cholera vibrio in artificially infected samples of raw Thames, Lea and New River water concluded the vast majority of vibrios died within one week, with cholera germs more susceptible than typhoid bacillus. The results indicated that by adequately storing raw impure river water, antecedent to their filtration, the safety of London, as regarded water-borne epidemics, was "almost, if not quite, assured."

In 1882 Herbert C. Foote presented a study done on American spring waters, finding that the total quantity of dissolved impurities to be 1–2 grains to 80–90 grains in 1 U.S. gallon (231 cubic inches). Lime salts made water hard but could be softened by boiling, the action of which liberated carbonic acid gas and formed insoluble calcium carbonate that settled to the bottom or formed incrustations around teakettle spouts. When the people of Glasgow substituted the pure water of Lock Katrine in place of hard well water, they saved $180,000 per annum, as hard water required much more soap in washing.[34]

Where Are We Now?

In March 1860 the British registrar-general issued statistics for the previous year. The mortality in 100,000 living was 2,229 deaths from all causes, of which 592 were by diseases of the zymotic class. Compared to the 20-year period between 1660 and 1679, mortality was 7:100,000, of which 3,400 were by zymotic diseases.

Life Statistics of London

Disease	Mortality per 100,000 1660–1679	Mortality per 100,000 1859
Small-pox	357	42
Measles	40	47
Fever	749	59
Scarlatina, croup	759	227
Childbirth	86	17
Dysentery	763	8
Diarrhea	120	11
Cholera	130	7
Syphilis	21	12
Scurvy, purpura	142	2
Dropsy	298	26
Apoplexy, paralysis, epilepsy, suicide	57	151
Consumption	1,079	611
Disease of digestive organs	146	95
Stone, diseases of the urinary organs	21	30
Childhood convulsions and teething	1,175	136
Fractures and wounds	19	25
Poison	1	2
Burns	3	13
Drowning, suffocation	23	10
Execution	5	1

In addition, during 1660–1679, an average of 1,132 lives were destroyed by plague. It was also noted "the high rates of mortality which then prevailed still attend cholera and current epidemics in certain localities. The nature of disease and the climate are still the same as they were in London before the Revolution.... Cholera was on an average then as fatal as it has been recently, and probably much more fatal than it will be again if London [not] be supplied with pure water."[35]

The Fourth Cholera Pandemic, 1863–1879

Isolated cholera cases were reported in Great Britain in 1865, but despite improved sanitary measures, 1866 represented a year of horrific loss of life.

Health of the Metropolis, 1865–1866

Date	Deaths from Diarrhea	Deaths from Cholera
July 22, 1865	280	18
October 7	83	5
May 5, 1866	16	1
July 14	150	32
July 21	221	346
July 28	347	904

Date	Deaths from Diarrhea	Deaths from Cholera
August 4	354	1,053
August 11	264	781
August 18	194	455
August 25	129	265
September 1	128	198
September 8	132	157
September 15	110	182
September 22	98	150
September 29	67	177
October 6	69	182
October 13	47	207
October 20		199 (cholera and diarrhea)
October 27	32	112
November 3	28	73
November 10	33	67
November 17	22	32
November 24	26	8
December 1	15	3
December 8	—	1[36]

The distribution of cholera in 1866 was nearly the same as in previous epidemics. The spike in deaths during three successive weeks in July was attributed to the East London Water Company, which drew water from the reservoirs at Old Ford, strengthening the "circumstantial inference" that part of the water drawn was taken from uncovered (as opposed to covered) reservoirs. The registrar-general's report concluded: "The difficulties of supplying twenty-one million gallons of pure water daily from the Lea, with only one small reservoir, holding a third part of the day's supply, below, and in close juxtaposition to the tidal portion of that river full of foul sewage, in all seasons of the year, are immense; and, in the conditions given, casualties, which no skill can entirely avoid, are almost inevitable."[37] The final tally indicated that cholera had been excessively fatal in Liverpool (42:1,000) and that the epidemic proved extraordinarily fatal for a short time, "from causes that favoured the diffusion of its elements." The entire mortality rate for London was 26:1,000, or 2 above the average; the eastern districts ranked highest in mortality, with 34:1,000 among 607,945 inhabitants. Mortality was lower than in 1865 in Manchester, Salford, Birmingham, Hull, Edinburgh and Glasgow.[38]

A report to the New York Metropolitan Board of Health, September 25, 1866, indicated the death rate in that city was 40:1,000 per annum and in Brooklyn it was 31:1,000; compared to other cities, Vienna's death rate was 40:1,000, London and Dublin, 24:1,000, Liverpool, 64:1,000. Zymotic diseases caused 62.5 percent of all deaths in New York; specifically, diarrheal disorders constituted 75.5 percent of the zymotic deaths.[39]

Cholera Mortality by Month, New York City, 1861–1865

Jan	Feb	March	April	May	June	Total
236	190	125	273	304	721	1,849

Of 22 wards, the sixth had the highest rate of cholera deaths (including those sent to cholera hospitals) in 1866 with 125; the 22nd ward followed with 76. The second and third wards had the least mortality with two each. Between June and September, 342 persons died; among those, 65 were listed as domestics, 33 as laborers and 15 as housekeepers. The board of health concluded, "We are warranted in asserting that there was abundant evidence of such infective influence of the 'rice-water' excrement." With few exceptions, the board said, cholera was limited to the tenant-house districts, adding, "not a respectable hotel or commercial visitor in the city was reached by the infection."[40]

There is no question that sanitary improvement in drainage, sewerage, water supply and cleaning greatly reduced fatalities in Great Britain. By 1867 in Cardiff, mortality was reduced from 33.2 per 1,000 per annum to 22.6; in Newport, the ratio of 31.8 was reduced to 21.6. In Salisbury, Croydon, Macclesfield and Merthyr, numbers were reduced by one-fifth; in Ely, the reduction was 14 percent. In his annual report, John Simon used these facts to justify in the public eye the preventability of disease.[41]

Dr. Farr's report on the London cholera epidemic of 1866 stated that 14,378 deaths were attributable to cholera, as compared to 20,097 in 1854, and 53,293 during the epidemic of 1849. The report bore out the generally accepted theory as to the close connection between epidemics and the quality of water and offered proof that sanitary measures could be effective. The third quarter of 1869 ending October 2 revealed increased mortality from zymotic diseases, reaching 7,316, or 848 above the 10 years' average, corrected for population growth. Scarlet fever proved the most deadly, killing 1,770, while "summer diarrhea" carried off 2,644 victims, with "simple cholera" accounting for 193 more. Of the 19,207 deaths for the quarter, 10,208 were children under 5 years.[42]

UNITED STATES STATISTICS OF MORTALITY
(FROM THE 1870 CENSUS)

(The total population was 38,558,371; of these, there were more people between the ages of 5 and 10 than any other period of life. Of every 1,000 children born, 170 died before their first birthday.) Fatalities from the most dangerous diseases were:

Consumption	69,896	Dropsy	7,856
Pneumonia	40,012	Debility	11,457
Enteric fever	22,187	Old age	7,986
Cholera infantum	20,255	Sill-born	9,060
Scarlet fever	20,320	Alcohol	1,410
Diarrhea	14,195	Accident	22,740
Convulsions	12,751	Suicide	1,345
Encephalitis	13,701	Homicide	2,057
Croup	10,692	Executions	31

Massachusetts had the highest number of deaths from consumption; Texas had the highest number of deaths from pneumonia; Arizona had the highest percentage of deaths from small-pox; Louisiana was the least healthful state, while Wisconsin had the smallest proportion of deaths. Native-born deaths were 424,730 to 65,963 foreign-born. The percentage of deaths to population ranked Massachusetts highest at 1.77, followed by Missouri, 1.63; California, 1.61; New York, 1.58; District of Columbia, 1.53 and Pennsylvania, 1.49.[43] For the year 1871, there were 27,000 deaths in New York City, of which 7,006 were infants under 2 years of age:

Accidents	2,294	Smallpox	210
Diarrheal diseases	1,880	Diphtheria	199
Other zymotics	954	Typhoid	169
Scarlatina	646	Suicide	105
Cholera morbus	444	Typhus fever	82
Whopping cough	360	Homicide	61
Croup	357	Cholera	2
Measles	300	Yellow fever	2[44]

The Great Cholera Epidemic of 1873 struck Hungary particularly hard. Statistics revealed that for the year, 433,295 cases were recorded, with 247,718 recoveries, 182,549 deaths and 2,978 still sick. The population of the countries of the crown of St. Stephen (as defined in the Croatian-Hungarian Settlement of 1868 as the Kingdom of Hungary and Triune Kingdom of Croatia, Slavonia and Dalmatia) amounted to 16,000,000 and it was estimated that 200,000 (or 1:30) souls were felled by cholera.[45] The same scourge struck Buenos Ayres: by February 1874, between 30 and 40 were daily falling victim, with a death total at 307.[46]

Statistics supplied by Elisha Harris, London Registrar, between July 5 and September 20, 1873 revealed the following:

Cholera Mortality

Week Ending	Total Mortality	Vienna	Peath, Hungary	Berlin	Paris, France
July 5	—	33	50	—	—
July 12	800	60	77	—	—
July 19	881	81	189	—	—
July 26	415	78	187	12	—
August 2	481	93	216	16	—
August 9	671	290	274	16	—
August 16	693	394	243	82	—
August 23	651	239	184	86	1
August 30	718	307	152	75	2
September 6	778	418	134	101	3
September 13	697	326	61	134	107
September 20	486	219	—	—	125[47]

Cholera deaths in Munich from November 15, 1873 (the reappearance of the disease) through mid–January 1874 were 2,138 cases and 988 deaths.[48]

The Sacrifice of Human Life

During the first six months of 1875, international mortality statistics from other than natural causes reveal the various modes by which people died:

Epidemics	50,000	Marine disasters	1,303
Earthquakes	20,070	Tornadoes	944
Famine	20,000	Fires	944
Floods	3,606	Explosions	207

These numbers reflect only those large disasters and do not include suicide, murder, war, massacre or other violent forms of death. The article concluded "it does not seem that there is any danger that the world will be overcrowded with population."[49]

The annual abstract of the London Sanitary Commissioner with the government of India seemed to bear out that prediction. Of the nine years for which statistics of European troops were compiled, 1879 presented the highest mortality from cholera at 11.07 per 1,000. In 1878 the ratio was 4.00, which was the highest since 1872 when it was 7.25. In all, 883 cases of cholera occurred among the troops, of which 654 proved fatal. The proportion of deaths in Bengal—16.18—was due to outbreaks among those on field service, accounting for more than half the casualties.[50]

Cholera appeared at Damietta, Egypt, on June 25, 1883. Statistics painted a grim picture of its spread and devastation.

Total Cholera Cases in Egypt
During a 70-day Epidemic Beginning June 25, 1883

Cairo	7,143	Mehalieh	342
Damietta	1,696	Samanoud	293
Mansurah	1,141	Menzalch	191
Shirbin	845	Tantab	164
Alexandria	733	Chober	101
Ghizeh	503		

Mortality per Week

1st week	747	6th week	4,607
2nd week	1,003	7th week	4,545
3rd week	1,124	8th week	2,093
4th week	3,176	9th week	832
5th week	4,693	10th week	481

The greatest mortality was at Cairo, where the disease commenced July 15 and lasted 36 days, with an average daily death rate of 198. The greatest number of deaths in one week (July 25–30) was 4,693 and the greatest in one day (August 3) was 1,693.[51]

The United States was relatively free from cholera in 1882: on a list issued by the Michigan Board of Health for the week ending June 17, 1882, cholera morbus ranked 20th out of 28 diseases, while the generic "intermittent fever" ranked first, "diarrhea" seventh, "dysentery" 21st and "cholera infantum 28th. Neuralgia, rheumatism, consumption and bronchitis rounded out the top five.[52]

In 1886 the Sanitary Board of Japan published a history of cholera in the empire, acknowledging that as the disease raged in China in 1822 it first appeared at Nagasaki, the only port open to foreign commerce. Another epidemic occurred in 1858, but after the country opened its ports to international commerce it became more frequent. During 1876–1877 there were 7,967 deaths; another epidemic followed in 1879 when 105,786 fatal attacks were recorded. After a lull of six years, cholera appeared again in 1885. By the time the report was published in 1886, the death toll had reached 7,152.[53]

Chapter Notes

Preface

1. *Courier (London)*, August 13, 1832.
2. Myron Echenberg, *Africa in the Time of Cholera* (Cambridge, NY: Cambridge University Press, 2011), 3.

Chapter 1

1. Samuel Taylor Coleridge, *The Rime of the Ancient Mariner*, http://www.online-literature.com/coleridge/646/.
2. "Epidemiology and Risk Factors," http://www.cdc.gov/cholera/epi.html.
3. Donald Venes, ed., *Taber's Cyclopedic Medical Dictionary* (Philadelphia: F.A. Davis, 2005, 1605), hereinafter cited as *Taber's*.
4. Kenneth Todar, "Vibrio cholerae and Asiatic cholera," http://textbookofbacteriology.net/cholera.html.
5. Ibid.
6. "Epidemiology and Risk Factors."
7. *Evansville (IN) Daily Enquirer*, April 26, 1855.
8. Todar, "Vibrio cholera."
9. Echenberg. *Africa*, 29–30.
10. "Cholera," http://www.nlm.gov/medlineplus/encv/article/000303htm; "Disease" http://cdc.gov/cholera/disease.html.
11. "General Information," http://www.cdc.gov/cholera/general.
12. Todar, "Vibrio cholera."
13. "Cholera," http://www.medicinenet.com/cholera/article.htm.
14. "General Information."

Chapter 2

1. *Monthly (London) Review*, June 1765.
2. *London Courier*, April 28, 1832.
3. *Taber's*, 648, 2056, 2256, 2365.
4. Todar, "Vibrio cholera."
5. Robert Hooper, *Lexicon Medicum; or Medical Dictionary* (New York: Harper, Brothers, 1842), hereafter cited as *Lexicon*.
6. *Dublin Journal*, December 9 to December 13, 1746.
7. *Monthly Review*, June 1765.

8. *St. James Chronicle, or The British Evening-Post (London)*, May 24, 1764.
9. *Monthly Review*, October 1766.

Chapter 3

1. *Monthly (London) Magazine*, October 1, 1799.
2. *Taber's*, 998.
3. "Thomas Sydenham," http://wikipedia.org/wiki/Thomas_Sydenham.
4. *London Chronicle*, June 10 to June 13, 1769.
5. *Monthly (London) Review*, May 1770.
6. Ibid., December 1, 1773.
7. *Penny London Post*, June 3–6, 1748.
8. *London Evening-Post*, December 24–27, 1763.
9. *Edinburgh Adviser*, August 30, 1776.
10. Matthew L. Lim, Gerald S. Murphy, Margaret Calloway, and David Tribble, "History of U.S. Military Contributions to the Study of Diarrheal Diseases," *Military Medicine* 170, April Supplement, 2005.
11. *Monthly (London) Magazine*, September 1798.
12. Ibid., November 1, 1799.

Chapter 4

1. *Monthly (London) Magazine*, March 1, 1800.
2. *Courier (London)*, February 8, 1832.
3. *Philosophical (London) Magazine*, July 1, 1799.
4. *Monthly Magazine*, March 1, 1800.
5. *Morning Chronicle and London Advertiser*, March 1, 1786.
6. *Times (London)*, August 16, 1794.
7. *Edinburgh Advertiser*, July 19 to July 23, 1799.
8. *Adams (PA) Centinel*, September 26, 1804.
9. *Weekly (PA) Advertiser*, August 10, 1811.
10. *Lycoming (PA) Gazette*, November 11, 1812.
11. *Anti-Jacobin Review and Magazine (London)*, May 1, 1805
12. *A New Review with Literary Curiosities (London)*, March 1, 1783.
13. *British Critic (London)*, September 1, 1800.
14. *Monthly Magazine*, November 1, 1800.
15. "Vis medicatrix naturae," http://medical-diction ary.the freedictionary.com.
16. Echenberg, *Africa*, 10.
17. *Monthly Magazine*, October 1, 1800.
18. Ibid., November 1, 1800.

19. Ibid., September 1, 1802.
20. Ibid., October 1, 1803.
21. Ibid., September 1, 1807.
22. Ibid., October 1809.

Chapter 5

1. *Monthly (London) Magazine*. October 1, 1810.
2. Ibid., August 1, 1812.
3. *Monthly (London) Review*, June 1815.
4. "Cholera's seven pandemics," http://www.cbc.ca/news/health/story/2008/05/09/f-cholera-outbreaks.html.
5. *Monthly Magazine*, April 1, 1817.
6. "The New Annual Register, or, General Repository of History, Politics, and Literature," January 1818.
7. *Gentleman's (London) Magazine*, April 1, 1818.
8. *Edinburgh Advertiser*, March 30, 1819.
9. Ibid., April 28, 1818.
10. *Evangelical (London) Magazine, and Missionary Chronicle*, May 1, 1820.
11. Ibid., January 1, 1820. (The word "Hindu" was spelled "Hindoo" in the 19th century and that spelling is used in the text.)
12. *Torch Light and Public Advertiser (MD)*, April 10, 1821.
13. *Baldwin's London Weekly Journal*, Februay 2, 1822.
14. *Republican (PA) Compiler*, May 30, 1821.
15. *Courier (London)*, July 15, 1823.
16. Ibid., December 13, 1821.
17. *Republican Compiler*, January 19, 1820.
18. "Cholera's seven pandemics."
19. *Saturday Clarion (OH)*, September 25, 1824.
20. *Courier*, June 16, 1831.
21. *Times (London)*, October 19, 1825, from the *Carlisle Journal*.
22. A.D. Cliff, *War Epidemics: An Historical Geography of Infectious Diseases in Military Conflict and Civil Strife, 1850–2000* (New York: Oxford University Press, 2004), 111.
23. *Baldwin's Journal*, May 13, 1826.
24. *Wilmington and Delaware Advertiser*, August 23, 1827.
25. *Trades' (London) Free Press*, January 19, 1828.
26. *Weekly (London) Free Press*, November 22, 1828.
27. *Morning (London) Journal*, December 17, 1828.

Chapter 6

1. *Times (London)*, July 4, 1831.
2. *Courier (London)*, November 18, 1830.
3. Ibid., November 25, 1830.
4. Ibid., November 5, 1830.
5. Ibid., November 25, 1830.
6. *Adams (PA) Sentinel*, December 7, 1830; *Christian (London) Advocate*, December 26, 1831.
7. *Daily Morning Advocate (WI)*, May 1; *Janesville (WI) Daily Gazette*, August 21; *Democratic Pharos (IN)*, December 6, 1854; *Morning Chronicle (London)*, June 2, 1855; *Evening Star (London)*, March 18, 1856; *Bucks County (PA) Gazette*, June 18, 1885.

8. *Courier*, November 3, 1830.
9. Ibid., November 5, 1830.
10. *Baldwin's London Weekly Journal*, November 29, 1830.
11. *Evans and Ruffy's (London) Farmer's Journal*, November 29, 1830.
12. *Baldwin's Weekly*, November 13, 1830.
13. *Courier*, November 25, 1830.
14. *Age (London)*, November 14, 1830.
15. *Albion (London)*, November 15, 1830.
16. *Courier*, November 29, 1830.
17. Ibid., December 1, 1830, from *Gazette de France*, November 17, 1930.
18. *Frederick (MD) Town Herald*, January 1, 1831.
19. *Albion*, January 11, 1831.
20. Ibid., January 18, 1831.
21. *Christian Advocate*, January 31, 1831.
22. *Albion*, January 22, 1831.
23. Ibid., January 31, 1831.
24. A.D. Cliff, *War Epidemics*, 109.
25. *Kent and Essex Mercury (London)*, February 1; *Baldwin's Weekly*, February 5, 1831.
26. "November Uprising," http://en.wikipedia.org/wiki/November_Uprising.
27. *Albion*, May 9, 1831.
28. Ibid., May 2, 1831.
29. Ibid., May 9, 1831.
30. *Courier*, March 11, 1831.
31. Ibid., July 23, 1831, from the *Medical Gazette*.
32. *Christian Advocate*, June 6, 1831.
33. *Albion*, June 14, 1831.
34. *Courier*, June 23, 1831.
35. *Times (London)*, July 4; *Courier*, July 5, 1831.
36. *Albion*, July 18, 1831.
37. Ibid., July 11, 1831.
38. *Christian Advocate*, June 6, 1831.
39. *Sandusky (OH) Clarion*, July 20, 1831.
40. *Courier*, July 23, 1831.
41. *Albion*, July 26, 1831.
42. *Age*, June 26, 1831.
43. *Times (London)*, July 4, 1831.
44. *Albion*, July 18, 1831.
45. *Times (London)*, July 4; *Courier*, July 5, 1831
46. *Courier*, June 28, 1831.
47. Ibid., July 20, 1831.
48. "November Uprising."
49. *Albion*, August 16, 1831.
50. Ibid., September 1, 1831.
51. *Courier*, September 13, 1831.
52. *Albion*, July 26, 1831.
53. *Kent and Essex Mercury*, August 2, 1831.
54. *Albion*, August 6, 1831.
55. *Country (London) Times*, August 22, 1831, from the *Medical Gazette*.
56. *Country Times*, November 14, 1831.
57. *Edinburgh Medical and Surgical Journal* 38, Edinburgh (1832), 455–459.
58. *British Banner (London)*, August 1, 1849.
59. *Country Times*, November 14, 1831.
60. Ibid., November 14, 1831.
61. *Christian Advocate*, January 30, 1832.
62. *Albion*, August 16, 1831.

63. Ibid.
64. Ibid.
65. *Country Times*, September 12, 1831.
66. A.D. Cliff, *War Epidemics*, 109.
67. *Adams (PA) Sentinel*, March 13, 1832, from a report by M. Jomard, dated Alexandria, November 18, 1831, and sent to the Paris Academy of Medicine.
68. *Evans and Ruffy*, September 19, 1831.
69. *Christian Advocate*, November 28, 1831.
70. Ibid., November 21, 1831.
71. *Times (London)*, December 9, 1831.
72. *Adams Sentinel*, December 6, 1831.

Chapter 7

1. *Courier (London)*, August 13, 1832.
2. Ibid., June 16, 1831.
3. Ibid., January 30, 1841.
4. Ibid., July 11, 26, 1831.
5. Ibid., August 17, 1831.
6. *Bells' (London) New Weekly Messenger*, February 19, 1832.
7. *Courier*, June 16, 1831.
8. *Christian Advocate (London)*, June 6, 1831.
9. *Albion (London)*, September 15, 1831.
10. *Courier*, June 27, 1831.
11. *Circular to Bankers (London)*, June 24, 1831.
12. *Courier*, October 19, 1831.
13. *Age (London)*, September 18, 1831.
14. Ibid., November 20, 1831.
15. *Times (London)*, October 17, 1831.
16. *Courier*, November 7, 1831.
17. *Times*, November 10, 1831.
18. *Patriot (London)*, May 30, 1832.
19. *Bell's Messenger*, July 8, 1832.
20. *Bell's Life in London and Sporting Chronicle*, November 27, 1831.
21. *Country Times (London)*, November 14, 1831.
22. *Courier*, November 14, 1831.
23. *Country Times*, November 14, 1831.
24. *Albion*, June 7, 1831.
25. *Baldwin's London Weekly Journal*, June 18, 1831.
26. *Courier*, July 23, 1831.
27. *Albion*, July 22, 1831.
28. *Times (London)*, July 29, 1831.
29. *Courier*, November 14, 1831.
30. *True Sun (London)*, March 5, 1832.

Chapter 8

1. *Age (London)*, December 25, 1831.
2. *Evans and Ruffy's Farmers' Journal (London)*, February 6, 1832.
3. *True Sun (London)*, March 5, 1832.
4. *Albion and The Star (London)*, March 29, 1832.
5. *True Sun*, March 5, 1832.
6. Ibid., March 20, 1832.
7. *Albion and Star*, March 2; *British Traveller and Commercial and Law Gazette (London)*, March 24, 1832.
8. *Albion and Star*, February 11, 1832.
9. *True Sun*, March 26, 1832.

10. *Courier (London)*, February 25, 1832.
11. *Bell's New Weekly Messenger (London)*, February 26, 1832; italics added.
12. S.L. Kotar and J.E. Gessler, *Smallpox: A History* (Jefferson, NC: McFarland, 2013), 103, 319.
13. *Evans and Ruffy's*, November 21, 1831.
14. *Albion (London)*, December 16, 1831.
15. *Courier*, November 26, 1831.
16. *Baldwin's London Weekly*, December 3, 1831.
17. *Courier*, December 8, 17, 21, 24, 28, 30; *Times (London)*, December 5, 16, 20, 23; *Albion*, December 16, 22; *Kent and Essex Mercury (London)*, December 20, 1831; *Christian Advocate (London)*, January 2, 1832.
18. *Albion*, December 16, 22; *Courier*, December 17, 21, 28, 30, 31; *Times*, December 23, 1831; *Christian Advocate*, January 2; *Courier*, January 2, 1832.
19. *Courier*, December 24, 28, 30, 31, 1831.
20. *Baldwin's London Weekly*, December 31, 1831.
21. (London) *Times*, November 10, 1831.
22. *Courier*, November 14, 1831.
23. *Age*, December 11, 1831.
24. *Times*, December 15, 1831.
25. *Courier*, December 20, 1831.
26. *Age*, December 11, 1831.
27. *Christian Advocate*, November 28, 1831.
28. *Courier*, December 20, 1831.
29. *Times*, December 16, 1831.
30. *Lexicon*.
31. *Albion and Star*, February 29, 1832.
32. Ibid., February 3, 1832.
33. *Bell's New Weekly*, February 26, 1832.
34. *Courier*, February 11, 1832.
35. *Evans and Ruffy's*, November 21, 1831.
36. *Bell's New Weekly*, February 19, 1832.

Chapter 9

1. *Bell's New Weekly Messenger (London)*, February 19, 1832.
2. *Courier (London)*, April 3, 1817.
3. *Philosophical Magazine and Journal (London)*, July 1, 1818.
4. *Champion and Sunday Review (London)*, August 17, 1818.
5. *Edinburgh Advertiser*, August 18, 1818.
6. *Law Chronicle Commercial and Bankruptcy Register (London)*, April 14, 1831.
7. *Courier*, January 17, 1832
8. Ibid., August 27, 1824.
9. *British Press (London)*, August 19, 1825.
10. *Kent and Essex Mercury (London)*, April 10, 1831.
11. *Evans and Ruffy's (London)*, September 19, 1831.
12. *Courier*, November 7, 1831.
13. *Albion and Star (London)*, January 20, 1832.
14. *Courier*, January 23, 1832.
15. *Bell's New Weekly*, February 19, 1832.
16. *Times (London)*, March 12, 1832.
17. "Poisoning Is a Fine Art," *Janesville (WI) Gazette*, September 7, 1876, from the *London Examiner*.
18. *Evans and Ruffy's*, June 4, 1832.
19. *Logansport (IN) Chronicle*, February 6, 1886.
20. *Washington (DC) Post*, March 7, 1907.

21. *San Antonio (TX) Light and Gazette*, February 19, 1911.

22. *Albion and Star*, February 24, 1832.

23. *Glasgow Courier*, March 6, 1832.

Chapter 10

1. *Reviewer (London)*, January 8, 1832.

2. *Bell's New Weekly (London)*, February 26, 1832.

3. *Christian Advocate*, January 23, February 13; *Courier*, January 26, February 9, 16, 21, 23; *Times (London)*, February 2; *Patriot (London)*, February 29, 1832.

4. *Kent and Essex Mercury (London)*, February 28, 1831.

5. *Courier (London)*, February 16, 1832.

6. *Bell's New Weekly*, February 19, 1832.

7. *True Sun (London)*, March 14, 1832.

8. *Reviewer*, January 15, 1832.

9. *Courier*, January 24, 1832.

10. *True Sun*, March 20, 1832.

11. *Bell's New Weekly*, February 19, 1832.

12. Ibid., February 5, 1832.

13. *Albion and Star*, March 2, 22, 27, 28, 29, 30, April 7, 12, May 3, 5, 8, 10, 11, 12, 14, 18; *Courier*, March 3, 12, 14, 15, 19, 23, April 4, 21, 25, May 7; *True Sun*, March 6, 7, 8, 9, 10, 13, 16, 19, 24, 31, April 2, 3, 6, 9, 16, 17, 18, 23, 27, 28, 30, May 1, 2, 16, 19, 22, 23, 24, 25; *Bell's New Weekly*, March 11; *Bell's Life in London*, March 25; *Evans and Ruffy's*, March 19; *British Traveller*, May 9; *Patriot*, May 16, 1832.

14. *Patriot*, May 16, 1832.

15. *Evans and Ruffy's*, March 12, 1832.

16. *Courier*, April 26, 1832

17. *Christian Advocate*, April 30, 1832.

18. *Albion and Star*, May 8, 1832.

19. *Courier*, May 7, 1832.

20. *Christian Advocate*, March 12; *Baldwin's London Weekly Journal and Surrey and Sussex Gazette*, March 31, 1832.

21. *Courier*, March 15, 1832.

22. *Albion and Star*, June 9, 12, 1832.

23. Ibid., June 19; *Christian Advocate and World*, June 25, 1832.

24. *Times*, July 3, 1832.

25. *Albion and Star*, July 6, 1832.

26. Ibid., June 24, 1832.

27. *Age*, June 24, 1832.

28. *Age*, April 1, 1832.

29. *True Sun*, March 6, 1832.

30. *Baldwin's Weekly and Surrey and Sussex*, March 31, 1832.

31. *Bell's New Weekly*, April 1, 7, 1832.

32. Ibid., June 3, 1832.

33. *True Sun*, June 28, 1832.

34. *Adams (PA) Sentinel*, April 10; *Star and Republican Banner (PA)*, July 17; *Christian Advocate*, April 30; *Courier*, July 7, 1832.

Chapter 11

1. *Bell's New Weekly*, January 8, 1832.

2. *Times (London)*, January 24, 1832.

3. *Patriot (London)*, February 22, 1832.

4. *Christian Advocate*, April 2, 1832.

5. *Times*, April 3, 1832.

6. *Courier (London)*, April 2, 1832.

7. *Albion and Star*, April 3, 1832.

8. *Times*, April 4, 1832.

9. *Courier*, April 10; *British Traveller*, April 27; *Patriot*, April 25, 1832.

10. *True Sun*, April 5; *Albion and Star*, April 5; *Courier*, April 6; *Evans and Ruffy's*, April 9, 1832.

11. *True Sun*, April 13, 1832.

12. *Baldwin's Weekly*, April 28, 1832.

13. *Age*, April 22, 1832.

14. *British Traveller*, April 21, 1832.

15. *Albion and Star*, April 19, 1832.

16. *Bell's New Weekly*, April 22, 1832.

17. *Age*, March 25, 1832.

18. *Courier*, July 17, August 15, 1832.

19. *Times*, April 6, 1832.

20. *Albion and Star*, September 28, 1832.

21. *Reno (NV) Evening Gazette*, March 21, 1887.

22. *Adams (PA) Sentinel*, August 14; *Courier*, August 8, 1832.

23. *Republican Compiler (PA)*, January 3; *Albion and Star*, February 1; *Times (London)*, January 16; *True Sun*, May 28, 1832.

24. *Courier*, April 25; *True Sun*, March 29; *Age*, April 15, 1832

25. *Austrian Observer*, January 19; *Times*, February 2, 1832.

26. *True Sun*, April 28, June 16; *Albion and Star*, July 26, 1832.

27. *Courier*, June 28, 1832.

28. Ibid., April 2; *Albion and Star*, May 9, 1832

29. *Albion and Star*, June 25, 1832.

30. *British Traveller*, May 1; *Christian Advocate*, April 2, 1832.

31. *True Sun*, June 21, 1832.

Chapter 12

1. *Age*, May 6, 1832.

2. *True Sun*, June 15; *Times (London)*, June 16; *Albion and Star*, June 22; *Adams (PA) Sentinel*, July 31, 1832.

3. *True Sun*, July 9, 1832.

4. John C, Peters, "Conveyance of Cholera," *Leavenworth Medical Herald*, October 1867.

5. *Huron (OH) Reflector*, July 10, 1832.

6. *Montreal Gazette*, June 19, 1832.

7. *Adams Sentinel*, July 10, 1832.

8. *Herald (Frederick, MD)*, June 30, 1832.

9. *Adams Sentinel*, July 3, 1832.

10. Ibid., March 10, 1834.

11. *Galveston (TX) Daily News*, January 13, 1887.

12. *Adams Sentinel*, July 3, 1832.

13. Ibid., July 10, 1832.

14. Ibid.

15. *Huron (OH) Reflector*, August 7, 1832.

16. B.A. Foex, "How the cholera epidemic of 1831 resulted in a new technique for fluid resuscitation," http://emj.bmj.com/content/20/4/316.full; Michael R. Aldrich, "The Remarkable W. B. O'Shaughnessy,"

http://antiquecannabisbook.com/chap1/Shaughnessy.htm; James, Philip B., "Hyperbaric Oxygen Treatment: The Last Frontier," http://www.hyperbaric-oxygen-info.com/hyperbaric-oxygen-therapy-frontier-philip-james; W. Gibson, "The Bio-Medical Pursuits of Christopher Wren," 331–341 (cited from Foex; notes 17–26 from Foex).

17. *Lancet (London)*, 1831; I, 366–371.

18. T. Murphy, "Character and Treatment of the Malignant Cholera at Liverpool Trial of Venous Injections," *Lancet* (London, 1832), ii, 368–369.

19. A. Masson, "Latta: Pioneer in Saline Infusion," *British Journal of Anaesthesia*, London (1971), 43; 681–686.

20. *Lancet*, 1831, i, 366–371.

21. Ibid., 490.

22. *Lancet*, 1832, i, 505–506.

23. Ibid., 490.

24. "Report to the Central Board of Health," May 23, 1832.

25. *Lancet*, June 2, 1832; i, 274–277.

26. *Lancet*, 1832, ii, 281.

27. *Courier*, July 3, 1832.

28. *Age*, July 22, 1832

29. "William Brooke O'Shaughnessy," http://en.wikipedia.org/wiki/William_Brooke_O'Shaughnessy).

30. *Huron Reflector*, January 14, 1832.

31. *Star, and Adams County Republican Banner (PA)*, January 31, 1832.

32. *Star and Adams County*, February 21, 1832.

33. *Huron Reflector*, March 20; *Mail (MD)*, March 23, 1832.

34. *Star and Adams County*, April 3, 1832, from the *Portland Daily Courier*, March 24, 1832.

35. *Huron Reflector*, April 24, 1832.

36. *Republican Compiler(PA)*, March 6; *Huron Reflector*, July 3, 1832.

37. *Albion and Star*, June 2, 1832.

38. *Huron Reflector*, August 7, 1832.

39. *Mail*, June 29; *Adams Sentinel*, June 26, July 3, 1832.

40. *Frederick Herald (MD)*, July 14, 1832.

41. *Mail*, July 27, 1832.

42. *Adams Sentinel*, July 31, 1832.

43. *Republican Compiler*, July 17, August 7; *Frederick Herald*, July 21, 28, August 4; *Mail*, August 17, 24; *Star and Republican Banner*, August 21; *Adams Sentinel*, August 7, 28, September 4, 1832.

44. *Adams Sentinel*, August 14, 1832.

45. S.L. Kotar and J.E. Gessler, *The Steamboat Era* (Jefferson, NC: McFarland, 2009), 47–48.

46. John Peters, "Conveyance of Cholera."

47. *Star and Republican Banner*, June 26, 1832.

48. *Huron Reflector*, August 7, 1832.

49. *Star and Republican Banner*, June 26; *Mail*, July 27; *Adams Sentinel*, July 10, 31, August 7, 28; *Republican Compiler*, August 7; *Frederick Herald*, July 28, 1832; "United States Army Report for 1832" (Washington, D.C., 1833), 81, 86, 90, 159.

50. *Huron Reflector*, September 25; *Republican Compiler*, October 18, from the *Washington Globe*; *Adams Sentinel*, November 13, 1832.

51. *Adams Sentinel*, December 4; *Sandusky Clarion*, September 12, 1832; *Huron Reflector*, January 8, 1833; *Star and Republican Banner*, December 11, 1832.

Chapter 13

1. John Williamson Nevin, *The Scourge of God* (Pittsburgh: Johnston and Stockton, 1832), 17.

2. *Adams Sentinel*, July 10, 1832.

3. *Frederick Herald*, August 4, 18; *Republican Compiler*, August 7; *Adams Sentinel*, August 7, 28, September 4; *Mail*, August 17, 24, 1832.

4. *Sandusky Clarion*, August 22, 1832.

5. *Adams Sentinel*, August 7, 14, 1832.

6. *Frederick Herald*, August 18, 1832.

7. *Mail*, July 27, 1832.

8. *Republican Compiler*, July 10; *Frederick Herald*, July 21, August 4, 18; *Adams Sentinel*, August 7, 1832.

9. Reprinted in the *Sandusky Clarion*, October 3, 1832.

10. *Adams Sentinel*, September 18, 1832.

11. *Huron Reflector*, September 4, 1832.

12. *Frederick Herald*, September 22, 1832.

13. Ibid., October 13, 1832, from the *Baltimore Republican*.

14. *True Sun (London)*, March 19, 1834.

15. *Adams Sentinel*, August 7, 14, September 4, 1832.

16. Ibid., September 11, 1832.

17. *Mail*, August 17, 1832.

18. *Adams Sentinel*, August 28, September 4; *Mail*, August 31, 1832.

19. *Frederick Herald*, September 29, 1832.

20. *Adams Sentinel*, December 25, 1832.

21. *Mail*, November 16; *Star and Republican Banner*, November 13, 1832.

22. *Sandusky Clarion*, October 3; *Huron Reflector*, October 9; *Adams Sentinel*, October 9; *Patriot (London)*, September 5, 1832.

23. *Adams Sentinel*, November 20, 1832.

24. Ibid., September 11, October 2, 9; *Frederick Herald*, September 22, 1832.

25. *Republican Compiler*, November 20; *Sandusky Clarion*, November 21; *Star and Republican Banner*, November 27; *Mail*, December 1; *Adams Sentinel*, October 9, December 4, 1832.

26. *Star and Republican Banner*, April 22, 1833.

27. *Adams Sentinel*, January 29; *Star and Republican Banner*, February 25, March 11, April 22; *Republican Compiler*, January 29; *Huron Reflector*, June 18, 1833.

28. Reprinted in the *Patriot (London)*, September 12, 1832.

Chapter 14

1. *Courier (London)*, July 13, 1832.

2. *Patriot*, July 11, 1832.

3. *True Sun*, September 8, 1832.

4. *Bell's New Weekly*, July 22, 1832.

5. *Courier*, July 28; *Albion and Star*, July 27; *Age*, July 29; *Commercialist and Weekly Advertiser*, July 29; *Baldwin's London Weekly*, September 1; *True Sun*, September 22; *Bell's New Weekly*, August 19, 1832.

6. *Courier*, July 12; *Circular to Bankers*, September 7; *Albion and Star*, August 10; *British Traveller*, July 27, 1832.

7. *British Traveller*, August 1; *Adams Sentinel (PA)*, September 25, 1832.

8. *True Sun*, July 20, 23, 26; *Times (London)*, August 22; *Kent and Essex Mercury*, September 11; *Courier*, July 30; *Bell's New Weekly*, September 16, 1832.

9. David Armstrong and Elizabeth Metzger Armstrong, *The Great American Medicine Show* (New York: Prentice Hall, 1991), 31–33.

10. Ibid., 34–35.

11. *Courier*, July 26, 1832.

12. *True Sun*, July 13; *Evans and Ruffy's*, July 16; *Christian Advocate*, July 16, 1832.

13. *British Traveller*, July 16, 26, August 2; *Albion and Star*, July 30, August 9, 1832.

14. *Courier*, July 24; *British Traveller*, August 4; *Star and Republican Banner*, November 6, 1832.

Chapter 15

1. *Adams Sentinel*, July 1, 1833, from a letter dated June 10.

2. *Sandusky Clarion*, April 17; *Huron Reflector*, April 16, 1833.

3. *Sandusky Clarion*, June 26, from the *Cincinnati Gazette*; *Adams Sentinel*, April 1, 1833.

4. *Republican Compiler*, July 2, 1833.

5. *Star and Republican Banner*, July 9, 1833.

6. *Star and Republican Banner*, June 3; *Mail*, May 10, June 7, 21, August 30; *Lycoming Gazette*, May 29, June 5; *Republican Compiler*, June 4, 18; *Adams Sentinel*, June 10, 17; *Huron Reflector*, June 11, 1833.

7. *Adams Sentinel*, June 24, 1833.

8. *Adams Sentinel*, July 1, 15; *Huron Reflector*, July 16; (London) *Mail*, July 19, 1833.

9. *Adams Sentinel*, June 3, 1833.

10. *Adams Sentinel*, July 29, August 5, 19, 26; *Republican Compiler*, August 20; *Sandusky Clarion*, August 28, 1833.

11. *Republican Compiler*, July 9; *Adams Sentinel*, July 15; *Huron Reflector*, July 16, 1833.

12. *Adams Sentinel*, July 1; *Mail*, July 5; *Huron Reflector*, July 16, 1833.

13. *Huron Reflector*, July 16; *Adams Sentinel*, July 22, 29, 1833; *Mail*, August 15, 1834.

Chapter 16

1. *Huron Reflector*, September 9, 1834, obituary of Captain Zebah Phillips, Berlin, August 21, 1834.

2. *Albion and Star*, January 23, 1833.

3. *Mail*, September 6, 1833.

4. *Adams Sentinel*, January 27, 1834.

5. *Albion and Star*, January 29, 1834.

6. *Times (London)*, February 8, 1833.

7. *Atlas (London)*, March 23, 1833.

8. *Adams Sentinel*, September 2, 1833.

9. *Patriot*, October 8, 1834.

10. *Albion and Star*, January 29, 1834.

11. *Republican Compiler*, March 26, April 2, 23, 30, May 4; *Star and Republican Banner*, April 1; *Adams Sentinel*, April 8, 22; *Lycoming Gazette*, April 24, July 3; *Mail*, April 26, May 3, 1833.

12. *Adams Sentinel*, July 1, 1833.

13. *Republican Compiler*, September 17, 1833.

14. *Adams Sentinel*, September 2, 1833, from the *Baltimore Gazette*.

15. *Mail (MD)*, September 6, November 1; *Adams Sentinel*, September 30, October 7, 28; *Republican Compiler*, November 5, 1833.

16. *Huron Reflector*, December 18, 1846; *Defiance Democrat*, June 23, 1849.

17. *Sandusky Clarion*, June 18; *Adams Sentinel*, July 28; *Torch Light*, July 31; *Huron Reflector*, August 5; *Republican Compiler*, August 26, September 2, 30; *Star and Republican Banner*, October 14, 1834.

18. *Huron Reflector*, July 16, 1833; *Republican Compiler*, March 25, 1834.

19. *Mail (MD)*, November 1, 8, 29; *Adams Sentinel*, November 25, 1833.

20. *Torch Light*, May 29, 1843.

21. *Adams Sentinel*, September 8, 1834.

22. *Mail (MD)*, November 7, 1834.

23. *Torch Light*, November 13, 1834.

24. *Mail*, January 17; *Republican Compiler*, November 18, 1834.

25. *Republican Compiler*, October 28; *Adams Sentinel*, October 27, 1834.

Chapter 17

1. *Adams Sentinel*, August 31, 1835.

2. *Hagerstown Free Press*, March 26, May 28; *Torch Light*, March 13; *Mail*, April 4; *Adams Sentinel*, January 27, May 12, 1834.

3. *Torch Light*, May 22; *Adams Sentinel*, June 9, 1834.

4. *Republican Compiler*, July 22; *Hagerstown Free Press*, July 23, 1834.

5. *Adams Sentinel*, August 18, 1834.

6. *Torch Light*, July 24, 31; *Adams Sentinel*, July 28, August 4, 11; *Republican Compiler*, July 29, 1834.

7. *Huron Reflector*, August 5, 1834.

8. *Torch Light*, April 3; *Adams Sentinel*, September 8, 29; *Star and Republican Banner*, September 9, 23, October 14, December 16; *Republican Compiler*, September 16, 1834.

9. *Torch Light*, August 28, October 16; *Republican Compiler*, September 30, 1834.

10. *Adams Sentinel*, June 1, 1835.

11. *Republican Compiler*, June 9, 1835.

12. *Bangor Daily Whig and Courier*, November 5, 1841.

13. *Republican Compiler*, May 26, June 23; *Mail*, June 5, 1835.

14. *Adams Sentinel*, August 10; *Huron Reflector*, September 8, 1835.

15. *Huron Reflector*, June 23, September 8; *Republican Compiler*, July 13, August 25; *Adams Sentinel*, July 13; *People's Press (PA)*, July 24, 1835.

16. *Adams Sentinel*, July 27, 1835.

17. *Huron Reflector*, August 11; *Republican Compiler*, September 8, 1835; *Bangor Daily Whig and Courier*, September 21, 1839.

18. *Republican Compiler*, September 13, 27, October 18, November 8, 15; *Hagerstown Mail*, September 23; *Baldwin's London Weekly Journal*, October 8; *Adams Sentinel*, November 7, 1836 (italics added); *Alton Observer*, January 26, 1837.

19. *Republican Compiler*, September 13, 1836 from the *Eastport Sentinel*.

20. *Huron Reflector*, July 28, 1835; *Hagerstown Mail*, January 27, 1837, July 13, 1838.

21. *Settler and Pennon*, September 14, 1844; *Western Statesman*, March 30, 1843, October 22, 1840; *Huron Reflector*, November 22, 1836; *Star and Republican Compiler*, August 1, 1836; *Adams Sentinel*, August 10, 1835; *Republican Compiler*, September 8, 1835.

Chapter 18

1. *Star and Republican Banner*, November 2, 1835.

2. *Courier*, October 31, 1835, December 30, 1836, August 29, 1837; *True Sun*, July 14, 1836, October 13, 1837; *Republican Compiler*, September 6, 1836, August 1, September 5, 1837; *Adams Sentinel*, January 16, 1837; *Hagerstown Mail*, February 3, 1837; *Alton Observer*, August 10, 1837; *Bell's New Weekly Messenger*, August 27, 1837; *Bangor Daily Whig and Courier*, September 7, 1837; *Gardeners' Gazette (London)*, August 20, 1837.

3. *Age*, August 28, 1836; *Gardeners' Gazette*, August 26, September 16; *True Sun*, October 13, 1837; *Hagerstown Mail*, January 26, 1838; *Adams Sentinel*, January 30, 1837.

4. *Republican Compiler*, October 13, November 10, 1835; *Adams Sentinel*, February 1, 1836; *Adams Sentinel*, October 10, 1842; *Nonconformist*, July 5; *Colonial Gazette (London)*, November 11, 1943; *Indian Mail (London)*, August 3, 1844.

5. *Republican Compiler*, August 1, 22; *Adams Sentinel*, September 11, 1837; *Patriot (London)*, November 8, 1838; *Bangor Daily Whig and Courier*, February 24, 1842.

6. *Bell's New Weekly Messenger*, July 5, 1840.

7. *Gardeners' Gazette*, November 28, 1840.

8. *Weekly Chronicle*, May 4, 1850.

9. *Atlas*, February 25, 1843.

10. *Miners' Free Press (WT)*, July 11, 1837.

11. *Republican Compiler*, September 1, 1835.

12. *Adams Sentinel*, August 31, November 16, 1835.

13. *Wisconsin Argus*, July 15; *Court Gazette (London)*, August 23; *Indian Statesman*, September 27, 1845; *Allen's Indian Mail*, July 4, 1836, June 24, 1837; *Weekly Chronicle (London)*, August 22; *Atlas*, September 5; *Alton (IL) Telegraph and Democratic Review*, October 9, 1836.

14. *Allen's Indian Mail*, April 5, 1845.

15. *Atlas*, September 19, 1846.

16. *Adams Sentinel*, April 27, 1846.

17. *Nonconformist*, October 15; *Huron Reflector*, November 18, 1845; *Milwaukee Daily Courier*, May 1, 7, 1846; *Patriot*, August 17; *Circular to Bankers*, September 18, October 2, 1846; *Atlas*, December 13, 1846.

18. *Lloyd's Weekly London*, December 13, 1846.

19. *Democratic Pharos (IN)*, July 8, 1846; *Bell's Life in London*, November 14, 1847; *Weekly Chronicle*, May 27, 1848; *Nonconformist*, December 29, 1847.

20. *Nautical Standard*, July 25; *Nonconformist*, September 16; *Star and Republican Banner (PA)*, October 9; *Bell's Life in London*, November 22, 1846; *Adams Sentinel*, January 4, 1847.

21. *Weekly Wisconsin*, January 5, 1848; *Nonconformist*, December 29, 1847.

22. *Atlas*, June 24; *Nautical Standard*, July 8; *Weekly Chronicle*, July 15, 1848.

23. *Guardian*, August 9, 1848.

24. *Atlas*, July 29; *Sandusky Clarion*, August 7, 1848.

Chapter 19

1. *Wisconsin Herald*, September 26, 1846.

2. *Nonconformist*, April 29, 1846; *Church and State Gazette*, January 8, November 5, 1847.

3. *Lloyd's Weekly*, July 12, 1846.

4. *Patriot*, May 26, 1845.

5. *Atlas*, August 29, 1846.

6. *Patriot*, December 13, 1847.

7. Ibid., August 10, 1848.

8. *Bell's Life in London*, August 13; *Church and State*, August 18, 1848.

9. *Rock River (WI) Pilot*, September 20, 1848.

10. Craig Foreback, "Blood Gases: Why? Where? And What Else?," http://www.clpmap.com/issues/articles/2012–07_02.asp.

11. *Cleave's Penny Gazette (London)*, December 28, 1839.

12. *Church and State*, August 7, 1846.

13. *Nonconformist*, October 1, 1845; *Weekly Chronicle*, June 27; *Atlas*, July 25, 1846.

14. *Daily News*, October 17, 1848.

15. *Church and State*, September 11, 1846.

16. Judy Pearsall, ed., *Concise Oxford Dictionary* (Oxford: Oxford University Press, 1999), 522.

17. *Weekly Chronicle*, September 19, 1846.

18. *Nonconformist*, April 7, 1847.

19. *Atlas*, July 22, 1848.

20. Reprinted in the *Nonconformist*, October 18, 1848.

21. *Atlas*, August 14, 1847.

22. *Patriot*, October 12, 30, 1848.

23. *Weekly Chronicle*, November 5, 1848.

24. *Nonconformist*, November 15; *Patriot*, November 23, December 7; *Guardian*, December 28, 1848.

25. *Patriot*, February 1, 26, March 15, July 19, September 6, November 5; *British Banner*, July 25, August 22, September 12, 26, October 31; *Nonconformist*, August 8, 15, 29, September 5, October 17, 24; *Christian Times*, August 17; *Atlas*, September 22; *Lloyd's Weekly*, October 7; *Church and State*, October 12, 1849.

26. *Christian Times*, September 28, 1849.

27. *Atlas*, February 17, 24, September 1, 1849.

28. *Nonconformist*, October 3, 1849.

29. *Daily News*, December 9, 1848.

30. Ibid., January 6, 1849.

31. *Atlas*, January 13; *Lloyd's Weekly*, January 14;

Daily News, January 8, 20; *Spirit of the Age*, January 27, 1849.

32. *Bell's Life in London*, June 10, September 16; *Lloyd's Weekly*, July 15; *Nonconformist*, October 10, 1849.

Chapter 20

1. *Patriot*, September 24, 1849.
2. *British Banner*, January 9, 1850.
3. *Nonconformist*, October 3, 1849.
4. *Guardian*, October 10, 1849.
5. *Patriot*, September 24, 1849.
6. *Daily Sanduskian*, October 30, 1849, from the *Cincinnati Gazette*.
7. Steven Johnson, *The Ghost Map* (New York: Riverhead Books, 2006), 57–71.
8. *Guardian*, October 10, 1849.
9. *Daily Sanduskian*, October 16, 1849.
10. *Guardian*, October 31, 1849.
11. *Bell's Life in London*, October 14, 1849 (italics added).
12. *Guardian*, October 10, 1849.
13. *Daily Sanduskian*, November 1, 1849, from the *Cincinnati Gazette*.

Chapter 21

1. *Sandusky Clarion*, December 25, 1848.
2. *Wisconsin Express*, November 30, 1848.
3. *Star and Banner*, December 8, 22, 1848.
4. *Republican Compiler*, December 25, 1848, January 1, 1849; *Bangor Daily Whig and Courier*, December 28; *Zanesville Courier*, December 28; *Adams Sentinel*, January 8; *Burlington Hawk-Eye*, January 11, from the *Missouri Republican; Fort Wayne Sentinel*, January 13; *Star and Banner*, February 2, 1849.
5. *Daily Sanduskian*, June 5; *Bangor Daily Whig and Courier*, June 13, 1849.
6. *Zanesville Courier*, May 26, 1849.
7. *Green Bay Advocate*, June 14, 1849.
8. *Fort Wayne Sentinel*, August 11; *Star and Banner*, June 1, 1849.
9. *Lima Argus*, March 20, 1849.
10. *Prairie du Chien Patriot*, June 13, 1849.
11. *Milwaukee Sentinel and Gazette*, January 13; *Huron Reflector*, May 22; *Daily Sanduskian*, June 1; *Zanesville Courier*, June 2; *Weekly Wisconsin*, May 30, 1849.
12. *Adams Sentinel*, June 4, 1849.
13. Israel Shipman Pelton Lord (Necia Dixon Liles, ed.), *At the Extremity of Civilization* (Jefferson, NC: McFarland, 1995), 15, 17, 23, 28.
14. *Weekly Wisconsin*, February 14; *Fort Wayne Times*, March 8, 1849.
15. Kotar and Gessler, *Steamboat Era*, 255–257.
16. *Adams Sentinel*, June 4; *Huron Reflector*, June 5, August 14; *Sheboygan Mercury*, June 30; *Wisconsin Argus*, August 7; *Alta California*, August 23, 1849.
17. *Burlington Hawk-Eye*, July 12, 1849.
18. *Davenport Gazette*, July 19, 1849.
19. *Southport (WI) American*, June 20, 1849.
20. *Adams Sentinel*, September 10, October 8, 1849
21. *Adams Sentinel*, June 11, September 17; *Daily Sanduskian*, June 27; *Weekly Wisconsin*, May 30; *Bangor Daily Whig and Courier*, June 9; *Logansport Journal*, September 8; *Patriot (London)*, October 4; *Huron Reflector*, October 9, 1849.
22. *Green Bay Advocate*, February 8, 1849; *Star and Banner*, April 26; *Waukesha Democrat*, May 28; *Fort Wayne Times*, June 6, 1850; *Daily News (London)*, October 19, 1852; *Republican Compiler*, November 14, 1853.
23. *Daily News (London)*, January 20; *Atlas*, July 23, 1853.
24. *Times (NY)*, October 4; *Star and Banner*, October 14, 1853.
25. *Defiance Democrat*, July 28, 1849, from the *Detroit Free Press*.
26. *Zanesville Courier*, June 12; *Star and Banner*, June 15; *Daily Sanduskian*, June 16, 26, 27; *Republican Compiler*, June 18; *Adams Sentinel*, June 18, September 17; *Weekly Wisconsin*, June 27, 1849.
27. *Janesville Gazette*, June 14, 1849, from the *New York Day Book*.
28. *Adams Sentinel*, August 6, 1849.
29. *Southport American*, August 8, 1849.
30. *Daily Sanduskian*, November 6, 1849.
31. *Zanesville Courier*, June 14, 1849.
32. *Adams Sentinel*, July 16, 1849.
33. "Caleb Quotem," http://www.infoplease.com/dictionary/brewers/caleb-quotem.html.
34. *Huron Reflector*, July 24, 1849.
35. *Fort Wayne Times*, September 20, 1849.
36. *Danville Weekly Advertiser*, July 14, 1849.
37. *Daily Sanduskian*, July 27, 1849.
38. *Adams Sentinel*, July 23, 1849, from the *Philadelphia Spirit of the Times*.
39. *Daily Sanduskian*, September 17, 1849.
40. *Milwaukee Sentinel and Gazette*, January 13, 1849.
41. *Republican Compiler*, June 22, 1846, July 29, 1850; *Star and Republican Banner*, September 18; *Burlington Hawk-Eye*, September 24, 1846; *Adams Sentinel*, August 9, 1847.
42. *Zanesville Gazette*, October 23, 1849.

Chapter 22

1. *Nonconformist*, November 1, 1849, from the *Times (London)*.
2. *Daily News*, September 8, 1853, from the *Globe (London)*.
3. *Patriot*, July 7, 1851.
4. *Weekly News and Chronicle*, June 11, 1853; *British Banner*, August 1. 1849, June 15, 1853; *Patriot*, July 14; *Atlas*, October 1, 1853; *Gleaner*, July 27, 1868.
5. *Allen's Indian Mail*, October 29, 1849, from the *Telegraph and Courier*, September 3, 1849.
6. *Allen's Indian Mail*, February 21, 1850.
7. Ibid., August 1, 1850.
8. *Nonconformist*, July 2, 1851.
9. *Allen's Indian Mail*, June 1, 1852.

10. *Lloyd's Weekly*, April 25, 1852.

11. *Bell's Life in London*, July 7, 1850.

12. *North-China Herald*, October 23, 1852.

13. *Lloyd's Weekly*, November 25, 1849.

14. *Sandusky Clarion*, September 18, 1848, from the *New York Sun*.

15. *Southport (WI) Telegraph*, November 10, 1848.

16. *British Banner*, January 31, 1849.

17. *Patriot*, September 6, 1849.

18. "Cholera epidemic strikes Cartagena," http://www.cartagenacaribe.com/en/history/republic/cholera.htm.

19. *Nonconformist*, August 7, 1850.

20. *Adams Sentinel*, April 8; *Daily Sanduskian*, July 3, 1850; *Defiance Democrat*, January 31, 1852.

21. *Atlas*, November 24, 1849.

22. *Church and State Gazette*, January 7, 1853.

23. *Bell's New Weekly Messenger*, April 25, October 10; *Freeholder and Commercial Advertiser*, May 22; *Lloyd's Weekly*, August 8, 15; *Patriot*, August 23, September 2; *Weekly News and Chronicle*, August 28; *Nonconformist*, September 1, 8; *Guardian*, September 7; *Nautical Standard*, December 18; *Morning Chronicle*, November 10, 1852.

24. *Patriot*, January 6, 1850.

25. *Patriot*, November 25; *Bell's Life in London*, December 15; *Guardian*, December 24, 1850; *British Banner*, March 12, 1851; *Nonconformist*, June 9; *Freeholder and Commercial Advertiser*, August 28, 1852.

26. *Weekly Wisconsin*, January 25, 1854.

27. *Daily Times (NY)*, March 2, 1854.

28. *British Banner*, July 16, 1851.

29. *Atlas*, July 23; *Daily News*, August 4; *Morning Chronicle*, August 9, 24, 30; *Star and Banner (PA)*, August 26, 1853.

Chapter 23

1. *Weekly News and Chronicle*, October 16, 1852.

2. Ibid., August 7, 1852.

3. *Daily News*, March 9; *Christian Times*, September 14, 1849; *Weekly Guardian*, March 10, 1850.

4. *Lloyd's Weekly*, September 30, 1849.

5. *British Banner*, January 24, 1849.

6. *Freeholder and Commercial Advertiser*, June 25; *Morning Chronicle*, September 15, 1852; *Daily News*, September 17, 1853.

7. *Bell's New Weekly*, December 16, 1849.

8. *Lloyd's Weekly*, December 16, 1849.

9. Ibid., January 13, 1850.

10. *Christian Times*, September 28, 1850.

11. Ibid., March 8, 1851.

12. *Press*, December 17, 1853.

13. *British Banner*, December 19, 1849.

14. *Nautical Standard*, July 20, 1850.

15. *Christian Times*, September 28, 1850.

16. *Daily News*, August 25, 1854.

17. *Christian Times*, September 28, 1850.

18. *Nonconformist*, December 17, 1851.

19. *Church and State*, September 16, 1853.

20. *Patriot*, September 19, November 14; *Press*, September 24; *Church and State*, September 30; *Weekly*

News and Chronicle, October 1, November 5; *Atlas*, October 15; *Nonconformist*, October 26, 1853.

21. *Weekly News and Chronicle*, October 15, 1853.

Chapter 24

1. *Times (NY)*, June 14, 1854.

2. *Danville (IN) Weekly Advertiser*, February 9, 1850.

3. *Milwaukee Sentinel and Gazette*, April 8; *Daily Sanduskian*, April 16. *Republican Compiler*, December 23, 1850; *Daily Times (NY)*, December 5, 1851, December 1, 1853; *Daily Alton (IL) Telegraph*, December 15, 1853.

4. *Adams Sentinel*, December 5; *Danville Advertiser*, December 10; *Sheboygan (WI) Lake Journal*, December 21, 1853; *Delaware State Reporter*, February 21, 1854.

5. *Danville Weekly*, December 1, 1849, February 9, 1850; *Daily Sanduskian*, December 20, 1849, April 5, 15, May 3; *Alton (IL) Telegraph and Democratic Review*, May 13, 1850.

6. *Milwaukee Sentinel*, May 13; *Danville Advertiser*, June 1; *Huron Reflector*, July 2; *Zanesville Courier*, July 9; *Weekly Wisconsin*, July 10, 1850.

7. *Danville Advertiser*, August 24; *Daily Sanduskian*, November 8, 1849.

8. *Alton Telegraph*, January 17, 1851.

9. *Star and Banner*, December 20; *Weekly Wisconsin*, December 25, 1850; *Wisconsin Statesman*, January 28; *Burlington (IA) Hawk-Eye*, May 22; *Watertown Chronicle*, June 11; *Prairie du Chien Patriot*, June 18, 1851.

10. *Weekly Wisconsin*, June 25; *Alton Telegraph*, July 11; *Huron Reflector*, July 15; *Burlington Hawk-Eye*, July 17; *Oshkosh Democrat*, July 18, 1851; *Weekly Wisconsin*, January 25; *Daily Zanesville Courier*, March 16, 1854.

11. *Fond du Lac Journal*, December 7, 1849; *Tioga Eagle*, June 26; *Weekly Wisconsin*, June 25; *Evening Times (NY)*, October 25, 1951.

12. *Galveston Daily News*, May 13, 1866.

13. *Daily Sanduskian*, November 15, 1849, from the *Cincinnati Gazette*; *Democratic Banner (IA)*, July 30; *Democratic Expounder (MI)*, October 7, 1852; *Janesville Gazette*, February 5; *Daily News (London)*, November 8; *Adams Sentinel*, December 5; *Daily Free Democrat*, December 13; *Daily Times (NY)*, December 15; *Independent American*, December 23; *Weekly News and Chronicle (London)*, December 31, 1853.

14. *Janesville Gazette*, July 12, August 5; *Oshkosh Courier*, July 12; *Daily Times (NY)*, July 18, 26; *Weekly Wisconsin*, July 26, 1854.

15. *Daily Times (NY)*, July 19, 24; *Weekly Wisconsin*, August 2, 1854.

16. *Daily Argus and Democrat*, August 14, 1854.

17. *Republican Compiler*, June 26; *Lima (OH) Argus*, October 21, 1854.

18. *Milwaukee Daily News*, September 1, 1855.

19. *Herald (NY)*, June 1, 1857.

Chapter 25

1. *Morning Chronicle (London)*, August 24, 1858.

2. *Morning Chronicle (London)*, March 7; *Church and State Gazette*, March 10, 17, 1854.

3. *Weekly News and Chronicle*, January 21, 28, February 4, 11, 18, 25, March 4, 11, 18, April 1, 1854.

4. *Bell's New Weekly Messenger*, August 6, 1854.

5. *Bell's New Weekly Messenger*, August 13; *Patriot*, August 14, 1854.

6. Steven Johnson, *The Ghost Map* (New York: Riverhead Books, 2006), 16–22.

7. *Nonconformist*, September 20, 1854; Harrison's name from *Ghost Map*, 54.

8. *Christian Weekly News*, September 26, 1854.

9. *Press (London)*, September 9; *Nonconformist*, September 13, 27, 1854.

10. *Christian Times*, September 8, 1854.

11. *Daily News (London)*, September 2, 21; *Nonconformist*, September 13, 1854.

12. *Daily News*, September 7, 25, 27, 1854.

13. *Morning Chronicle*, September 13, 20, 1854.

14. *Patriot*, September 25, 1854.

15. *Morning Chronicle*, October 4, 1854.

16. *Daily News*, September 29; *Atlas*, September 30, 1854.

17. *Morning Chronicle*, January 15, February 5, 1855.

18. Where not otherwise indicated, details were drawn from *The Ghost Map*, 19–22, 58–62, 151–152, 178–179, and Sandra Hempel, *The Strange Case of the Broad Street Pump* (Berkley: University of California Press, 2007), 226–227, 231–234, 273.

19. *Weekly Chronicle*, January 6, 1855.

20. *Daily News*, September 17, 1855 (italics added).

21. *Evening Star (London)*, June 14, 1856.

22. *Morning Chronicle*, August 24, 1858.

23. *Morning Chronicle*, June 29, 1858; Hempel, *Strange Case*, 246–247.

Chapter 26

1. *Nonconformist*, September 6, 1854.

2. "The Crimean War," http://en.wikipedia.org/wiki/Crimean_War.

3. *Weekly News and Chronicle*, April 22, 1854.

4. *Church and State Gazette*, July 28; *British Banner*, August 2; *Bell's New Weekly Messenger*, August 6; *Weekly News and Chronicle*, August 12; *Nonconformist*, August 30; *Christian Times*, September 1, 1854.

5. *British Banner*, August 16; *Weekly News and Chronicle*, August 5, 1854.

6. *Morning Chronicle*, August 26, 30; *Patriot*, August 24, 28, 31, 1854.

7. *Guardian (Manchester)*, September 6, 1854.

8. *Weekly Chronicle*, August 25, 1855.

9. *Bell's Life in London and Sporting Chronicle*, December 2; *Weekly Christian News*, December 18, 1855.

10. *Lloyd's Weekly*, March 16, 1856.

11. *Church and State Gazette*, July 28, August 18; *Weekly News and Chronicle*, August 5, 1854.

12. *Mail (London)*, September 25, 1854.

13. *Nonconformist*, September 19, 1855.

14. *Adams (PA) Sentinel*, October 15, 1855.

15. *Daviess County (IN) Democrat*, August 7, 1869.

16. *Evening Star (London)*, August 15; *Weekly Chronicle and Register (London)*, August 16, 1856;

Morning Chronicle, September 22; *Guardian*, October 28, 1857; *Alton (IL) Courier*, February 11, 1858.

17. *Christian Weekly News*, October 24, 31, November 7; *Daily Globe (Washington, DC)*, November 24; *Press*, December 23, 1854; *British Banner*, April 11; *Morning Chronicle*, June 1; *Nonconformist*, August 1, 1855; *Guardian*, August 13, 1856; *Christian Times*, December 15, 1854.

18. *Weekly Chronicle and Register*, October 16; *Guardian*, June 23, 1858.

19. *Morning Chronicle*, June 25, 1858.

20. *Weekly Chronicle and Register*, September 22, 1860.

21. *Penny Newsman (London)*, August 11, 1861.

22. *Miner and Workman's Advocate (London)*, April 15, 1865.

Chapter 27

1. *Nonconformist*, March 1, 1865.

2. *Daily Milwaukee News*, November 7, 1866.

3. *Allen's Indian Mail (London)*, May 28, 1863.

4. *Illustrated Times (London)*, June 13, 1868.

5. *Allen's Indian Mail*, July 14, 1864.

6. *London and China Telegraph*, October 29, 1863.

7. *Illustrated Times*, September 2; *British Standard (London)*, September 22; *Lloyd's Weekly*, October 22, 1865; Dhiman Barua, *Cholera* (New York: Plenum, 1992), 12.

8. *Watchman and Wesleyan Advertiser (London)*, July 19, 1865.

9. *Janesville Gazette*, August 16, 1865.

10. *Englishman (London)*, August 26, 1865.

11. *Bell's Life and Sporting Chronicle*, April 1; *Guardian*, April 12; *Miner and Workman's Advocate*, April 15, 1865.

12. Lim, "Military Contributions."

13. January 3, 1982.

14. *Patriot*, September 28, 1865.

15. *Weekly Chronicle*, August 4; *Elyria (OH) Independent Democrat*, October 17; *West Eau Claire (WI) Argus*, October 31, 1866.

16. *Illustrated Times (London)*, October 21, 1865.

17. Ibid., October 21, 1865.

18. *Guardian*, May 16; *Patriot*, July 26; *Poor Law Chronicle (London)*, August 7, 1866.

19. *Lloyd's Weekly*, September 16, 1866.

20. Charles E. Rosenberg, *The Cholera Years: The United States in 1832, 1849 and 1866* (Chicago: University of Chicago Press, 1987), 191.

21. *Fort Wayne (IN) Daily Gazette*, August 20; *Times (NY)*, August 21, 1866.

22. *Times (NY)*, August 20, 1866.

23. *Davenport Daily Gazette*, August 30, 1866.

24. *Times (NY)*, September 3; *Semi-Weekly Wisconsin*, September 29; *Hillsdale Standard*, September 18; *Daily Arkansas Gazette*, September 27, 1866.

25. *Waukesha (WI) Freeman*, October 9; *West Eau Claire Argue*, November 7; *Waukesha (WI) Plaindealer*, November 20, 1866; *Semi-Weekly Wisconsin*, January 12, 1867.

26. *Times (NY)*, "First Annual Report to the Gov-

ernor of the State," January 3 (another installment of
the report appeared on January 23, 1867).

27. Echenberg, *Africa*, 35–36.

28. *Dubuque Daily Herald*, October 4, 22; *West Eau
Claire Argus*, October 16, 1867.

29. *Janesville Gazette*, October 10, 1867, from the
NY Evening Post; "The Communicability of Cholera,"
from the *Lancet*, October 19, 26, 1867.

30. *Anglo-American Times (London)*, June 15; *Nonconformist*, May 15; *Times (NY)*, April 19, July 12; *Edinburgh Evening Courant*, May 13, September 24; *West
Eau Claire Argus*, July 3, 1867.

31. *Daily Milwaukee News*, September 27, 1867.

32. *Lloyd's Weekly*, August 25, 1867.

33. *Edinburgh Evening Courant*, September 3; *Atlas*,
September 23; *Decatur Republican*, September 26; *Nonconformist*, August 28, 1867.

34. *London and China Telegraph*, September 10,
1867; *Allen's Indian Mail*, January 9, 1868.

35. *Guardian*, February 12; *Alton (IL) Weekly Telegraph*, February 15, 1868.

36. *Allen's Indian Mail*, July 28, 1869.

37. *Atlas*, October 16, November 27, 1868; *Allen's
Indian Mail*, October 14, 1868, October 6, 1869; *Connersville (IN) Examiner*, November 10, 1869.

38. *London and China Telegraph*, May 9, 1870.

39. Echenberg, *Africa*, 45–46.

40. Reprinted in *Echo*, September 17, 1869.

41. *Herald (NY)*, September 18, 1869.

42. Echenberg, *Africa*, 50; *Bangor Daily Whig and
Courier*, April 21; *Echo*, March 15, 1870.

43. *Edinburgh Evening Courant*, December 9, 1869;
Nonconformist, February 9; *Marshall Statesman (MI)*,
March 6, 1870.

Chapter 28

1. *Echo*, March 16, 1869.

2. *Nonconformist*, October 6, 1869

3. *Week's News (London)*, September 23, 1871.

4. *Church Herald (London)*, July 29; *Sun and Central Press (London)*, August 1; *Herald (NY)*, August 1;
Republican Daily Journal (KS), August 8; *Edwardsville
(IL) Intelligencer*, August 10; *Lorain (OH) Constition-
alist*, August 16; *Orville (OH) Crescent*, August 16; *Nonconformist*, August 16; *Echo*, August 24, September 11;
Illustrated Times, September 2; *Janesville Gazette*, September 18; *Rochester (IN) Sentinel*, September 23, 1871.

5. *Church Herald*, August 3, 1872.

6. *Boston Daily Globe*, October 1, 1873.

7. *London and China Telegraph*, October 13, 1873;
Rochester (IN) Union Spy, February 19, 1875; *Sterling
(IL) Standard*, May 28, 1874.

8. "Dr. Francis Julius LeMoyne," http://www.wchspa.
org/crematory.html.

9. *Sullivan (IN) Democrat*, November 30, 1881;
Wellsboro (PA) Agitator, December 2, 1884.

10. *Republican Daily Journal*, July 18, 1873, from the
Cincinnati Enquirer.

11. *Democratic (IN) Union*, August 8; *Burlington
(IA) Daily Hawk-Eye*, August 13; *World (NY)*, August
14, 1873.

12. *Atlanta Constitution*, May 25 (italics added);
Cambridge City (IN) Tribune, August 5; *Palo Alto (IA)
Pilot*, September 23, November 11; *Jackson (IA) Sentinel*,
October 28; *Upper Des Moines (IA)*, December 16, 1875.

13. *World*, June 11, July 16, 1873.

14. *Sandusky Daily Register*, November 21; *World*,
July 7; *Salt Lake (UT) Daily Tribune*, July 30; *Janesville
Gazette*, December 9, 1873.

15. *Jefferson (IA) Bee*, August 2, 1873, from the
Chicago Tribune.

16. *World*, August 20, 29; *Echo*, October 24, 1874.

17. *Jackson (IA) Sentinel*, September 3, 1874; *Janesville
Gazette*, September 14, 1875.

18. *Echo*, June 19, 1876; *Colonies and India (Lon-
don)*, May 5; *Davenport (IA) Daily Gazette*, May 16;
Lebanon (PA) Daily News, May 16; *Evening Mirror
(PA)*, May 16; *Boston Daily Globe*, May 16, 1877;
Colonies and India, December 3, 1881.

19. *London and China Telegraph*, September 2, 1880.

20. *Freeborn County (MN) Standard*, November 7,
1878.

21. *Boston Daily Globe*, September 2, 1872; *World*,
August 29; *Hour (London)*, September 11, 1873.

22. *Hour*, June 9; *Steubenville Daily Herald and
News*, July 31, 1874.

23. *Herald (NY)*, September 27, 1871.

24. *Logansport (IN) Daily Star*, February 24; *Echo*,
July 18, 1874.

25. *Lowell (MA) Weekly Sun*, January 28, 1882; *Iowa
State Reporter*, September 6; *Belleville (KS) Telescope*,
October 4; *London and China Telegraph (Shanghai)*,
December 11, 1883; Richard J. Evans, *Death in Ham-
burg: Society and Politics in the Cholera Years* (New
York: Penguin, 2005), 264–265.

26. *Fort Wayne Daily Gazette*, September 18, 1881.

27. Ibid., May 16; *Freeport Republican*, May 20, 1882.

28. Evans, *Death in Hamburg*, 264–265; *British
Mail (London)*, May 1; *Warren (PA) Ledger*, May 26;
Centaur (London), October 6, 1883.

Chapter 29

1. *Nonconformist and Independent (London)*, October 25, 1883.

2. *Restitution (IN)*, October 19; *Echo*, November
12, 1881.

3. *London and China Telegraph (Shanghai)*, July 8,
1882, *Oshkosh Daily Northwestern*, June 30; *Lloyd's
Weekly*, July 1, 1883; *Boston Daily Globe*, July 22, 1882,
June 30, 1883; *Manitoba Free Press*, July 2, 1883.

4. *Times (NY)*, July 18, 24, 1883.

5. *Advocate (IN)*, June 16; *Warren (IN) Republic*,
September 14; *Centaur (London)*, September 9; *London
and China Telegraph*, November 14; *Weekly Wisconsin*,
December 20, 1882.

6. *Guardian*, August 1, 1883.

7. Evans, *Death in Hamburg*, 265–266.

8. *Nonconformist and Independent*, October 25;
Salt Lake Daily Tribune, November 11; *Independent
(IA)*, November 29, 1883.

9. Echenberg, *Africa*, 5.

10. Evans, *Death in Hamburg*, 266.

11. Ibid., 268–271.

12. *Times (NY)*, August 23; *Atlanta Constitution*, August 28; *Clerkenwell Press (London)*, October 1; *Wellsboro (PA) Agitator*, September 30, 1884.

13. *Times (NY)*, August 24, 1884.

14. *Fort Wayne Daily Sentinel*, September 5; *Fort Wayne Daily Gazette*, September 25, 1883, from the *Scientific American*.

15. *Logansport Chronicle*, May 27, 1882; *Janesville Daily Gazette*, March 4, 1885.

16. *Fort Wayne Daily Gazette*, October 15, from the *Times (NY)*; *Times (NY)*, October 16; *Lawrence (KS) Gazette*, November 1, 1883.

17. *Argus (OH)*, November 1, 1883.

18. *Galveston Daily News*, August 8, 1879; *Times (NY)*, July 26; *Echo*, July 20; *Daily Miner (MT)*, July 28; *Boston Daily Globe*, August 1, 1883.

19. *North-China Herald (Shanghai)*, June 6, 1884.

20. *Boston Daily Globe*, July 5, 1885.

21. *St. Joseph Traveler Herald (MI)*, April 19; *Colonies and India*. May 2; *Chester (PA) Times*, October 31; *Centaur*, November 8; *Echo*, December 19; *London and China Telegraph*, November 18; *Burlington Hawk-Eye*, October 2; *Times (NY)*, September 10, October 5, 1884; *Boston Daily Globe*, October 20, 1884, from the *Norristown Herald; Coshocton (OH) Age*, February 21; *Titusville Morning Herald*, March 25, December 29; *Palo Alto Reporter*, May 29, 1886,

22. *British Mail*, September 2, 1884,

23. *Hendricks County (IN) Republican*, September 18, 1884,

24. *London and China Telegraph*, April 7; *North-China Herald*, February 20; *Monticello (IA) Express*, April 24, 1884; *Colonies and India*, May 30; *Evening Gazette (Cedar Rapids, IA)*, June 23; *Atlanta Constitution*, June 25; *Times (NY)*, June 25, 29; *Lloyd's Weekly*, June 29; *Manitoba Daily Free Press*, June 30, 1884.

25. *Boston Daily Globe*, July 1; *Manitoba Daily Free Press*, July 8, 1884.

26. *Marshall Statesman*, August 1; *Galveston Daily News*, August 1; *San Antonio Light*, August 1; *Times (NY)*, August 3; *Clerkenwell Press (London)*, August 6; *Atlanta Constitution*, August 26, 1884.

27. *Times (NY)*, August 10, 18; *Burlington Hawk-Eye*, August 10; *Guardian*, August 27, 1884.

28. *Guardian*, October 1; *Daily Gazette (Colorado Springs, CO)*, August 28; *British Mail*, October 2; *National Advocate (IA)*, October 2; *Salt Lake Daily Tribune*, October 7; *Times (NY)*, September 7; *Manitoba Daily Free Press*, November 13, 1884; *Decatur Weekly Republican (IL)*, February 12, 1885.

29. *London and China Telegraph*, October 19, 1885, September 20, 1886; *North-China Herald*, May 28, August 27; *Warren (IN) Republican*, November 4, 1886.

30. *Daily Herald (IA)*, October 22, 1889; *Evening Express (PA)*, September 8; *Echo*, September 11, 1893; *Times (NY)*, November 24, 1895.

31. *Times (NY)*, September 13, 1895; *Eau Claire Daily Free Press*, January 6; *Galveston Daily News*, January 27; *Daily Gleaner (Jamaica)*, January 22; *Evening Gazette (Cedar Rapids, IA)*, March 15; *Daily Northwestern (WI)*, March 31; *Morning Oregonian*, April 1, 1887.

32. *Ohio Democrat*, April 29, 1886.

33. *Salt Lake Daily Tribune*, July 24, 1884; *Times (NY)*, April 7, July 11; *Atchison Daily Globe (KS)*, May 19; *Monticello Express (IA)*, July 23, 1885; *Malvern Leader (IA)*, May 28, 1885, from the *Boston Transcript*.

34. Thorne, R. Thomas, "The Present State of Our Knowledge as to the Significance of the Comma-Bacillus in Cholera," *Journal of the Incorporated Society of Medical Officers of Health*, vol. 7 (London: E.W. Allen, 1895), 324–325; *World (NY)*, September 10, 1893.

35. "Elie Metchnikoff," http://www.britannica.com/print/topic/378080; *Daily Gleaner*, July 29, 1920.

Chapter 30

1. *Daily Mail (London)*, January 13, 1897.

2. *London and China Telegraph*, August 24, 1888; *Times (NY)*, September 2, 1900; *Daily Mail*, April 18, 1899.

3. Evans, *Death in Hamburg*, 292–293.

4. *Evening Gazette (IA)*, July 23, 1901.

5. P.J.A. Maignen, "Ozone Treatment of Water Supply," *Cedar Rapids Evening Gazette*, August 29, 1904; Bruno Langlais, David A. Reckhow, Deborah R. Brink, eds., *Ozone in Water Treatment: Application and Engineering* (Boca Raton, FL: Lewis, 1991), 2–4.

6. Kirk T. Mosley, "Cholera," U.S. Army Medical Department, Office of Medical History, http://history.amedd.mil/booksdocs/wwii/PM4/CH21.Cholera.htm; "Philippine-American War," http://en.wikipedia.org/wiki/Philippine-American-War; "Spanish American War," http://en.wikipedia.org/wiki/Spanish%E2%80%93American_War.

7. *Fort Wayne News*, October 7, 1903.

8. "Simon Flexner Biography," http://www.faqs.org/health/bio/26/Simon-Flexner.html.

9. "Origin and development of health cooperation," http://www.who.int/global_health_histories/background/en.

10. *Francesville (IN) Tribune*, July 14, 1904; *Oakland (CA) Tribune*, September 2; *Ogden (UT) Standard*, September 2, 1905; *Racine (WI) Journal*, July 6, 1906; *San Antonio Light*, March 8, 1908.

11. *Lethbridge (Alberta) Daily Herald*, September 11; *Van Wert (OH) Daily Bulletin*, September 19; *Titusville Morning Herald*, September 22; *Times (NY)*, September 24; *Indiana (PA) Democrat*, October 7; *Daily Gleaner*, October 13; *Billings (MT) Daily Gazette*, November 4, 1908; *Logansport (IN) Pharos*, August 27, 1909.

12. *Logansport (IN) Daily Tribune*, May 28, 1910.

13. *Logansport (IN) Semi-Weekly Reporter*, July 1, 1910; *Newark (OH) Advocate*, July 18; *Indianapolis (IN) Sunday Star*, September 10, 1911.

14. *Oakland Tribune*, November 15; *Laredo (TX) Weekly Times*, November 17; *Atlanta Constitution*, November 18, 1912; *Middletown (NY) Times-Press*, February 15, 1913.

15. *Milford (IA) Mail*, October 1, 1914.

16. *Manitoba Free Press*, September 28; *Burlington (IA) Hawk-Eye*, August 4, October 14, 1914.

17. *Fort Wayne Sentinel*, October 5; *Bismark (ND) Daily Tribune*, November 15; *Altoona (PA) Mirror*, No-

vember 25; *Des Moines (IA) News*, December 2, 1914; *LeMans (IA) Semi-Weekly Sentinel*, March 23; *Jeffersonian (KS) Gazette*, July 14; *Galveston Daily News*, August 2, 1915; *San Antonio Light*, October 10, 1918.

18. *Washington (D.C.) Post*, September 5; *Fairbanks (AK) Daily Times*, October 12, 1915.

19. *Fort Wayne Journal-Gazette*, September 9; *Mansfield (OH) News*, August 18, 1915.

20. *North-China Herald*, August 12; *Washington (IN) Democrat*, August 15, 1916; *Laurel (MS) Leader*, July 17; *Twin Falls (ID) Daily News*, July 27, 1918; *Manitoba Free Press*, April 23; *Beatrice (NE) Daily Sun*, December 25, 1920; *Tyrone (PA) Daily Herald*, August 1; *Atlanta Constitution*, August 1; *Hamilton (OH) Evening Journal*, August 27; *News-Palladium (MI)*, September 29; *Oakland Tribune*, October 26, 1921; *Connersville (IN) News-Examiner*, February 18; *Monessen (PA) Daily Independent*, July 18; *Olean (NY) Evening Herald*, April 13, 1922; *Oxnard (CA) Daily Courier*, May 29, 1923; "Origin and development of health cooperation." www.who.int/global_health_histories/background/en

21. *Des Moines (IA) News*, March 17; *North-China Herald*, August 23, September 13; *Landmark (NC)*, November 7, 1919; *Lethbridge Daily Herald*, October 19; *Roswell (NM) Daily Record*. November 20; *Indianapolis Sunday Star*, November 21, 1920.

22. *North-China Herald*, July 31, September 4, October 9, November 6; *Evening Independent (OH)*, August 7; *Kokomo (IN) Daily Tribune*, August 7; *Roswell Daily Record*, August 10, 1926.

23. *Chronicle-Telegram (OH)*, August 25, 1924; *Dubois (PA) Courier*, December 2; *Manitoba Free Press*, December 22, 1927; *Muscatine (IA) Journal*, June 20, 1929.

24. *Lima (OH) News*, July 10; *Bakersfield Californian*, September 8, 1930; *Bismark (ND) Tribune*, April 14, 1931.

25. *Waterloo (IA) Evening Courier*, September 15, 1928.

26. *Salt Lake Tribune*, November 10, 1929.

27. *Oakland Tribune*, September 26, 1926.

28. *San Antonio Express*, August 3, 1931.

29. *San Mateo (CA) Times*, June 21, 1928; *Oneonta (NY) Daily Star*, August 18; *Bismark Tribune*, October 30, 1930; *Chester (PA) Times*, March 10, 1933; *Oakland Tribune*, May 30, 1941; Dottore Emiliano Fruciano, "Phage as an antimicrobal agent: d'Herelle's heretical theories and their role in the decline of phage prophylaxis in the West," http://www.ncbi.nlm.nih.gov/pmc/articles/PMC2542891/.

30. *Edwardsville (IL) Intelligencer*, August 24; *LaCrosse (WI) Tribune*, December 15, 1931; *San Antonio Express*, August 3; *Evening News-Journal (NM)*, August 23; *Van Wert Daily Bulletin (OH)*, October 13; *Monessen (PA) Daily Independent*, October 17, 1932; *Salamanca (NY) Republican-Press*, July 19, 1933; *LeGrand (IA) Reporter*, March 23, 1934.

Chapter 31

1. *Monessen (PA) Daily Independent*, September 26, 1947.

2. Mosley, "Cholera," 452–462; *Santa Fe New Mexican*, February 7; *Lethbridge Herald (Alberta)*, December 18, 1942.

3. *Charleston (WV) Gazette*, April 28, 1941; *Del Rio (TX) News-Herald*, July 4; *Billings (MT) Gazette*, October 25, 1943; *Salt Lake Tribune*, January 5; *Daily Gleaner (Jamaica)*, September 21; *Lethbridge Herald*, September 9, 1944; *San Antonio Light*, May 2, 1945; *Hope(AZ) Star*, September 13, 1947; *Amarillo (TX) Daily News*, February 20, 1948.

4. *Sandusky (OH) Register Star-News*, December 18; *Daily Register (IL)*, December 19, 1950; *Beatrice (NE) Daily Sun*, February 5; *Daily Mail (MD)*, April 25, 1951.

5. *Daily Gleaner*, July 22; *Ludington (MI) Daily News*, September 16, 1940; *Lebanon (PA) Daily News*, January 13; *Bee (VA)*, March 17, 1941; *Racine Journal*, May 16; *Port Arthur (TX) News*, June 14; *Van Wert (OH) Times-Bulletin*. August 20; *Joplin (M) News Herald*, August 20, 1942; *Big Strings (TX) Daily Herald*, September 16; *Cullman (AL) Banner*, December 9, 1943; *San Antonio (TX) Express*, February 1, 1944, June 25, 1945; *Biloxi (MS) Gulfport Herald*, October 4, 1944; *Herald Press (MI)*, July 24, 1945.

6. "Origin and development of health cooperation," WHO: http://www.who.int/global_health_histories/background/en/.

7. *Tucson Daily Citizen*. March 29; *Reno (NY) Evening Gazette*, April 26; *Iowa City Press-Citizen*, May 17; *Wisconsin State Journal*, August 25, 1946.

8. *Monessen (PA) Daily Independent*, September 26; *Charleston (WV) Gazette*, October 24, 1947; *Syracuse (NY) Post-Standard*, January 4, 1948.

9. *El Paso (TX) Herald-Post*, October 11, 1947; *Vidette (IN) Messenger*, January 16, 1948.

10. *Mt. Pleasant (IA) News*, June 29, 1953; *Pacific Stars and Stripes (Tokyo)*, September 9, 1953, December 30, 1957; *Panama City (FL) News*, August 19; *New Castle (PA) News*, October 8, 1954; *Oshkosh (WI) Daily Northwestern*, June 20, 1955; *Daily Herald (UT)*, May 16; *Independent Press-Telegram (CA)*, May 27, 1956; *Indiana (PA) Evening Gazette*, August 2, 1956, May 31, 1958; *Harrison (AR) Daily Times*, August 13, 1956; *Winnipeg Free Press*, November 27, 1957; *Montana Standard*, April 18; *Lethbridge Herald*, April 22; *Daily Chronicle (WA)*, May 12, 1958.

11. *Pacific Stars and Stripes (Tokyo)*, June 28, 1958, March 9, 1959; *Statesville (NC) Record and Landmark*, August 2, 1958; *Florence (SC) Morning News*, February 8; *Bakersfield Californian*, August 23; *Southern Illinoisan*, September 11; *Daily Gleaner*, September 17; *Montana Standard*, September 19, 1960.

12. G. Balakrish Nair and Jai P. Narain, "From endotoxin to exotoxin: De's rich legacy to cholera," http://www.who.int/bulletin/volumes/88/09-072504/en/.

13. *Manitowoc (WI) Herald-Times*, May 26, 1943.

14. *News (MD)*, June 1, 1944; *Times-Recorder (OH)*, May 28, 1940.

15. *Winona (MN) Republican-Herald*, May 4; *Portsmouth (OH) Times*, May 17; *San Antonio Sunday Light*, September 26, 1948.

16. *Hammond (IN) Times*, February 24, 1943.

17. *Reno Evening Gazette*, August 9, 1945.
18. Lim, "Military Contributions," 30–32; "Fighting Asia's Illness," *Pacific Stars and Stripes (Tokyo)*, December 22, 1960.
19. *Sunday Independent Press-Telegram (CA)*, November 16, 1952; *Anniston (AL) Star*, October 3; *Del Rio News-Herald*, September 24; *Pampa (TX) Daily News*, November 6, 1956; *Alton (IL) Evening Telegraph*, September 11, 1957; *News (MD)*, July 31; *Paris (TX) News*, August 2; *Corpus Christi (TX) Caller-Times*, August 2; *Pacific Stars and Stripes (Tokyo)*, August 7, 1959; Rashmi Khare, Shanta Banerjee and Kanika Kundu, "Coleus Aromaticus Benth: A Nutritive Medicinal Plant of Potential Therapeutic Value," *International Journal of Pharma and Bio Sciences* 2, no. 3 (July-September 2011): 488–489.

Chapter 32

1. William J. Drummond, "Cholera Marching on World Health Scene," *Times (Los Angeles)*, March 26, 1972, from the *Sunday Gazette-Mail (WV)*.
2. *Charlestown (WV) Gazette*, August 22; *Corpus Christi Times*, August 23, 1961; *Pacific Stars and Stripes*, August 23, 1961, January 18, 1962.
3. *Pacific Stars and Stripes*, November 6, 1969.
4. *Star-News (CA)*, August 5; *Corpus Christi Times*, August 8, 1972.
5. *Winnipeg Free Press*, August 30, 1961; *Oakland (CA) Tribune*, January 12, 1963, January 12, 1966; *Beckley (WV) Post-Herald*, April 29, 1963; *Lethbridge Herald*, July 10; *Amarillo (TX) Globe-Times*, November 24, 1965; *Wisconsin State Journal*, August 30, 1966; *Lubbock (TX) Avalanche-Journal*, April 6, 1967; *Progress-Index (VA)*, May 6, 1968; *Daily Review (CA)*, August 28; *Daily Gleaner*, September 1; *Star-News (CA)*, September 2, 1970.
6. *Titusville (PA) Herald*, October 19, 1970.
7. *Anniston (AL) Star*, November 25, 1971.
8. *Des Moines (IA) Register*, March 8, 1976.
9. *Lethbridge Herald*, September 22, 1976; *Stars and Stripes (Germany)*, July 6, 1977.
10. *Register*, July 7, 1979.
11. *Press-Telegram (CA)*, June 18; *Star-News (CA)*, July 20, 1965; *Victoria (TX) Advocate*, March 3, 1977.
12. *Monday Advocate (OH)*, September 24; *Brownwood (TX) Bulletin*, October 21; *Arizona Republic*, October 28; *Stars and Stripes (Germany)*, October 21, 1973.
13. *Evening Capital (MD)*, December 23, 1977; *Del Rio (TX) News-Herald*, September 21; *Stars and Stripes (Germany)*, September 22; *Galveston Daily News*, September 26; *Register (CA)*, November 11, 1978; *Iola (KS) Register*, June 21, 1979.
14. *Lethbridge Herald*, April 6, 1979; *Galveston Daily News*, September 30, 1980, September 1, 1983, October 23, 27, 1984; *New Mexican*, December 20, 1980; *Port Arthur (TX) News*, May 21, 26, June 30, July 8, August 21, October 14, 1981; *Altoona Mirror*, October 13, 1981, May 3, 1991; *Sequin Gazette-Enterprise*, June 6, 1982; *Baytown Sun*, October 25, 1984; *Pacific Stars and Stripes (Japan)*, February 4; *Progress (PA)*, May 16, 1987; *Daily Republican Register (IL)*, January

20; *Daily Herald (PA)*, September 25; *Paris News*, October 1, 1989; *Syracuse Herald-Journal*, January 8, 1990, September 27, 1991; *Stars and Stripes (Germany)*, December 20, 1991; *Winnipeg Free Press*, September 12, 1983.
15. *Beckley Post-Herald/Raleigh Register (WV)*, November 12; *Arizona Republic*, November 12, 1972; *Lethbridge Herald*, November 18, 1972, December 21, 1978; *Chronicle Telegram (OH)*, July 18, 1979; *Daily Gleaner*, February 12, 1982, July 30, 1990; *Titusville Herald*, March 20, 1990.
16. *Cedar Rapids (IA) Gazette*, April 6, 1979; *Stars and Stripes (Germany)*, July 26, 1983; *Herald-Zeitung (TX)*, July 24; *Ironwood (MI) Daily Globe*, December 18, 1980; *Register (CA)*, September 16, 1984.

Chapter 33

1. *Morning Chronicle (London)*, September 8, 1854.
2. Lim, "Military Contributions," 31–32.
3. Lim, "Military Contributions," 31–32; *Hutchinson (KS) News*, November 28, 1963, April 17, 1964; *Lowell (MA) Sun*, December 19, 1963; *Des Moines Register*, November 7, 1967.
4. *Southern Illinoisan*, February 9; *Corpus Christi Times*, February 19; *Pacific Stars and Stripes*, February 22, 1964.
5. *Cumberland (MD) News*, August 12, 1969; *Independent Press-Telegram (CA)*, July 31; *Sandusky Register*, November 8, 1971; *Star-News*, February 18, 1974; *Florence (SC) Morning News*, August 27, 1979.
6. *Galveston Daily News*, August 26, 1962, November 10, 1966.
7. "Miracle cure for an old scourge: An interview with Dr. Dilip Mahalanabis," http://www.who.int/bulletin/volumes/87/2/09-060209/en.
8. "From endotoxin to exotoxin"; *Derrick (PA)*, January 6, 1972; *Ukiah (CA) Daily Journal*, December 26, 1977; *Kokomo Tribune*, February 21, 1987.
9. "The Global Task Force on Cholera Control," http://www.who.int/cholera/task_force/en/.
10. "Prevention and control of cholera outbreaks: WHO policy and recommendations," http://www.who.int/cholera/prevention_control/recommendations/en/index.html.
11. G.B. Nair, "Vibrio cholerae," Geneva: WHO, 1993.
12. *Pharos-Tribune (IN)*, August 3, 2000.
13. Nair, "Vibrio Cholerae."
14. *Daily News (TX)*, January 15, 2003.
15. Barua, *Cholera*, 287–289.
16. Ibid., 287–308.
17. *News (MD)*, December 9, 1995.
18. *Frederick (MD) Post*, July 1, 1996.
19. "High Hopes for Oral Cholera Vaccine: A Trial of a New Oral Cholera Vaccine in Kolkata Is Promising but, as Patralekha Chatterjee Reports, a Vaccine Is Only One Weapon in the Battle Against Disease," WHO Bulletin, www.questia.com/read/1G1-225073858/high-hopes-for-oral-cholera-vaccine.
20. Barua, *Cholera*, 287–308.
21. *Gaston (NC) Gazette*, June 12, 2007.

22. "Immunization, Vaccines and Biologicals," http://www.who.int/immunization/topics/Cholera/en/index.html.

23. "Cholera,":http://www.who.int/cholera/prevention_control/recommendations/en/index4.html.

Chapter 34

1. M.J. Wilson, "Scientists err on cholera prediction," Newsweek Feature Service, *Arizona Republic*, September 11, 1970.

2. Nair, "Vibrio Cholerae."

3. "High Hopes for Oral Cholera Vaccine."

4. "Factsheets," http://www.who.int/mediacentre/factsheets/fs107/en/index/html.

5. Nair, "Vibrio Cholerae"; *New Mexican*, February 20, 1993.

6. *Daily News-Record (VA)*, March 10; *New Mexican*, August 6, 1992.

7. *European Stars and Stripes (Germany)*, August 15, 1993; *Orange (TX) Leader*, August 22; *Lawrence (KS) Journal-World*, March 30, 1994.

8. *Sunday Santa Fe New Mexican*, June 11, 1995; *Wisconsin State Journal*, June 12, 1995, June 8, 1996.

9. *Syracuse Herald-Journal*, November 23, 1995.

10. *Winchester (VA) Star*, November 9; *Winnipeg Free Press*, November 13, 1996; *Wisconsin State Journal*, February 18; *Texas City Sun*, October 15, 1997; *Gleaner*, December 20, 1997, January 28, 1998; *Daily Herald (IL)*, November 7, 1998.

11. *Wisconsin State Journal*, March 15; *Gleaner*, April 25; *Lima (OH) News*, April 30; *Lethbridge Herald*, October 6, 2000; *Herald American Post-Standard (NY)*, January 7; *Lawrence Journal-World*, June 5, 2001; *Garden City (KS) Telegram*, April 12, 2002; *Pharos-Tribune (IN)*, March 7; *Post-Standard (NY)*, June 9; *Progress (PA)*, August 27, 2003; *Capital Times (WI), June 30, 2004; Daily Globe (MI)*, April 20; *News Herald (FL)*, September 2, 2005; *Daily News-Record (VA)*, May 18, 2006, February 22, 2007; *Post-Standard*, September 15, 2007; *Gazette (IA)*, November 11; *Roswell (NM) Daily Record*, December 3, 2008; *Post-Standard*, January 7, 17, 2009; *Clovis (NM) News Journal*, September 12; *Daily Southerner (NC)*, October 25; *Gleaner*, November 18, December 12; *Bakersfield Californian*. December 25, 2010; *Facts (TX)*, May 5; *Winchester Star (VA)*, May 5, 2011; *Gleaner*, April 4, 2012.

12. Barua, *Cholera*. 330–333, 335, 339–340, 344–345; Nair, "Vibrio Cholerae"

13. "Cholera: International Health Regulations," http://www.who.int/cholera/health_regulations/en/.

14. *Gleaner*, April 26, 1974.

15. "Cholera: Fact Sheet," .\http://www.who.int/mediacentre/factsheets/fs107/en/index.html.

16. *Stars and Stripes (Japan)*, October 4, 1963.

17. *Post-Standard (NY)*, November 23, 1978.

18. Barua, *Cholera*, 210, 216–217, 224, 253, 256, 268–269, 272; "From endotoxin to exotoxin."

19. *Oakland (CA) Tribune*, December 24, 1949.

20. *Hutchinson (KS) News*, August 9, 1982.

21. *Independent Record (MT)*, February 27; *Waterloo (IA) Daily Courier*, February 27; *Albuquerque Tribune*, February 28; *Rocky Mountain (NC) Sunday Telegram*, April 13; *El Paso (TX) Herald-Post*, July 18, 1952; *Delta-Democrat-Times (MS)*, August 21, 1961; *Chronicle-Telegram (OH)*, January 5, 1982; *Hutchinson News*, November 18, 1986.

22. "Bioterrorism and Military Health Risks," http://www.who.int/dg/bruntland/speeches/2003/DAVOS/en; "Prevention and control of cholera outbreaks: WHO policy and recommendations," http://www.who.int/cholera/prevention_control/recommendations/en/index6.html and http://www.who.int/cholera/prevention_control/recommendations/en/index2.html; "Cholera," http://www.who.int/mediacenter/factsheets/fs107/en/index/html; Lim, "Military Contributions."

23. *Daily Herald (IL)*, June 12, 1998.

24. *Post-Standard*, December 19, 2008.

25. *St. Louis (MO) Post-Dispatch*, May 8, 2013.

Chapter 35

1. "Cholera," http://www.who.int/mediacentre/factsheets/fs107/en/index/html.

2. *Jackson County (IN) Democrat*, August 8, 1854.

Glossary

1. *News (MD)*, December 9, 1995.

2. *Taber's*, 53.

3. Ibid., 135.

4. *North-China Herald*, April 1, 1892.

5. Ibid.

6. *Chester Times*, February 19, 1940.

7. *Waterloo Courier*, June 28, 1876.

8. *Ironwood Daily Globe*, August 30, 1924.

9. "Dengue," http://www.merriam-webster.com/dictionary.

10. *Fort Wayne World*, March 28, 1885.

11. *Taber's*, 678.

12. Ibid., 794.

13. Ibid., 818.

14. *Fort Wayne World*, March 28, 1885.

15. *Courier*, February 17, 1837.

16. *North-China Herald*, April 1, 1892.

17. Ibid.

18. *Adams Sentinel*, July 30, 1838.

19. *Star and Sentinel*, August 1, 1883.

20. *London and China Telegraph*, November 22, 1883.

21. *Taber's*, 1,480.

22. Ibid., 1,598.

23. *Echo*, June 10, 1869.

Appendix I

1. *Star and Banner (PA)*, November 10, 1848.

2. *Hagerstown Mail*, July 1, 1836.

3. *Adams (PA) Sentinel*, August 25, 1834.

4. *Weekly Chronicle (London)*, December 31, 1842.

5. *True Sun (London)*, March 13, 1832.

6. *Commercialist and Weekly Advertiser (London)*, March 4, 1832.

7. *Cherokee Advocate (Indian Territory-OK)*, April 29, 1876.

8. *Huron Reflector.* May 22, 1849.

9. *Courier*, April 2, 1832.

10. Ibid., April 23, 1832.

11. *Age*, April 29; *Frederick (MD) Herald*, June 2, 1832.

12. *Huron (OH) Reflector*, July 10, 1832.

13. Ibid., July 3; *Adams Sentinel*, July 3, 1832.

14. *Patriot (London)*, March 7, 1832.

15. *Courier*, June 9, 1832.

16. *Evans and Ruffy's Farmers' Journal (London)*, April 30, 1832.

17. *Courier*, May 8, 1832.

18. *Albion and the Star*, May 3, 1832.

19. *Bell's New Weekly Messenger (London)*, November 4, 1832.

20. *Courier*, April 27, 1832.

21. *Adams Sentinel*, September 18, 1832.

22. *Lycoming Gazette*, May 8, 1833.

23. *Star and Republican Banner*, October 16, 1832; *Huron Reflector*, September 3, 1833.

24. *Morning Chronicle (London)*, September 9, 1852.

25. *Galveston (TX) Daily News*, May 13, 1866.

26. *Sun and Central Press (London)*, September 15, August 30, 1871.

27. *Indiana (PA) Democrat*, September 8, 1881.

28. *Torch Light*, October 16, 1834 (italics added).

29. *True Sun*, April 21, 1832.

30. *Courier*, May 3, 1832.

31. *Church and State Gazette (London)*, September 30; *Republican Compiler (PA)*, December 19; *New-York Daily Times*, October 24, 1853

32. *Allen's Indian Mail (London)*, October 20; *Nonconformist (London)*, October 27, 1869; *Warren (IN) Republican*, May 26, 1870; *Seymour (IN) Times*, February 8, 1872.

33. *Nonconformist*, August 15, 1849.

34. *Daily Wisconsin Patriot*, July 16, 1855.

35. *Christian Advocate (London)*, April 10, 1832 (from the *Scottish Guardian*).

36. *Sandusky (OH) Clarion*, August 21, 1833.

37. *Mail (London)*, August 16, 1833.

38. Ibid., August 16, 1833.

39. Ibid.

40. *Lycoming Gazette*, August 7, 1833.

41. *Echo (London)*, March 18, 1869.

42. *Atlas (London)*, November 4, 1848.

43. *Weekly News and Chronicle (London)*, September 11, 1852.

44. Steven Johnson, *The Ghost Map* (New York: Riverhead Books, 2006), 66–67, 145–146.

45. *Courier*, January 8, 1848.

46. *Nonconformist*, November 8, 1854; *Lloyd's Weekly Newspaper (London)*, December 30, 1866.

47. *Nonconformist*, September 13, 1865; *Dubuque Daily Herald*, September 3, 1867.

48. *Patriot*, October 26, 1848.

49. *Courier*, January 1, 1848.

50. *Church and State Gazette*, October 27, 1848.

51. *Allen's Indian Mail*, August 13, 1846.

52. *Nonconformist*, September 13, 1848.

53. *Weekly Chronicle*, November 6, 1847.

54. *Nonconformist*, October 4, 1848.

55. *Guardian (Manchester)*, September 27, 1848.

56. *Atlas*, August 26, 1854.

57. *Morning Chronicle*, September 14, 1852.

58. *Sandusky Clarion*, January 7, 1849.

59. *Allen's Indian Mail*, May 18, 1852.

60. *British Standard (London)*, September 15, 1865.

61. *British Workman (London)*, September 1; *Anglo-American Times*, August 25, 1866.

62. Barua, *Cholera*, 280.

63. *Lethbridge Herald*, August 30, 1932.

64. *Sandusky Clarion*, December 25, 1848; *Illustrated Times (London)*, April 28, 1866; *Star and Republican Banner*, May 4, 1835; *Danville Weekly Advertiser*, February 10; *Christian Times (London)*, July 20; *Nautical Standard and Steam Navigation Gazette (London)*, October 27, 1849; *Newport Daily News*, June 28, 1847; *Torch Light*, September 4, 1834; *Christian Weekly News*, September 26, 1854.

65. *Reviewer*, April 22, 1832.

66. *Courier*, June 29, 1832.

67. *Adams Sentinel*, November 13, 1848; *Allen's Indian Mail*, August 13, 1846; *Fort Wayne (IN) Sentinel*, August 11, 1849.

68. *Republican Compiler*, November 11, 1834.

69. *Patriot*, October 12, 1848.

70. *British Banner*, January 18; *Nonconformist*, January 18; *Empire (London)*, January 28; *Patriot*, February 27, 1854.

71. *Sun, Central Press*. July 4, 1873.

72. David Armstrong and Elizabeth Metzger Armstrong, *The Great American Medical Show* (New York: Prentice Hall, 1991), 31–32; Donald Venes, ed., *Taber's Cyclopedic Medical Dictionary*, 20th ed. (Philadelphia: F.A. Davis, 2005), 77, 1007.

73. *Sandusky Clarion*, February 4, 1849.

74. *Bangor Daily Whig and Courier*, May 31, 1849.

75. *Lloyd's Weekly Newspaper*, October 14; *Bell's Life in London and Sporting Chronicle*, October 14; *Nonconformist*, October 17, 1849.

76. *Daily Sanduskian*, August 16; *Patriot*, September 10, 1849.

77. *Janesville Gazette*, December 27, 1849, February 14, 1850.

78. *Echo*, "The Air-Dust Question," Parts 1 and 2, February 24, 25, 1870; *Edinburgh Evening Courant*, April 5, 1869.

79. *Defiance (OH) Democrat.* July 21, 1849.

80. *British Standard*, September 15, 1865.

81. *Hornellsville (NY) Tribune*, March 8, 1872.

82. *Herald, Torch Light* (MD), November 1, 1875.

83. *Indiana (PA) Progress*, June 10, 1875.

84. *Edinburgh Evening Courant*, April 5, 1869; *Lebanon (PA) Daily News*, April 24, 1874.

85. *New York Times*, March 6, 15, 21, 1867.

86. *New York Times*, August 5, 1867; *Jones County (IA) Liberal*, March 12, 1874.

87. *Lloyd's Weekly Newspaper*, August 2, 1868.

88. (Dr.) Farquharson, "Disinfectants and How to Use Them," *Daily Davenport (IA) Gazette*, July 6, 1880.

89. *British Standard*, September 1; *Illustrated Times*,

September 9; *Patriot*, October 19, 1865; *Nonconformist*, October 18, 1865, May 29, 1867; *Galveston Daily News*, July 19, 1872,from the *Pittsburg Commercial*.

90. *Daily Sanduskian*, August 31, 1849; "Broussais, Francois Joseph Victor," http://encyclopedia2.thefree dictionary.com; "Francois-Joseph-Victor Broussais," http://britannica.com/print/topic/81446.

91. *La Crosse Independent Republican*, July 25, 1855; *Christian Times*, October 26, 1855.

92. *Weekly News and Chronicle*, September 30, 1854; *Patriot*, September 1, 1859; *Daily News (London)*, January 26, 1849, from the *Glasgow Chronicle*.

93. *Daily Free Democrat (WI)*, November 30, 1854; *Appleton (WI) Crescent*, September 29, 1855.

94. *Sun*, Central Press, September 25, 1871.

95. *Anglo-American Times*, June 30, 1866.

96. *British Workman*, July 2, 1866.

97. *New York Herald*, September 15, 1869; *St. Joseph Herald (MI)*, February 29, 1868.

98. *Indiana (PA) Democrat*, July 21, 1870.

99. *Rockingham (VA) Register*, April 21; *Monticello (IA) Express*, May 12, 1870.

100. *Dubuque Herald*, July 2, 1872; *Titusville Morning Herald*, July 15, 1873.

101. *Indiana (PA) Progress*, January 23; *Rochester (IN) Union Spy*, May 1, 1873, from the *St. Louis Globe*.

102. *Decatur Republican*, June 19, 1873.

103. *New York Herald*, May 27; *Coshocton (OH) Democrat*, July 9, 1872; *New York Times*, July 16, 1873; *Marshall (MI) Statesman*, July 1, 1880.

104. *American Settler (London)*, February 7, 1885.

105. *World*, July 15, 1873.

106. *Guardian (Manchester)*, May 20, July 15; *Newark (OH) Daily Advocate*, May 22; *Belleville (KS) Telescope*. July 9; *Daily Index-Appeal* (VA), July 7, from the *New York Herald; Daily Herald-Tribune* (Lawrence, KS), July 22, 1885; Baura, *Cholera*, 286.

107. Baura, *Cholera*, 286–287.

108. *Manitoba Free Press*, July 17; *Boston Daily Globe*, July 26; *Fort Wayne Daily Gazette*, August 8; *Sioux County (IA) Herald*, July 27, 1882; *Jackson Sentinel*, August 26; *Cambridge Jeffersonian*. August 12, 1880.

109. *Oakland (CA) Tribune*, May 24, 1914.

110. *Galveston (TX) Daily News*, March 24, 1906; *North-China Herald* (Shanghai), August 7, 1909, August 24, 1912; *Racine (WI) Journal*, April 6, 1909; *New York Times*, September 26, 1909; *Lowell (MA) Sun*, October 7, 1914.

111. *Daily News Standard* (PA), April 25, 1921.

112. *Indiana (PA) Gazette*, September 29, 1986.

113. *Winnipeg Free Press*, January 21, 1984.

Appendix II

1. *Echo*, June 10, 1969.

2. *Evening Herald (London)*, January 11, 1865.

3. *Patriot (London)*, April 25, 1832.

4. *Albion and Star*, April 25, 1832.

5. *Republican Compiler (PA)*, April 3, 1832.

6. *Patriot*, April 18; *British Traveller*, April 4; *Albion and Star*, April 5, 10, 12; *Evans and Ruffy's*, April 9; *Times (London)*, April 9, 1832.

7. *Patriot*, May 30; *Courier*, June 1, July 2, 3, 7, 18, 24, August 31; *Albion and Star*, June 4, 5, 7, 8, 9, 11, 12, 13, 14, 16, 20, 21, 23, 27, July 20, 25, 31, August 2, 9; *True Sun*, May 4, June 18, 20, 22, 24, 26, 27, 28, 29, July 5, 11, 12, 13, 14, 16, 18, 19, 23, 26, 30, August 1, 3, 4, 6, September 22; *Commercialist*, July 1, 1832.

8. *Courier*, September 13, 1838.

9. *Allen's Indian Mail*, July 26, 1848.

10. *Logansport Journal*, September 8, 1849.

11. *Defiance Democrat*, July 21, 1849.

12. *Adams Sentinel*, July 16, 1849.

13. Ibid., July 16, 1849.

14. *Western Star*, June 22, 1849.

15. *Atlas*, December 29, 1849.

16. *British Banner*, January 9, 1850, January 8, 1851.

17. *Patriot*, July 3, 1851.

18. *British Banner*, January 31, 1849.

19. *Nautical Standard*, January 21; *Press*, February 11; *Atlas*, February 18, 1854; *Connersville Times*, December 1, 1886.

20. *Week's News*, April 22, 1876.

21. *Sioux Country Herald*, March 12, 1885; *Adams County Union-Republican*, December 19, 1906.

22. *Patriot*, July 27; *Weekly News and Chronicle*, July 29, August 12, 23, November 11; *Nonconformist*, August 2, 9, 23, 30, September 27, November 1; *Press*, August 12, September 2; *Guardian*, August 16; *British Banner*, September 6, October 4, 18, 25; *Morning Chronicle*, September 13, November 15, December 6; *Church, State*, September 15; *Christian Times*, October 13, 1854.

23. *Christian Weekly News*, November 21, 1854.

24. *Morning Chronicle*, November 1, 1854.

25. *Press*, December 30, 1854, from the *Medical Times*.

26. *Morning Chronicle*, May 16, July 13, 25, August 2; *Daily News*, August 15; *Weekly Chronicle*, August 25; *Lloyd's Weekly*, September 2; *Patriot*, September 5; *Guardian*, October 10, 31, 1855.

27. *Morning Chronicle*, March 1, 8, 1855.

28. *Janesville Gazette*, August 7; *Times (NY)*, August 14, 1854.

29. *Times (NY)*, August 15, 26, 1854.

30. *Patriot*, August 28, 1854.

31. *Evening Herald*, August 17, 1859.

32. *Morning Chronicle*, April 18, 1860.

33. *Evening Herald*, October 15, 1863.

34. *Goshen (IN) Times*, February 2, 1882; *Shoreditch Observer (London)*, July 10, 1909.

35. *Morning Chronicle*, March 15, 1860.

36. *Lloyd's Weekly*, July 30, October 5, 1865, September 2, 30, October 7, November 11, December 16, 1866; *Illustrated Times*, May 12, August 18, October 13; *Guardian*, August 1, October 17, December 5; *Watchman and Wesleyan Advertiser*, August 9, October 17, November 21; *Patriot*, August 23; *Weekly Chronicle*, September 8, 15, 22, November 3, 17, December 1; *Bell's Life in London*, November 10, 1866.

37. *Weekly Chronicle*, September 22, 1866.

38. *Lloyd's Weekly*, January 13, 1867.

39. *Times (NY)*, September 26, 1866.

40. Ibid., January 23, 1867.

41. *Nonconformist*, September 25, 1867.

42. *Edinburgh Courant*, August 17, 1868; *Lloyd's Weekly*, October 17, 1869.

43. *Jefferson Bee*, June 14, 1873.

44. *Wisconsin State Journal*, January 3, 1872.

45. *Central Press (London)*, January 1, 1874, from the *London Medical Record*.

46. *Logansport Daily Star*, February 23, 1874.

47. *World*, October 15, 1873.

48. *Nonconformist*, January 21, 1874.

49. *Chicago Tribune*, July 10, 1875.

50. *Week's News*, December 31, 1881.

51. *Manitoba Free Press*, September 12, 1883.

52. *Marshall Statesman*, June 29, 1882.

53. *Monticello Express*, December 30, 1886.

Bibliography

Acland, Henry Wentworth (M.D.). *Memoir on the Cholera at Oxford, in the Year 1854, with Considerations Suggested by the Epidemic.* London: Churchill, 1856.

Aldrich, Michael R. "The Remarkable W. B. O'Shaughnessy." http://antiquecannabisbook.com/chap1/Shaughnessy.htm.

Allan, Thomas (M.R.C.S.). *Plain Directions for the Prevention and Treatment of Cholera.* 5th ed. London: Henry Renshaw, 1854.

Armstrong, David, and Elizabeth Metzger Armstrong. *The Great American Medical Show, Being an Illustrated History of Hucksters, Healers, Health Evangelists and Heroes from Plymouth Rock to the Present.* New York: Prentice Hall, 1991.

Arnott, James (M.D.). "On the Remedial and Anaesthetic Uses of Intense Cold." *Edinburgh Monthly Journal of Medical Science,* 1854.

Barua, Dhiman, and William B. Greenough III. *Cholera.* New York: Plenum Medical, 1992.

Blane, Sir Gilbert, "Observations on the Comparative Prevalence, Mortality, and Treatment of Different Diseases," *The Monthly Review.* London: June 1815.

"Broussais, Francois Joseph Victor." http://encyclopedia2.thefreedictionary.com.

Buchanan's Journal of Man. "Cholera," April, 1849.

Bushman, Stephenson (M.D.). *Cholera and Its Cures: An Historical Sketch.* London: Orr, 1850.

"Caleb Quotem." http://www.infoplease.com/dictionary/brewers/caleb-quotem.html.

Carpenter, William B. (M.D.). "On Cholera and Its Preventibility." 10-part series. *Weekly News and Chronicle,* January 21–April 1, 1854.

Chapman, John (M.D.). *Cases of Diarrhoea and Cholera.* London: Bailliere, Tindall, and Cox, 1871.

Chapman, John (M.D.). *Diarrhoea and Cholera: Their Nature, Origin, and Treatment Through the Agency of the Nervous System.* London: Trubner, 1865.

Chatterjee, Patraleka. "High Hopes for Oral Cholera Vaccine: A Trial of a New Oral Cholera Vaccine in Kolkata Is Promising, but as Patralekha Chatterjee Reports, a Vaccine Is Only One Weapon in the Battle Against the Disease." WHO Bulletin. www.questia.com/read/1G1-225073858/high-hopes-for-oral-cholera-vaccine.

"Cholera." http://www.medicinenet.com/cholera/article.htm.

"Cholera." http://www.nlm.goc/medlineplus/encv/article/000303htm.

"Cholera epidemic strikes Cartagena." http://www.cartagenacaribe.com/en/history/republic/cholera.htm.

"Cholera's seven pandemics." http://www.cbc.ca/mews/health/story/2008/05/09/f-cholera-outbreaks.html.

Cliff, A.D. *War Epidemics: An Historical Geography of Infectious Diseases in Military and Civil Strife, 1850–2000.* New York: Oxford University Press, 2004.

"The Crimean War." http://en.wikipedia.org/wiki/Crimean_War.

"Disease." http://cdc.gov/cholera/disease.html.

"Dr. Francis Julius LeMoyne." http://www.wchspa.org/crematory.html.

Drury, Dr. *Cholera, Diarrhoea, Dysentery.* London: Headland, 1866.

Echenberg, Myron. *Africa in the Time of Cholera: A History of Pandemics from 1817 to the Present.* New York: Cambridge University Press, 2011.

Edinburgh Medical and Surgical Journal 38, no. 3. "Medical Intelligence." Edinburgh: Adam Black, 1832.

The Edinburgh Practice of Physic and Surgery. 8 vols. Edinburgh: Kearsley, 1800.

"Elie Metchnikoff." http://www.britannica.com/print/topic/378080.

"Epidemiology and Risk Factors." http://www.cdc.gov/cholera/epi.html.

Foex, B.A. "How the cholera epidemic of 1831 resulted in a new technique for fluid resuscitation." http://emj.bmj.com/content/20/4/316.full.

Fordyce, George (M.D.). *Elements of the Practice of Physic: Part II, Containing the History and Methods of Treating Fevers and Internal Inflammations.* London: Johnson, 1768.

Foreback, Craig. "Blood Gases: Why? Where? And What Else?" http://www.clpmag.com/issues/articles/2012-07_02.asp.

"Francois-Joseph-Victor Broussais." http://britann
ica.com/print/topic/81446.

Fruciano, Dottore Emiliano, *Phage as an antimicrobal agent: D'Herelle's heretical theories and their
role in the decline of phage prophylaxis in the West.*
http://www.ncbi.nlm.nih.gov/pmc/articles/
PMC2542891/.

"General Information." http://www.cdc.gov/cholera/
general.

Gibson, W. "The Bio-medical Pursuits of Christopher Wren," *Medical History.* Vol. 14. No. 4, 1970:
331–341.

Gordon, L.D.B., and C. Liddell. *Exposition of a Plan
for a Metropolitan Water Supply.* London: Hip-
polyte Bailliere, 1849.

Grant, William (M.D.). *Observations on the Nature
and Cure of Fevers.* 2 vols. London: Cadell, 1773.

Granville, Dr. *Sudden Death,* London: Churchill,
1854.

*Half-Yearly Abstract of the Medical Sciences, Being a
Digest of British and Continental Medicine and of
the Progress of Medicine and the Collateral Sciences.*
Vol. 46 (July-December). Philadelphia: 1868,
Henry C. Lea.

Hamlin, Christopher. *Cholera: The Biography.* New
York: Oxford University Press, 2009.

Hassall, Richard (M.D) *Cholera: Its Nature and
Treatment, and the Preventive Measures Commu-
nities and Individuals Should Adopt.* London:
Henry Renshaw, 1854.

Hempel, Sandra. *The Strange Case of the Broad Street
Pump.* Berkley: University of California Press,
2007.

Hooper, Robert. *Lexicon Medicum, or, Medical Dictionary.* New York: Harper, 1842.

James, Philip B. "Hyperbaric Oxygen Treatment: The
Last Frontier." http://www.hyperbaric-oxygen-info.
com/hyperbaric-oxygen-therapy-frontier-philip-
james.

Johnson, Steven. *The Ghost Map.* New York: Riverhead Books, 2006.

Kennedy, Hartley. *Notes on the Epidemic Cholera.*
London: Smith, Elder, 1846.

Khare, Rashmi Sahay, Shanta Banerjee, Kanika
Kundu. "Coleus Aromaticus Benth: A Nutritive
Medicinal Plant of Potential Therapeutic Value."
International Journal of Pharma and Bio Sciences
2, no. 3 (July-Sept 2011).

Kotar, S.L., and J.E. Gessler, *Smallpox: A History.* Jefferson, NC: McFarland, 2013.

_____. *The Steamboat Era: A History of Fulton's Folly
on American Rivers, 1807–1860.* Jefferson, NC:
McFarland, 2009.

Langlais, Bruno, David A. Reckhow and Deborah
R. Brink, eds. *Ozone in Water Treatment: Application and Engineering.* Boca Raton: Lewis, 1991.

Lim, Matthew L., Gerald S. Murphy, Margaret Calloway and David Tribble. "History of U.S. Military

Contributions to the Study of Diarrheal Diseases."
Military Medicine 170 (April Supplement, 2005).

Lord, Israel Shipman Pelton. *At the Extremity of Civilization.* Edited by Necia Dixon Liles. Jefferson,
NC: McFarland, 1995.

Macomb, (Major General) Alexander: "United
States Army Report for 1832."

Maignen, P.J.A. "Ozone Treatment of Water Supply."
Cedar Rapids Evening Gazette, August 29, 1904.

Masson, A. "Latta: Pioneer in Saline Infusion."
British Journal of Anaesthesia. London: 1971.

Monro, Donald (M.D.). *An Account of the Diseases
Which Were Most Frequent in the British Military
Hospitals in Germany, from January 1761, to the
Return of the Troops to England in March 1763.*
London: Millar, 1766.

Mosley, Kirk T. "Cholera." U.S. Army Medical Department, Office of Medical History. http://
history.amedd.mil/booksdocs/wwii/PM4/CH21.
Cholera.htm.

Murphy, T. "Character and Treatment of the Malignant Cholera at Liverpool Trial of Venous Injections." *Lancet.* London: 1832.

Nevin, John Williamson. *The Scourge of God.* Pittsburgh: Johnston and Stockton, 1832.

*New Annual Register, or, General Repository of His-
tory, Politics, and Literature for the Year 1818.* London: Printed for William Stockdale, 1819.

"November Uprising." http://en.wikipedia.org/
wiki/November_Uprising.

O'Shaughnessy, William Brooke. *Report on the
Chemical Pathology of the Malignant Cholera.*
London: Highley, 1832.

Parkin, John (M.D.). *The Prevention and Treatment
of Diseases in the Potato and Other Crops.* London:
W. Wood, 1847.

Pearsall, Judy, ed. *Concise Oxford Dictionary.* 10th
ed. New York: Oxford University Press, 1999.

Peters, John C. (M.D.). "Conveyance of Cholera."
Leavenworth Medical Journal, October 1867.

Pedestrian. *Plague Cradles of the Metropolis.* London:
Thomas Bosworth, 1855.

"Philippine-American War." http://en.wikipedia.
org/wiki/Philippine-American-War.

Reece, Richard (M.D.). *The Domestic Medical Guide,
in Two Parts.* 3d. ed. London: Longman, 1805.

Rosenberg, Charles E. *The Cholera Years: The United
States in 1832, 1849 and 1866.* Chicago: University of Chicago Press, 1987.

Ruddy, John (M.D.). *A Chronological History of the
Weather and Seasons, and of the Prevailing Diseases
in Dublin.* London: Robinson and Roberts, 1770.

"Sickness and Death in the Old South: King Cholera."
http://www.tngen.org/darkside/cholera.html.

"Simon Flexner Biography." http://www.faqs.org/
health/bio/26/Simon-Flexner.html.

Smith, Robert Angus. *Disinfectants and Disinfection.*
Edinburgh: Edmonston & Douglas, 1869.

Smith, Southwood (M.D.). "Results of Sanitary Improvement: Illustrated by the Operation of the Metropolitan Societies for Improving the Dwellings of the Industrious Classes, the Working of the Common Lodging-Houses Act, &c." London: Knight, 1854.

Snow, John, *On the Mode of Communication of Cholera.* 2d ed. London: John Churchill, 1855.

"Spanish American War." http://en.wikipedia.org/wiki/Spanish%E2%80%93American_War.

Stedman, John (M.D.). *Physiological Essays and Observations.* London, 1769.

Stephens, Henry (M.R.C.S.). *Cholera: An Analysis of Its Epidemic, Endemic, and Contagious Character.* London: Henry Renshaw, 1854.

Stevens, William (M.D.). *Dr. Stevens's Treatise on the Cholera.* London: G. & C. & H. Carvill, 1832.

_____. *Observations on the Nature and the Treatment of the Asiatic Cholera.* London: Bailliere, 1853.

"Thomas Sydenham." http://wikipedia.org/wiki/Thomas_Sydenham.

Thorne, R. Thomas. "The Present State of Our Knowledge as to the Significance of the Comma-Bacillus in Cholera." *Journal of the Incorporated Society of Medical Officers of Health* 7 (October 1894–September 1895). London: E.W. Allen, 1895.

Todar, Kenneth. "Vibrio cholerae and Asiatic cholera." http://textbookofbacteriology.net/cholera.html.

Venes, Donald, ed. *Taber's Cyclopedic Medical Dictionary.* 20th ed. Philadelphia: F.A. Davis, 2005.

"Vis medicatrix naturae." http://medical-dictionary.the.

Von Orlich, (Captain) Leopold. *Travels in India, Including Sinde and the Punjab.* Translated from the German by H. Evans Lloyd. London: Longman, Brown, Green and Longmans, 1845.

White, W. *A Treatise on Inflammation, and other Diseases of the Liver, Commonly Called Bilious.* Bath: Cadell and Davies, 1808.

Wilkinson, James John Garth (M.D.). *The Cholera and the Minister of Health.* London: Theobald, 1855.

"William Brooke O'Shaughnessy." http://en.wikipedia.org/wiki/William_Brooke_O'Shaughnessy.

Wilson, Andrew (M.D.). *Short Remarks Upon Autumnal Disorders of the Bowels, and on the Nature of Some Sudden Deaths, Observed to Happen at the Same Season of the Year.* London: Wilson and Fell, 1765.

Wood, George Bacon, and Franklin Bache. *The Dispensatory of the United States of America.* 6th ed. Grigg & Elliot, 1845.

World Health Organization Publications

"Bioterrorism and Military Health Risks." http://www.who.int/dg/bruntland/speeches/2003/DAVOS/en/.

"Cholera." http://www.who.int/mediacentre/factsheets/fs107/en/index.html.

"Cholera: Cholera Country Profiles." http://www.who.int/cholera/countries/en/index.html.

"Cholera: The Global Task Force on Cholera Control. http://www.who.int/cholera_task_force/en/.

"Cholera: Immunization, Vaccines and Biologicals." http://www.who.int/immunization/topics/Cholera/en/index.html.

"Cholera: International Health Regulations." http://www.who.int/cholera/health_regulations/en/.

"Cholera: Prevention and control of cholera outbreaks: WHO policy and recommendations." http://www.who.int/cholera/prevention_control/en/.

"Cholera: Prevention and control of cholera outbreaks: WHO policy and recommendations: Cholera vaccines." http://www.who.int/cholera/prevention_control/recommendations/en/index4.html.

Cholera: Prevention and control of cholera outbreaks: WHO policy and recommendations: Control." http://www.who.int/cholera/prevention_control/recommendations/en/index2.html.

"Cholera: Prevention and control of cholera outbreaks: WHO policy and recommendations: Diagnosis." http://www.who.int/cholera/prevention_control/recommendations/en/index.html.

"Cholera: WHO position paper on Oral Rehydration Salts to reduce mortality from cholera." http://www.who.int/cholera/technical/en/index.html.

"Miracle cure for an old scourge. An interview with Dr. Dilip Mahalanabis." http://www.who.int/bulletin/volumes/87/2/09–060209/en/.

Nair, G. Balakrish, and Jai P. Narain. "From endotoxin to exotoxin: De's rich legacy to cholera." http://www.who.int/bulletin/volumes/88/3/09–072504/en/.

Nair, G.B., et al., "Vibrio cholerae." Geneva: World Health Organization, 1993.

"Origin and development of health cooperation." http://www.who.int/global_health_histories/background/en.

Newspapers and Magazines

Adams (PA) Centinel/Sentinel
Adams County (IA) Union-Republican
Advocate (IN)
Age (London)
Albion (London)
Albion and The Star (London)
Albuquerque (NM) Tribune
Allen's Indian Mail (London)
Alta California
Alton (IL) Evening Telegraph
Alton (IL) Observer

Alton (IL) Telegraph & Democratic Review
Alton (IL) Weekly Courier
Alton (IL) Weekly Telegraph
Altoona (PA) Mirror
Amarillo (TX) Daily News
Amarillo (TX) Globe-Times
American Settler (London)
Anglo-American Times (London)
Anniston (AL) Star
Anti-Jacobin Review and Magazine (London)
Appleton (WI) Crescent
Argus (OH)
Arizona Republic
Atchison (KS) Daily Globe
Atlanta Constitution
Atlas (London)
Austrian Observer
Bakersfield Californian
*Baldwin's London Weekly Journal and Surrey and
    Sussex Gazette*
Baltimore Republican
Bangor (ME) Daily Whig and Courier
Baytown (TX) Sun
Beatrice (NE) Daily Sun
Beckley (WV) Post-Herald
Beckley (WV) Post-Herald/Raleigh Register
Bee (VA)
Belleville (KS) Telescope
Bell's Life in London and Sporting Chronicle
Bell's (London) New Weekly Messenger
Big Spring (TX) Daily Herald
Billings (MT) Daily Gazette
Biloxi (MS) Gulfport Daily Herald
Bismark (ND) Daily Tribune
Boston Daily Globe
Boston Transcript
British Banner (London)
British Critic
British Journal of Anaesthesia (London)
British Press
British Standard (London)
British Traveller
Brownwood (TX) Bulletin
Burlington (IA) Hawk-Eye
Carlisle (London) Journal
Cedar Rapids (IA) Gazette
Centaur (London)
Central Press (London)
Champion and Sunday Review (London)
Charleston (WV) Gazette
Cherokee Advocate (Indian Territory, OK)
Chester Times (PA)
Christian Advocate (London)
Christian Times (London)
Christian Weekly News (London)
Chronicle-Telegram (OH)
Church & State Gazette (London)
Church Herald (London)

Cincinnati Gazette
Circular to Bankers (London)
Cleave's Penny Gazette (London)
Clerkenwell (London) Press
Clovis (NM) News Journal
Colonial Gazette (London)
Colonies and India (London)
Commercialist & Weekly Advertiser (London)
Connersville (IN) Examiner
Connersville (IN) News-Examiner
Connersville (IN) Times
Corpus Christi (TX) Caller-Times
Corpus Christi (TX) Times
Coshocton (OH) Age
Country (London) Times
Courier (London)
Court Gazette (London)
Cullman (AL) Banner
Cumberland (MD) News
Daily Alton (IL) Telegraph
Daily Argus and Democrat (WI)
Daily Arkansas Gazette
Daily Chronicle (WA)
Daily Free Democrat (WI)
Daily Gazette (Colorado Springs, CO)
Daily Globe (MI)
Daily Herald (IA)
Daily Herald (IL)
Daily Herald (PA)
Daily Herald (UT)
Daily Index-Appeal (VA)
Daily Milwaukee News
Daily Miner (MT)
Daily News (London)
Daily News (TX)
Daily News-Record (VA)
Daily News Standard (PA)
Daily Northwestern (WI)
Daily Register (IL)
Daily Republican Register (IL)
Daily Review (CA)
Daily Sandusky/Sanduskian (OH)
Daily Times (NY)
Danville (IN) Weekly Advertiser
Davenport (IA) Gazette
Daviess County (IN) Democrat
Decatur (IL) Republican
Defiance (OH) Democrat
Delaware State Reporter
Del Rio (TX) News-Herald
Delta-Democrat-Times (MS)
Democratic Banner (IA)
Democratic Expounder (MI)
Democratic Pharos (IN)
Democratic Union (IN)
Des Moines (IA) News
Des Moines (IA) Register
Detroit Free Press

Dublin Journal
Dubois (PA) Courier
Dubuque (IA) Daily Herald
Eastport (MA) Sentinel
Eau Claire (WI) Daily Free Press
Edinburgh Advertiser
Edinburgh Adviser
Edinburgh Evening Courant
Edinburgh Medical and Surgical Journal
Edwardsville (IL) Intelligencer
El Paso (TX) Herald-Post
Elyria (OH) Independent Democrat
Empire (London)
Englishman (London)
Evangelical (London) Magazine, and Missionary Chronicle
Evans and Ruffy's (London) Farmer's Journal
Evansville (IN) Daily Enquirer
Evening Capital (MD)
Evening Express (PA)
Evening Gazette (Cedar Rapids, IA)
Evening Independent (OH)
Evening Mirror (PA)
Evening News-Journal (NM)
Evening Star (London)
Facts (TX)
Fairbanks (AK) Daily Times
Florence (SC) Morning News
Fond du Lac (WI) Journal
Fort Wayne (IN) Daily Gazette
Fort Wayne (IN) Journal-Gazette
Fort Wayne (IN) News
Fort Wayne (IN) Sentinel
Fort Wayne (IN) Times
Francesville (IN) Tribune
Frederick (MD) Herald
Frederick (MD) Post
Frederick (MD) Town Herald
Freeborn County (MN) Standard
Freeholder and Commercial Advertiser (London)
Freeport (IL) Republican
Galveston (TX) Daily News
Garden City (KS) Telegram
Gardeners' Gazette (London)
Gaston (NC) Gazette
Gazette de France
Gazette (IA)
Gentleman's (London) Magazine
Glasgow Courier
Gleaner (Jamaica)
Globe (London)
Globe (Washington, DC)
Goshen (IN) Times
Green Bay (WI) Advocate
Guardian (Manchester)
Hagerstown (PA) Free Press
Hamilton (OH) Evening Journal
Hammond (IN) Times

Harrison (AR) Daily Times
Hendricks County (IN) Republican
Herald (NY)
Herald American Post-Standard (NY)
Herald Press (MI)
Herald-Zeiting (TX)
Hillsdale (MI) Standard
Hope Star (AR)
Hornellsville (NY) Tribune
Hour (London)
Huron (OH) Reflector
Hutchinson (KS) News
Independent (IA)
Independent American (WI)
Independent Press-Telegram (CA)
Independent Record (MT)
Illustrated Times (London)
Independent Press-Telegram (CA)
Indian Mail (London)
Indian Statesman (London)
Indiana (PA) Democrat
Indiana (PA) Evening Gazette
Indianapolis (IN) Sunday Star
Iola (KS) Register
Iowa City (IA) Press-Citizen
Iowa State Reporter
Ironwood (MI) Daily Globe
Jackson County (IN) Democrat
Jackson (IA) Sentinel
Janesville (WI) Gazette
Jefferson (IA) Bee
Jeffersonian (KS) Gazette
Joplin (MO) News Herald
Kent & Essex (London) Mercury
Kokomo (IN) Daily Tribune
La Crosse (WI) Independent Republican
La Crosse (WI) Tribune
Lancet (London)
Landmark (NC)
Laredo (TX) Weekly Times
Laurel (MS) Leader
Law Chronicle Commercial, and Bankruptcy Register (London)
Lawrence (KS) Gazette
Lawrence (KS) Journal-World
Lebanon (PA) Daily News
Le Grand (IA) Reporter
Le Mans (IA) Semi-Weekly Sentinel
Lethbridge (Alberta) Daily Herald
Lima (OH) Argus
Lima (OH) News
Lloyd's Weekly London Newspaper
Logansport (IN) Chronicle
Logansport (IN) Pharos
Logansport (IN) Daily Star
Logansport (IN) Daily Tribune
Logansport (IN) Semi-Weekly Reporter
London and China Telegraph (Shanghai)

London Chronicle
London Evening Post
London Examiner
London Medical Record
Lorain (OH) Constitutionalist
Lowell (MA) Weekly Sun/Sun
Lubbock (TX) Avalanche-Journal
Ludington (MI) Daily News
Lycoming (PA) Gazette
Mail (MD)
Mail/British Mail (London)
Malvern (IA) Leader
Manitoba Daily Free Press
Manitowoc (WI) Herald-Times
Mansfield (OH) News
Marshall (MI) Statesman
Medical Gazette (London)
Medical Times (London)
Middletown (NY) Times-Press
Milford (IA) Mail
Milwaukee Daily Courier
Milwaukee Daily News
Milwaukee Sentinel and Gazette
Miner and Workman's Advocate (London)
Miners' Free Press (WT)
Missouri Republican
Monday Advocate (OH)
Monessen (PA) Daily Independent
Montana Standard
Monthly (London) Magazine
Monthly (London) Review
Monticello (IA) Express
Morning Chronicle, and London Advertiser
Morning (London) Journal
Morning Oregonian
Mt. Pleasant (IA) News
Muscatine (IA) Journal
National Advocate (IA)
Nautical Standard and Steam Navigation Gazette
   (London)
New Castle (PA) News
New Mexican
New Review with Literary Curiosities (London)
New York Daily Times
New York Day Book
New York Evening Post
New York Evening Times
Newark (OH) Advocate
News (MD)
News Herald (FL)
News-Palladium (MI)
News-Record (VA)
Nonconformist (London)
Nonconformist and Independent (London)
Norristown (MA) Herald
North-China Herald (Shanghai)
Oakland (CA) Tribune
Ogden (UT) Standard

Ohio Democrat
Olean (NY) Evening Herald
Oneonta (NY) Daily Star
Orange (TX) Leader
Orville (OH) Crescent
Oshkosh (WI) Courier
Oshkosh (WI) Daily Northwestern
Oshkosh (WI) Democrat
Oxnard (CA) Daily Courier
Palo Alto (CA) Reporter
Pampa (TX) Daily News
Panama City (FL) News
Paris (TX) News
Patriot (London)
Penny London Post
Penny Newsman (London)
People's Press (PA)
Pharos-Tribune (IN)
Philosophical (London) Magazine/and Journal
Pittsburg (PA) Commercial
Poor Law Chronicle (London)
Port Arthur (TX) News
Portland (OR) Daily Courier
Portsmouth (OH) Times
Post (Washington DC)
Prairie du Chien (WI) Patriot
Press (London)
Press-Telegram (CA)
Progress (PA)
Progress-Index (VA)
Racine (WI) Journal
Register (CA)
Reno (NV) Evening Gazette
Republican (PA) Compiler
Republican Daily Journal (KS)
Restitution (IN)
Reviewer (London)
Rochester (IN) Sentinel
Rochester (IN) Union Spy
Rockingham (VA) Register
Rock River (WI) Pilot
Rocky Mountain (NC) Telegram
Roswell (NM) Daily Record
St. James Chronicle, or, the British Evening-Post
St. Joseph (MI) Herald
St. Joseph (MI) Traveler Herald
St. Louis (MO) Globe
St. Louis (MO) Journal
St. Louis (MO) Post-Dispatch
Salamanca (NY) Republican-Press
Salt Lake (UT) Daily Tribune
San Antonio (TX) Express
San Antonio (TX) Light
San Antonio (TX) Light and Gazette
Sandusky (OH) Clarion
Sandusky (OH) Register
Sandusky (OH) Register Star-News
San Mateo (CA) Times

Santa Fe New Mexican
Saturday Clarion (OH)
Scientific American
Seguin (TX) Gazette-Enterprise
Semi-Weekly Wisconsin
Settler & Pennon (PA)
Seymour (IN) Times
Sheboygan (WI) Lake Journal
Sheboygan (WI) Mercury
Shoreditch (London) Observer
Sioux County (IA) Herald
Southern Illinoisan
Southport (WI) American
Spirit of the Age (London)
Spirit of the Times (Philadelphia)
Star and (Adams County) Republican Banner (PA)
Star and Republican Compiler (PA)
Star-News (CA)
Stars and Stripes (European; Germany)
Stars and Stripes (Pacific; Tokyo)
Statesville (NC) Record & Landmark
Sterling (IL) Standard
Steubenville (OH) Daily Herald & News
Sullivan (IN) Democrat
Sun (New York)
Sun and Central Press (London)
Syracuse (NY) Herald-Journal
Syracuse (NY) Post-Standard
Telegraph and Courier (London)
Texas City (TX) Sun
Times (London)
Times (New York)
Times Recorder (OH)
Tioga (PA) Eagle
Titusville (PA) Morning Herald
Torch Light & Public Advertiser (MD)
Trades' (London) Free Press
Tribune (Chicago)
True Sun (London)
Tucson (AZ) Daily Citizen

Twin Falls (ID) Daily News
Tyrone (PA) Daily Herald
Ukiah (CA) Daily Journal
Van Wert (OH) Daily Bulletin
Van Wert (OH) Times-Bulletin
Victoria (TX) Advocate
Vidette (IN) Messenger
Warren (IN) Republic
Warren (PA) Ledger
Washington (IN) Democrat
Watchman and Wesleyan Advertiser (London)
Waterloo (IA) Daily Courier
Waterloo (IA) Evening Courier
Watertown (WI) Chronicle
Waukesha (WI) Democrat
Waukesha (WI) Freeman
Waukesha (WI) Plaindealer
Weekly (PA) Advertiser
Weekly Chronicle (London)
Weekly Chronicle and Register (London)
Weekly (London) Free Press
Weekly News and Chronicle (London)
Weekly Wisconsin
Week's News (London)
Wellsboro (PA) Agitator
West Eau Claire (WI) Argus
Western Home Journal (KS)
Western Statesman (MI)
Wilmington and Delaware Advertiser
Winchester (VA) Star
Winnipeg Free Press
Winona (MN) Republican-Herald
Wisconsin Argus
Wisconsin Express
Wisconsin Herald
Wisconsin State Journal
Wisconsin Statesman
World (NY)
Zanesville (OH) Courier

Index